Atlas of Technics in Surgery

Thoracic and Cardiovascular

By JOHN L. MADDEN, M.D., F.A.C.S.

Director of Surgery, St. Clare's Hospital, New York City;
Clinical Professor of Surgery, New York Medical College

With 63 Contributing Authors
Discussing the Illustrated Surgical Technics

Illustrations By

Alfred Feinberg & Robert Wabnitz

With

Frank Robinson Neil Hardy Don Johnson
Elizabeth H. Brödel Harriet E. Phillips
William Didusch Leonard Dank

APPLETON-CENTURY-CROFTS/New York
A Publishing Division of Prentice-Hall, Inc.

JOHN L. MADDEN'S

Atlas of Technics In Surgery

Second Edition

Volume 2: Thoracic and Cardiovascular

75 76 77 78 79 / 10 9 8

Library of Congress Catalog Card Number 64-25234

PRINTED IN THE UNITED STATES OF AMERICA 0-8385-0132-X

To my wife
Birdie
and children
Pam
John
Brian
Michael
Tommy
Kathy

CONTRIBUTING AUTHORS

WILLIAM G. ANLYAN
Professor of Surgery and Dean, Duke University Medical Center

HENRY T. BAHNSON
Professor and Chairman, Department of Surgery, The University of Pittsburgh School of Medicine; Surgeon-in-Chief, Presbyterian-University Hospital, Pittsburgh

JOHN M. BEAL
Professor and Chairman, Department of Surgery, Northwestern University Medical School; Chief of Surgery, Passavant Memorial Hospital, Chicago

CLAUDE S. BECK
Professor of Cardiovascular Surgery, Western Reserve University School of Medicine

BRIAN BLADES
Professor and Chairman, Department of Surgery, George Washington School of Medicine; Surgeon-in-Chief, The George Washington University Hospital, Washington, D.C.

ARTHUR H. BLAKEMORE
Associate Professor Clinical Surgery Emeritus, Columbia University, College of Physicians and Surgeons; Associate Attending Surgeon Emeritus, Presbyterian Hospital, Columbia University, College of Physicians and Surgeons

* ALFRED BLALOCK
Professor and Director, Department of Surgery, The Johns Hopkins University School of Medicine; Surgeon-in-Chief, Johns Hopkins Hospital

SIR RUSSELL BROCK
Lecturer in Surgery, University of London; Surgeon, Guy's Hospital and Brompton Hospital, London, England

JOHN ROBINSON BROOKS
Senior Associate in Surgery, Peter Bent Brigham Hospital; Assistant Clinical Professor in Surgery, Harvard Medical School

O. THERON CLAGETT
Head of a Section of Surgery, Mayo Clinic; Professor of Surgery, The University of Minnesota, Rochester, Minnesota

HERBERT CONWAY
Attending Surgeon in Charge of Plastic Surgery, The New York Hospital; Professor of Clinical Surgery, Department of Surgery, Cornell Medical Center

DENTON A. COOLEY
Professor of Surgery, Baylor University College of Medicine; Chief, Cardiovascular Service, Texas Children's Hospital; Attending Surgeon, Methodist, St. Luke's Episcopal, and Ben Taub General Hospitals, Houston

PHILIP COOPER
Chief, Surgical Service, Veterans' Administration Hospital, Bronx, New York; Professor of Clinical Surgery, Albert Einstein College of Medicine

JAMES T. DANIELS
Chief of Neurological Surgery, St. Clare's Hospital, New York; Associate Professor, Clinical Neurosurgery, New York University Post-Graduate Medical School

MICHAEL E. DeBAKEY
Professor and Chairman, Cora and Webb Mading Department of Surgery, Baylor University College of Medicine; Surgeon-in-Chief, Jefferson Davis Hospital; Chief Consultant in Surgery, Veterans' Administration Hospital; Senior Attending Surgeon, Methodist Hospital, Houston

PAUL T. DeCAMP
Active Staff Surgeon, Ochsner Foundation Hospital, New Orleans; Associate Professor of Clinical Surgery, Tulane University School of Medicine

RALPH A. DETERLING, JR.
Professor and Chairman, Department of Surgery, Tufts University School of Medicine; Surgeon-in-Chief, Tufts-New England Medical Center; Director, First (Tufts) Surgical Service, Boston City Hospital

LESTER R. DRAGSTEDT
Thomas D. Jones Distinguished Service Professor of Surgery Emeritus, The University of Chicago; Research Professor of Surgery, University of Florida, Gainesville

CHARLES DUBOST
Professor, Faculty of Medicine, Chair of Cardiovascular Surgery, Broussais Hospital, Paris, France

* Deceased

BEN EISEMAN
Professor and Chairman, Department of Surgery, The University of Kentucky Medical School; Chief Surgeon, University Hospital, Lexington

JOHN H. GARLOCK
Professor of Surgery, Columbia University, College of Physicians and Surgeons; Senior Surgeon, Mt. Sinai Hospital

EDGAR L. FRAZELL
Attending Surgeon and Chief of the Head and Neck Service, Memorial Hospital for Cancer and Allied Diseases, New York

CAMERON HAIGHT
Professor of Surgery, Surgeon-in-Charge, Section of Thoracic Surgery, The University of Michigan Medical Center, Ann Arbor

C. ROLLINS HANLON
Professor and Director, Department of Surgery, St. Louis University School of Medicine; Surgeon-in-Chief, St. Louis University Hospitals, St. Louis

STANLEY O. HOERR
Staff Surgeon and Chairman of the Division of Surgery, Cleveland Clinic, Cleveland

CRANSTON W. HOLMAN
Director, Second Surgical Division (Cornell), Bellevue Hospital; Attending Surgeon, The New York Hospital; Associate Professor of Clinical Surgery, Cornell University Medical College

EMILE HOLMAN
Professor of Surgery, Emeritus, Stanford University School of Medicine

CHARLES A. HUFNAGEL
Professor of Surgery and Director of Surgical Research Laboratories, Georgetown University Medical Center; Attending in Surgery, Georgetown University Hospital, Washington, D.C.

GEORGE H. HUMPHREYS, II
Valentine Mott Professor of Surgery, Columbia University, College of Physicians and Surgeons; Director of Surgical Service, Presbyterian Hospital

ELLIOTT S. HURWITT
Chief, Surgical Division, Montefiore Hospital and Medical Center; Professor of Surgery, Albert Einstein College of Medicine

JULIAN JOHNSON
Professor of Surgery, The University of Pennsylvania School of Medicine and Graduate School of Medicine; Associate Chief and Chief of Surgical Division I, Department of Surgery, Hospital of the University of Pennsylvania

JOHN C. JONES
Senior Attending Surgeon, Los Angeles County Hospital, Hospital of the Good Samaritan; Chief of Thoracic Surgery, Los Angeles Children's Hospital; Clinical Professor of Surgery, The University of Southern California School of Medicine, Los Angeles

ORMAND C. JULIAN
Department of Surgery, The University of Illinois School of Medicine

JOHN L. KEELEY
Professor and Chairman, Department of Surgery, Stritch School of Medicine, Loyola University, Hines, Illinois; Chairman, Department of Surgery, Mercy Hospital, Chicago; Consulting Surgeon, Veterans Administration Hospital, Hines

* CHARLES K. KIRBY
Late Professor of Surgery, School of Medicine and Graduate School of Medicine, The University of Pennsylvania

CONRAD R. LAM
Surgeon-in-Charge, Division of Thoracic Surgery, Henry Ford Hospital, Detroit

ROBERT R. LINTON
Senior Visiting Surgeon, Massachusetts General Hospital; Assistant Clinical Professor of Surgery, Harvard University

WILLIAM P. LONGMIRE
Professor and Chairman, Department of Surgery, University of California Medical Center, School of Medicine, Los Angeles

* Deceased

JERE W. LORD, JR.
Visiting Surgeon, Fourth Surgical Division, Bellevue Hospital; Attending Surgeon, University Hospital; Professor of Clinical Surgery, New York University Post-Graduate Medical School

EARLE B. MAHONEY
Professor of Surgery, The University of Rochester School of Medicine and Dentistry; Surgeon, Strong Memorial Hospital, Rochester, New York

HERBERT C. MAIER
Director of Surgery, Lenox Hill Hospital; Visiting Surgeon, Bellevue Hospital; Associate Attending Surgeon, Presbyterian Hospital; Associate Clinical Professor of Surgery, Columbia University, College of Physicians and Surgeons

FERDINAND F. McALLISTER
Associate Attending Surgeon, Presbyterian Hospital; Assistant Professor of Clinical Surgery, Columbia University, College of Physicians and Surgeons

WILLIAM H. MULLER, JR.
Stephen H. Watts Professor and Chairman, Department of Surgery, The University of Virginia School of Medicine; Surgeon-in-Chief, University of Virginia Medical Center, Charlottesville

MERLE M. MUSSELMAN
Professor and Chairman, Department of Surgery, The University of Nebraska College of Medicine; Chairman, Department of Surgery, University of Nebraska Hospital, Omaha

ALTON OCHSNER
Director of Surgery, Ochsner Foundation Hospital and Ochsner Clinic; Emeritus Professor of Surgery, Tulane University, New Orleans

RICHARD H. OVERHOLT
Director of the Overholt Thoracic Clinic, Boston; Clinical Professor of Surgery (Thoracic), Tufts University School of Medicine

JOHN L. POOL
Associate Attending Surgeon, Memorial Hospital for Cancer and Allied Diseases, Clinical Assistant Professor of Surgery, Cornell University Medical College

GERALD H. PRATT
Attending Surgeon and Chief of Cardiovascular Surgical Section, Department of Surgery, The St. Vincent's Hospital and Medical Center; Attending Surgeon, St. Clare's Hospital, Polyclinic Hospital; Associate Clinical Professor of Surgery, New York University School of Medicine

MARK M. RAVITCH
Associate Professor of Surgery, The Johns Hopkins University School of Medicine; Surgeon, Johns Hopkins Hospital

WILLIAM F. RIENHOFF, JR.
Surgeon, Johns Hopkins Hospital, Professor Emeritus of Surgery, The Johns Hopkins University School of Medicine

CHARLES B. RIPSTEIN
Professor of Surgery, Albert Einstein College of Medicine; Chief of Thoracic Surgery, Bronx Municipal Hospital Center; Director of Surgery, Brookdale Hospital Center, Brooklyn

CHARLES ROB
Professor and Chairman, Department of Surgery, The University of Rochester School of Medicine and Dentistry; Surgeon-in-Chief, Strong Memorial Hospital, Rochester, New York

LOUIS M. ROUSSELOT
Director of Surgery, The St. Vincent's Hospital and Medical Center; Professor of Clinical Surgery, New York University School of Medicine

PAUL C. SAMSON
Associate Clinical Professor of Surgery, Stanford University School of Medicine; West Coast Area Consultant in Thoracic and Cardiac Surgery, Veterans' Administration

GARDNER W. SMITH
Surgeon, University of Virginia Hospital, Charlottesville; Instructor in Surgery, Department of Surgery, The University of Virginia School of Medicine

FRANK SPENCER
Professor of Surgery, The University of Kentucky College of Medicine; Surgeon, University of Kentucky Medical Center, Lexington

* RICHARD H. SWEET
Visiting Surgeon, Massachusetts General Hospital; Associate Clinical Professor of Surgery, Harvard Medical College

* Deceased

SAMUEL ALCOTT THOMPSON
Associate Professor of Surgery, New York Medical College; Attending Surgeon, Flower and Fifth Avenue Hospitals; Director of Thoracic Surgery, Metropolitan Hospital; Consulting Surgeon, St. Clare's Hospital, New York

ARTHUR S. W. TOUROFF
Consulting Surgeon, The Mount Sinai Hospital; Formerly: Clinical Professor of Surgery, Columbia University, College of Physicians and Surgeons

ARTHUR B. VOORHEES, JR.
Instructor in Surgery, Columbia University, College of Physicians and Surgeons; Assistant Attending Surgeon, Presbyterian Hospital

KENNETH W. WARREN
Surgeon, Lahey Clinic, New England Baptist and New England Deaconess Hospitals, Boston

C. STUART WELCH
Professor of Surgery, Albany Medical College; Attending Surgeon, Albany Medical Center Hospital

JOHN P. WEST
Attending Surgeon, St. Luke's Hospital; Associate Attending Surgeon, The New York Hospital; Associate Professor of Clinical Surgery, Cornell University Medical College

CONTENTS

OPERATIVE TECHNICS

The Anterior Thoracic Incision 2

The Posterior (Prone) Thoracic Incision 6

The Posterolateral Thoracic Incision 10

The Thoracoabdominal Incision 16

Discusser: CHARLES B. RIPSTEIN

Scalenotomy 24

Discusser: JAMES T. DANIELS

Tracheostomy 28

Discusser: EDGAR L. FRAZELL

Excision of Cylindroma of the Trachea 32

Discusser: JOHN L. POOL

Pulmonary Lobectomy: Right Upper Lobe 36

Discussers: JULIAN JOHNSON, BRIAN BLADES

Pulmonary Lobectomy: Combined Right Middle and Lower Lobes 42

Discussers: JULIAN JOHNSON, BRIAN BLADES

Total Pneumonectomy: Right 50

Discussers: WILLIAM F. RIENHOFF, JR., ALTON OCHSNER, SIR RUSSELL BROCK

Pulmonary Lobectomy: Left Upper Lobe 58

Discussers: CHARLES K. KIRBY, JOHN C. JONES

Pulmonary Lobectomy: Left Lower Lobe 66

Discussers: JOHN C. JONES, CHARLES K. KIRBY

Total Pneumonectomy: Left 72

Discussers: ALTON OCHSNER, SIR RUSSELL BROCK, WILLIAM F. RIENHOFF, JR.

Thymectomy 80

Discussers: MERLE M. MUSSELMAN, O. THERON CLAGETT

Congenital Atresia of the Esophagus with Tracheoesophageal Fistula 88

Discussers: JOHN M. BEAL and CRANSTON W. HOLMAN, CAMERON HAIGHT

Congenital Atresia of the Esophagus with Hypoplasia of the Lower Esophageal Segment 92

Discussers: JOHN M. BEAL and CRANSTON W. HOLMAN, CAMERON HAIGHT

Resection of Pharyngoesophageal Diverticulum 94

Discusser: KENNETH W. WARREN

Esophagocardiomyotomy—Transabdominal Approach 100

Discussers: RICHARD H. SWEET, MARK M. RAVITCH, C. ROLLINS HANLON

Esophagocardiomyotomy—Transthoracic Approach 104

Discussers: MARK M. RAVITCH, C. ROLLINS HANLON

Esophagectomy. Left Transpleural, Transdiaphragmatic Approach with Supraaortic and Infraaortic Esophagogastrostomy 110

Discusser: JOHN H. GARLOCK

Esophagectomy. Combined Right Cervical, Right Thoracic, and Left Abdominal Approach with Cervical Esophagogastrostomy 118

Discusser: JOHN H. GARLOCK

Esophagectomy—Right Transpleural Approach 134

Esophagectomy and Colon Transplant 138

Discusser: EARLE B. MAHONEY

The Transthoracic Repair of an Esophageal Hiatus Hernia 162

Discussers: PAUL C. SAMSON, RICHARD H. SWEET, DENTON A. COOLEY, JOHN ROBINSON BROOKS

The Transabdominal Approach for the Repair of an Esophageal Hiatus Hernia . . 178

Discussers: DENTON A. COOLEY, RICHARD H. SWEET

Eventration of the Diaphragm 182

Infradiaphragmatic Resection of the Vagus Nerves and Antecolic Gastrojejunostomy . 188

Discussers: LESTER R. DRAGSTEDT, STANLEY O. HOERR

Patent Ductus Arteriosus 196

Discussers: HERBERT C. MAIER, ARTHUR S. W. TOUROFF

Tetralogy of Fallot 202

Discusser: ALFRED BLALOCK

Coarctation of the Aorta 212

Discussers: RALPH A. DETERLING, JR., CHARLES DUBOST

Pulmonary Valvotomy 224

Discusser: GEORGE H. HUMPHREYS, II

Mitral Commissurotomy 232

Discusser: ELLIOTT S. HURWITT

Cardiopericardiopexy 238

Discusser: SAMUEL A. THOMPSON

Coronary Thromboendarterectomy 242

Discussers: CLAUDE S. BECK, WILLIAM P. LONGMIRE, JR.

Cardiac Resuscitation 246

Pericardiectomy 248

Discussers: EMILE HOLMAN, CONRAD R. LAM, WILLIAM H. MULLER, JR., and GARDNER W. SMITH

Aortic Embolectomy 258

Discusser: FERDINAND F. MCALLISTER

Excision of an Aneurysm of the Thoracic Aorta and the Insertion of a Preserved Homologous Aortic Graft 264

Discusser: MICHAEL E. DE BAKEY

Excision of an Aneurysm of the Abdominal Aorta and the Insertion of a Preserved Homologous Aortic Graft 276

Discusser: MICHAEL E. DE BAKEY

Excision of an Aneurysm of the Popliteal Artery and the Insertion of an Alcohol (70 Per Cent) Preserved Homologous Aortic (Thoracic) Graft 290

Discussers: ORMAND C. JULIAN, ROBERT R. LINTON

Excision of an Aneurysm of the Common Carotid Artery and the Insertion of an Autogenous Vein Graft 298

Discusser: HENRY T. BAHNSON

Carotid Thromboendarterectomy 304

Discussers: B. EISEMAN and FRANK SPENCER, CHARLES ROB

Carotid Arterial Bypass Graft (Dacron) 312

Discussers: B. EISEMAN and FRANK SPENCER, CHARLES ROB

Carotid Glomectomy 318

Discusser: RICHARD H. OVERHOLT

Restoration of Peripheral Arterial Continuity by Resection and Graft (Vein) Replacement or a Shunt Bypass 322

Discusser: JOHN P. WEST

Surgical Exposure of the Popliteal Vessels and Posterior Tibial Nerve in the Upper Third of the Leg 328

Femoral Thromboendarterectomy 330

Discusser: JOHN P. WEST

Renal Thromboendarterectomy 336

Discusser: PAUL T. DE CAMP

Aortorenal Bypass Graft 342

Discusser: PAUL T. DE CAMP

Segmental Resection of Renal Artery and Primary Anastomosis; Splenorenal Arterial Anastomosis 346

Discusser: PAUL T. DE CAMP

Ligation of the Superficial Femoral Vein 348

Discusser: W. G. ANLYAN

Ligation of the Inferior Vena Cava 352

Discussers: JERE W. LORD, W. G. ANLYAN

Repair of Traumatic Laceration of the Inferior Vena Cava 360

Discusser: JOHN L. KEELEY

Splenectomy and End-to-Side Splenorenal Shunt 364

Discussers: ARTHUR H. BLAKEMORE and ARTHUR B. VOORHEES, JR., C. STUART WELCH, LOUIS M. ROUSSELOT

End-to-Side Portacaval Shunt 376

Discussers: ARTHUR H. BLAKEMORE and ARTHUR B. VOORHEES, JR., C. STUART WELCH

Side-to-Side Portacaval Shunt 386

Discusser: C. STUART WELCH

Right Transaxillary, Transpleural Thoracic Sympathetic Ganglionectomy 390

Discusser: CHARLES A. HUFNAGEL

Left Transaxillary, Transpleural Thoracic Sympathetic Ganglionectomy 396

Left Lumbar Sympathetic Ganglionectomy 398

Discusser: GERALD H. PRATT

Right Lumbar Sympathetic Ganglionectomy 404

Modified Kondoléon Operation 406

Discussers: HERBERT CONWAY, GERALD H. PRATT

Transthoracic, Supradiaphragmatic Resection of the Vagus Nerves 418

References 423

Index 455

Atlas of Technics in Surgery

Thoracic and Cardiovascular

In the preparation of the Second Edition of the *Atlas of Technics in Surgery,* it was immediately apparent that two volumes would be required for its publication. This was necessitated by the large number of new operative procedures, the increase in the reference lists, and the additional discussers, not only for the new operations but also for those previously published in the First Edition.

This Volume 2 contains the thoracic and cardiovascular operations which are generally performed. Accordingly, open heart operations are purposely not included because of the limited experience of the author and the highly specialized nature of these operations.

It is believed important to reemphasize that each of the operations illustrated was witnessed in the operation room at least once by the artist as it was being performed by the author. It is sincerely believed that this is the best way to obtain both anatomic realism and originality of presentation.

THE ANTERIOR THORACIC INCISION

A. The right inframammary curvilinear incision, extending from the midline of the sternum to the right midaxillary line, is depicted.

B. By blunt dissection with a pledget of gauze on a ring clamp, the pectoralis major muscle is separated from the underlying pectoralis minor muscle, and the proposed line of transection of its fibers is shown by the dotted line.

C. Close-up to show the compression of the fibers of the pectoralis major concomitant with their severance. This particular technic is considered a valuable adjunct in the prevention of excessive blood loss. Intermittent release of the digital compression permits the visualization of bleeding points within the muscle which are clamped as the severance of the muscle fibers proceeds.

D. The fibroareolar tissue layer overlying the serratus anterior muscle is divided, and the transection of the fibers of the pectoralis minor muscle is begun with a scalpel.

E. The transection of the pectoralis major and minor muscles is completed, and the underlying second and third ribs and the intervening external intercostal muscle layer are visible.

F, G, H. A longitudinal incision is made through the periosteum overlying the third rib (F), and the lower half of the incised periosteum is separated from the inferior border of the rib with a periosteal elevator (G, H).

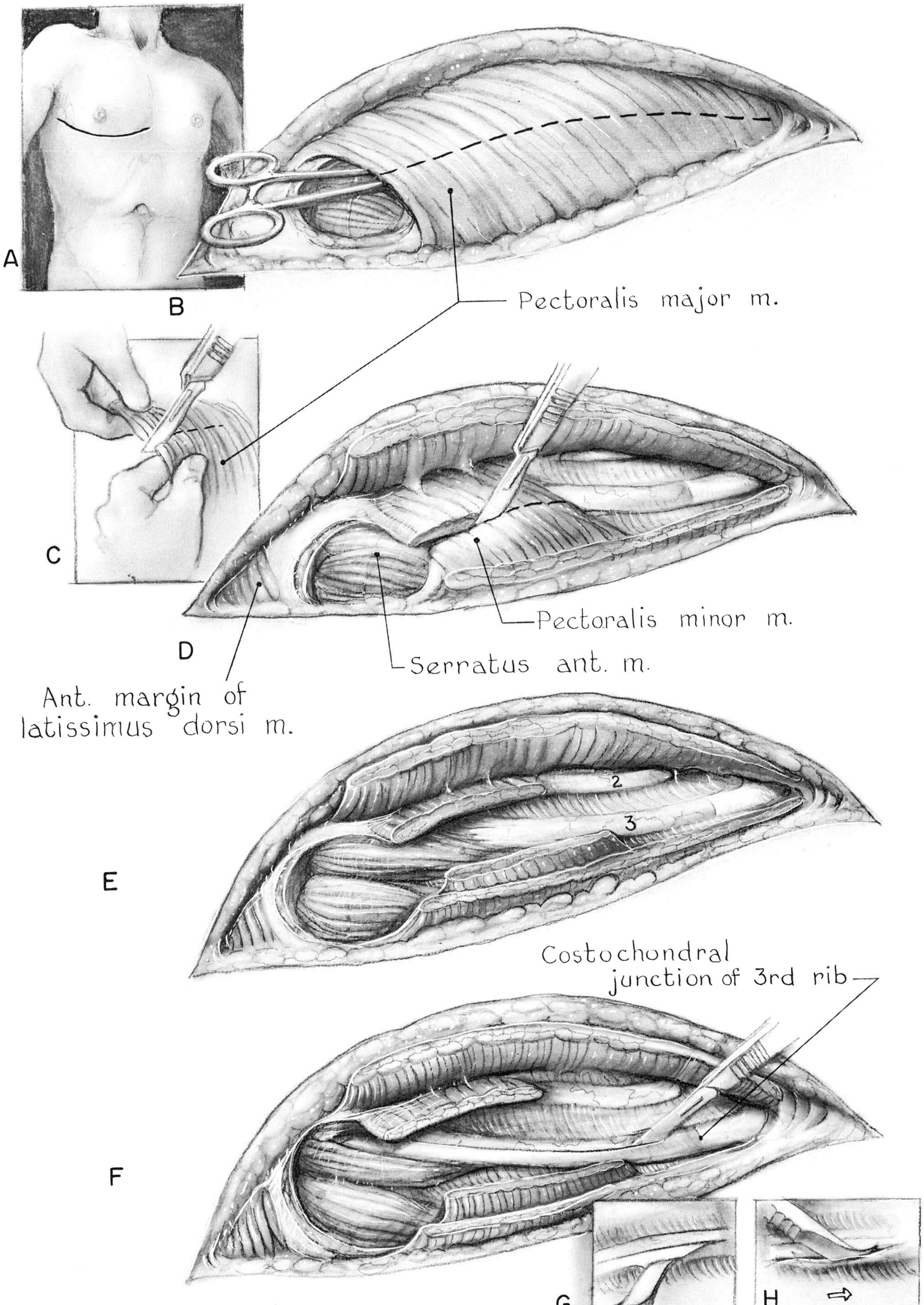
A
B
Pectoralis major m.
C
Pectoralis minor m.
D
Serratus ant. m.
Ant. margin of latissimus dorsi m.
2
3
E
Costochondral junction of 3rd rib
F
G
H

I, J, K, L. A subperichondrial resection of a small segment (2 cm.) of the cartilage of the third rib is done (I, J), and the adjacent internal mammary vessels are doubly clamped and severed preliminary to ligation with ligatures of 00 silk (K, L).

M. The mobilization of the third rib is completed, and the detached but intact external and internal intercostal muscle layers and the related neurovascular bundle are shown. The third rib is retracted upward and the opening into the right pleural cavity is extended anteriorly by scissor dissection.

N. In the closure of the incision, double strands of No. 2 chromic catgut are inserted through periosteal "windows" along the inferior border of the fourth rib as pericostal approximating sutures. The severed fibers of the latissimus dorsi muscle are united with interrupted sutures of silk (00).

O. The rib cage is approximated by tying the previously inserted pericostal sutures, and the transected fibers of the pectoralis minor muscle are sutured with interrupted sutures of 00 silk. In the approximation of the rib cage, the intact intercostal muscle layers may be seen overlying the lower half of the anterior surface of the third rib.

P. The fibroareolar tissue layer and the cut margins of the pectoralis major muscle are sutured with interrupted sutures of 00 silk. In this approach, as in all other types of thoracic incisions, water-seal drainage of the pleural cavity, using a No. 16 Foley catheter, is routinely performed.

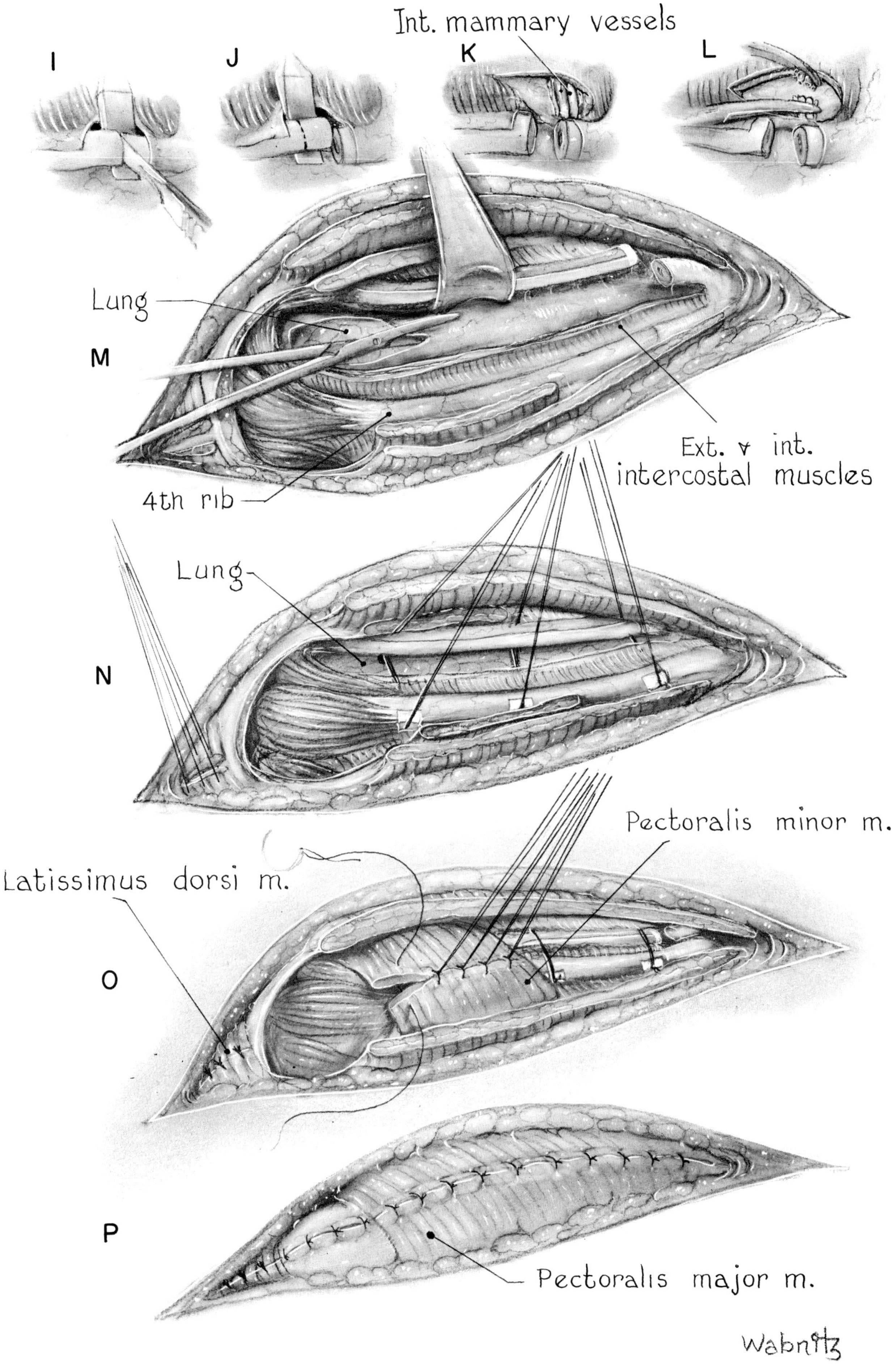
Int. mammary vessels
I
J
K
L
Lung
M
Ext. & int.
intercostal muscles
4th rib
Lung
N
Pectoralis minor m.
Latissimus dorsi m.
O
P
Pectoralis major m.
Wabnitz

THE POSTERIOR (PRONE) THORACIC INCISION

A. The position of the patient and the outline of the incision are shown.

B. The latissimus dorsi muscle is mobilized by blunt gauze dissection, and the direction for transection of the fibers of this muscle is indicated.

C. Bleeding points in the severed margins of the latissimus dorsi muscle are clamped and the clamps are subsequently replaced by suture ligatures of 000 silk. The exposed portion of the trapezius muscle is severed and the intact serratus anterior and rhomboideus major muscles are visible.

D. The fibers of the serratus anterior and rhomboideus major muscles are severed, the mobilized lateral border of the sacrospinalis muscle is retracted posteriorly, and the line of incision in the periosteum overlying the anterior surface of the fifth rib is shown. This incision extends from a point 3 to 4 cm. beyond the angle of the rib, anteriorly to the midaxillary line.

DISCUSSION—DR. CHARLES B. RIPSTEIN. *Anterior Incision.* The chief advantages of this incision are speed, ease of closure, and minimal disturbance of respiratory and circulatory function. It also has the minor advantages of not interfering with scapular muscles and of having an excellent cosmetic scar.

The anterior incision can be used for resections of most segments of the lung, although lower lobe segments may be difficult to expose. It is useful in cardiac surgery, and particularly good exposure is obtained when a combined right and left anterior incision are joined by a transverse sternal incision.

I have used this incision with complete satisfaction in a wide variety of thoracic procedures. Exposure can be widened by combining a unilateral anterior incision with a vertical sternal-splitting incision.

In the illustration, a right anterior thoracic incision is shown. I prefer to elevate the chest to a 45 degree angle with a sandbag and suspend the arm from the ether screen. The submammary skin incision is usually extended upward in the midline. There is no advantage to resecting a rib in this incision; such a maneuver leaves a large defect anteriorly and does not provide added exposure. If the latissimus dorsi is mobilized laterally and the fibers of the serratus anterior are split in the desired intercostal space, a wide exposure can be obtained.

Closure can be accomplished with interrupted sutures as illustrated or, alternatively, with a continuous suture. In females, when the breast has been elevated from the chest wall, a submammary drain is advisable to prevent a collection in the submammary space. I feel strongly that, although it is not shown, intercostal tube drainage to an underwater seal is mandatory in all thoracotomies.

Posterolateral Incision. This is the standard thoracotomy incision in most clinics. It offers the widest exposure for unilateral lesions. Its only disadvantage is the dependant position of the nonoperated side which makes respiratory exchange more difficult in poor risk patients. Where high exposure is required, the posterior limb of the incision must be extended into the parascapular area and the scapula mobilized by dividing the trapezius and rhomboid muscles. This step is not necessary if the chest is entered below the sixth rib.

The illustrations show resection of the sixth rib, but this incision may enter the chest anywhere from the third to the tenth rib. Removal of a rib is optional. This is seldom necessary in children where wide re-

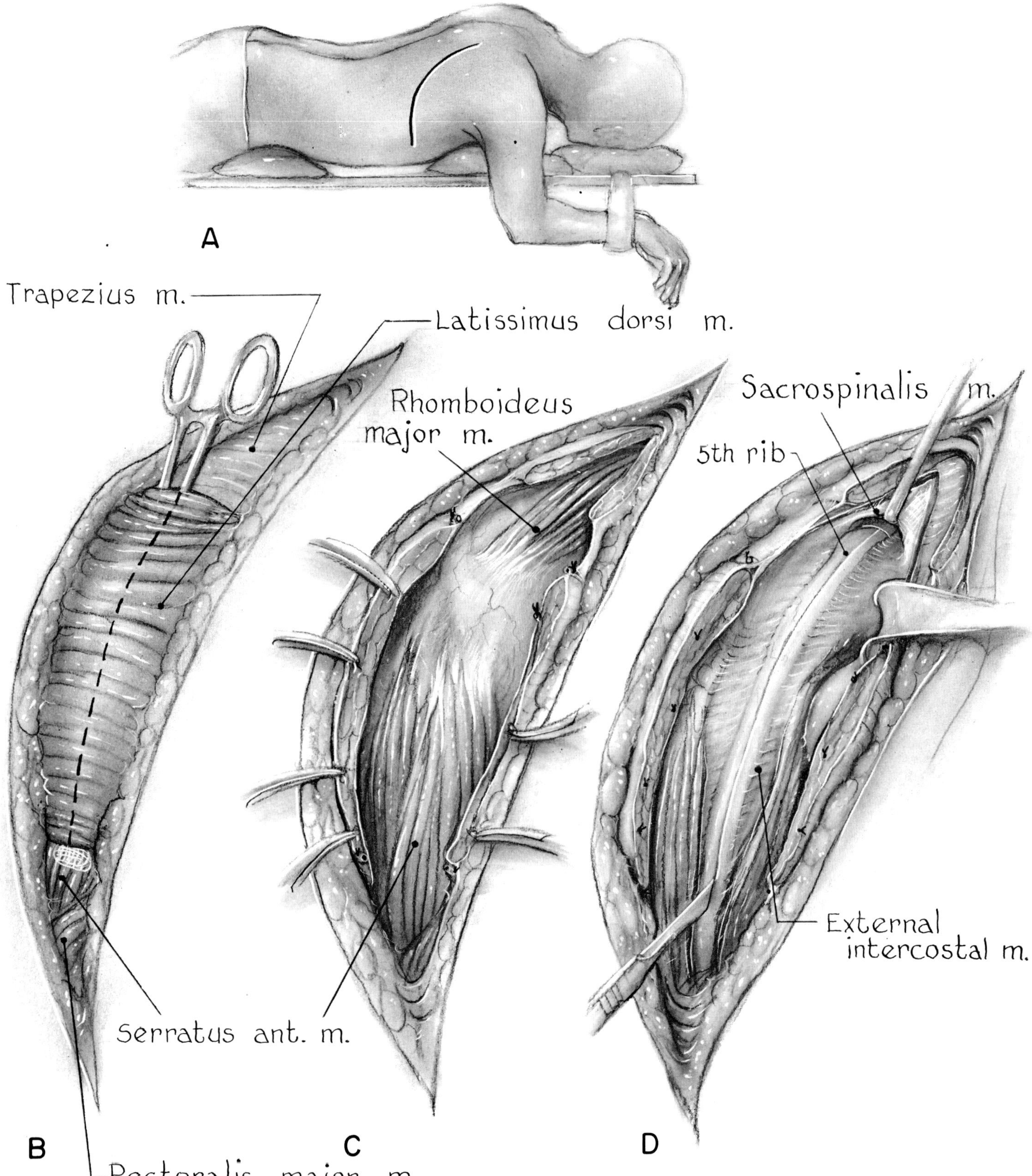
A
Trapezius m.
Latissimus dorsi m.
Rhomboideus major m.
Sacrospinalis m.
5th rib
External intercostal m.
Serratus ant. m.
B
C
D
Pectoralis major m.

E, F, G, H, I. Close-up views to show the separation of the periosteum from the rib prior to its resection.

J. The rib is transected posteriorly and elevated from its bed prior to its transection anteriorly.

K. The right pleural cavity is entered through the bed of the fifth rib, and, with a scalpel, the incision in the endothoracic fascia and parietal pleura is extended anteriorly.

L, M. The rib margins and the soft tissues of the incisional wound are covered with moist gauze pads (L) and protective moist toweling (M) prior to the insertion of a self-retaining rib retractor for the exposure of the intrapleural viscera. In the closure of this incision, the same basic principles of technic as previously described are followed.

Discussion—Dr. Ripstein (cont.)

traction is possible without producing fracture. In adults, I prefer to enter the chest through an intercostal space and divide the posterior portions of adjacent ribs to permit wide retraction.

Closure is well illustrated; again I recommend intercostal tube drainage.

Thoracoabdominal Incision. Combined thoracoabdominal incisions offer magnificent exposure in dealing with lesions involving lower thoracic, upper abdominal, and retroperitoneal organs. On the left side, the lower esophagus, diaphragm, stomach, spleen, colon, kidney, adrenal aorta, and sympathetic chain are well exposed. On the right side, the diaphragm, liver, biliary tract, duodenum, vena cava, kidney, and adrenal are readily accessible.

The right thoracoabdominal incision is well illustrated. The abdominal portion may be extended to the midline and the right rectus muscle completely divided to obtain maximum exposure. The details of closure are most important, and a meticulous anatomic reconstruction is desirable. I have found it advantageous to leave a covering of fascia and areolar tissue over the costal arch and to approximate the divided cartilage by fine interrupted sutures through this layer.

Posterior Incisions. The advantages of this approach are two: first, it permits the operated side to be dependent, an advantage when there is a great deal of tracheobronchial secretion or exudate, and second, it does not interfere with expansion of the nonoperated lung. The disadvantages are the inconvenience of posturing the patient and the inadequate exposure of certain areas in the anterior chest and mediastinum.

This incision is used chiefly in resection for tuberculosis, but it has not attained the widespread popularity of the posterolateral approach.

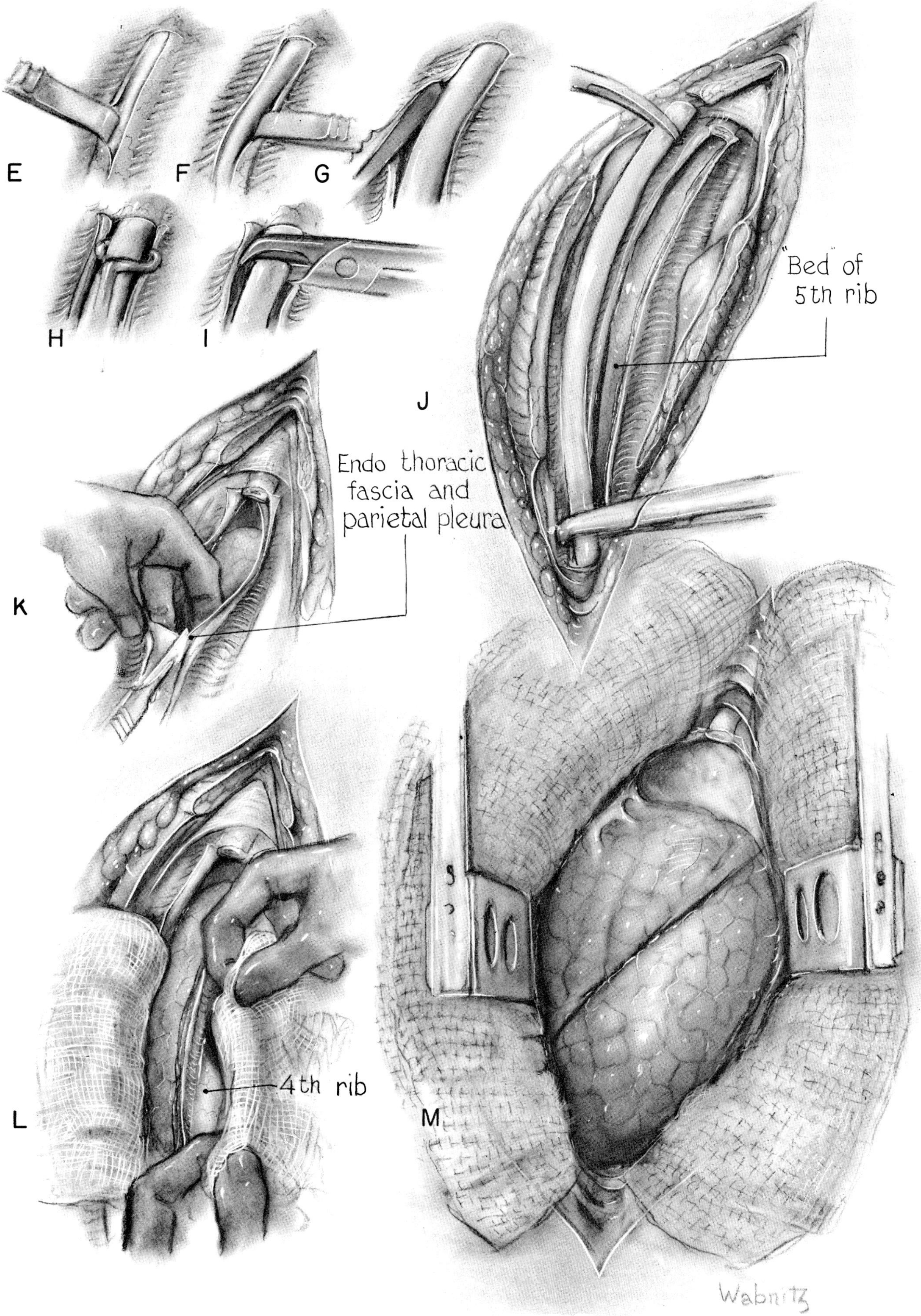
E
F
G
H
I
"Bed" of
5th rib
J
Endo thoracic
fascia and
parietal pleura
K
4th rib
L
M
Wabnitz

THE POSTEROLATERAL THORACIC INCISION

A. The curvilinear posterolateral incision, extending from the anterior axillary line, posteriorly and upward, to a point midway between the vertebral border of the scapula and the thoracic spine, is outlined and crosshatched to facilitate later closure.

B. The latissimus dorsi muscle is mobilized by blunt gauze dissection, and the line of transection of its fibers is indicated by the dotted line.

C. The transection of the latissimus dorsi muscle is completed, and the right hand of the surgeon is inserted upward beneath the mobilized portion of the serratus anterior muscle to identify the fifth rib. In this maneuver the uppermost rib readily palpable is the second. The site of severance of the trapezius muscle is depicted by the dotted line.

D. The fifth rib is identified, and the fibers of the serratus anterior muscle overlying this rib are severed with a scalpel as demonstrated. To avoid minor technical difficulties, the serratus magnus (anterior) muscle should always be severed over the length of the rib that is either mobilized or resected. The site of division of the fibers of the rhomboideus major muscle and the adjacent fibroareolar tissue is indicated.

E. A portion of the rib cage and the intervening intercostal muscle layers are shown. A longitudinal incision through the periosteum overlying the exposed portion of the anterior surface of the fifth rib is begun.

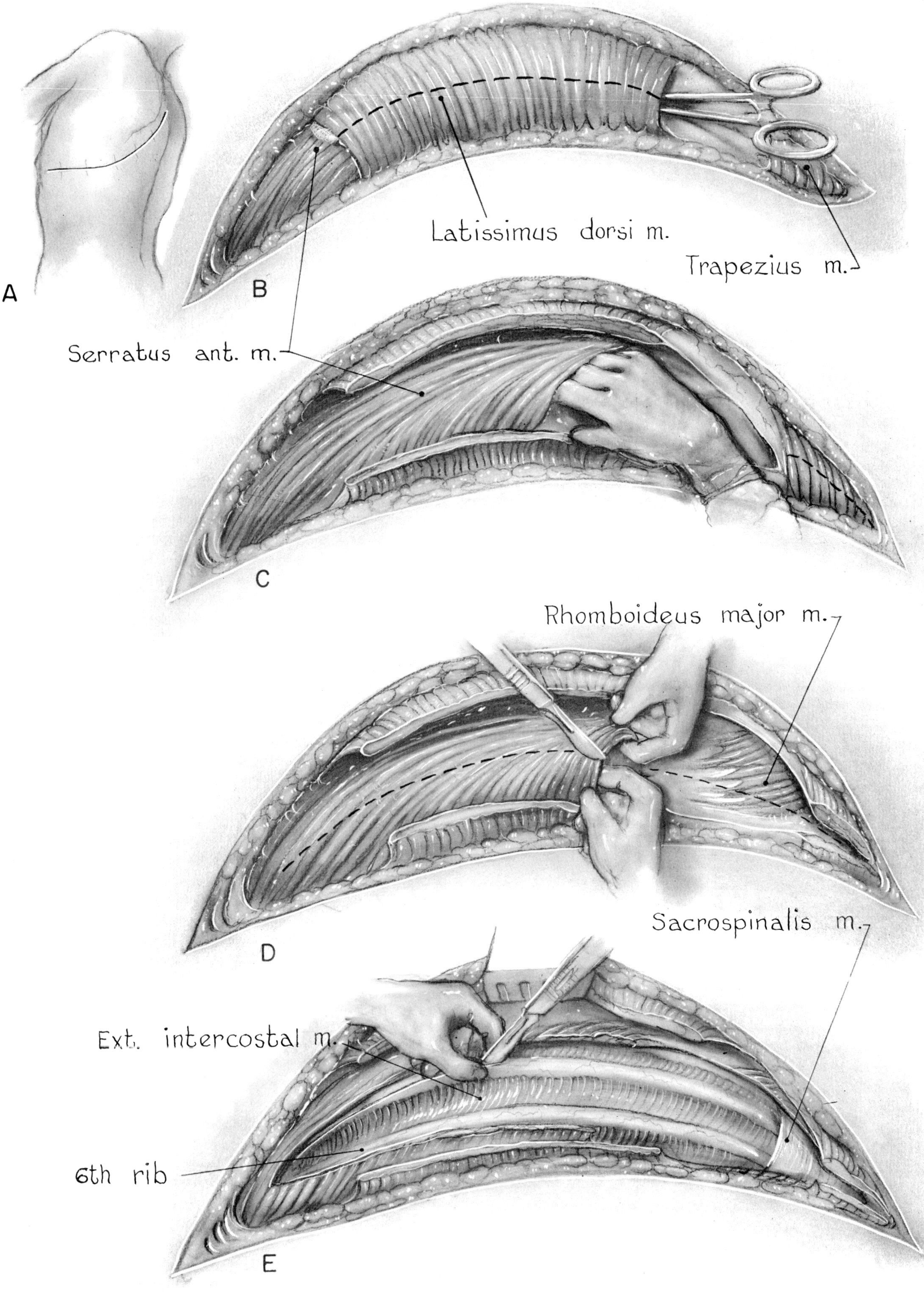
Latissimus dorsi m.
Trapezius m.
A
B
Serratus ant. m.
C
Rhomboideus major m.
D
Sacrospinalis m.
Ext. intercostal m.
6th rib
E

F. The mobilized lateral border of the sacrospinalis muscle is retracted posteriorly, and the angle of the fifth rib is visible.

G, H, I, J. The periosteum is removed from the lower half of the anterior surface of the fifth rib (G, H), and the posterior surface of the rib is separated from the subjacent endothoracic fascia and parietal pleura by both instrumental (I) and digital (J) dissection. The dissection in the plane beneath the rib is continued cephalad under the fourth and third ribs respectively. This method, originally described by Sir Russel C. Brock of England, permits free mobility of the rib cage and obviates the need of performing a rib resection. Furthermore, transection of the related intercostal muscle layers is unnecessary. These muscle layers, the external and internal intercostals, and the accompanying neurovascular bundle remain intact and are an aid in securing an air tight closure of the chest wall.

K. The fifth rib is rotated upward, and the incision in the subjacent parietal pleura is extended posteriorly by scissor dissection.

L_1, L_2, L_3. These illustrations depict the formation of periosteal "windows" to prevent the impingement of the pericostal sutures upon the periosteum in an attempt to lessen the incidence of post-thoracotomy pain.

L_4. The closure of the incision is commenced by the insertion of multiple pericostal sutures consisting of double strands of No. 2 chromic catgut.

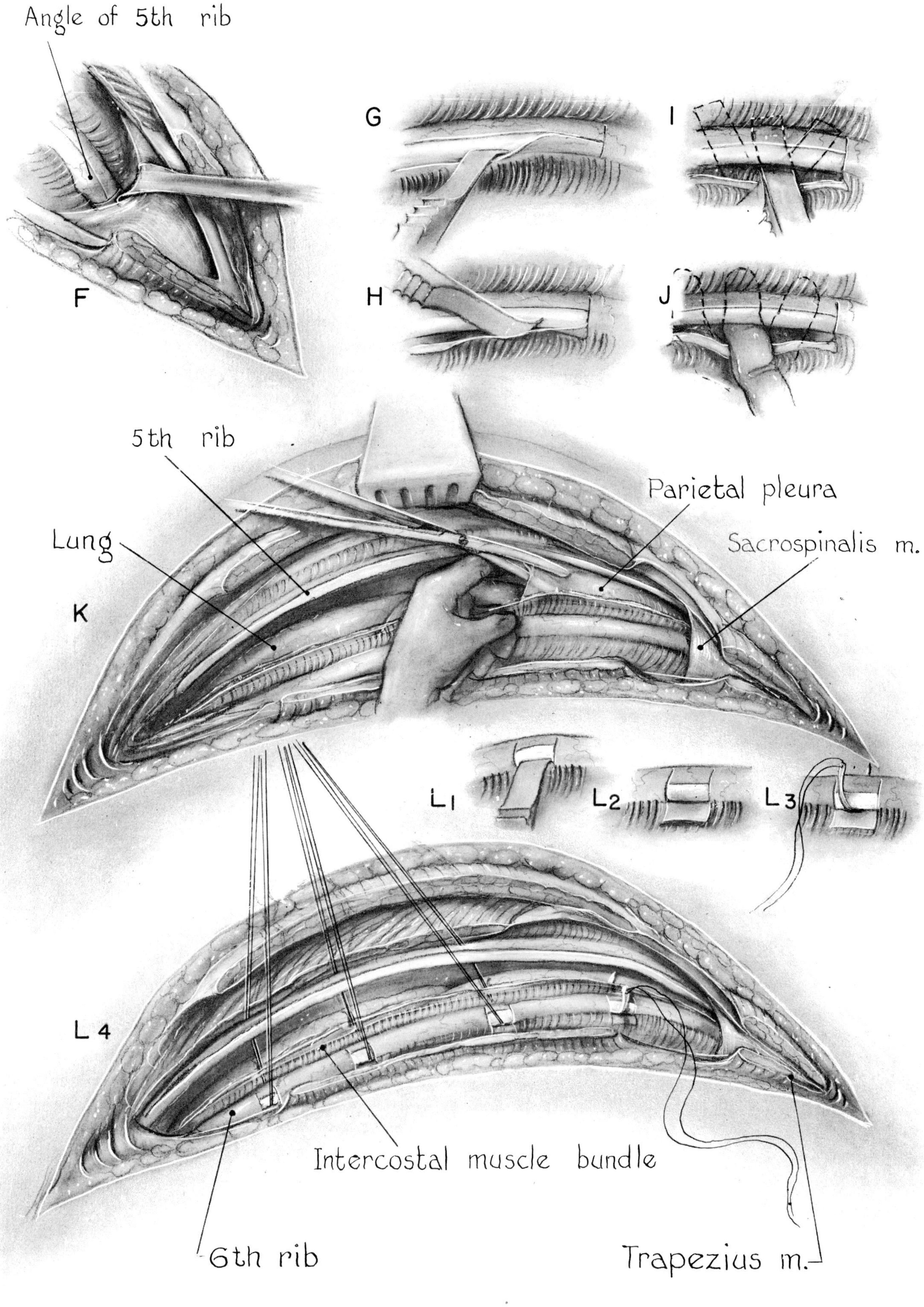
Angle of 5th rib
F
G
H
I
J
5th rib
Parietal pleura
Lung
Sacrospinalis m.
K
L1
L2
L3
L4
Intercostal muscle bundle
6th rib
Trapezius m.

M, N. The pericostal sutures are tied, and the overlap of the lower half of the anterior surface of the fifth rib by the subjacent intact intercostal muscle layers is visible. To secure an air tight closure of the pleural cavity, the lateral margin of the sacrospinalis muscle is approximated to the subjacent intercostal muscle layers with a mattress suture of 00 silk (M) and two simple interrupted sutures of 00 silk (N).

O. The approximation of the rib cage is completed, and the severed fibers of the serratus anterior and the rhomboideus major muscles are sutured with interrupted sutures of 00 silk.

P, Q. The latissimus dorsi muscle and the fibroareolar tissue layer overlying the "angle of auscultation" between this muscle and the trapezius muscle, and the transected fibers of the trapezius muscle are sutured with interrupted sutures of 00 silk (P). The skin layer is closed with interrupted sutures of 000 silk (Q). Although not demonstrated, in all thoracic incisions in which an entrance into the pleural cavity is made, water-seal drainage of the pleural cavity is routinely employed.

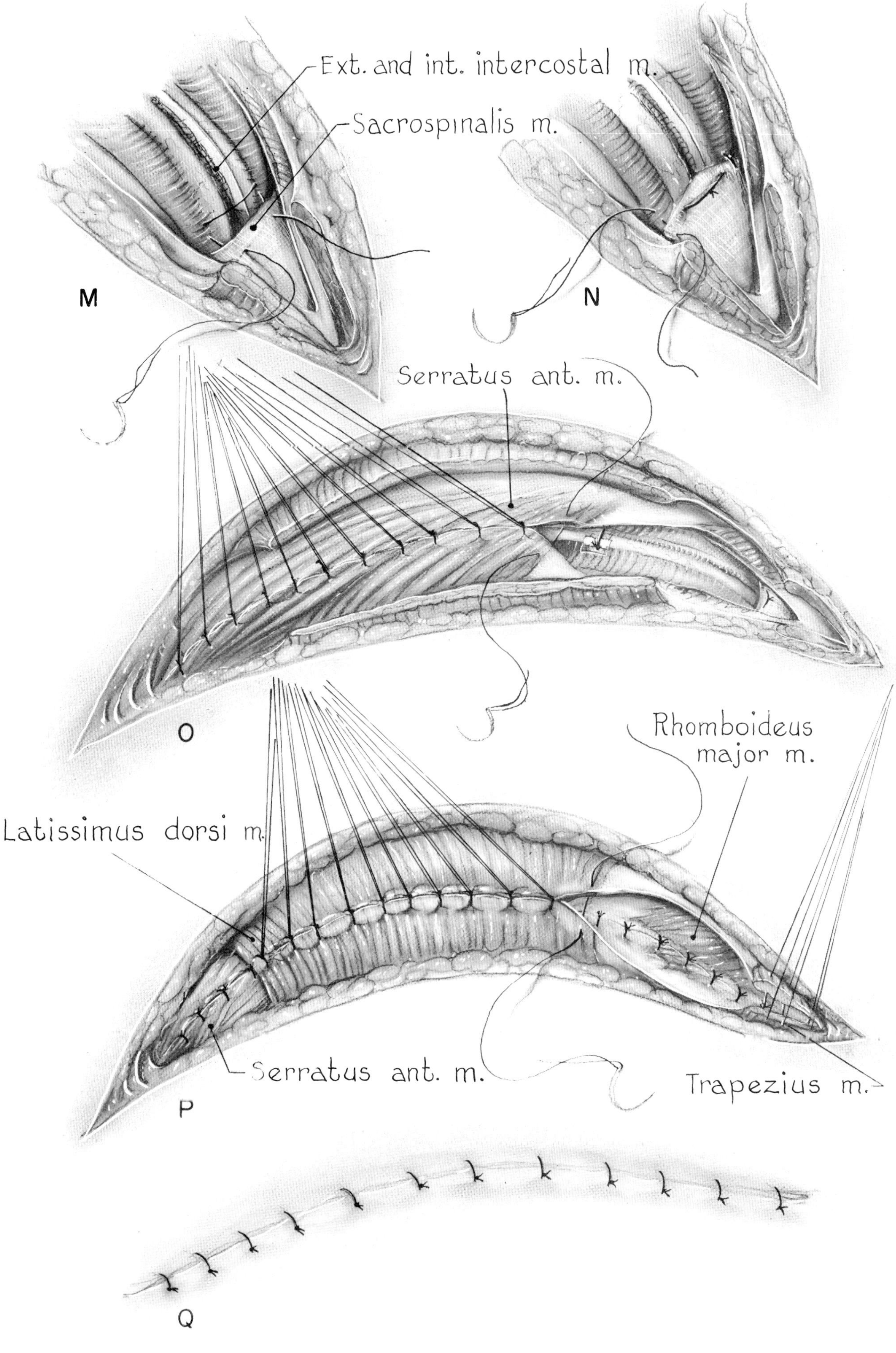
Ext. and int. intercostal m.
Sacrospinalis m.
M
N
Serratus ant. m.
O
Rhomboideus major m.
Latissimus dorsi m.
Serratus ant. m.
Trapezius m.
P
Q

THE THORACOABDOMINAL INCISION

The thoracoabdominal incision, either right or left, is of distinct value if used when properly indicated. It converts the pleural and the peritoneal cavities into one main cavity and thereby gives excellent exposure of the operative area. However, closure of the wound is time-consuming and there is a predisposition to more frequent postoperative complications. Furthermore, it is believed that this type of incision is employed too frequently as a routine when either an abdominal or a thoracic incision alone would suffice for the operation that is planned.

The right thoracoabdominal incision, as depicted in the artist's illustrations, may be particularly useful in reconstructive operations upon the common duct, total excision of the right lobe of the liver, and shunt operations between the portal vein and the inferior vena cava. The left thoracoabdominal incision may be used effectively in resections of the lower end of the esophagus, total gastrectomy, the removal of large and adherent spleens, and in the performance of shunt operations between the splenic and the left renal veins.

A. The incision overlying the eighth interspace and extending across the right costal margin onto the anterior abdominal wall is shown.

B. The incision is deepened through the skin and the subcutaneous fatty tissue layers to expose the underlying musculature of the anterolateral thoracic and the anterior abdominal walls.

C. The exposed muscles—the latissimus dorsi, the serratus magnus, and the external oblique muscle and its aponeurosis—are severed with a scalpel to expose the eighth and ninth ribs and the intervening external intercostal muscle.

D. The incision is continued through the external intercostal muscle layer, and the fibers of the internal intercostal muscle which course in a different plane are depicted.

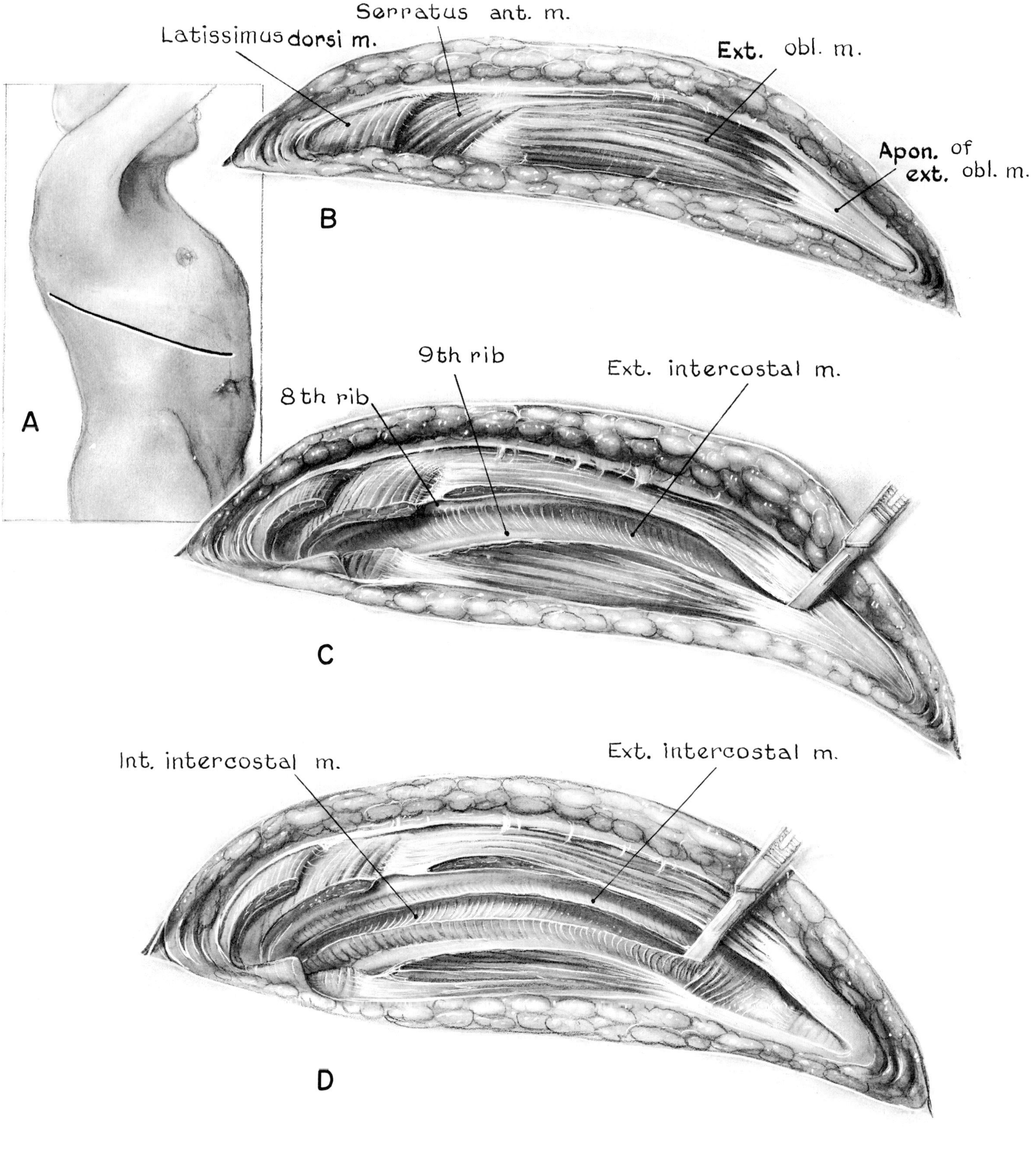
Serratus ant. m.
Latissimus dorsi m.
Ext. obl. m.
Apon. of ext. obl. m.
A
B
9th rib
8th rib
Ext. intercostal m.
C
Int. intercostal m.
Ext. intercostal m.
D

E. The incision is deepened posteriorly through the internal intercostal muscle, the endothoracic fascia, and the parietal pleura to enter the right pleural cavity. This incision is then extended anteriorly to the costal arch severing the fibers of the internal intercostal muscle and the underlying fibers of the right leaflet of the diaphragm.

F. The incision is continued across the costal arch and through the musculature of the anterior abdominal wall to enter the peritoneal cavity.

G. The incision is completed, and the adequacy of the exposure of the operative field obtained by the conversion of the pleural and peritoneal cavities into a common cavity is shown.

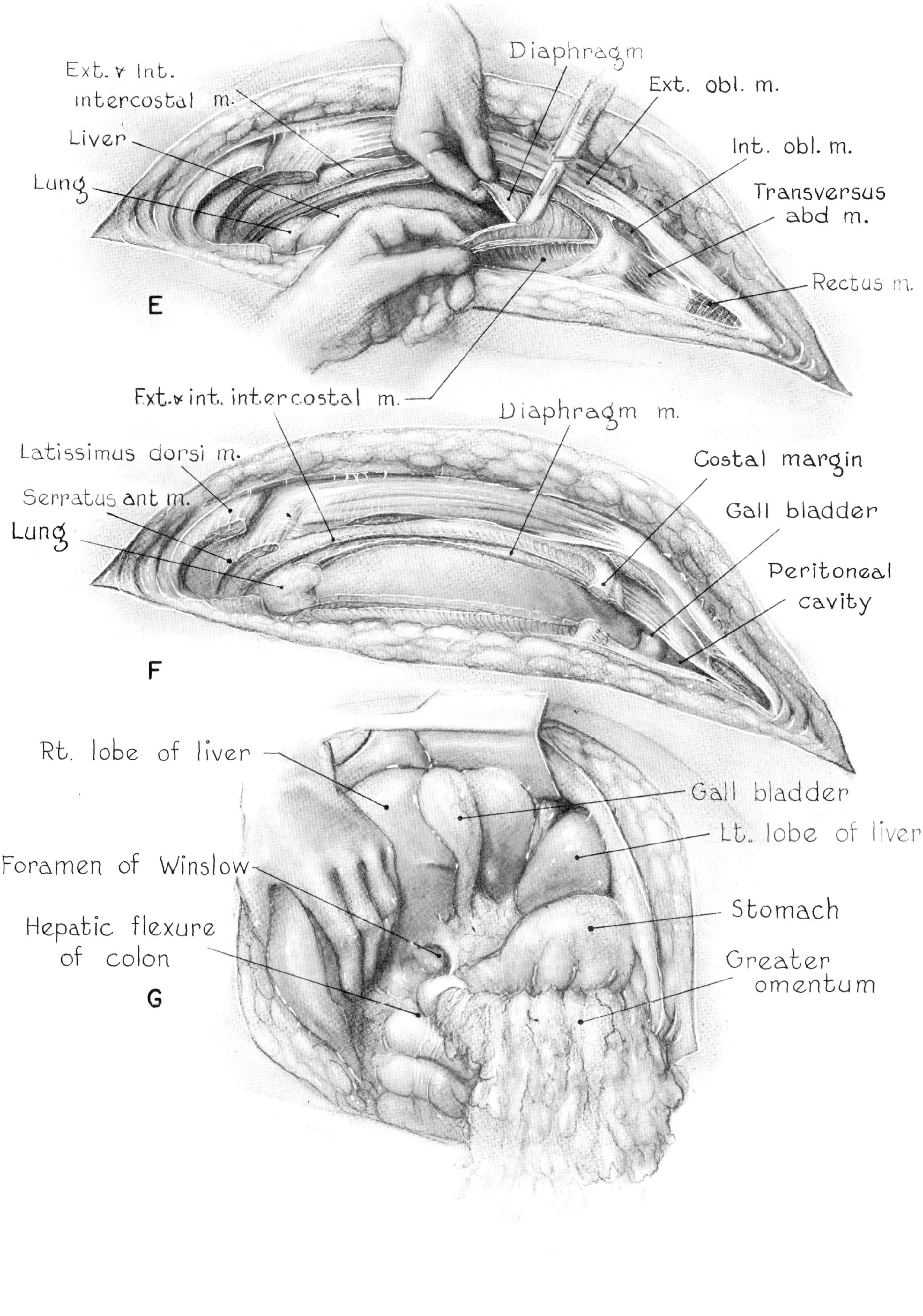
Ext. & Int. intercostal m.
Liver
Lung
Diaphragm
Ext. obl. m.
Int. obl. m.
Transversus abd m.
Rectus m.
E
Ext. & int. intercostal m.
Diaphragm m.
Latissimus dorsi m.
Serratus ant m.
Lung
Costal margin
Gall bladder
Peritoneal cavity
F
Rt. lobe of liver
Gall bladder
Lt. lobe of liver
Foramen of Winslow
Hepatic flexure of colon
Stomach
Greater omentum
G

H. The closure of the incision is begun by the approximation of the cut margins of the diaphragm with interrupted sutures of silk (00). The surrounding related structures are indicated.

I. Two pericostal sutures of double strands of No. 2 chromic catgut are inserted preliminary to the approximation of the eighth and ninth ribs. Prior to the insertion of these sutures periosteal "windows" are made along the inferior border of the lower or ninth rib. This is done to prevent the impingement of the sutures upon the periosteum and thereby possibly lessen both the incidence and/or the severity of post-thoracotomy pain.

J. The rib cage is approximated with a self-retaining Bailey–Gibbons rib approximator, and the pericostal sutures are tied and cut. The sutures of silk (000) in the intercostal muscle layers are first inserted and, after approximation of the ribs, they are then tied and cut. A figure of 8 mattress suture of No. 1 braided silk is inserted to unite the cut margins of the costal arch.

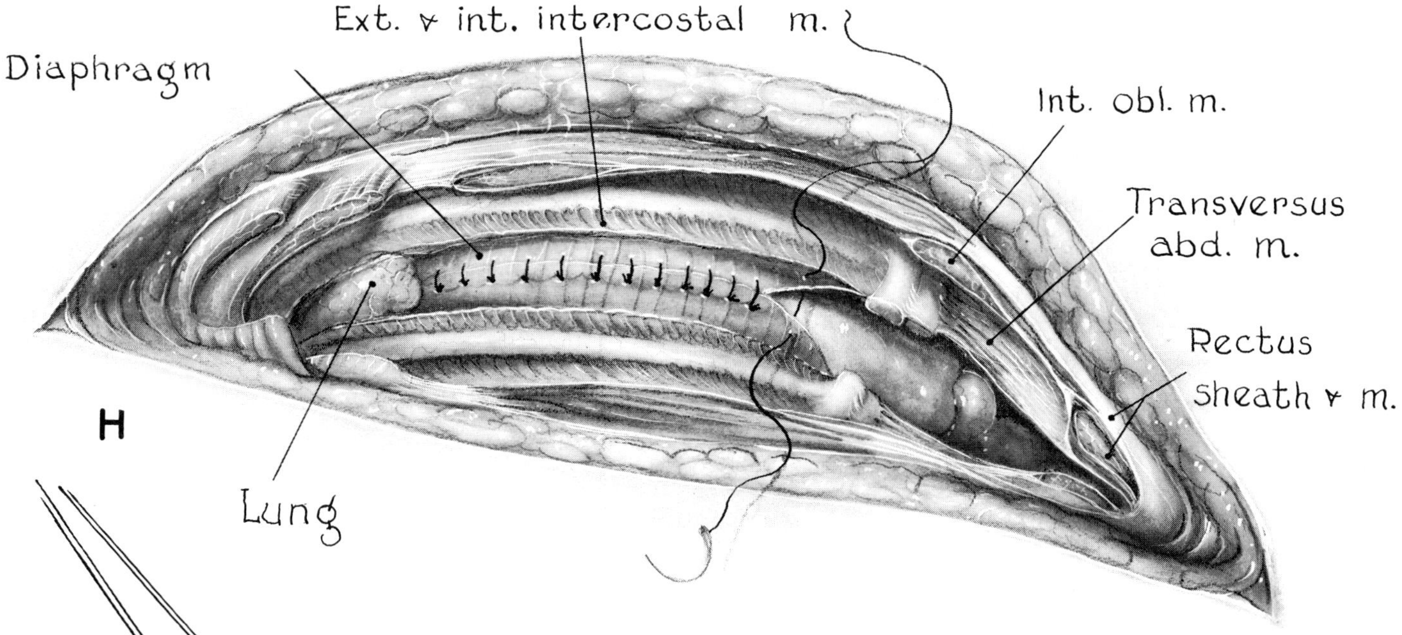
Ext. & int. intercostal m.
Diaphragm
Int. obl. m.
Transversus abd. m.
Rectus sheath & m.
Lung

H

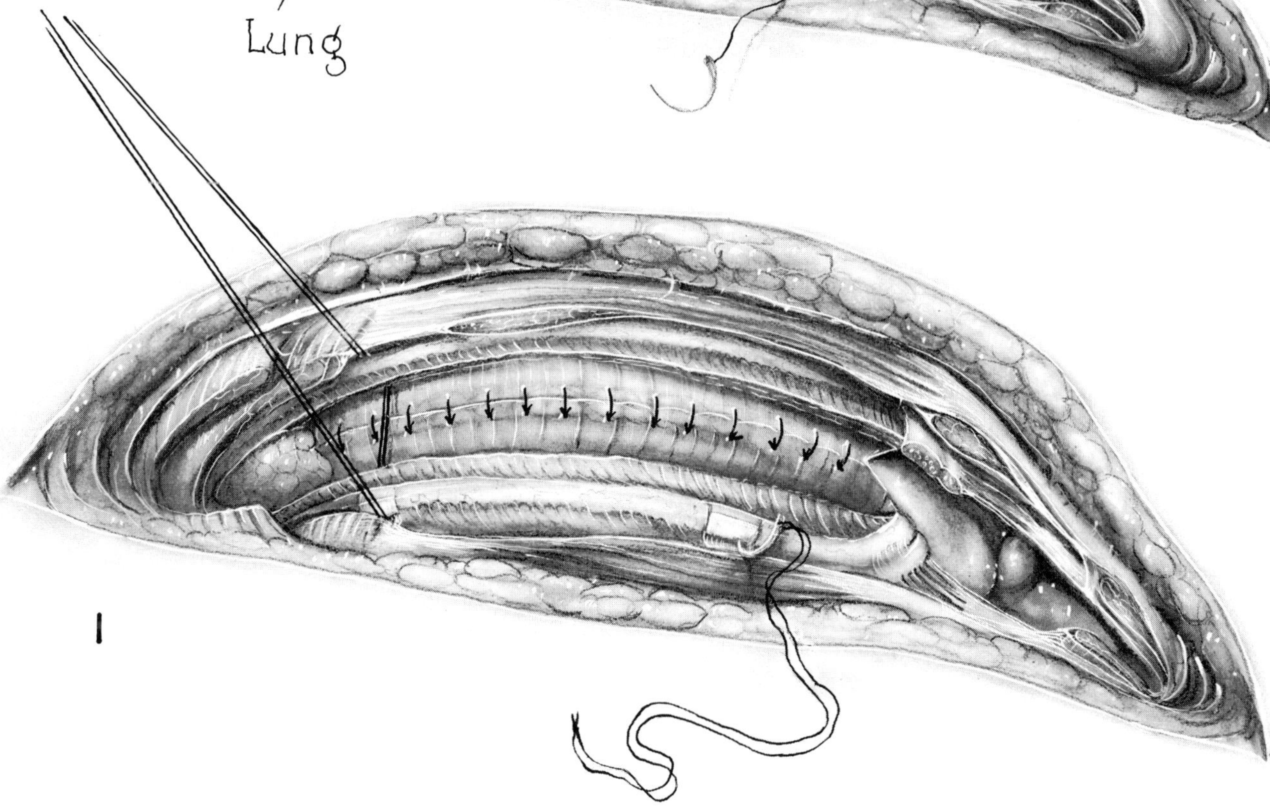

I

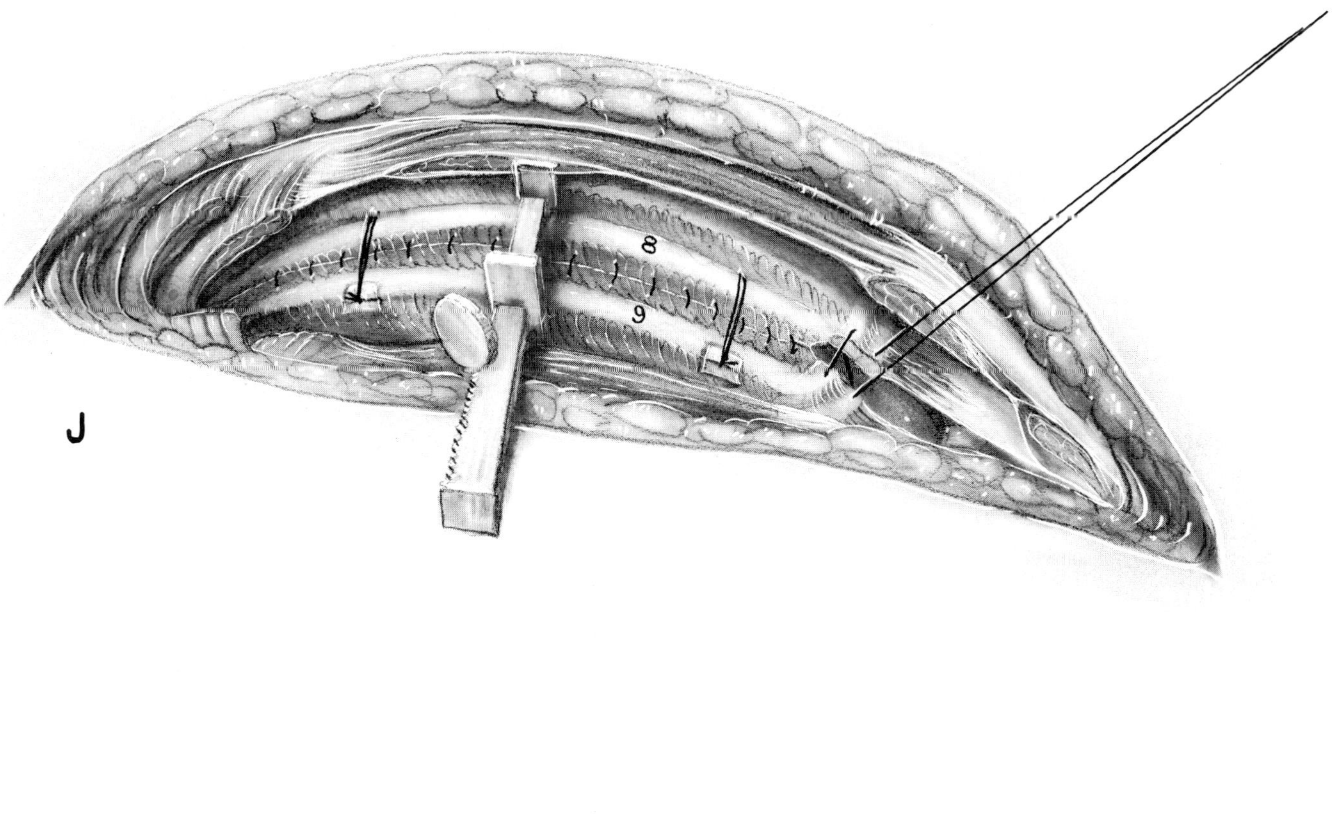
8
9

J

K. The closure of the rib cage is completed, and the cut margins of the serratus anterior and the external oblique muscles are sutured with interrupted sutures of silk (00).

L. Close-up showing the approximation of the severed fibers of the latissimus dorsi muscle with interrupted silk (00) sutures.

M. The transversus abdominis muscle layer is approximated with a series of interrupted sutures of silk (000), which are shown inserted but not tied.

N. The closure of the transversus abdominis muscle is completed, and the suturing of the internal oblique muscle is begun using sutures of silk (000).

O. The closure of the muscle layers is completed by suturing the aponeurosis of the external oblique muscle and the anterior rectus sheath. Although not illustrated in the drawings, water-seal drainage of the pleural cavity is routinely employed.

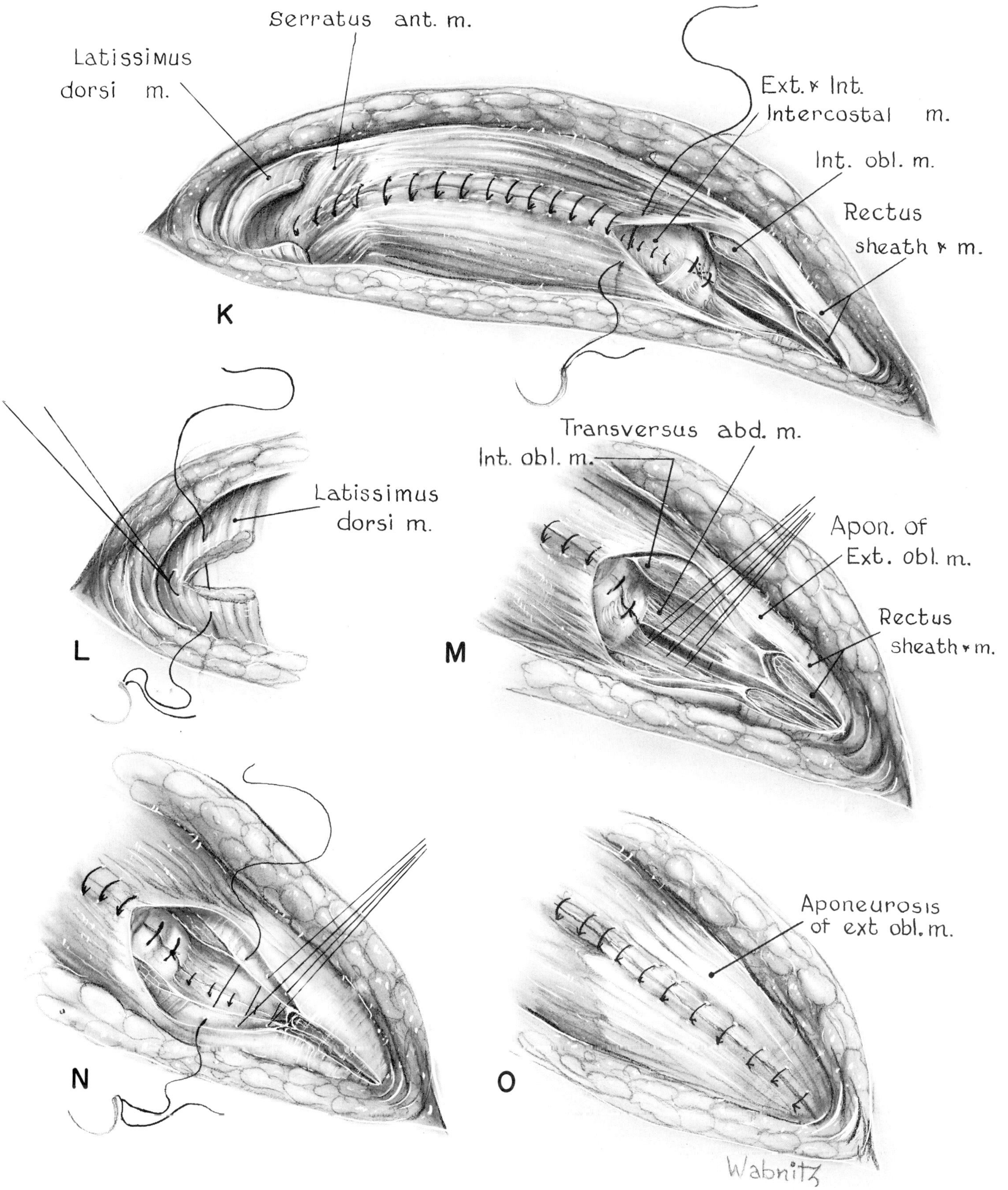
Serratus ant. m.
Latissimus dorsi m.
Ext. & Int. Intercostal m.
Int. obl. m.
Rectus sheath & m.
K
Latissimus dorsi m.
L
Transversus abd. m.
Int. obl. m.
Apon. of Ext. obl. m.
Rectus sheath & m.
M
N
Aponeurosis of ext obl. m.
O
Wabnitz

SCALENOTOMY

A. The site of the incision overlying the subclavian triangle of the neck is represented by a dotted line. This incision, located approximately 4 cm. cephalad to the clavicle, is bound anteriorly by the posterior border of the sternomastoid muscle and posteriorly by the external jugular vein.

B. The skin incision is deepened through the subcutaneous fatty tissue plane to expose the platysma muscle.

C. The fibers of the platysma muscle are severed transversely, and the incision in the anterior layer of the deep cervical fascia (investing layer) is visible.

D. The clavicular belly of the sternomastoid muscle is retracted anteriorly, and the incision in the middle layer of the deep cervical fascia between this muscle and the inferior belly of the omohyoid muscle is indicated by the dotted line.

E. The middle layer of the deep cervical fascia (omohyoid "fascial carpet") is incised, and the underlying fat pad, a characteristic anatomic landmark, is protruded into the incision.

F. A portion of the fat pad is held in tissue forceps and displaced posteriorly to expose portions of the scalenus anterior muscle and the phrenic nerve. A blood vessel accompanying the nerve may also be seen.

G. The lowermost portion of the scalenus anterior muscle is elevated on a clamp, and the transection of its fibers in layers is begun. The internal jugular vein, the transverse scapular vessels, and the phrenic nerve with its accompanying vessel are demonstrable.

DISCUSSION—DR. JAMES T. DANIELS. The apparently simple procedure of dividing a muscle such as the scalenus anticus can be appreciated as complex when the important structures lying in proximity to it are visualized. The illustrated technic of approach through the subclavian triangle to the scalenus anticus muscle demonstrates graphically the intricate relationship of these structures to the muscle. It is essential to recall that the entire nerve and blood supply to the upper extremity and one-half the nerve supply to the diaphragm are contained within this small area, lying much deeper than it is possible to indicate in a two dimensional illustration. The maneuvering within this confined space is conducted with care in order to avoid injuring the adjacent structures.

From the viewpoint of operative surgery alone, relief of disturbing neurovascular symptoms due to compression by scalenotomy is achieved by knowledge of the anatomic relationship of the local and adjacent structures, proper exposure, and careful technic. Illustrations designed to serve as a guide for this purpose can be expected to fulfill these requirements. A knowledge of the normal anatomic arrangement of the elements present in the vicinity of the scalenus anticus muscle is presumed. The need for this knowledge is obvious when consideration is given the fact that lying nearby the scalenus anticus muscle and the structures contained within the precise boundaries of the subclavian triangle are the pleura, the carotid sheath and its contents, and the subclavian and jugular veins. For the careless operator there are many opportunities for disaster.

Individual preferences based on experience suggest various considerations for slight alterations of technic. These variations present themselves by anticipating certain anomalies or abnormalities the surgeon may encounter in this region. For example, the anterior approach as illustrated is preferable to the lateral, particularly when a cervical rib of significant proportion is to be resected. In this instance a "collar" incision passing 5 to 6 cm. upward and backward from a point slightly above the sternoclavicular articulation is advantageous. This affords exposure of the tendinous clavicular attachment of the sternocleidomastoid muscle. Division of the clavicular attachment provides considerable space and exposure of the proximal portion of the subclavian artery and obviates difficult retraction. It is readily sutured with mattress sutures. The incision repre-

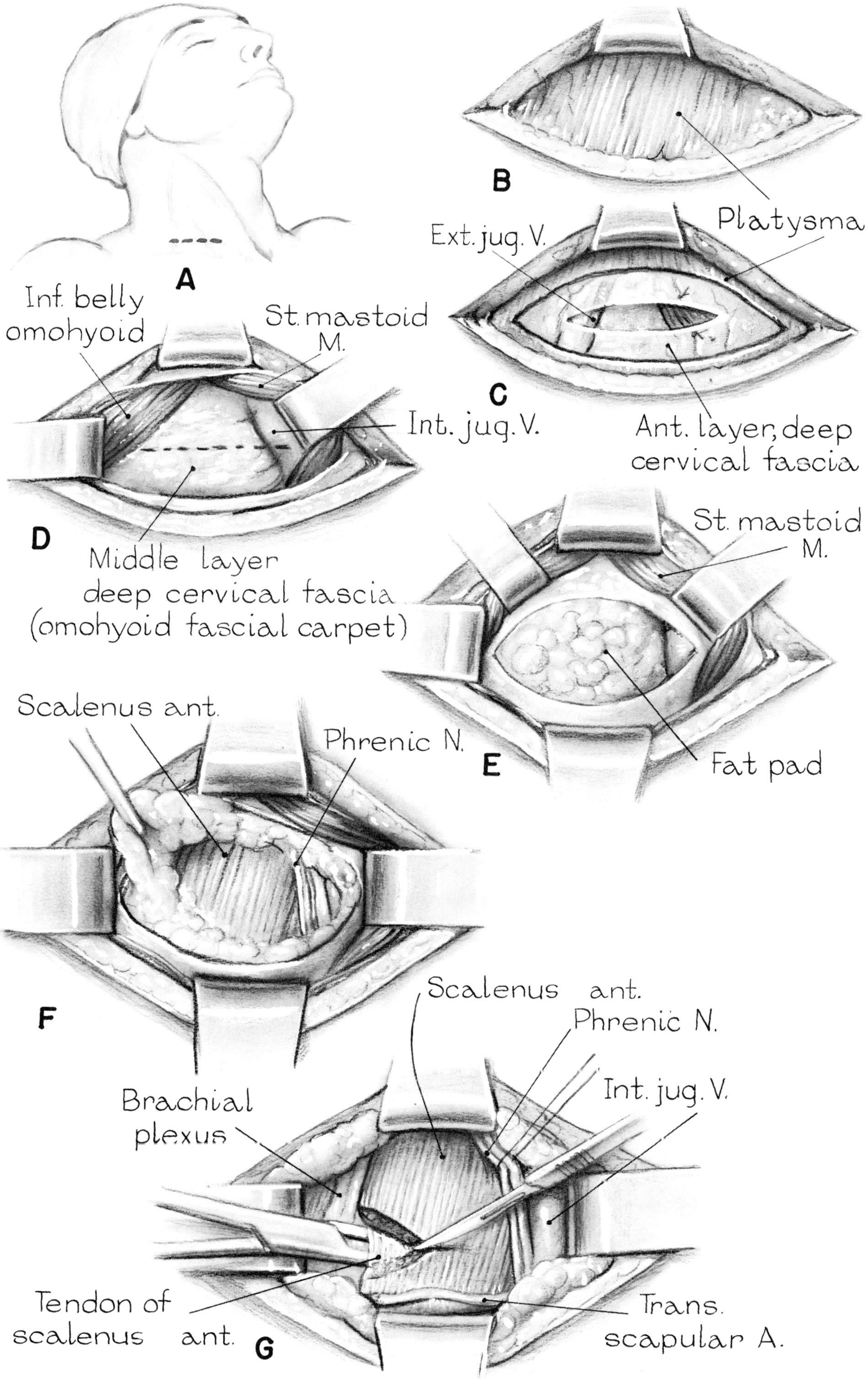
A
B
Platysma
Ext. jug. V.
C
Ant. layer, deep cervical fascia
Inf. belly omohyoid
St. mastoid M.
Int. jug. V.
D
Middle layer deep cervical fascia (omohyoid fascial carpet)
St. mastoid M.
E
Fat pad
Scalenus ant.
Phrenic N.
F
Scalenus ant.
Phrenic N.
Int. jug. V.
Brachial plexus
Tendon of scalenus ant.
G
Trans. scapular A.

H. The transection of the remaining tendinous portion of the scalenus anterior muscle is about to be completed. In this regard, it is most important to sever completely all of the muscle and tendinous fibers to obtain complete release of the compression effect upon the subjacent subclavian artery.

I. The scalenotomy is finished, and the relation of the ends of the completely transected muscle to the surrounding structures is visible.

J, K. The fat pad is replaced, and the middle (J) and the anterior (K) layers of the deep cervical fascia are approximated with interrupted sutures of fine (0000) silk.

L. The skin is being closed with interrupted sutures of 000 silk. Each suture is threaded on a straight cambric or milliner's needle.

Discussion—Dr. Daniels (cont.)

sented in A, Plate 12, is well suited to this purpose by slight extension anteriorly. The sternocleidomastoid and omohyoid muscles are retracted together as shown in Plate 12 (D). Only occasionally is it necessary to sever the omohyoid.

It may be suggested that, when the incision is made closer to the clavicle, the transverse cervical and suprascapular arteries will cross horizontally along the line of approach to the scalenus anticus muscle, particularly its tendinous insertion. These are readily isolated, clamped, severed, and ligated or electrocoagulated. At this low level, the phrenic nerve has, in coursing downward, obliquely crossed the scalenus anticus from its lateral to its medial border. The nerve lies medial and may be difficult to find beneath the sternocleidomastoid muscle. It is readily found higher up, and it should be identified, liberated, and displaced medialward where it can be protected for some distance.

In the lateral aspect of the exposure, the brachial plexus is found emerging from behind the scalenus anticus muscle at its lateral border. The surgeon must be aware that the distal portion of the subclavian artery lies inferior to the plexus, after arching posterior to the scalenus anticus muscle. This is illustrated in Plate 13 (I). Therefore it is signally important to anticipate possible injury to the subclavian artery. Occasionally, atheromatous plaques form on the vessel as the result of prolonged compression and irritation. Such plaques have been dislodged and fatal hemorrhage reported. If forceps are to be passed posterior to the muscle, it must be done with great care. My own preference is to free the plexus from the lateral border of the scalenus anticus muscle, to place a cotton strip upon the plexus, and to move it gently medialward as the muscle is divided in the same direction. Direct visualization is thus achieved and injury to the artery avoided. It is considered safer to sever the muscle in a piecemeal manner by grasping a few fibers in tissue forceps and carefully inspecting each group before sectioning with scissors.

Plate 13 (I) demonstrates the presence of a few fibrous adhesions attached to the inferior border of the arching subclavian artery. These are occasionally situated about the vasa vasorum. If they are injured, troublesome extravasation of blood will occur between the muscular and adventitial layers of the subclavian artery. This is best avoided by severing the fibrous adhesions some distance from the vessel.

The layers of the deep cervical fascia—the so-called "fat pad," which, incidentally, harbors Virchow's lymph node on the right side—contain many fine blood vessels. These are disrupted in this procedure, and care must be taken to avoid oozing which will stain the surrounding structures, making identification difficult. They can readily be electrocoagulated, or, if such a unit is not available, ligation may be necessary.

Irrigation of the operative area with warm saline, gentle suctioning, and the use of wet cotton strips or "paddies" used for sponging, quite satisfactorily serve the purpose of maintaining the normal appearance of tissues. When sectioning the scalenus anticus muscle, the oozing encountered can be minimized in this fashion, thus enabling the surgeon to identify precisely the structure he is about to divide.

In closing the wound, in addition to the readily recognized necessity for closing the deep cervical fascia over the "fat pad" to avoid a troublesome postoperative "lump" beneath the incision, two considerations are noteworthy. They are, first, that a deeply placed suture near the clavicle can perforate the subclavian vein, and second, that an attempt should be made to avoid a resultant ugly scar, especially in a female patient. The wound should, of course, be closed in layers, preferably with interrupted 0000 silk sutures as Doctor Madden suggests. This should include a subcuticular layer placed deeply enough to be well covered by the thin skin in this area.

A very careful skin closure with 000000 "arterial silk" and an "atraumatic needle" will afford accurate approximation of the wound edges and prevent an unsightly scar.

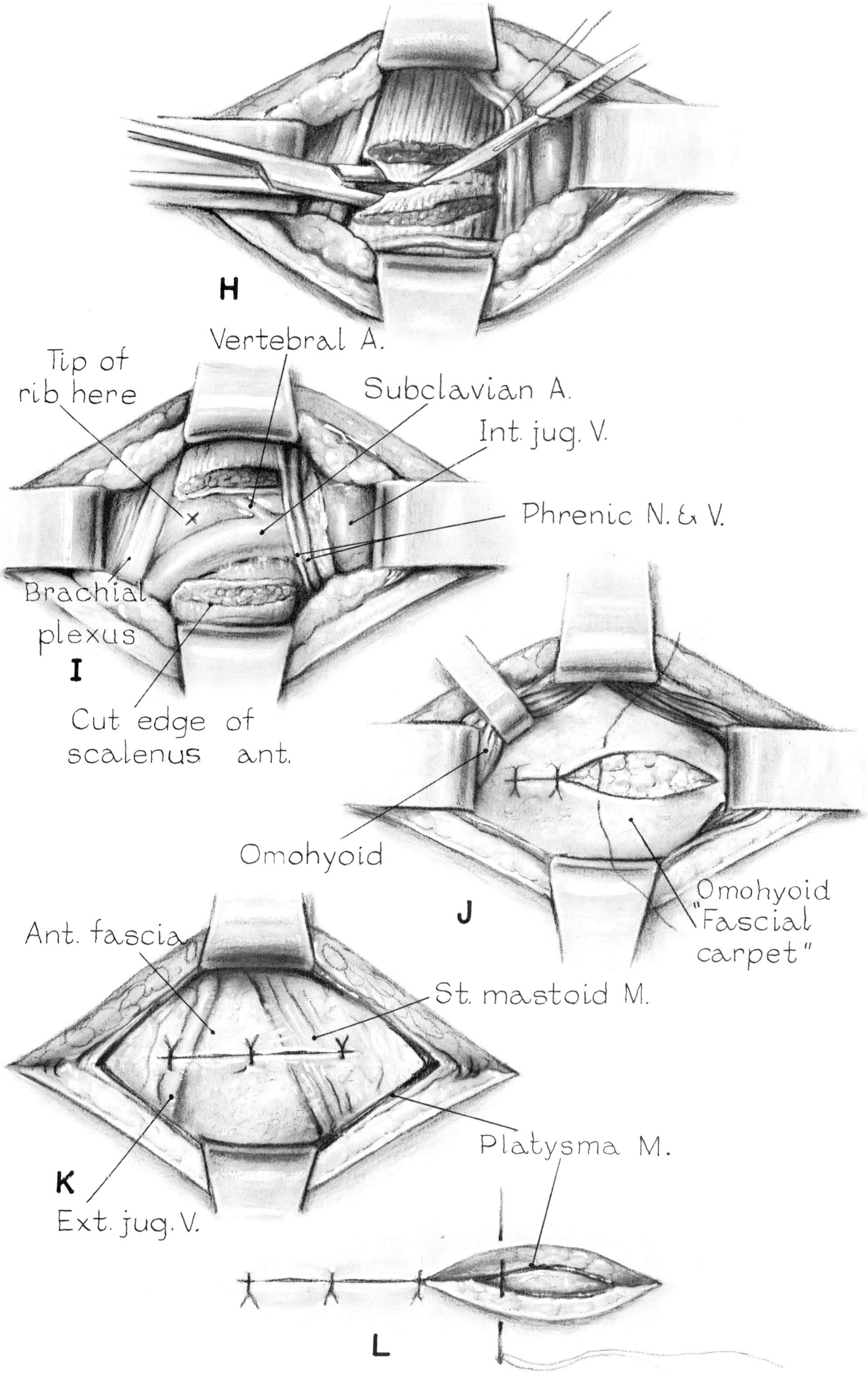
H
Vertebral A.
Tip of
rib here
Subclavian A.
Int. jug. V.
Phrenic N. & V.
Brachial
plexus
I
Cut edge of
scalenus ant.
Omohyoid
J
Omohyoid
"Fascial
carpet"
Ant. fascia
St. mastoid M.
Platysma M.
K
Ext. jug. V.
L

TRACHEOSTOMY

A tracheostomy may be performed either electively or as an emergency operation. Frequently it is done as an emergency procedure and, unfortunately, it is oftentimes performed too late. A good dictum to follow is that if the necessity for the performance of a tracheostomy is seriously questioned, it is usually a good indication for the operation. The technic for an elective tracheostomy is illustrated.

A. The two types of incision employed, the transverse and longitudinal, are indicated. The transverse incision is preferred.

B. The incision is deepened through the subcutaneous tissue plane, and its continuation through the fibers of the underlying platysma muscle is shown.

C. The upper and lower flaps of skin, subcutaneous fat, and platysma muscle are retracted and, with a scalpel, the anterior or investing layer of the deep cervical fascia is incised in the midline.

D. The sternohyoid muscles are retracted, and the underlying anterior borders of the sternothyroid muscles may be seen. An incision is made through the middle or pretracheal fascia layer of the deep cervical fascia to expose the isthmus of the thyroid gland.

E. The left finger of the surgeon is inserted downward beneath the pretracheal fascia, and the incision in this fascia is extended caudad by scissor dissection.

Discussion—Dr. Edgar L. Frazell. The choice of the skin incision for tracheostomy is usually dictated by the circumstances of the individual case. When performed electively it is usually done as an integral part of some other operative procedure about the head and neck region.

The type of incision must then conform to the necessities of the primary operation. As an emergency measure, tracheostomy is both dramatic and life-saving. Rapid exposure of the trachea with minimal dissection of skin flaps is imperative in such cases. I find this is facilitated by the use of the vertical midline incision as it minimizes blood loss from the distended veins in the area. Furthermore, the incision through subcutaneous tissue and fascia corresponds to the natural cleavage plane between the pretracheal muscles. Additional exposure is obtained by extension of the incision in either direction to allow for variations in the position of the thyroid isthmus. The latter structure may be retracted superiorly or inferiorly or rapidly divided between clamps to expose the second or third tracheal ring.

The important objective in an emergency tracheostomy is to establish an artificial airway in the shortest possible time. Simple incision of two or more tracheal cartilages is usually sufficient for introduction of the canula, though some surgeons prefer excision of a window. The latter technic tends to delay spontaneous closure of the fistula after the emergency is past. Suture of the wound about the tracheostomy may lead to troublesome subcutaneous emphysema in some cases and cellulitis in others.

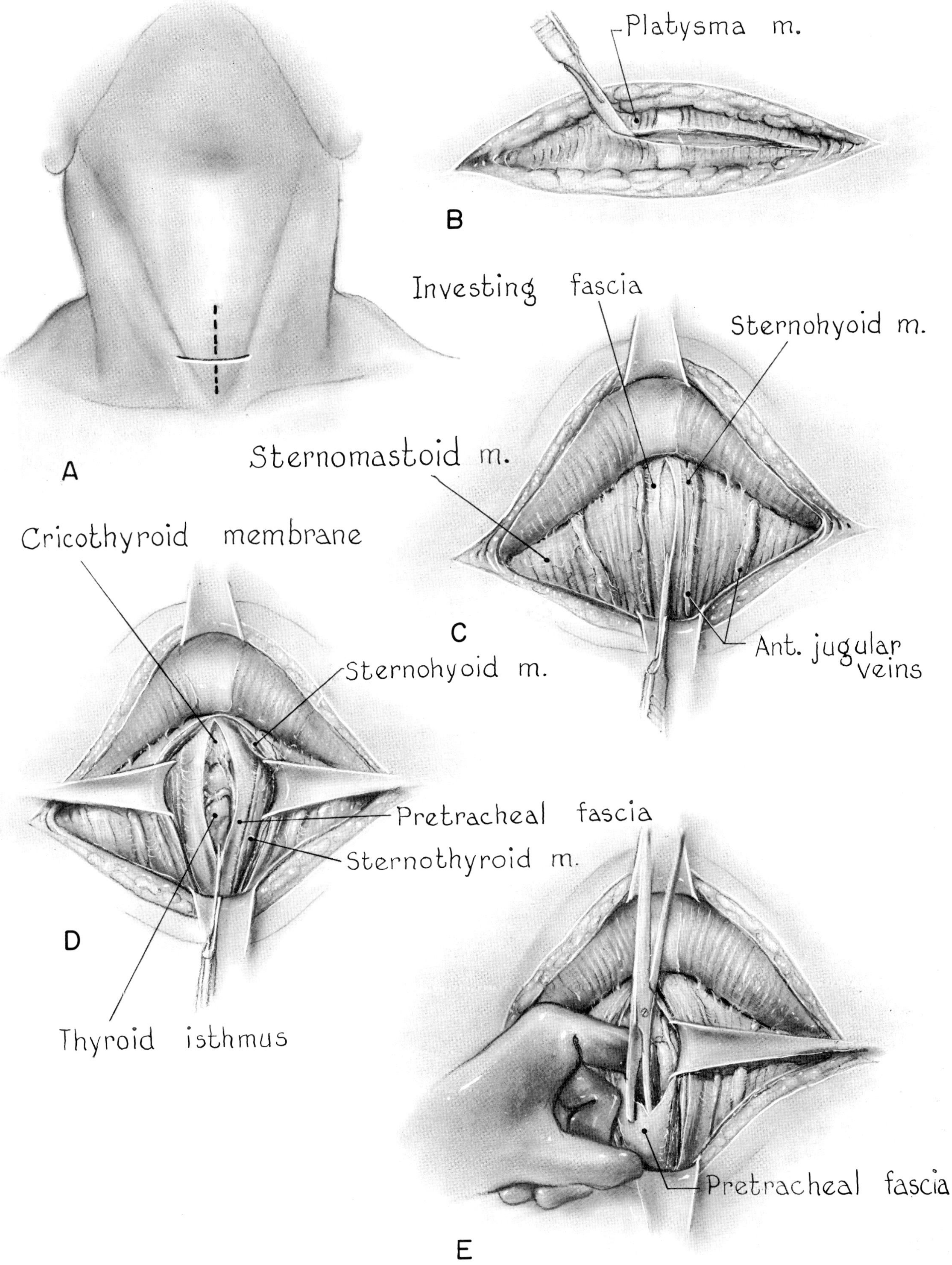
Platysma m.
B
Investing fascia
Sternohyoid m.
Sternomastoid m.
A
Cricothyroid membrane
C
Ant. jugular veins
Sternohyoid m.
Pretracheal fascia
Sternothyroid m.
D
Thyroid isthmus
Pretracheal fascia
E

F. The incision in the pretracheal fascia layer is completed, and a portion of the trachea is exposed. The inferior border of the isthmus of the thyroid gland is grasped in anatomic forceps, and its attachment to the anterior surface of the proximal portion of the trachea is freed by scissor dissection.

G. The isthmus of the thyroid gland is retracted upward, and the oval segment of the trachea to be incised is indicated in dotted outline. A segment of the third and frequently the fourth tracheal rings is included in this excision. Entrance into the trachea above this level is avoided to prevent the subsequent occurrence of laryngeal stenosis. Immediately prior to opening into the trachea, 8 to 10 minims of cocaine (10 per cent) is injected into its lumen as depicted. This maneuver, originally suggested by Sir St. Clair Thomson, lessens the cough as the tracheal lumen is entered.

H, I. The severance of the remaining attachment of the oval segment of the anterior portion of the trachea is being completed (H) prior to the insertion of the tracheostomy tube (I). In the adult, the No. 5 and No. 6 tubes are the two sizes most commonly employed. In the infant child and adolescent, tubes ranging in size from No. 0 to No. 4 may be used.

J. The tracheostomy tube is inserted and the obturator removed to complete the operation. One or two skin sutures to approximate loosely the skin margins may be inserted. This type of wound is always potentially infected and accordingly a layer or tight closure of the incision is avoided. In some instances no sutures are used, the wound being covered by a moistened sterile split piece of gauze.

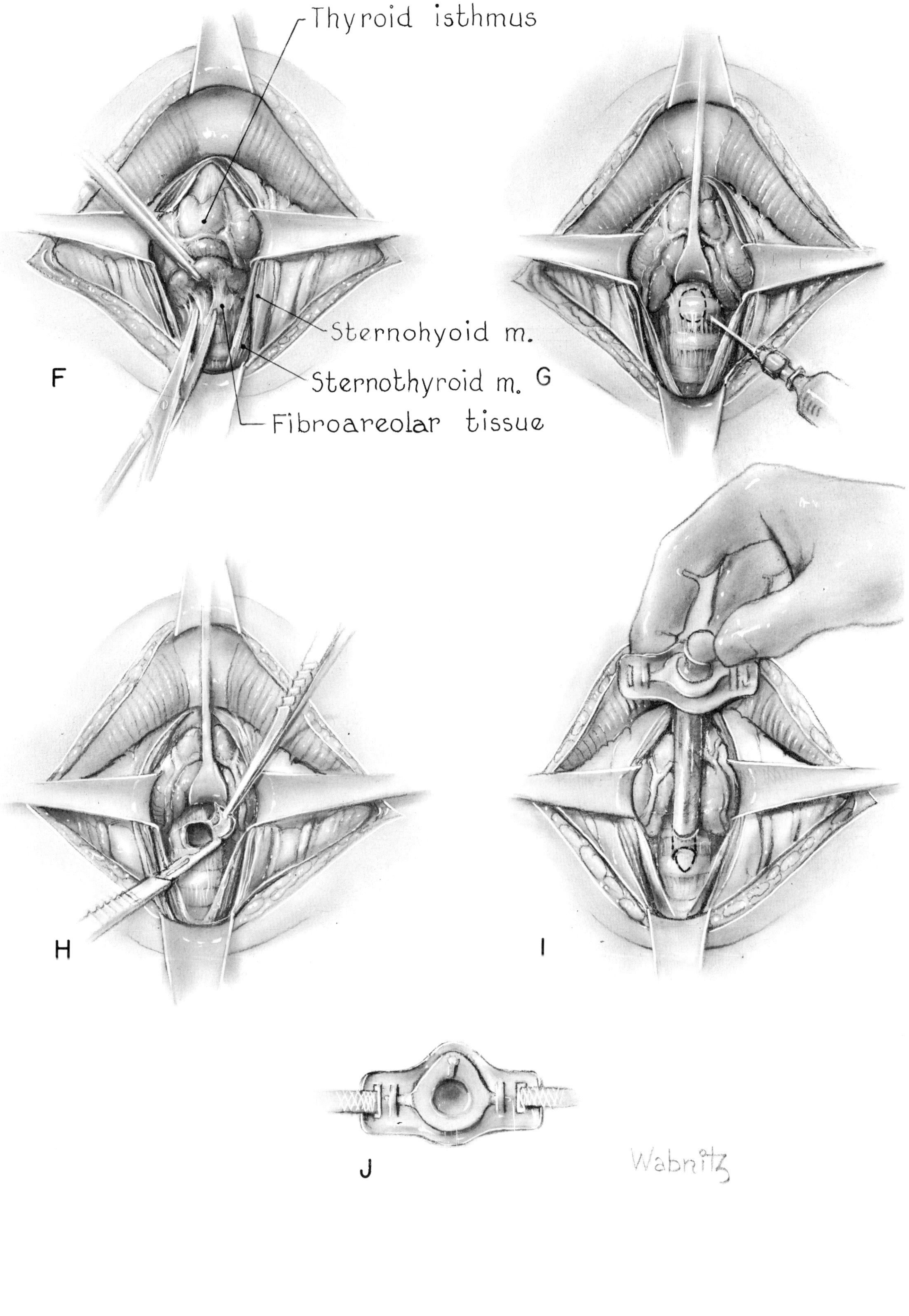
Thyroid isthmus
Sternohyoid m.
Sternothyroid m.
Fibroareolar tissue
F
G
H
I
J
Wabnitz

EXCISION OF CYLINDROMA OF THE TRACHEA

The patient, a 60-year-old white man, was admitted to the hospital because of progressively worsening inspiratory dyspnea. Three years previously a diagnosis of chronic lymphatic leukemia was established, and the response of the patient to the treatment prescribed was satisfactory.

The present symptoms were at first thought to be due to compression of the trachea by enlarged mediastinal lymph nodes. Accordingly, a course of nitrogen mustard therapy was prescribed without benefit. A bronchoscopy was done, and no gross abnormalities were detected. A bronchogram was then performed, and a constant filling defect in the upper third of the trachea was demonstrated. A repeat bronchoscopy was done, and on insertion of the bronchoscope, no gross abnormalities were observed; on its withdrawal, however, the smooth outline of the tumor which was attached to the left posterolateral wall of the trachea was readily visible.

It is now two years since the removal of the tumor (cylindroma), and the patient is completely without symptoms.

A, B. The transverse "collar" incision depicted (A) is deepened through the platysma muscle layer, and the sternohyoid muscle to either side of the midline is shown (B).

C, D. The isthmus of the thyroid gland is serially clamped and severed (C) to expose the trachea (D). The clamps on the isthmus are replaced with suture ligatures of 000 silk (D).

E. A long segment of the trachea is mobilized and encircled by a cotton tape. The location of the tumor within the lumen of the trachea is indicated in stippled outline.

Discussion—Dr. John L. Pool. Tumors of the trachea of all sorts are quite rare. The so-called bronchial adenomas are the most common, and of these the carcinoid type is found four or five times as frequently as the cylindroma. The usual symptoms, as in Dr. Madden's patient, are cough and strangulation. The diagnosis should be suspected in such patients when the chest roentgenogram is negative. Palpation of the neck is unrewarding unless nodal metastasis has occurred, which is unusual. Mirror laryngoscopy will only reveal a vocal cord paralysis in those instances where the tumor has extended into the tracheo-esophageal groove.

Sometimes mirror laryngoscopy will reveal the superior face of an upper tracheal adenoma, but the best evaluation of the size and exact location of these tracheal tumors is by radiographic technique, especially Bucky and tomographic films in two planes. Bronchoscopy will allow visualization, and biopsy may be attempted. When located on the posterior tracheal wall, esophagram and esophagoscopy should be included in the presurgical evaluation, since some growths transgress the party wall without involving the recurrent laryngeal nerves. Diagnosis by sputum cell study has been unrewarding.

Recent studies of adenomatous tumors of the trachea and bronchi, such as that by Dr. Goodner (1), suggest the probability that these lesions are in reality malignant though their rate of growth is slow and evidence of metastasis may be delayed many years. Wider excision than simple enucleation is, therefore, indicated.

Planning the approach that is most direct to the involved portion of trachea is aided by roentgenographic localization. A cervical approach, as illustrated, is certainly simpler than thoracotomy and can be extended if necessary by median sternotomy. Lesions in the distal third of the trachea are best approached by a right posterolateral thoracotomy. In any case, anesthesia by endotracheal tube is essential, and it is well to have a sterile duplicate set of anesthesia tubing available in case control of respiration distal to the tumor becomes necessary. In this case the sterile tube can be introduced into the distal trachea by the surgeon and the connection to the anesthesia apparatus handed off the field.

The careful exposure achieved by Dr. Madden (C, D, E) is essential prior to actually approaching the tumor. The recurrent laryngeal nerves should be dissected out in their entire course to avoid trauma, and the esophagotracheal wall dis-

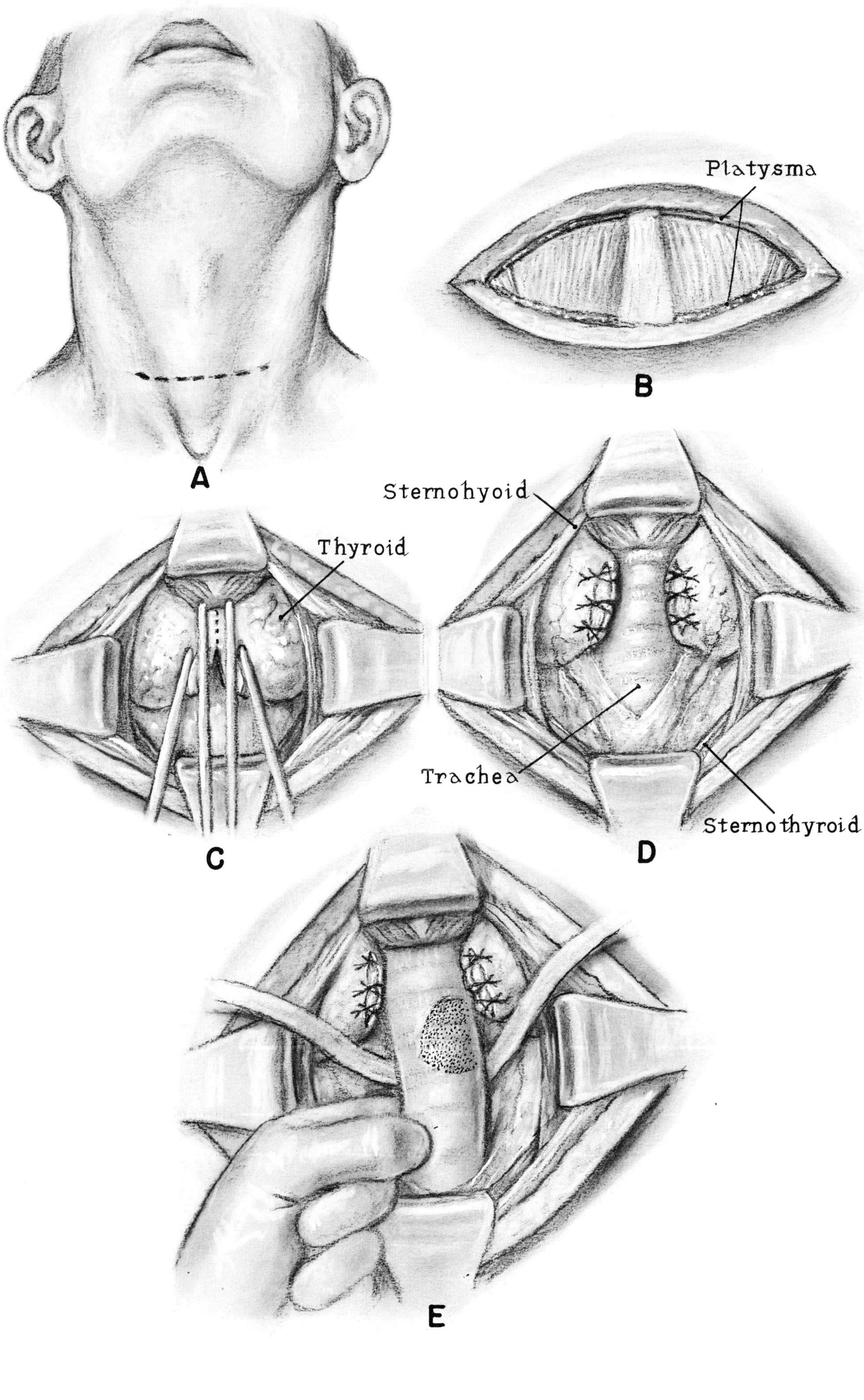
Platysma
A
B
Sternohyoid
Thyroid
Trachea
Sternothyroid
C
D
E

F. Ribbon retractors are inserted over protective moist gauze pads into the depths of the wound on either side of the trachea. The incision in the trachea and its subsequent extension are indicated by the solid and broken lines, respectively.

G, H. The incised margins of the trachea are retracted to show the tumor (G), which is better seen after enlarging the opening (H). The broken line (H) depicts the plane of dissection for the detachment of the tumor from the left posterolateral wall of the trachea.

I, J. The encapsulated tumor is held in a Babcock clamp, and as upward traction is maintained, it is freed by scissor dissection (I) and removed (J). The irregular circumscribed margin of its capsule is visible (J).

K. The site of attachment of the tumor to the wall of the trachea posteriorly is fulgurated both for its hemostatic and possible cancericidal effects.

L. The tracheal incision is partially closed, using interrupted sutures of 000 silk.

M. A tracheostomy tube (No. 6) is inserted through the center opening, and a drain is placed in the dependent portion of the wound.

N. The closure of the incision about the tube and drain completes the operation.

Discussion—Dr. Pool (cont.)

sected free, as illustrated, unless there is evidence of esophageal invasion requiring resection of the invaded portion of that organ.

Dr. Madden illustrates admirably the need for wide exposure within the trachea. I do not, however, believe in grasping these tumors, fearing cell dissemination, but prefer traction sutures through the adjacent tracheal wall. Also, it is wise because of the malignant potential of cylindromas to take a 1 cm. cuff of normal tissue beyond the visible growth and to remove the full thickness of the tracheal wall. In my experience this is best repaired by a wire reinforced dermal graft, after the method of Gebauer (2).

A tracheostomy is always essential to reduce pressure on the suture line, but I do not recommend drains adjacent to the tracheostomy because of the inevitable infection. Such an operation as the one illustrated probably does not require drainage, but if for reasons of "dead space" or continued ooze, drainage is necessary, it is more safely done through a lateral stab wound and into areas sealed off from the trachea. An operative or postoperative complication that may occur is pneumothorax. The mechanism is by suction of air from the open neck wound into the retrosternal space in a patient whose airway is partially obstructed. Rupture of the mediastinal pleura on one or both sides then occurs and would be apparent during or immediately after the procedure, as described by Bowden and Schweizer (3). Careful follow-up of these patients is mandatory because of the danger of recurrence.

References

1. Goodner, J. T., Berg, J. W., and Watson, W. L. The nonbenign nature of bronchial carcinoids and cylindromas, Cancer, 14:539, 1961.
2. Gebauer, Paul W. Bronchial resection and anastomosis, J. Thoracic Surg., 26:241, 1953.
3. Bowden, Lemuel, and Schweizer, Olga. Pneumothorax and mediastinal emphysema complicating neck surgery, Surg., Gynec. & Obst., 96: 81, 1950.

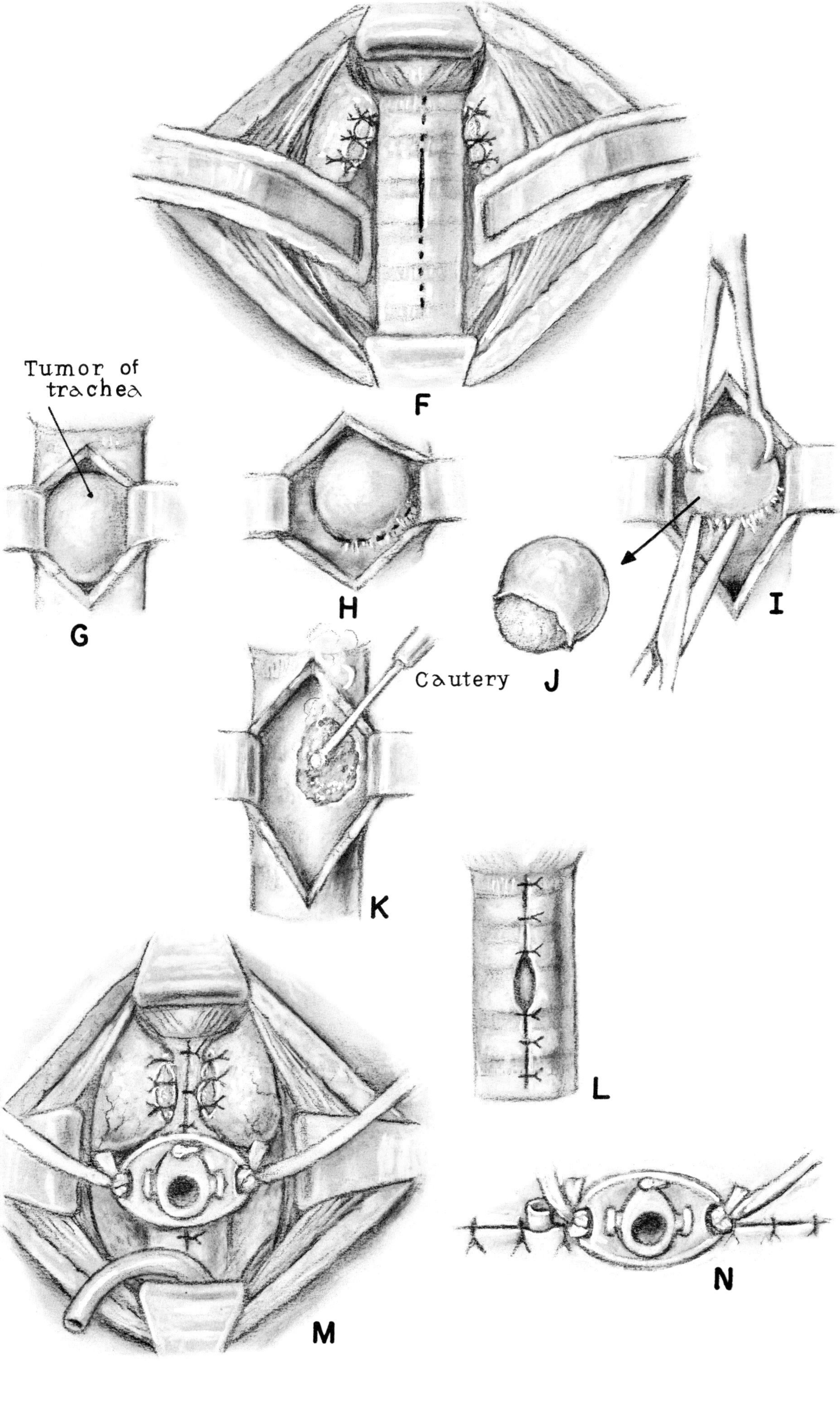
F
Tumor of trachea
G
H
I
J
Cautery
K
L
M
N

PULMONARY LOBECTOMY: RIGHT UPPER LOBE

A. The patient is placed in the direct left lateral prone position, and the right posterolateral thoracotomy incision overlying the fifth rib is indicated.

B. The right pleural cavity is entered, and the related structures are depicted. The right lung is displaced posteriorly, and the pleura overlying the hilar structures anteriorly is severed (broken line) by scissor dissection.

C, D. The pulmonary artery and superior pulmonary vein are exposed, and the mobilized apical branch of the pulmonary artery is being encircled by a silk (00) ligature (C). This artery, doubly ligated in continuity, is being severed between the ligatures (D).

DISCUSSION—DR. JULIAN JOHNSON. The technic of upper lobectomy described differs in no major way from that which I have utilized for many years. I will, however, point out minor variations in technic simply as a matter of interest to the reader.

The lateral position with a posterolateral incision is preferred for upper lobe lobectomy, since it is felt that this puts the operator in the best over-all position to approach the hilum of the lobe or lung from all directions. However, either the face-down position or the supine position can be used for right upper lobe resection. The face-down position is indicated in the event that an upper lobe resection is to be carried out in the presence of cavitary disease of the upper lobe when there is still an appreciable amount of secretion present; this places the anesthetist in a more favorable position to keep the other lobes and the other lung clear of secretions. Fortunately, with our present methods of preoperative preparation, the surgeon these days seldom finds himself in the position of having to use this position. While the anterior approach is perfectly feasible, I have not used it in a good many years, it being my thought that it leaves a bit less room for error in the performance of the lobectomy and places the surgeon in a more difficult position if he has inadvertently torn a major vessel or finds a good many adhesions present at the time of operation.

The resection of a rib during thoractomy has been largely abandoned by me, except in those instances where there is reason to believe that there is an obliteration of the pleural space, such as when an extrapleural pneumonectomy for tuberculous empyema is being performed. I normally use the fourth interspace incision for the right upper lobe, although the fifth is acceptable. If the fifth intercostal incision is made, it is preferable to cut the fifth rib posteriorly to gain adequate exposure. When the operation is being carried out on a young person, the intercostal incision usually gives satisfactory exposure, but when operating upon an older person, it is preferable to cut at least one rib posteriorly. Whether a rib is resected or not is probably of very little importance. I have thought if the rib is not resected it has allowed more rapid closure of the chest and also gives a nicer appearance on the postoperative roentgenograms.

The Burford modification of the Finochietto rib spreader or some similar modification has received wide acceptance, as opposed to the double rib spreaders illustrated.

Although there is considerable variation, the first branch of the right pulmonary artery is usually the apical anterior branch, which comes off as one artery and then bifurcates into the apical and the anterior branches shortly thereafter. If the artery referred to as the apical branch of the pulmonary artery in C is supposed to represent the joint trunk of the apical anterior artery as suggested by its bifurcation in D, it is unusually small in this particular patient and represents a smaller portion of the right pulmonary artery blood flow than one usually sees. It has been my custom in

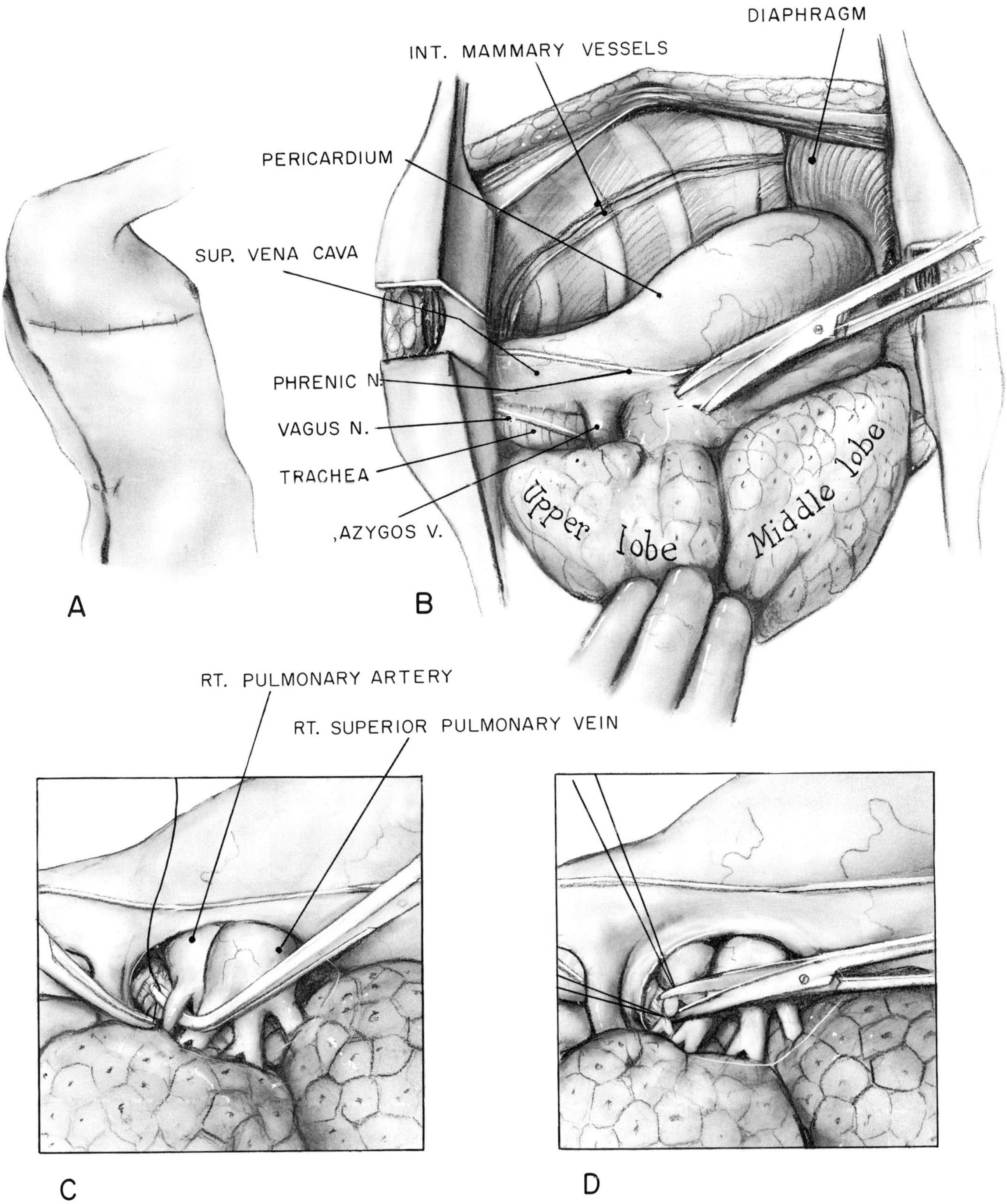
DIAPHRAGM
INT. MAMMARY VESSELS
PERICARDIUM
SUP. VENA CAVA
PHRENIC N.
VAGUS N.
TRACHEA
AZYGOS V.
Upper lobe
Middle lobe
A
B
RT. PULMONARY ARTERY
RT. SUPERIOR PULMONARY VEIN
C
D

E, F. The apical tributary of the superior pulmonary vein is doubly ligated (00 silk) in continuity and transected with scissors between the ligatures (E). The anterior tributary is treated in like manner (F).

G. The middle and lower lobes are retracted in opposite directions, and the visceral pleura lining the major interlobal fissure is cut (broken line) with scissors.

H. A segment of the pulmonary artery and its branches to the upper, middle, and lower lobes are visible. The posterior arterial branch is being mobilized by scissor dissection.

H_1. The posterior artery is doubly ligated (00 silk) in continuity and severed (broken line) between the ligatures.

H_2. In some patients two posterior arterial branches may be present, as indicated.

Discussion—Dr. Johnson (cont.)

the division of most of these arteries and veins in this area to back up the proximal ligature with a suture ligature in juxtaposition to it.

In the division of the venous supply to the right upper lobe I have frequently found it possible to identify the tributaries to the superior pulmonary vein coming from the middle lobe and then ligating the remaining portion of the superior pulmonary vein just distal to the point where the middle lobe tributary joins it. It may be necessary to put the distal ligatures on the branches, but the proximal ligature can frequently be placed around the remaining vein with a suture ligature in juxtaposition to it.

E and F show only two branch veins coming from the upper lobe, the apical and anterior tributaries. Much more commonly there is a vein coming from the posterior segment of the upper lobe. Also the apical anterior vein frequently joins to form one tributary and there is another tributary referred to by some as the inferior vein. Considerable care is indicated in placing the ligature around the distal portion of the posterior segmental vein, since it is in very close proximity to the pulmonary artery.

If, after the division of the major vessels on the anterior aspect of the hilum of the upper lobe, one has a situation where the major fissure is tightly fused, the upper lobe can be displaced posteriorly and downward and the upper lobe bronchus exposed in that manner and divided, rather than approached from the rear as shown. As the distal portion of the severed bronchus is then gently retracted, the fissure between the posterior part of the upper and lower lobes can be divided. The posterior segmental artery will then come into view and can be divided, and the minor fissure can be divided, separating the upper from the middle lobe.

Separation of the upper from the middle lobe is not illustrated in this series. This fissure is seldom complete and almost always has to be divided by sharp and blunt dissection, as illustrated in the section on lower and middle lobe lobectomy. In this instance, however, the upper lobe would be collapsed and the middle lobe inflated. Following the separation of this fissure, I feel that it is important to stop all of the air leaks if possible—certainly at least the major ones. The technic which I have found very useful is to clamp the area on the surface of the fissure that is leaking with a Babcock clamp and place a catgut tie behind it.

In the division of the bronchus it has been my custom to use two Sarot bronchus clamps and cut between them. The Sarot clamp is a noncrushing clamp. Silk sutures are placed behind the clamp with a short straight needle, and the clamp is removed before the ligatures are tied over the end of the bronchus. The bronchial stump can then be buried under the pleural flap containing the azygous vein.

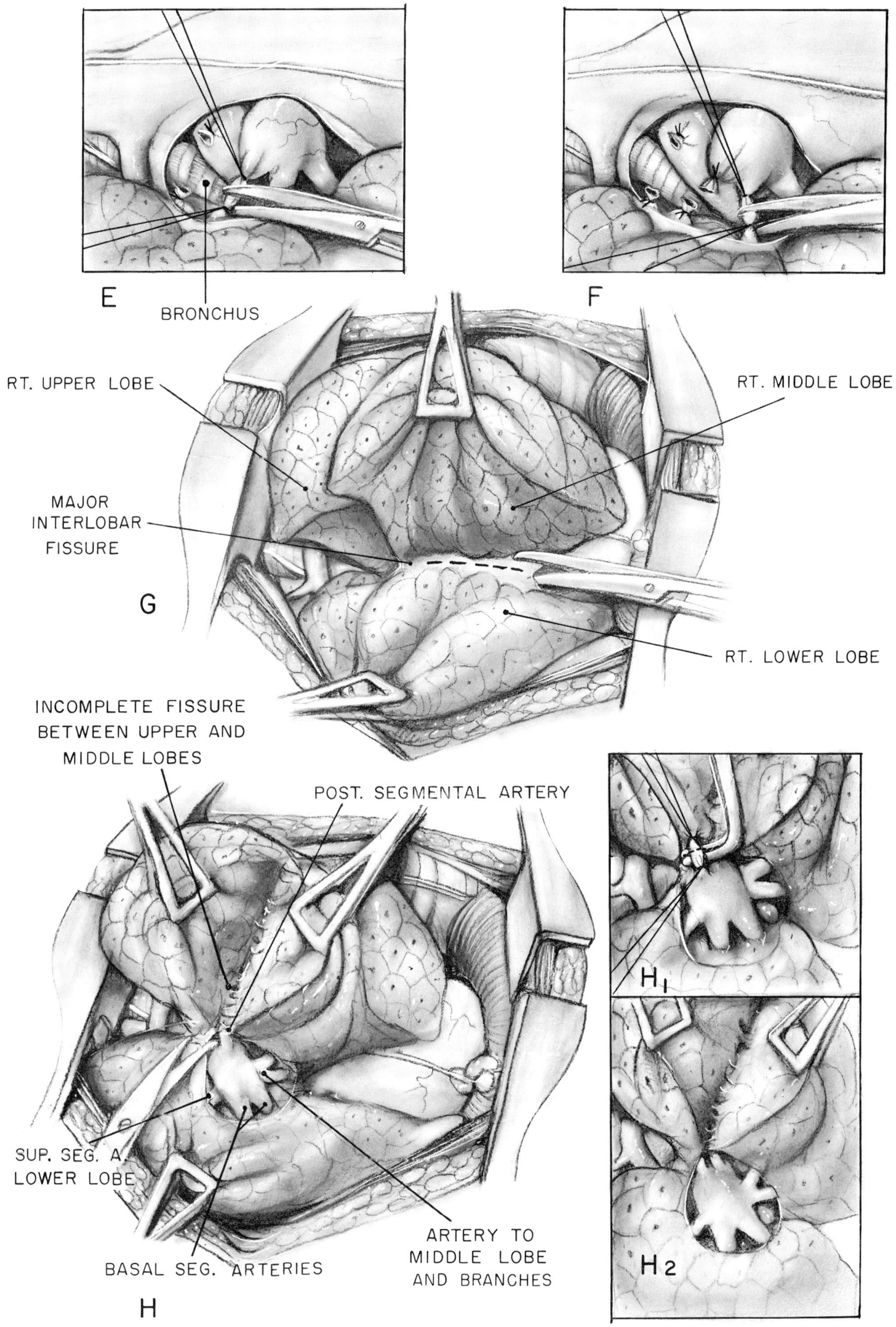
E
BRONCHUS
F
RT. UPPER LOBE
RT. MIDDLE LOBE
MAJOR
INTERLOBAR
FISSURE
G
RT. LOWER LOBE
INCOMPLETE FISSURE
BETWEEN UPPER AND
MIDDLE LOBES
POST. SEGMENTAL ARTERY
H_1
SUP. SEG. A.
LOWER LOBE
BASAL SEG. ARTERIES
ARTERY TO
MIDDLE LOBE
AND BRANCHES
H_2
H

I. The branch bronchus to the right upper lobe, occluded by a clamp (Sarot) distally, is being severed proximally with a scalpel.

I_1, I_2. The insets show an extended dissection of the upper lobe bronchus to expose its segmental branches (I_1) and the partially severed bronchus being occluded with sutures (000 silk) as its transection is continued (I_2).

J. The operative field on completion of the right upper lobe lobectomy is seen in relation to the surrounding structures. Before closure of the wound two catheters are inserted. One (18 F) is placed anteriorly as an air vent, and the other (24 F, Foley) posteriorly for the drainage of fluid. This is shown in the illustrated technic for removal of the lower lobe of the left lung.

Discussion—Dr. Brian Blades. Although some surgeons still employ an anterior approach for upper lobe lobectomy, the posterolateral approach has many advantages. Whether one resects a portion of the fifth rib or employs an intercostal incision between the fifth and sixth ribs will depend upon the age of the patient and general habitus. In older patients it is usually better to do a subperiosteal excision of the portion of the rib, since with the intercostal incision adequate exposure often results in multiple fractured ribs.

In C the apical branch of the pulmonary artery to the upper lobe is shown, but it would be an advantage if the anterior branch was labeled, since it is often possible to ligate the artery proximal to the division of anterior and apical branches.

If an upper lobe lobectomy is being performed for carcinoma, it is of great advantage to ligate and divide the major azygous vein. This insures better exposure of the mediastinum and any lymph nodes that may be involved.

In patients with suppurative disease in whom secretions are troublesome during the performance of the lobectomy, it is easy and possible to divide the bronchus first, approaching it from the posterior aspect.

If possible, it is desirable to separate the incomplete fissures between the upper and middle lobes, and often between the upper lobe and the superior division of the lower lobe after the hilar dissection has been completed. By doing so, the amount of bleeding from the incomplete fissure surfaces is minimized.

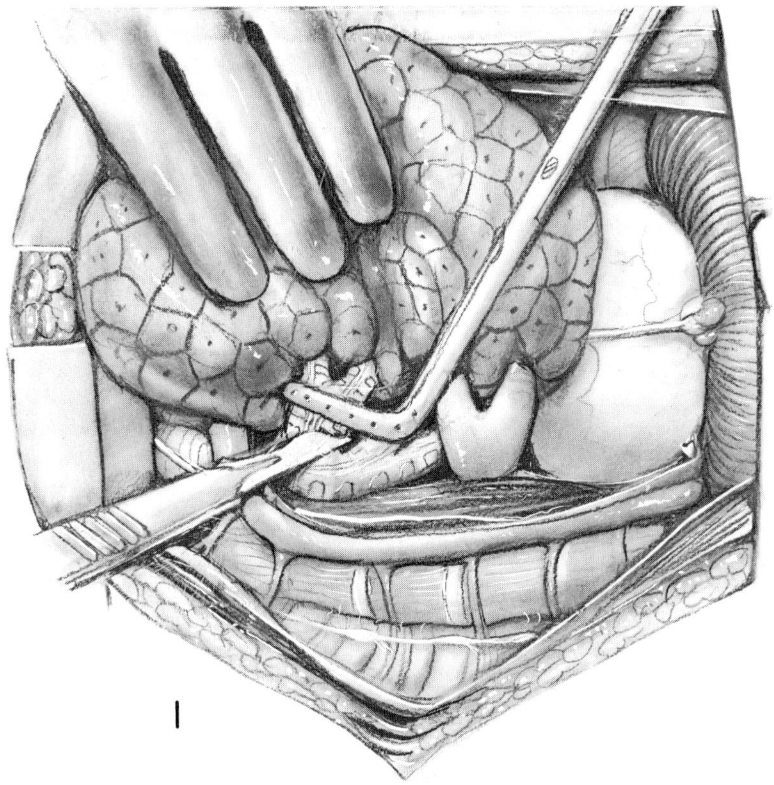

I

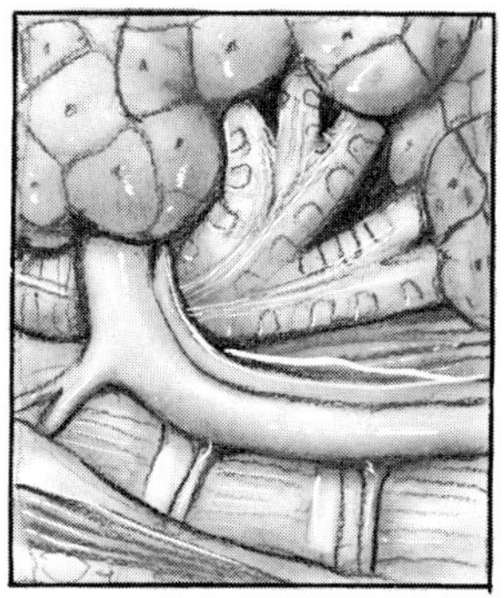

I_1

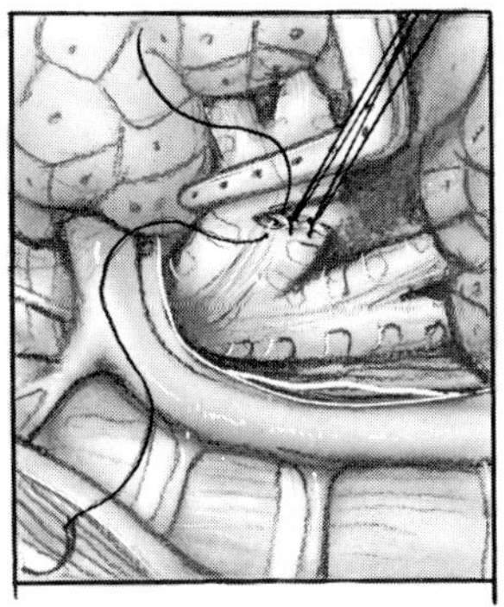

I_2

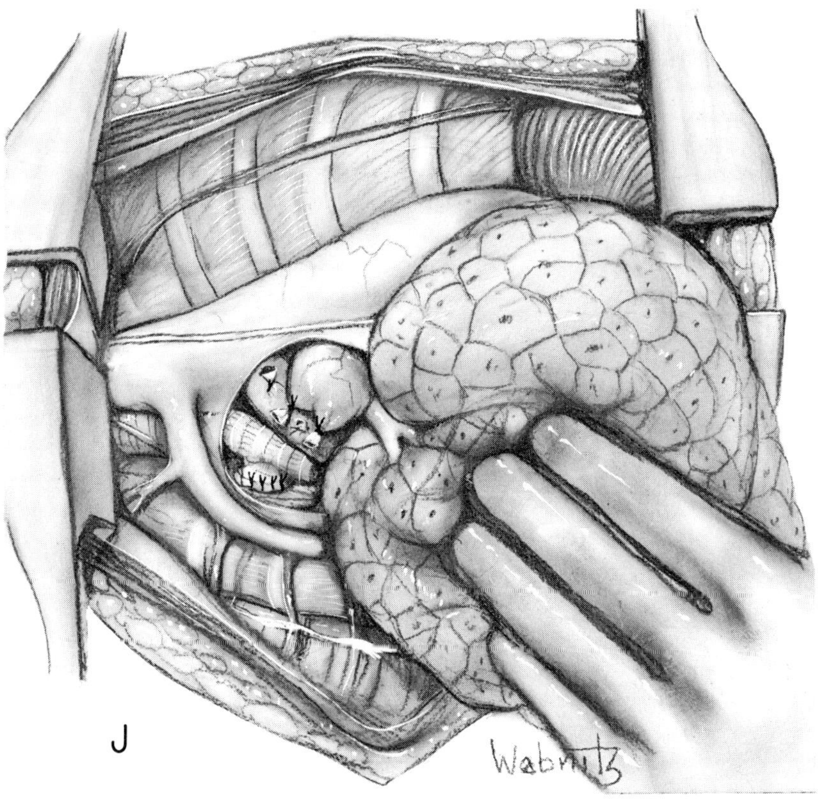

J

PULMONARY LOBECTOMY: COMBINED RIGHT MIDDLE AND LOWER LOBES

A. The patient is placed in the direct right lateral prone position, and the thoracotomy incision is outlined and cross-hatched to facilitate later closure.

B. Clamps (Duval) are applied to the right lung, and as traction is maintained, the visceral pleura overlying the major interlobar fissure is severed by scissor dissection.

C. The major fissure is opened, and the arterial branches to the lobes of the right lung are indicated. The incomplete fissure between the upper and middle lobes is being dissected with scissors.

D. The artery to the superior segment of the lower lobe is doubly ligated (000 silk) in continuity and severed (broken line).

E. Similarly, the arteries to the basal segments of the lower lobe and to the middle lobe are ligated and severed. The arterial branch to the posterior segment of the upper lobe remains intact.

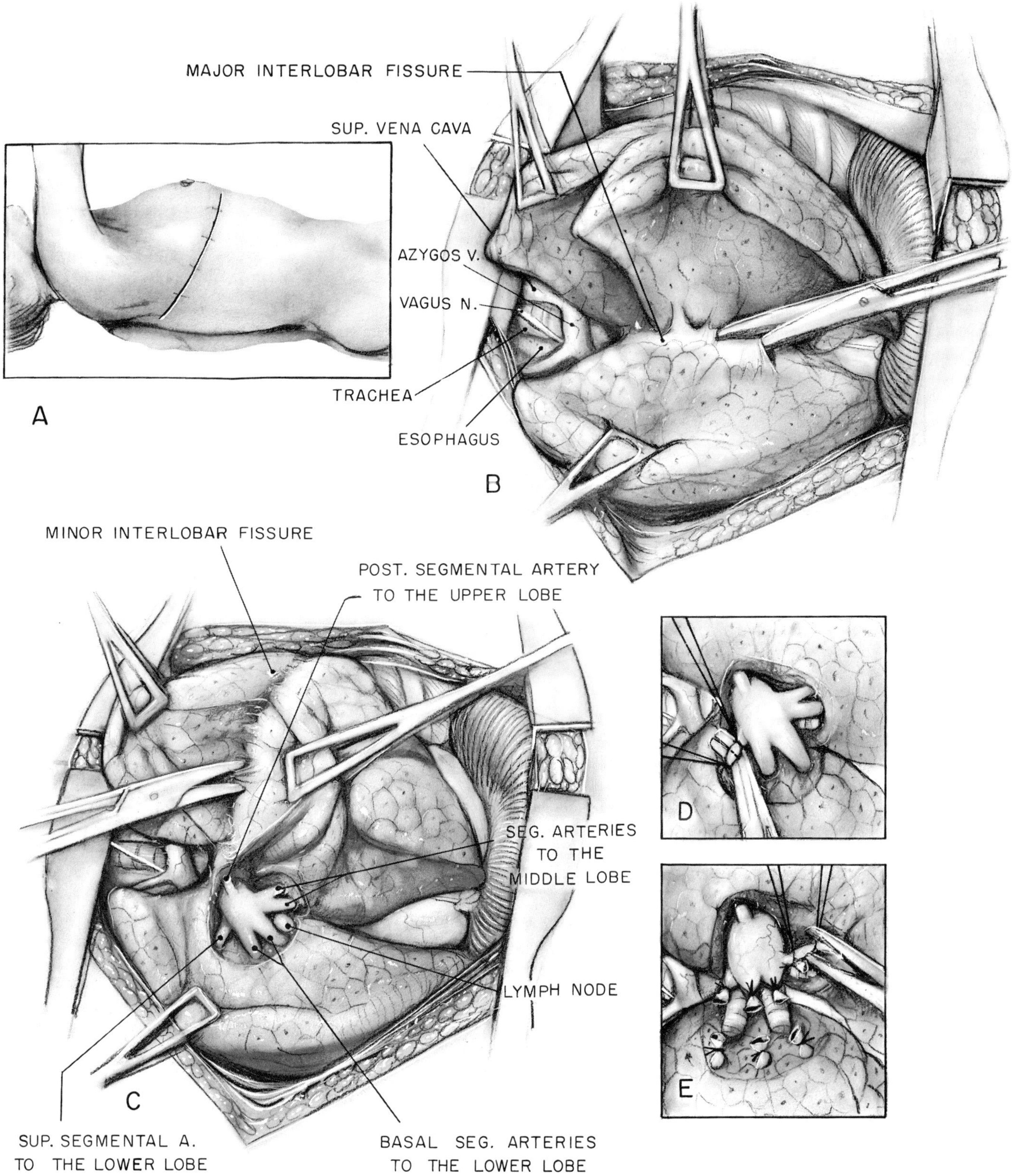
MAJOR INTERLOBAR FISSURE
SUP. VENA CAVA
AZYGOS V.
VAGUS N.
TRACHEA
ESOPHAGUS
A
B
MINOR INTERLOBAR FISSURE
POST. SEGMENTAL ARTERY TO THE UPPER LOBE
SEG. ARTERIES TO THE MIDDLE LOBE
LYMPH NODE
C
SUP. SEGMENTAL A. TO THE LOWER LOBE
BASAL SEG. ARTERIES TO THE LOWER LOBE
D
E

F. Upon completion of the ligation and severance of the arterial blood supply to the middle and lower lobes, the right lung is manually retracted upward and the inferior pulmonary ligament is doubly clamped and severed (broken line).

G, H. The anterior layer of the inferior pulmonary ligament is cut in a cephalad direction (G) to expose the inferior and superior pulmonary veins (H). The vein draining the middle lobe, a tributary of the superior pulmonary vein, is first doubly ligated (000 silk) in continuity, and then a transfixion suture ligature of 000 silk is inserted in juxtaposition to the proximal ligature (H).

I, J. The middle lobe vein is severed between the transfixion suture ligature and the distal ligature. The remaining intact tributaries of the superior pulmonary vein drain the upper lobe.

Discussion—Dr. Julian Johnson. The lateral position with the usual posterolateral approach is preferred for resection of the right middle and lower lobes. On the other hand, if the patient is being operated upon for suppurative disease or if there is a tumor present with suppuration behind it, it may be wise to use the face-down position. I seldom find this necessary at the present time with the modern means of preoperative preparation, but occasionally, particularly in the presence of bronchial stenosis, it is difficult to get the patient clear of secretions and the face-down position is advisable. In the lateral approach the incision is made in the fifth or sixth intercostal space. In a person of middle age or older the upper rib is divided posteriorly to give adequate exposure.

The Duval clamps shown in B have been widely used, but I prefer not to apply even this relatively atraumatic clamp to the lobe that is not to be removed, but rather to hold the lobe aside with a sponge stick. In the division of the arterial supply to the lower and middle lobes, it is sometimes possible to divide the pulmonary artery as one trunk right below the artery to the posterior segment of the upper lobe rather than as five separate branches as shown. Most often, even when a single ligature can be placed proximally, multiple ligatures will be placed distally in order to get an adequate cuff beyond the proximal ligature. It is my custom to back up the proximal ligature with a suture ligature in juxtaposition to it in all of the arterial branches in a manner similar to that shown in H for the pulmonary vein.

It is my custom to divide the inferior pulmonary ligament (F) up to the inferior pulmonary vein both in front and back at the beginning of the operation as a precautionary measure. If any of the great vessels at the hilum of the lung should be inadvertently torn, this places the surgeon in

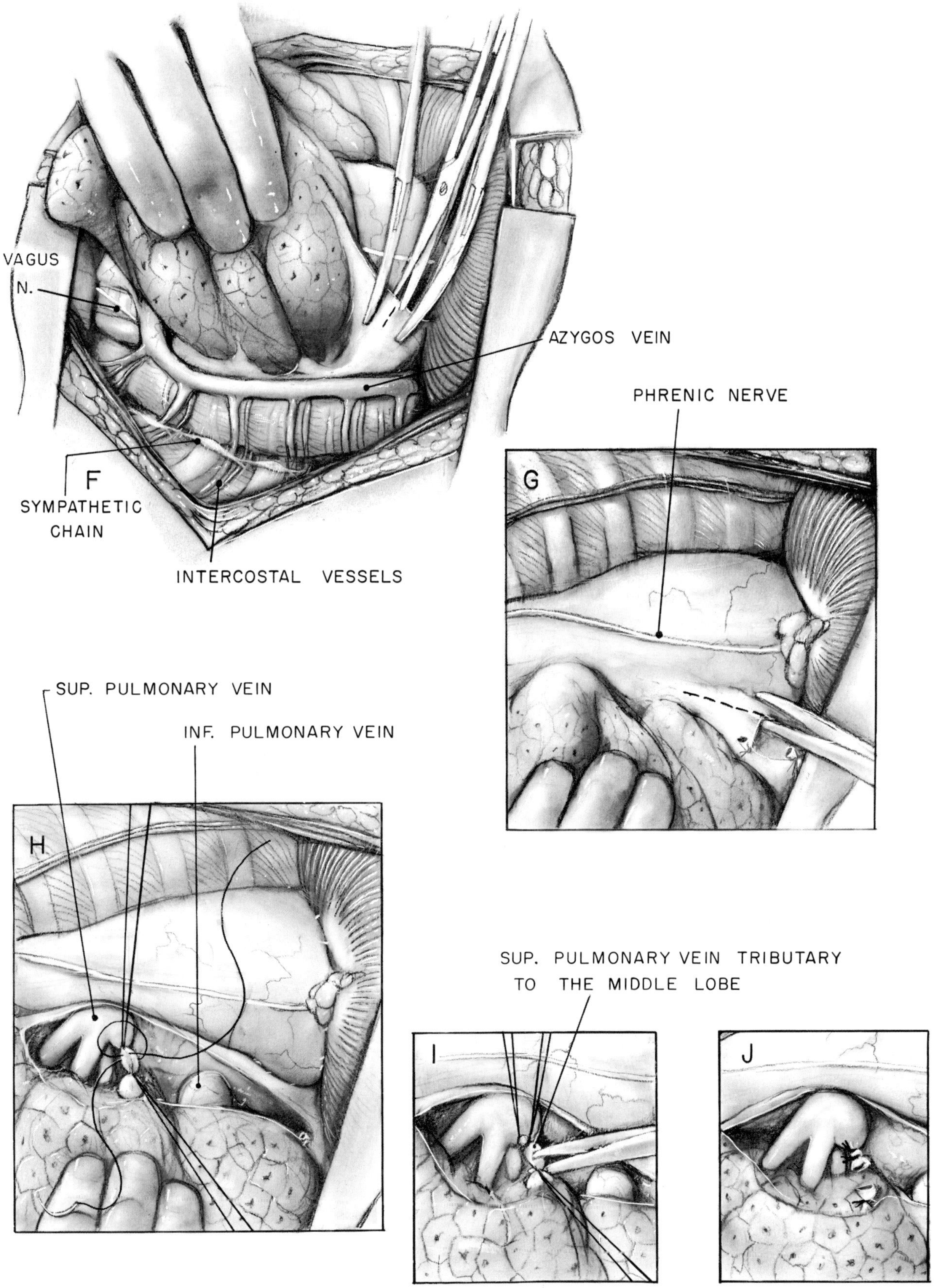
VAGUS
N.
AZYGOS VEIN
F
SYMPATHETIC
CHAIN
INTERCOSTAL VESSELS
PHRENIC NERVE
G
SUP. PULMONARY VEIN
INF. PULMONARY VEIN
H
SUP. PULMONARY VEIN TRIBUTARY
TO THE MIDDLE LOBE
I
J

K, L. The posterior layer of the inferior pulmonary ligament is severed (broken line in K) to expose the bronchus to the lower lobe and the inferior pulmonary vein, which is being encircled by a ligature of 00 silk (L).

M, N, O. Similarly, the superior and basal tributaries of the inferior pulmonary vein are encircled by ligatures of 000 silk (M), and after ligation of the inferior pulmonary vein, its tributaries are doubly ligated (000 silk) in continuity and severed (N, O).

P. The major interlobar fissure is re-entered, and the bronchus to the middle lobe is occluded preliminary to inflation of the upper lobe. This maneuver is a technical expediency to facilitate the recognition of the true cleavage plane between the upper and middle lobes.

Discussion—Dr. Johnson (cont.)

a much better position to get his hand around the vessels proximally and to control the bleeding.

If the pulmonary artery has been ligated as a single trunk below the branch to the posterior segment of the upper lobe, it will give one improved exposure to the bronchi to the middle and lower lobes. It is often possible to divide the bronchus at the intermediate bronchus immediately above the middle-lobe bronchus, thereby having one bronchial suture line rather than four as depicted.

In the technic for the division of the incomplete minor fissure (Q, R), when only the upper lobe is to remain in the right pleural space, it is probably doubly important to control any leak from the surface of the upper lobe so as to allow speedy filling of the right pleural space. If the residual right upper lobe seems unduly small and it appears unlikely that it will fill the right pleural space, a temporary crush of the phrenic nerve may be helpful if the patient's pulmonary function is good. The leaks on the surface of the upper lobe are most easily controlled by occluding them with Babcock clamps and tying with catgut ligatures.

In the division of the bronchi to the middle lobe (T), it is probably wise to place a clamp across the distal bronchi before these bronchi are divided to avoid any spill which may have collected distally. I make every effort possible to pull the pleural flap over the bronchial stump as an added precaution against a leak.

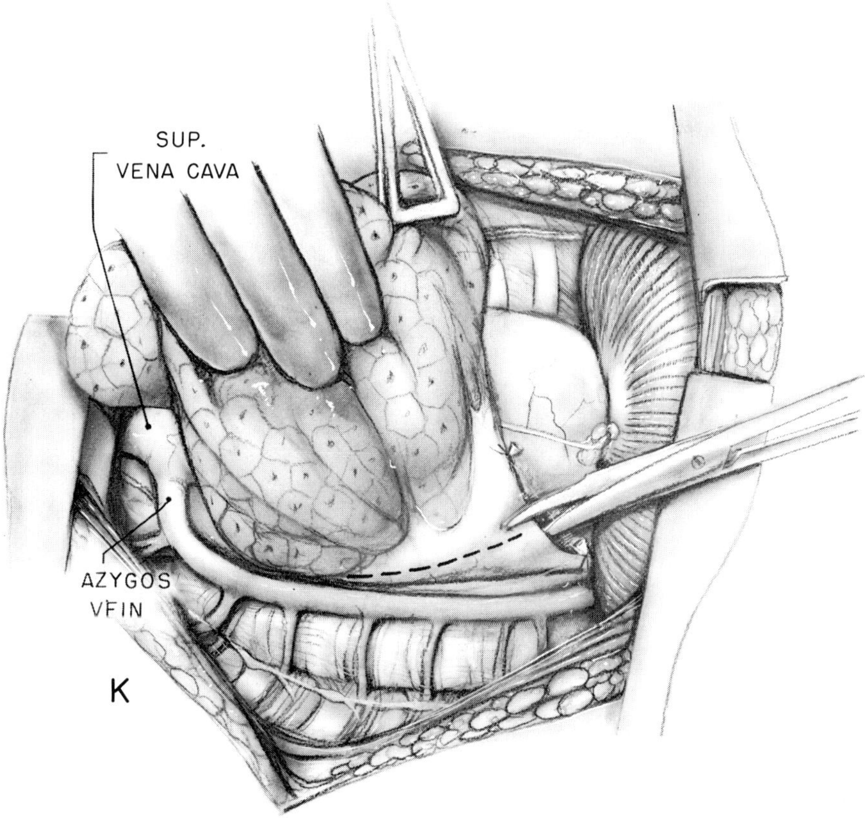
SUP.
VENA CAVA
AZYGOS
VEIN

K

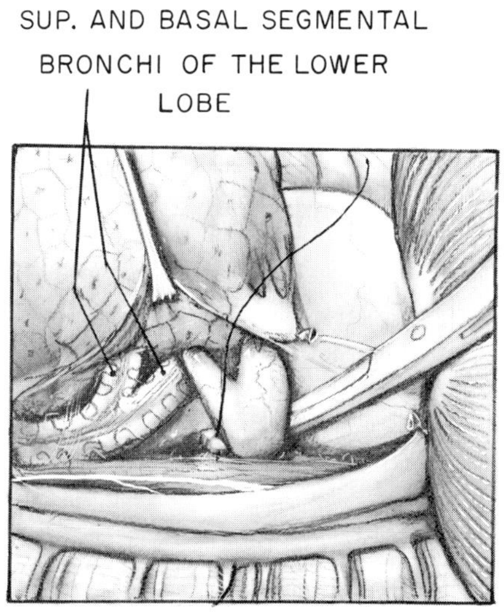
SUP. AND BASAL SEGMENTAL
BRONCHI OF THE LOWER
LOBE

L

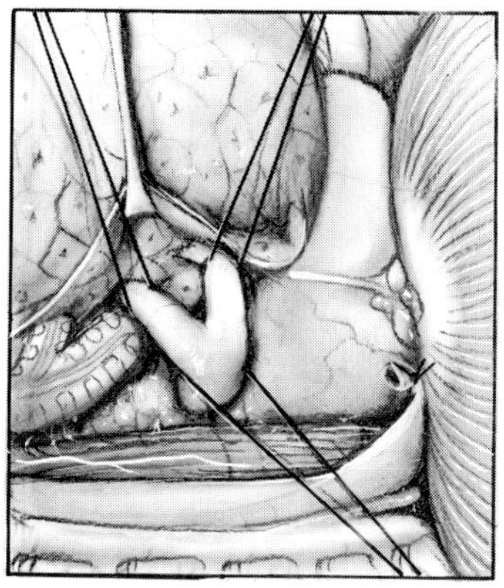

M

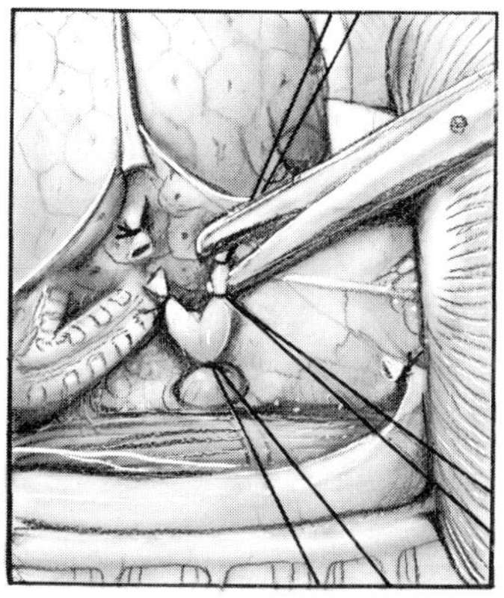

N

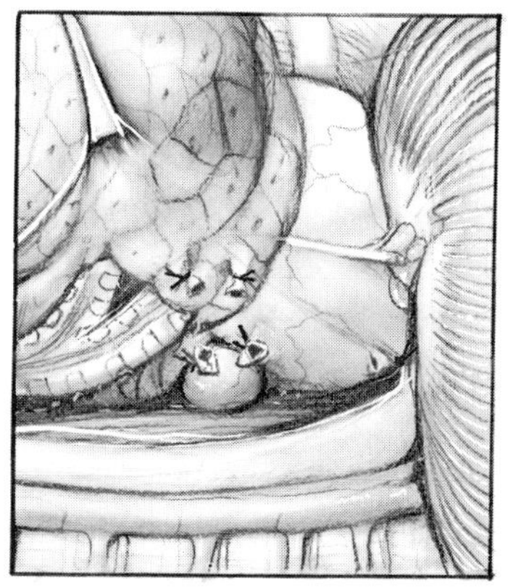

O

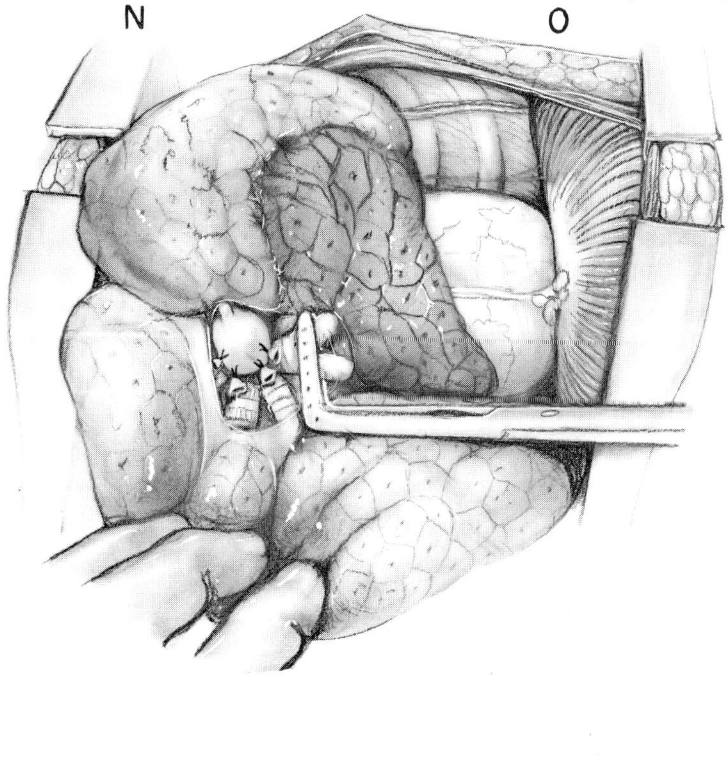

P

Q, R. The cleavage plane between the inflated upper and deflated middle lobe is developed by a continuation of blunt digital (Q) and scissor (R) dissection to separate the lobes completely.

S, T. The medial and lateral branch bronchi of the middle lobe bronchus are transected and occluded proximally with interrupted sutures of 000 silk, swedged on a minimum trauma needle.

U. Similarly, the superior and basal branch bronchi of the lower lobe bronchus are transected and occluded to complete the removal of the middle and lower lobes of the right lung. In this patient the indication for operation was extensive bronchiectasis. In patients with cancer, transection of the bronchus proximal to its branch bronchi is indicated.

V. The operative field on completion of the operation is shown. The occluded middle lobe bronchus is hidden from view by the pulmonary artery.

Discussion—Dr. Brian Blades. The same principles concerning the use of an intercostal incision or the subperiosteal resection of a portion of a rib apply for right middle and lower lobe lobectomy. For the combined lobectomy, an approach at the level of the sixth rib or an intercostal incision between the sixth and seventh ribs is desirable.

I prefer to divide the pulmonary ligament before proceeding with the hilar dissection. This makes it easier to manipulate the lobes and gives better exposure. It should be mentioned that there is usually at least one small arterial bleeder in the pulmonary ligament, which should be ligated. Moreover, as in the case of upper lobe lobectomy, it is preferable, if possible, to divide the incomplete fissures between the upper and middle lobes, and sometimes the superior division of the lower lobe after the hilar dissection has been completed.

If the resection of the bronchus is carried out from the posterior approach it is almost always possible to divide the intermediate bronchus to the middle and lower lobes and therefore have only one bronchial stump after removal of the lobe. The proximal bronchus should not be clamped to avoid crushing the bronchus.

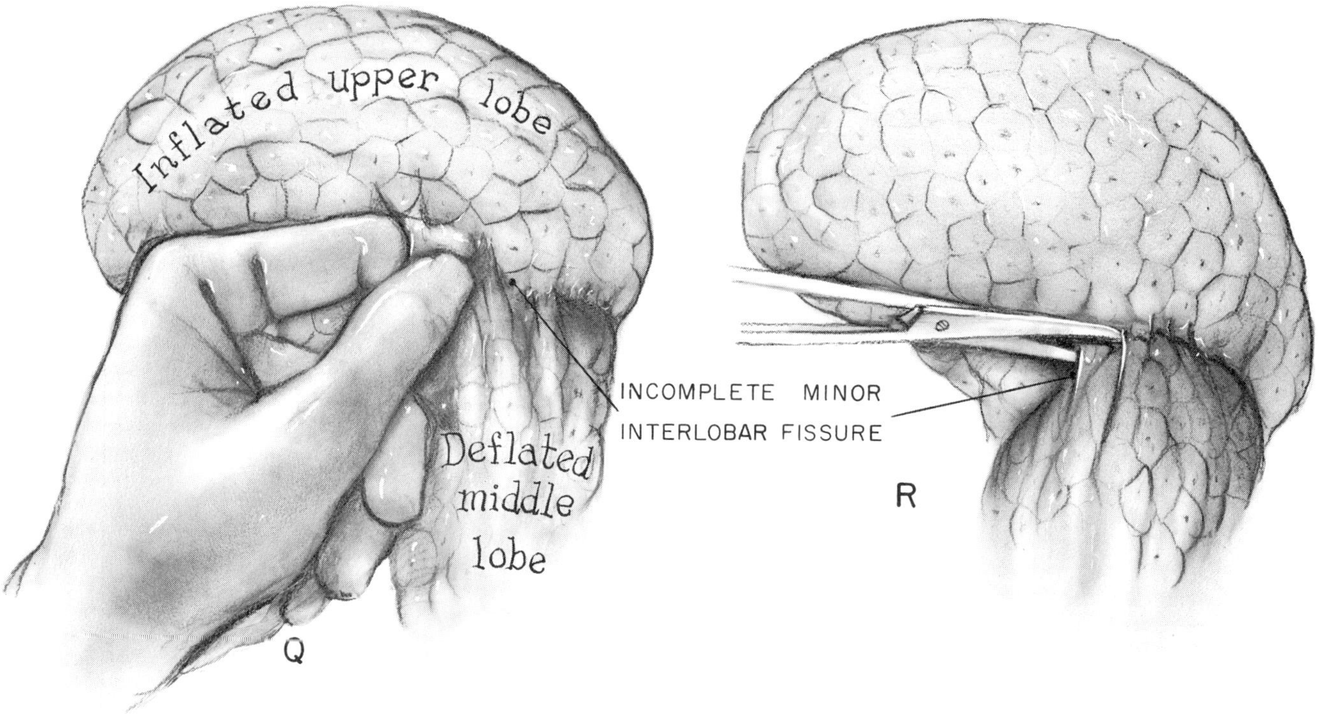
Inflated upper lobe
Deflated middle lobe
INCOMPLETE MINOR INTERLOBAR FISSURE

Q

R

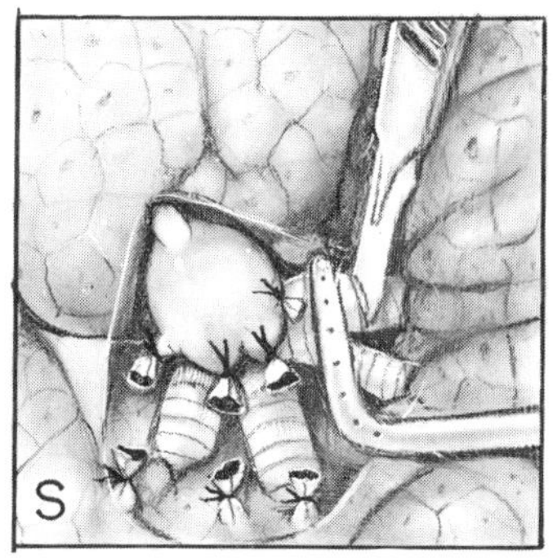

S

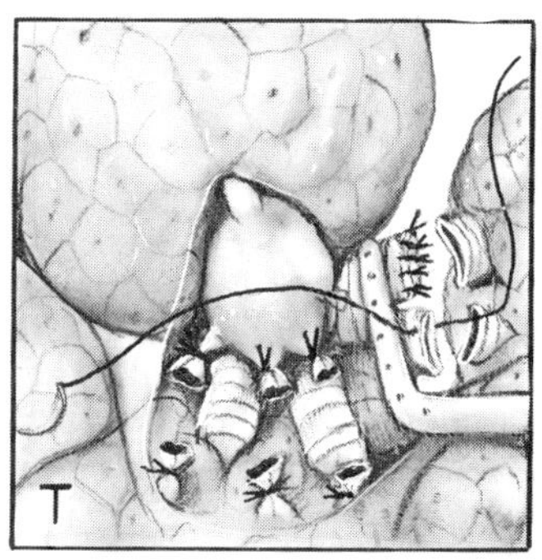

T

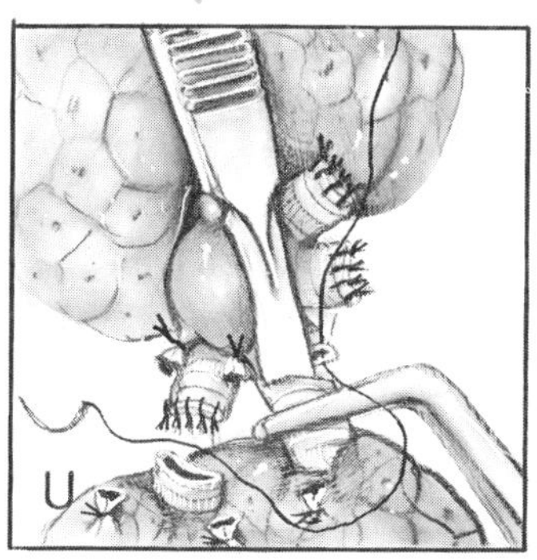

U

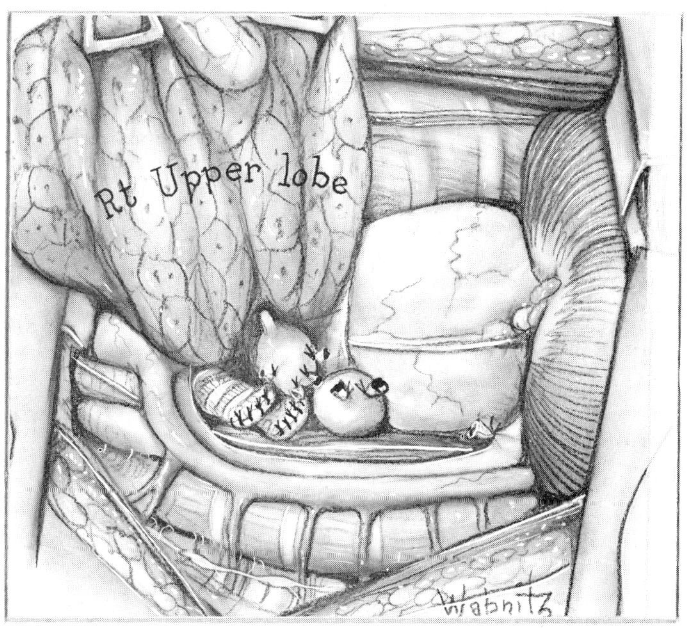
Rt Upper lobe
Wabnitz

V

TOTAL PNEUMONECTOMY: RIGHT

A. The patient is placed in the direct left lateral prone position, and the right posterolateral thoracotomy incision overlying the fifth rib is indicated.

B. The right pleural cavity is entered, and the related structures are depicted. The left lung is displaced posteriorly, and the pleura overlying the hilar structures anteriorly is severed (broken line) by scissor dissection.

C, D. The pulmonary artery and superior pulmonary vein are exposed, and the mobilized apical branch of the pulmonary artery is being encircled by a silk (00) ligature (C). This artery, doubly ligated in continuity, is being severed between the ligatures (D).

Discussion—Dr. William F. Rienhoff, Jr. The description of total pneumonectomy is, with minor exceptions, essentially the same technic as I originally described in 1933 and reported in the Bulletin of the Johns Hopkins Hospital.

In the case of right total pneumonectomy, I think the anterolateral incision, instead of the posterolateral as illustrated, is the one to be preferred. My reasons for this choice are (1) the patient breathes much better under anesthesia because he is flat on the table and (2) the postoperative discomfort is much less.

In C the apical posterior branch of the left pulmonary artery is ligated, but this step can be avoided by ligating the left pulmonary artery in the beginning as illustrated in E. The closure of the bronchus is as I described it in 1933, which I think is correct.

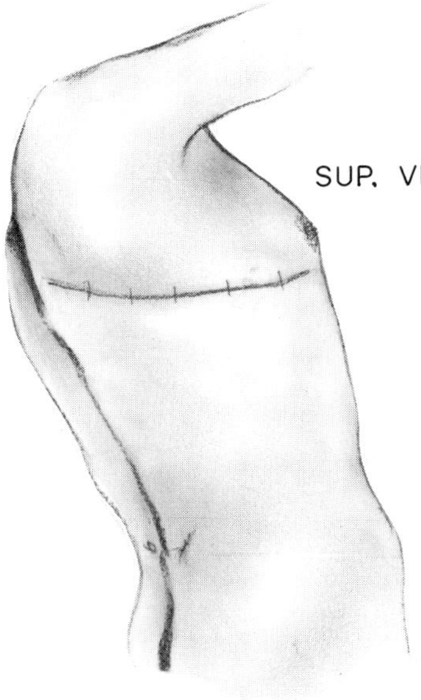

A

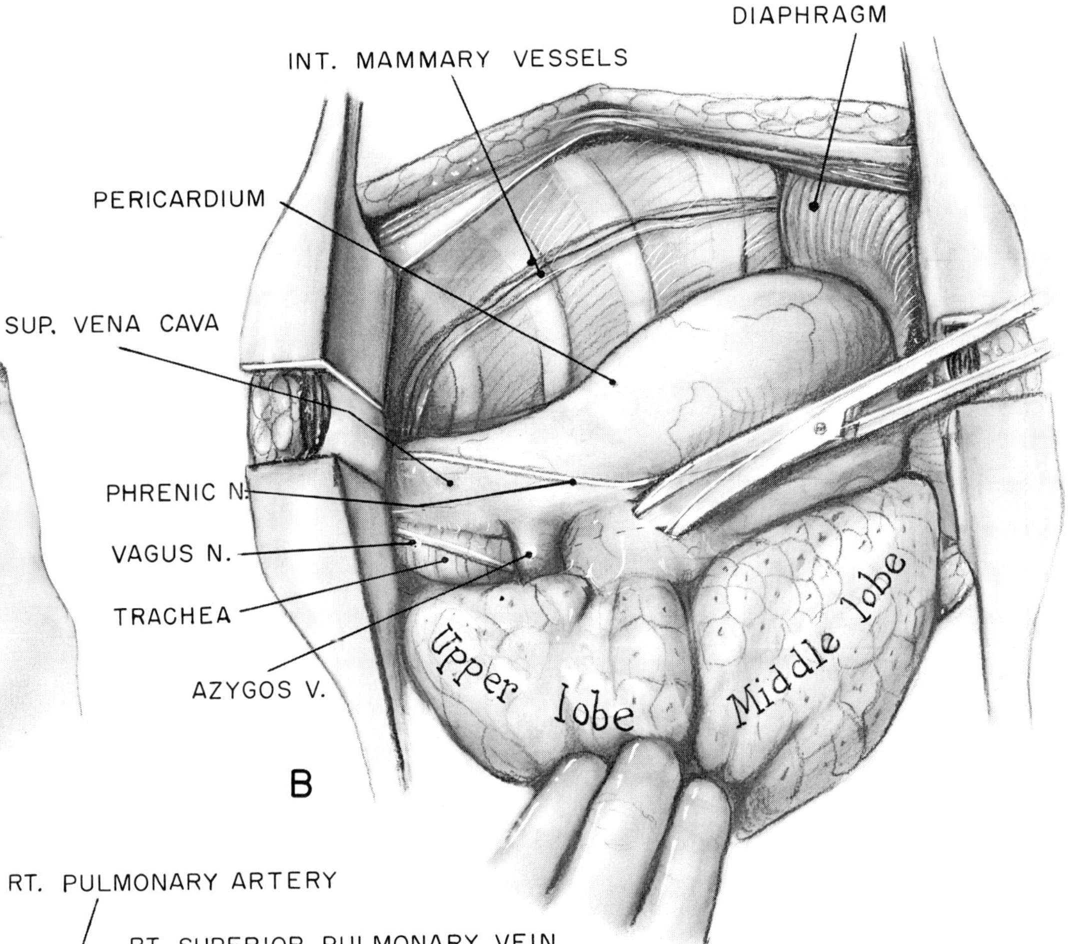
DIAPHRAGM
INT. MAMMARY VESSELS
PERICARDIUM
SUP. VENA CAVA
PHRENIC N.
VAGUS N.
TRACHEA
AZYGOS V.
Upper lobe
Middle lobe

B

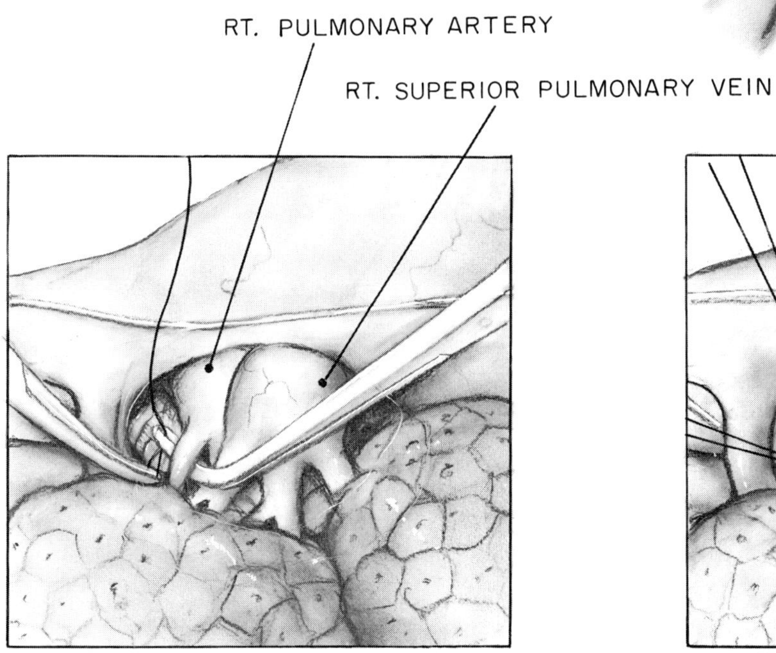
RT. PULMONARY ARTERY
RT. SUPERIOR PULMONARY VEIN

C

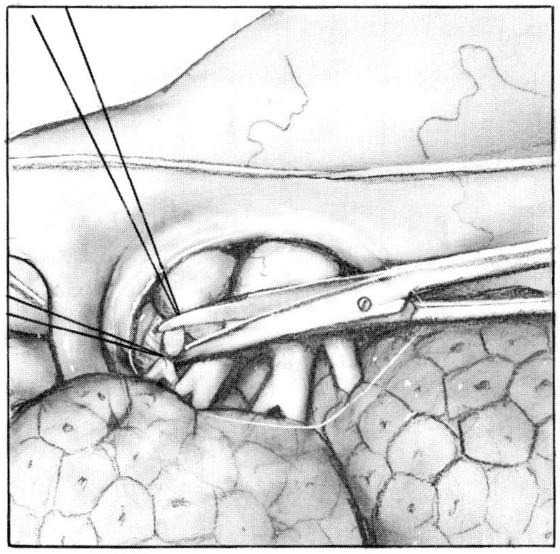

D

E. To facilitate the mobilization of the pulmonary artery, the anterior tributary of the superior pulmonary vein is doubly ligated in continuity (000 silk) and severed between the ligatures.

F. The retraction of the pulmonary vein exposes a larger surface area of the pulmonary artery, which is being mobilized posteriorly by blunt digital dissection. This is a safe and efficient method for the isolation of the large vessels in the pulmonary hilum.

F_1. A ligature of 00 silk is being withdrawn beneath the mobilized pulmonary artery.

G, H. The pulmonary artery is occluded in continuity with two ligatures (00) and two transfixion suture ligatures (000) of silk. One of the suture ligatures, which are inserted between the ligatures, is tied, and the other is being inserted (G). The artery is then severed with scissors between the transfixion suture ligatures (H).

I, J, J_1. The superior pulmonary vein, mobilized by blunt digital dissection (I), is being encircled by a ligature of 00 silk (J). The pulmonary vein is ligated, and its remaining tributary veins are triply ligated in continuity and transected (broken line) between the two distal ligatures (J_1).

Discussion—Dr. Alton Ochsner. On the right side, as on the left, it is my custom to extend the incision farther anteriorly than is shown in A. After the mediastinum is incised, as shown in B, it is often desirable to doubly ligate, transfix, and divide the venae azygos major, particularly if there are any nodes in this area; this step facilitates the dissection. The incision in the mediastinal pleura is extended up to the apex of the thorax to facilitate removal of the nodes in the superior mediastinum. On the right side, in contradistinction to the left, one need not fear involvement of the recurrent laryngeal nerve. Finger dissection of the pulmonary artery is accomplished, and it is my rule usually to isolate the pulmonary artery as a trunk and doubly ligate the artery as a single trunk together with transfixion, using two transfixions on the cardiac side placed in such a way as to incorporate the four quadrants of the artery. However, ligation of the branches of the pulmonary artery is permissible.

Whereas isolation, ligation, and division of the superior branch of the superior pulmonary vein may be desirable, usually this is not necessary, as the pulmonary artery can be freed and ligated, transfixed, and divided before the pulmonary vein is approached. This is a method that I have usually used. After satisfactory ligation, transfixion, and division of the pulmonary artery, leaving a stump long enough so there is no danger of slipping of the ligature, the superior pulmonary vein is freed by digital dissection. Subsequently the same method of ligation, transfixion, and division is accomplished either as a common trunk or, as

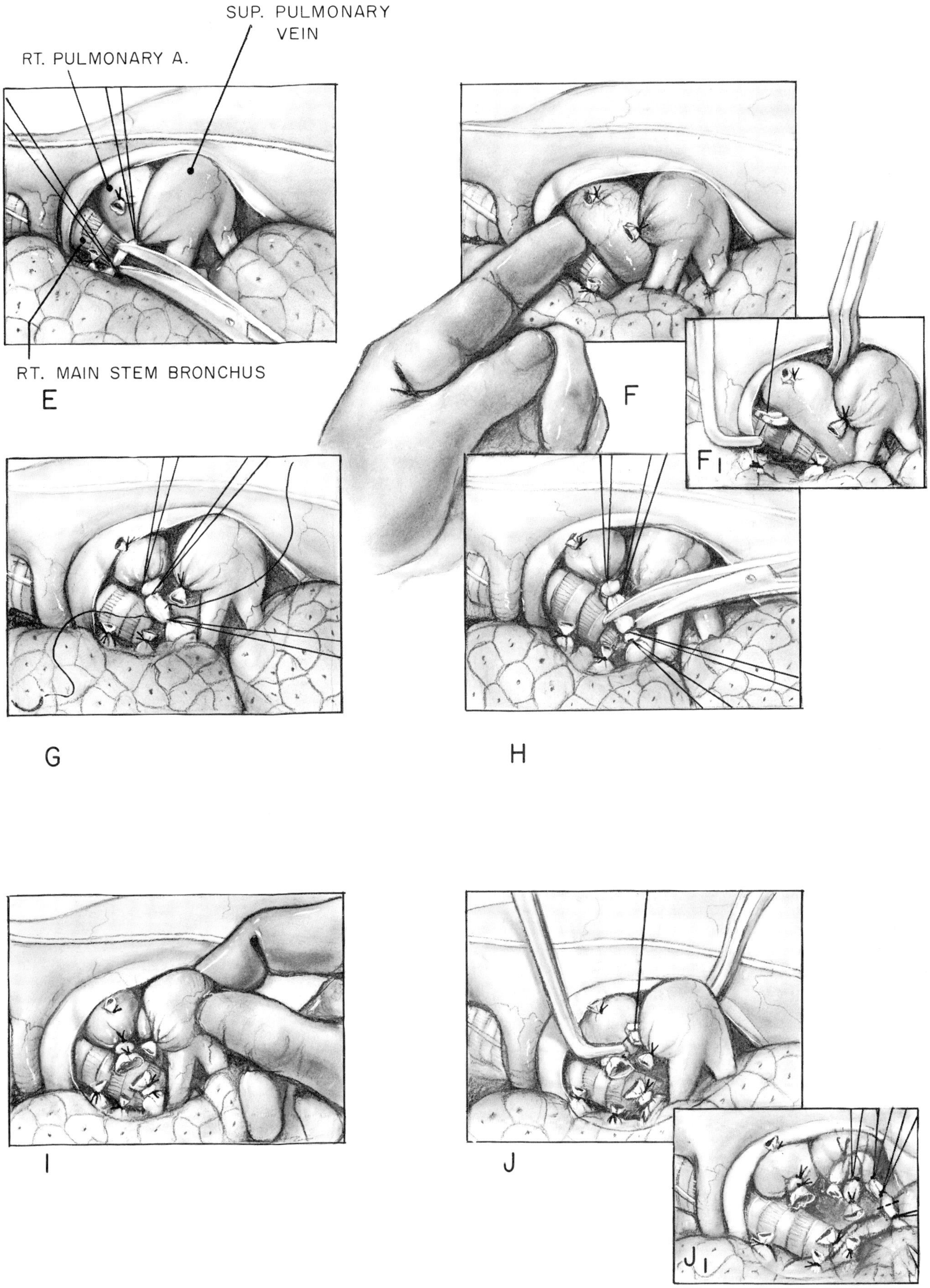
SUP. PULMONARY VEIN
RT. PULMONARY A.
RT. MAIN STEM BRONCHUS
E
F
F1
G
H
I
J
J1

K. The inferior pulmonary ligament, having been initially partially clamped, severed, and ligated, is mobilized farther by scissor dissection to expose the inferior pulmonary vein that is located at its apex.

L. The mobilized inferior pulmonary vein is being encircled by a ligature of 00 silk, which is subsequently tied. The relation of the inferior pulmonary vein to the surrounding structures is shown.

M. The inferior pulmonary vein is ligated, and its superior and basal tributaries are doubly ligated in continuity and transected (broken line) between the ligatures.

N. The right main stem bronchus is cross-clamped. Proximal to the clamp, it is serially severed (broken line) and closed, using interrupted sutures of 000 silk.

O. The operative field upon completion of the total removal of the right lung is shown in relation to the surrounding structures. The wound is closed in layers without drainage. Following the skin closure, air is aspirated from the pleural cavity until a slightly negative pressure is established.

Discussion—Dr. Ochsner (cont.)

shown in J and I, as individual branches of the trunk.

The inferior pulmonary ligament is incised, as shown in K, and by traction of the lower lobe branches anteriorly, the inferior pulmonary vein is easily identified and can either be ligated as a common trunk or, as shown in M, ligated and transfixed as a trunk from the cardiac side and as individual branches on the pulmonary side.

After the pulmonary artery and the superior and inferior pulmonary veins have been ligated, transfixed, and divided, the nodes are carefully dissected from around the carina to permit isolation of the bronchus. On the right side as well as the left, one can either use one bronchial clamp distally or two clamps, one proximally and one distally. If one is used proximally, it should be applied only tightly enough to compress the bronchus without crushing it. The bronchial sutures, as shown in N, should be tied only snugly enough to approximate the walls of the bronchus. On the right side it is usually not necessary to cover the bronchial stump with pleura, but this is desirable if it can be done. The stump is much more likely to retract into the mediastinum and is less likely to leak. On the right side, as on the left, a catheter is placed in the anterior end of the wound and left in until the wound has been completely closed and the patient returned to the supine position. Then the anesthetist expands the opposite lung, permitting egress of the trapped air in the right hemithorax. While the lung is kept expanded, the catheter is removed and the small opening covered with vaseline gauze.

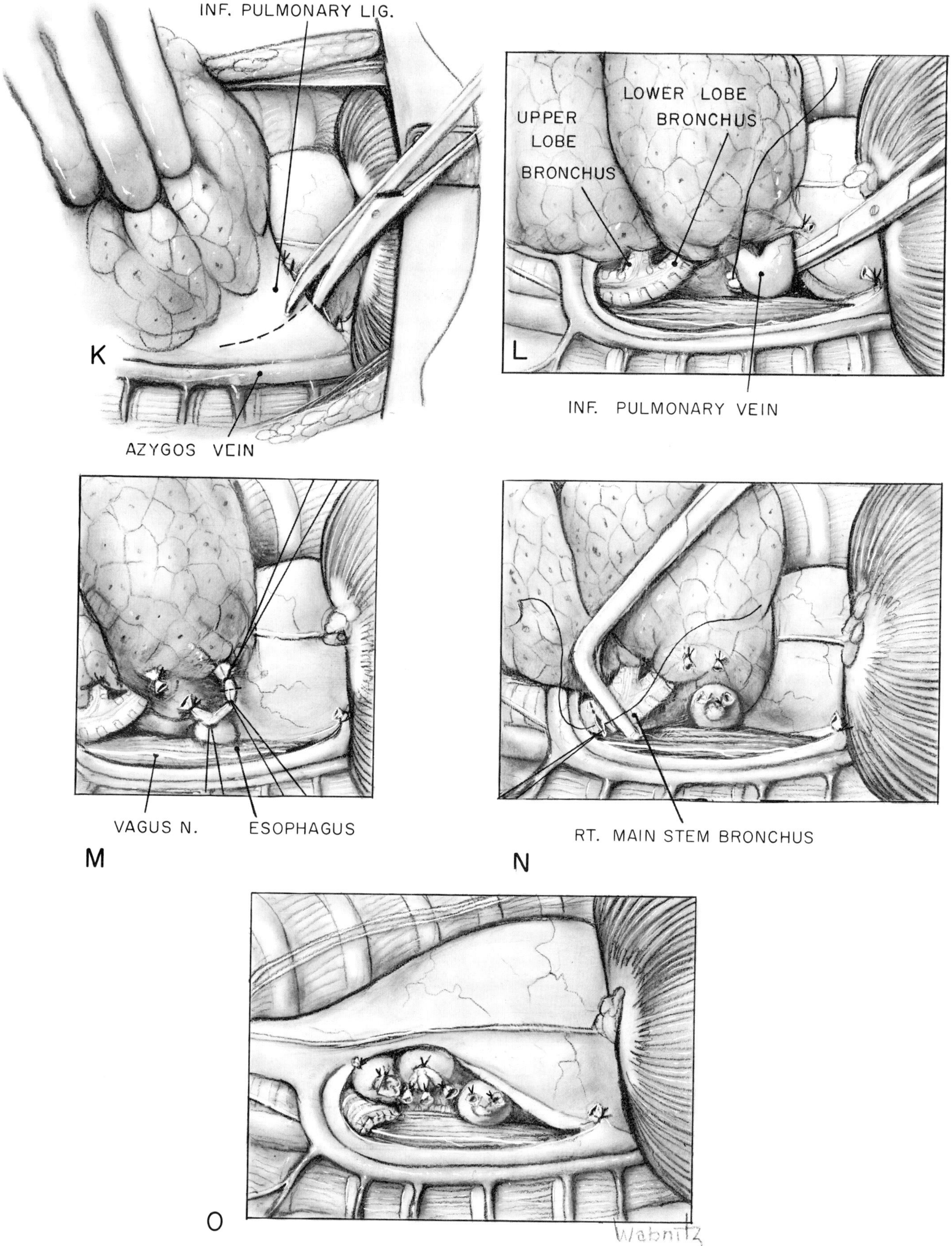
INF. PULMONARY LIG.
K
AZYGOS VEIN
UPPER LOBE BRONCHUS
LOWER LOBE BRONCHUS
L
INF. PULMONARY VEIN
VAGUS N.
ESOPHAGUS
M
RT. MAIN STEM BRONCHUS
N
O
Wabnitz

DISCUSSION—SIR RUSSELL BROCK. It is not enough to describe the operation as "total pneumonectomy," because a different type of procedure is needed for a nonmalignant disease such as tuberculosis or bronchiectasis than for cancer. Also, with cancer a different type of operation is needed in differing circumstances, such as age or frailty.

For the nonmalignant conditions the dissection and securing of the major vessels and bronchus may be done in the "hilum" proper—that is between the pericardium and the lung—but in cancer it is better to avoid opening or interfering with the true "hilum." In advanced cases frank growth is seen as an extension around the great vessels, often presenting as a collar around the hilum, adherent to the pericardium and frequently ulcerating through on to its serous surface. This gross extension may prevent resection and is obviously unfavorable. It is clear that before such gross involvement occurs there must be lesser degrees of extension scarcely detectable by macroscopic inspection, and to dissect within this zone would then be undesirable. It is therefore wiser to make a routine of not touching these tissues, not to open the "box" formed by pericardium medially and by lung laterally, but always to resect a rectangle or oval of pericardium related to the hilar vessels and to secure these vessels as far medially as possible. Even in elderly or frail subjects this may still be the only way in which a growth can be resected. There are, however, occasions in which the hilum appears so anatomic that it becomes reasonable to spare an elderly or ill patient the slight extra disturbance of an intrapericardial procedure.

With regard to incision, this should be a long posterolateral one and my own preference is to use the bed of the sixth rib rather than the fifth and to divide the posterior end of the sixth rib; if necessary, the posterior end of one rib above or below or both may be divided to give more exposure. In cases of tuberculosis, especially in which pleurectomy is also needed, it is often preferable to excise the sixth rib and to divide the posterior end of the rib above and below as required.

It may be unwise to enter the pleural cavity at once if the lung is adherent; the separation may be better in the extrapleural plane. Certainly this should be done in the area of adherence of a superficial growth; sometimes it may be necessary or safer to resect the relevant portion of the parietes to insure clearance of potentially invaded tissues.

A decision that must be made is whether to secure the veins or the bronchus first. In cancer there can be no doubt that in theory it is best to secure the veins at once so as to prevent vascular embolism from manipulation of the lung. In practice, however, it is often found that it is just not possible to dissect and ligate the veins safely without much undesirable manipulation of the lung and they must then be left until a later stage. There is also a good argument for securing the bronchus first in order to protect against inhalation of infected material into the opposite lung, even though the anaesthetist has used some form of balloon to block the bronchus and to prevent soiling. This can never be an absolute protection and is inferior to a clamp across the bronchus. If the veins are not secured first, the bronchus should be defined and clamped at once. It is quite dangerous to leave the securing of the bronchus until the last or until a late stage because of the danger of soiling, especially when the other hilar structures have been divided and the lung remains connected only by the bronchus. The preliminary clamping need not be in the final elective position, although with experience even this can usually be achieved as a rapid first step. The only justification for leaving the bronchus until last is when the growth extends so high that the division of the bronchus must be made as a precise, critical, almost tailored step.

Because of the need to secure the bronchus early, it is preferable to approach the hilum from behind—a step that in any case usually involves less disturbance of the lung than displacing it posteriorly.

Once the pleura on the back of the hilum has been incised, the vagus nerve should be identified and retracted backward, any bronchial vessels thus exposed being secured. The bronchus can then be easily isolated, encircled, and clamped at its origin from the trachea.

If a simple pneumonectomy is to be performed for nonmalignant disease, the pleural incision need not extend beyond the hilum and the main hilar structures can be secured as shown in the illustrations. If, however, the lesion is malignant, it is desirable to remove the associated lymph nodes, for actual experience with cancer of the lung has shown that, just as elsewhere in the body, the nodes may be involved microscopically even though not macroscopically, and it surely cannot be denied that a radical clearance of these potentially involved nodes is a thoroughly desirable surgical step.

The incision begun on the back of the hilum should be extended as far as the apex just anterior to the vagus nerve; en route the vena azygos is ligated and divided. It should be left long where it joins the superior vena cava, as the stump proves useful to rotate the vena cava forward in order to aid clearance of the right tracheobronchial fossa; the ligature should be applied close to the caval wall.

At the apex the pleural incision is carried forward for about 2 cm., to expose the phrenic nerve and its accompanying vessels; these and the nerve are ligated and divided, and the incision is carried downward anterior to the phrenic nerve in front of the hilum. The contents of the right tracheobronchial fossa are now exposed and can be dissected out. Often large nodes previously concealed are disclosed. The medial boundary of the fossa

DISCUSSION—SIR RUSSELL BROCK (cont.)

is formed by fascia covering the aortic arch; the posterior wall is the trachea, and the anterior is formed by the superior vena cava.

In the illustrations the hilar areolar space is opened to secure the upper lobe arteries as a first step. This is unnecessary, undesirable, and frequently impossible. It is preferable to incise the pericardium along the line of the displaced phrenic nerve. If the veins are to be secured, this can now be done. In this event the phrenic nerve and vessels should be freed down to the diaphragm, ligated, and divided and the pericardial incision continued to just below the inferior pulmonary vein.

It is the custom in standard textbooks of anatomy to describe the veins as joining the left atrium separately; the illustrations show them being individually secured and ligated. This again is unnecessary and undesirable. In the living subject it will be found that a common pulmonary vein always exists, or at any rate that it is possible to encircle a portion of the atrium where the veins join it, so that what is virtually a common trunk of entry is displayed. This can be defined by a very little dissection above and posteriorly, after the mesentery of the inferior vein has been divided. The finger or an instrument slips all the way round except for this one site above and behind. A single heavy ligature is then tied around this common trunk. Working from inside the pericardium and without disturbing the hilar areolar tissue, the pericardium can be gently and easily pushed laterally to expose the superior and inferior veins joining to form the common vein. Each is encircled by a transfixion ligature. In all of these large vessels a transfixion stitch should be used to guard against slipping but should be supported by a proximal ligature.

The pericardial incision is now continued upward, where it will be found that a small recess extends in front of the right pulmonary artery and lateral to the superior vena cava. This recess should be completely opened, and the operation field then joins the previous clearance of the right tracheobronchial fossa. It is now a simple matter to free the lower part of the superior vena cava and to rotate it medially, making use of the stump of the vena azygos left long for this purpose. The clearance of the lymph nodes can be carried a stage farther, and the pulmonary artery is now *widely exposed as it lies partly within the serous pericardium and partly outside it* and emerging from under cover of the superior vena cava. It is now encircled *well within the mediastinum,* behind the vena cava and medial to the hilar "box." A long length of artery is available for double ligation, the first ligature encircling the vessel and the more lateral one first transfixing it. The part of the artery adjacent to the lung is either ligated or secured with a clamp before being divided. If growth extends along or around the main right pulmonary artery, resection may be impossible without this maneuver, which allows dissection so deep within the mediastinum. In very difficult cases it may be necessary to leave the division of the artery as the last step of removal of the lung so that meticulous freeing from growth is possible, just as may be needed in similar circumstances with the division of the veins or of the main bronchus.

Once the artery is divided, lymph nodes are displayed lying in front of the lower end of the trachea, joining laterally and above with those in the right tracheobronchial fossa and medially with those within the concavity of the aortic arch. A deliberate clearance in continuity can be made. At this stage in a *right* radical pneumonectomy the *left* recurrent laryngeal nerve is displayed as part of a good operation.

Attention now should turn to the ligamentum latum previously partly opened when the phrenic nerve and vessels were ligated above the diaphragm. This fold of pleura should be ligated and cut from the diaphragm, and an incision should be made along its posterior surface to join the original pleural incision on the back of the hilum. The ligamentum latum is then carefully dissected from its medial relation, the esophagus, any vessels are secured, and the lymph nodes are meticulously excised with it. There is always a large well-defined "sentinel" node in the highest part of the ligament immediately below the inferior pulmonary vein. Once this has been swept from the adjacent pericardium, this structure can be divided horizontally below the inferior pulmonary vein and then vertically upward until the inferior tracheobronchial fossa is opened. If the veins have not been earlier secured, they may now be taken and divided. In this way the inferior tracheobronchial compartment is widely displayed for clearance of its lymph node group and for confirming that the bronchus clamp is placed at the very origin of the bronchus immediately below the carina.

A distal clamp is then applied, the bronchus is divided between the two clamps, and the lung is removed.

There are many ways of suturing the bronchus. A method that has proved very successful in my practice has been the use of interrupted stainless steel sutures passed as a figure of 8 around the clamp, which is removed before the individual sutures are tied.

It is preferable, but not essential, to cover the cut end of the bronchus. If the vagus nerve was preserved and displaced backward, it will be found that a fascial fold passes like a mesentery from it to the lateral surface of the esophagus. Two fine mattress sutures are passed through this fold and pick up fascia on the front of the bronchus stump; when tied, they cover the stump with the fascia, the vagus nerve being displaced harmlessly in front of the bronchus. Sometimes a long piece of parapericardial fat may be fashioned or mobilized from the anterior pericardiophrenic angle so as to be sutured over the bronchus stump.

PULMONARY LOBECTOMY: LEFT UPPER LOBE

The patient, an 80-year-old white man whose apparent good general condition belied his age, was admitted to the hospital with the chief complaint of constant pain in the left axillary region of two months' duration. The pain radiated downward along the lateral chest wall, was worse at night, and of progressively increasing severity. During the same period there was an associated weight loss of 25 pounds. Also, recurrent episodes of hemoptysis, never severe, occurred and persisted. A box of cigars was smoked weekly.

Bronchoscopy was essentially normal. A roentgenogram of the chest showed a circumscribed shadow of increased density, located peripherally in the left upper lobe, which merged indistinguishably with the adjacent pleura. Because of the constant chest pain and roentgenographic findings, infiltration of the overlying pleura and chest wall was suspected. This was confirmed at operation as shown. Death due to metastatic disease occurred nine months after operation.

A. The patient is placed in the direct right lateral prone position, and the posterolateral thoracotomy incision overlying the fifth interspace is outlined and crosshatched to facilitate later closure.

B, C. The incision is deepened into the pleural cavity, and a segment of the costal cage (second, third, and fourth ribs), infiltrated by the tumor, is resected as a part of the surgical specimen.

D. The mobilized segment of the costal cage is covered with a moist gauze sponge, and as manual traction downward is maintained, the areolar tissue attachments between the upper lobe and the pulmonary artery are freed by scissor dissection. The apical-posterior branch and its bifurcation just prior to its entrance into the lung parenchyma are visible.

E. The apical-posterior artery is doubly ligated (00 silk) and transected. An anterior branch, doubly ligated (00 silk) in continuity, is being severed with scissors between the ligatures.

E′. The upper lobe is retracted upward and medialward to show the interlobar visceral pleura being severed (broken line) for the further exposure of the pulmonary artery and its branches.

Discussion—Dr. Charles K. Kirby. Removal of the left upper lobe is usually carried out for the purpose of excising a tumor that is located peripherally. Ten years ago resection of the left upper lobe was performed with relative frequency for inflammatory lesions, tuberculous and nontuberculous. Lobectomy for inflammatory lesions has become much less common in my experience, and this has also been true of many other surgeons with whom I have discussed this subject.

When a bronchogenic carcinoma has invaded the chest wall, as in the patient presented, resection is often warranted for palliative purposes and for the purpose of attempting to obtain a prolonged survival. The long-term results are not as favorable, in my experience, when the pleura has been invaded by tumor cells and resection of a portion of the chest wall is necessary.

It is usually desirable to carry the skin incision farther anteriorly than is depicted in A. By extending the skin incision as far anteriorly as the nipple line, it is often possible to open the rib spreader to a somewhat greater extent without risking fracture of a rib. Rib fractures that occur as a complication of opening the rib spreader appear to increase the postoperative pain to a considerable extent in many patients.

One of the problems complicating left upper lobectomy in a significant percentage of patients is the presence of adhesions between the visceral and parietal pleura. Before beginning the dissection of the hilum in such patients, it is necessary to deal with these adhesions first, which may be an exceedingly difficult problem. Not uncommonly, the problem of freeing adhesions that bind the apex of the upper lobe to the apex of the pleural cavity is considerably more difficult from the technical standpoint than the problems encountered in dealing with the hilar structures. When possible, it is advisable to divide the adhesions intrapleurally, carrying the dissection a little closer to the upper lobe than to the chest wall. If the adhesions are vascular, this provides some tissue on the chest wall side that can be clamped and ligated, which is the simplest method of dealing with blood vessels which accompany adhesions. If the adhesions are very short, however, or if there is actual symphysis between the parietal and visceral pleura, the dissection may have to be carried out extrapleurally. Control of bleeding, particularly at the apex of the chest, is considerably more difficult when an extrapleural dissection is necessary. During such a dissection, the greatest risk is that of injuring the axillary vein. This is a very real hazard, and the most important factor in avoiding it is certain knowledge of the actual location of the axillary vein. By careful palpation of the axillary artery and the first rib, it is possible to localize the

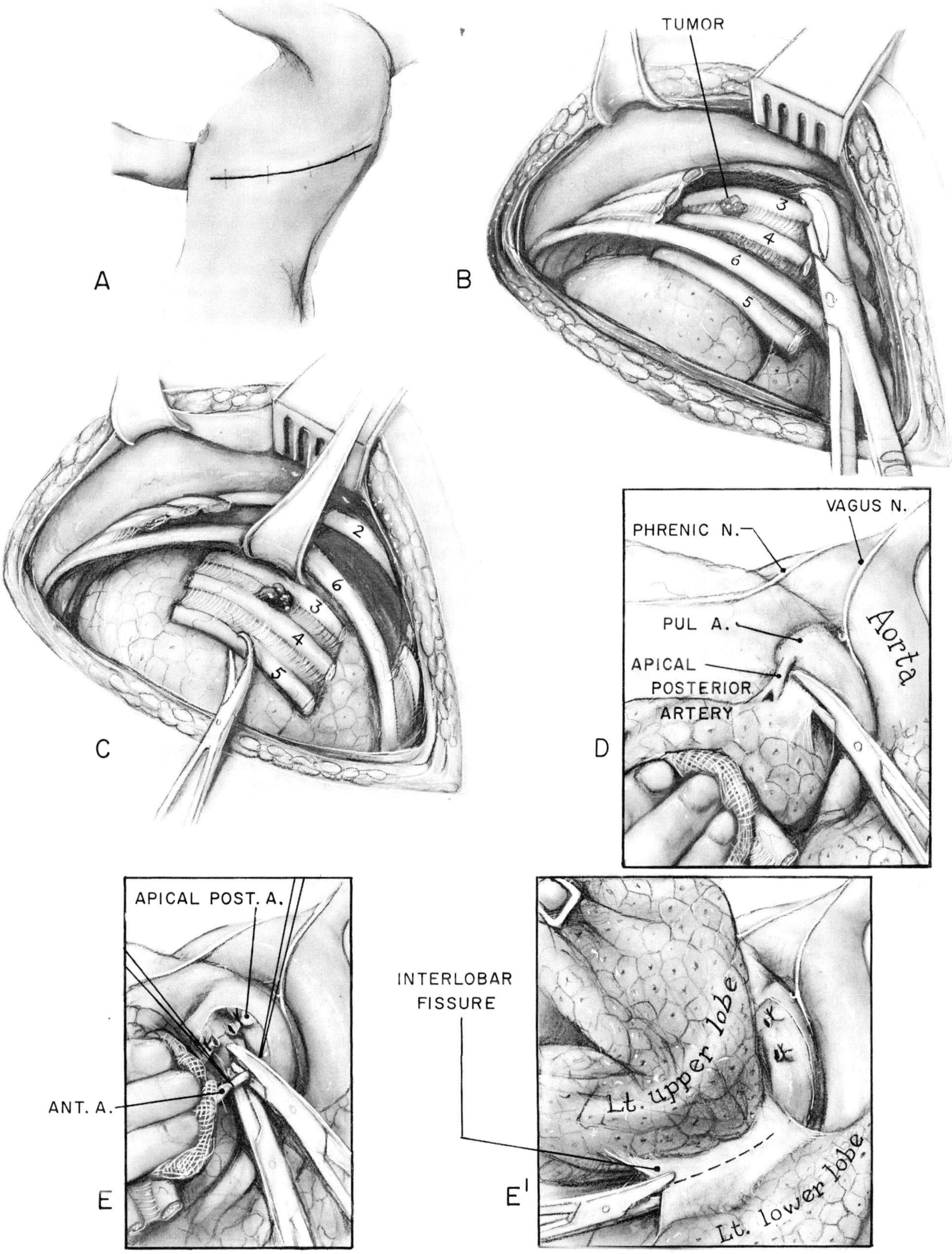
A
TUMOR
3
4
6
5
B
2
6
3
4
5
C
VAGUS N.
PHRENIC N.
PUL A.
Aorta
APICAL
POSTERIOR
ARTERY
D
APICAL POST. A.
ANT. A.
E
INTERLOBAR
FISSURE
Lt. upper lobe
Lt. lower lobe
E'

F, F′. The interlobar fissure is opened, and the relation of the pulmonary artery and its branches to the lobes of the lung and the relation of the stem bronchi to the left upper lobe are visible. In this patient there were two anterior branches (both ligated and severed). The lingular arteries arose separately from the pulmonary artery rather than from a common trunk (F′), which is more frequently found. The artery to the inferior segment of the lingula is being encircled with a ligature of 000 silk. The more common arrangement of the arterial branches to the left upper and lower lobes is shown in F′. In these two specimens (F, F′) there is a slight variation in the relation of the arterial branch to the superior segment of the lower lobe and the arterial supply to the lingula.

F″. The ligation and severance of the arterial branches to the left upper lobe is completed.

G. The upper lobe is manually retracted posteriorly, and the anterior mediastinal pleura is severed (broken line) by scissor dissection for the exposure of the superior pulmonary vein.

H. The superior pulmonary vein is mobilized by both clamp and digital dissection. The use of the index finger for dissection is an efficient, safe, and highly recommended method that minimizes the danger of injury to the vein and resulting hemorrhage.

H′. When its mobilization is completed, the superior pulmonary vein is encircled with a ligature of 00 silk, which is not immediately tied.

I. Two of the tributaries of the superior pulmonary vein are ligated and severed and the third one is doubly ligated in continuity before being severed (broken line).

I′. On completion of the ligation of the three tributary veins, the ligature encircling the superior pulmonary vein is tied. The retraction of the vein after severance of its tributaries exposes an additional branch of the pulmonary artery, the anterior mediastinal (I and I′), which arises opposite to, and in this patient is larger than, the apical-posterior branch, the ligated stump of which lies superiorly. The anterior mediastinal artery is now elevated on a clamp prior to being ligated in continuity and severed.

J. The ligation of the superior pulmonary vein and the double ligation and severance of its three tributary veins are completed. Also the anterior mediastinal artery has been ligated in continuity, and its branches have been doubly ligated and transected between the ligatures.

Discussion—Dr. Kirby (cont.)

position of the axillary vein so that the dissection can be carried out with unusual care in this region. When an extrapleural dissection is necessary at the apex of the chest, it is of great importance to be able to use the electrocautery. Bleeding points on the inner surface of the ribs and intercostal bundles cannot be clamped and often cannot be dealt with very satisfactorily by suturing. Use of the electrocautery is usually ideal for dealing with such bleeding points. The total operating time can often be greatly decreased. Without the electrocautery, more time can readily be spent in trying to control the bleeding from the chest wall than in carrying out all the maneuvers which are actually necessary for removal of the lobe.

Mobilization of the left pulmonary artery and the segmental branches to the upper lobe have been well illustrated (D through F″). Unfortunately, the dissection is rarely so straightforward and clear-cut because there is an "incomplete" fissure between the upper and lower lobe, or there are many adhesions between the two lobes, in more than half of the patients. In either event, extensive dissection may be necessary before the pulmonary artery can be exposed in the depths of the fissure. The safest approach in opening up the fissure, in my experience, is to work from above downward. The main trunk of the left pulmonary artery can be readily exposed where it curves around the left upper lobe bronchus before entering the fissure. A plane in the loose areolar tissue overlying the pulmonary artery can be readily entered, and dissection along this plane can be safely carried down into the fissure for a short distance without the risk of dividing segmental branches. This also provides the surgeon an opportunity of clarifying the precise location of the fissure. It can usually be readily ascertained which is the upper and which is the lower lobe. Dissection can then be carried out, preferably with the scissors, in the correct plane. Bleeders may be encountered, and, if so, they are clamped and ligated. Much of the dissection in the fissure can ordinarily be carried out without dividing bleeders, if the surgeon has identified the correct plane. Dissection is carried progressively downward along the pulmonary artery and in the fissure in this manner until the entire main trunk of the left pulmonary artery has been exposed.

It has been my practice to place suture ligatures distal to the free ligatures on the segmental branches of the pulmonary artery. Very little further time and effort is required. The security provided by the use of suture ligatures has seemed worthwhile to me.

The superior pulmonary vein is sufficiently long,

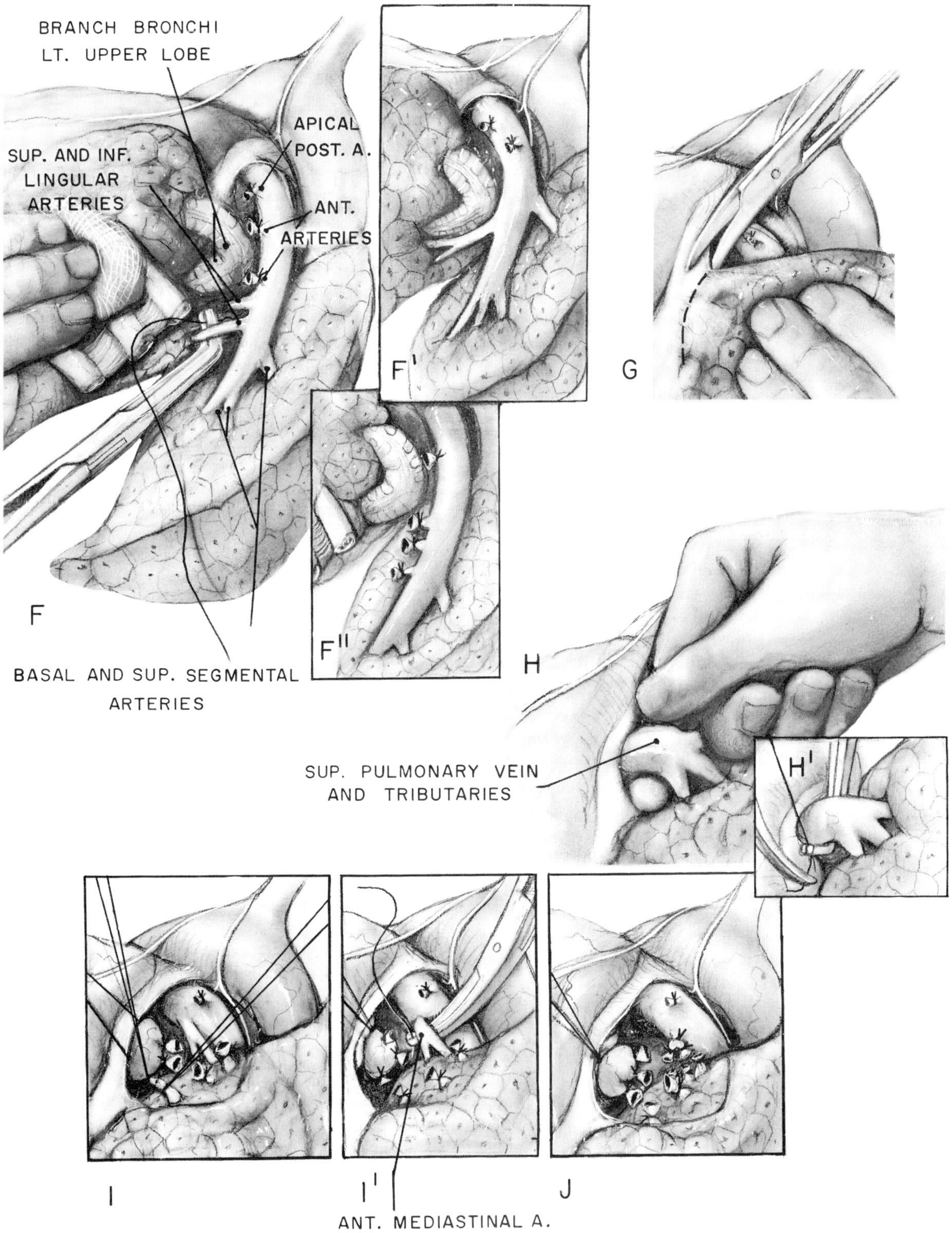
BRANCH BRONCHI
LT. UPPER LOBE
SUP. AND INF.
LINGULAR
ARTERIES
APICAL
POST. A.
ANT.
ARTERIES
F
F'
F''
G
BASAL AND SUP. SEGMENTAL
ARTERIES
H
H'
SUP. PULMONARY VEIN
AND TRIBUTARIES
I
I'
J
ANT. MEDIASTINAL A.

K. The left upper lobe is retracted anteriorly, and the interlobar fissure is again exposed. The main stem bronchi to the superior (apical-posterior and anterior) and lingula (superior and inferior) segments are mobilized and encircled by cotton tapes.

L. The superior branch bronchus, occluded by a clamp (Sarot) distally, is being partially transected by a scalpel on a right-angle handle.

M, N. The open proximal end of the partially transected bronchus is occluded seriatim by sutures of 000 silk as the bronchus is serially transected.

DISCUSSION—DR. KIRBY (cont.)

in most patients, to permit application of one free ligature and one suture ligature to the main trunk. Double ligatures on the tributaries of the superior pulmonary vein have not usually been necessary (I, J), but if a short main trunk of the superior pulmonary vein is encountered, ligation of the individual tributaries proximally and distally is undoubtedly a wise precaution. More extensive dissection of the individual tributaries must be carried out in order to obtain an adequate cuff. This dissection is not without risk and must be performed with great care.

A somewhat different method of dividing and suturing the bronchus (L through P) has seemed preferable to me. The upper and lower divisions of the upper lobe bronchus are dissected out for some distance beyond the bifurcation, as illustrated. It is useful to use a "wiping" maneuver with gauze sweeping adherent parenchyma, peribronchial lymph nodes, and other peribronchial tissues peripherally. Two Sarot clamps are then placed separately on both the superior and inferior divisions of the upper lobe bronchus, and both of these branch bronchi are then divided between the clamps with a scalpel. This permits removal of the entire upper lobe before bronchial suturing is commenced, and there is excellent exposure during bronchial suturing. The bronchial sutures are inserted with straight needles proximal to the bronchial clamps. After they have all been inserted beneath one of the clamps, the clamp is removed. Traction is applied to the sutures, which are neatly matched and handed to the operator serially by the first assistant, for tying.

Pleuralization of the bronchial stumps has been generally considered an important factor in preventing the development of a bronchopleural fistula. I have always pleuralized the bronchial stump, and the incidence of this complication in my hands has been so low that I have been convinced about the importance of this step. The left upper lobe bronchial stump is one of the most difficult to pleuralize because dissection of the superior pulmonary vein often causes lacerations in the portion of the mediastinal pleura that might potentially be the most readily available. I have avoided this difficulty by using a hinged flap of pericardium. The hinge is based just anterior to the phrenic nerve and a U-shaped incision is made up toward the anterior mediastinum. This incision is made through the entire thickness of the pericardial sac and the flap is rotated on its hinge 180° so that the pleural surface near the tip of the flap covers the bronchial stump. Sutures that are used to close the end of the bronchus are passed through the flap, anchoring it securely in position. It should be stressed that this is a flap of tissue with an adequate blood supply rather than a free graft. It is applied without tension in such a manner as to provide every opportunity for firm, early sealing of the bronchial stump.

After the left upper lobe is removed the apex of the left lower lobe still lies a considerable distance from the apex of the chest (Q, R). It is important to mobilize the left lower lobe so that it can rise to the top of the chest. In order to accomplish this, the pulmonary ligament must be completely divided from the diaphragm right up to the inferior pulmonary vein. It appears helpful also to divide the remaining portion of the pleura which is reflected on the hilum both anteriorly and posteriorly. After this has been done, as the chest is being closed, the lower lobe will be seen to occupy the desired position. One additional maneuver that is employed by many surgeons is to paralyze the diaphragm temporarily by pinching the phrenic nerve a short distance above the diaphragm. This undoubtedly decreases the likelihood that there will be a residual collection of air or fluid on top of the left lower lobe.

The use of an upper and lower tube, as illustrated, is strongly recommended. Rather than bringing the upper tube out through the anterior end of the incision, as is illustrated and as I used to do, it now seems preferable to me to bring this tube out one or two interspaces below the intercostal space which is actually opened.

It has seemed advisable to apply suction to both the upper and lower chest drainage tube, but particularly to the upper drainage tube, following left upper lobectomy. It is important to remove all air and fluid from the apex of the chest during the early postoperative period so that full expansion of the lower lobe can take place at the top of the left hemithorax. When suction has not been used, there has been a persistent effusion on top of the left lower lobe in some instances.

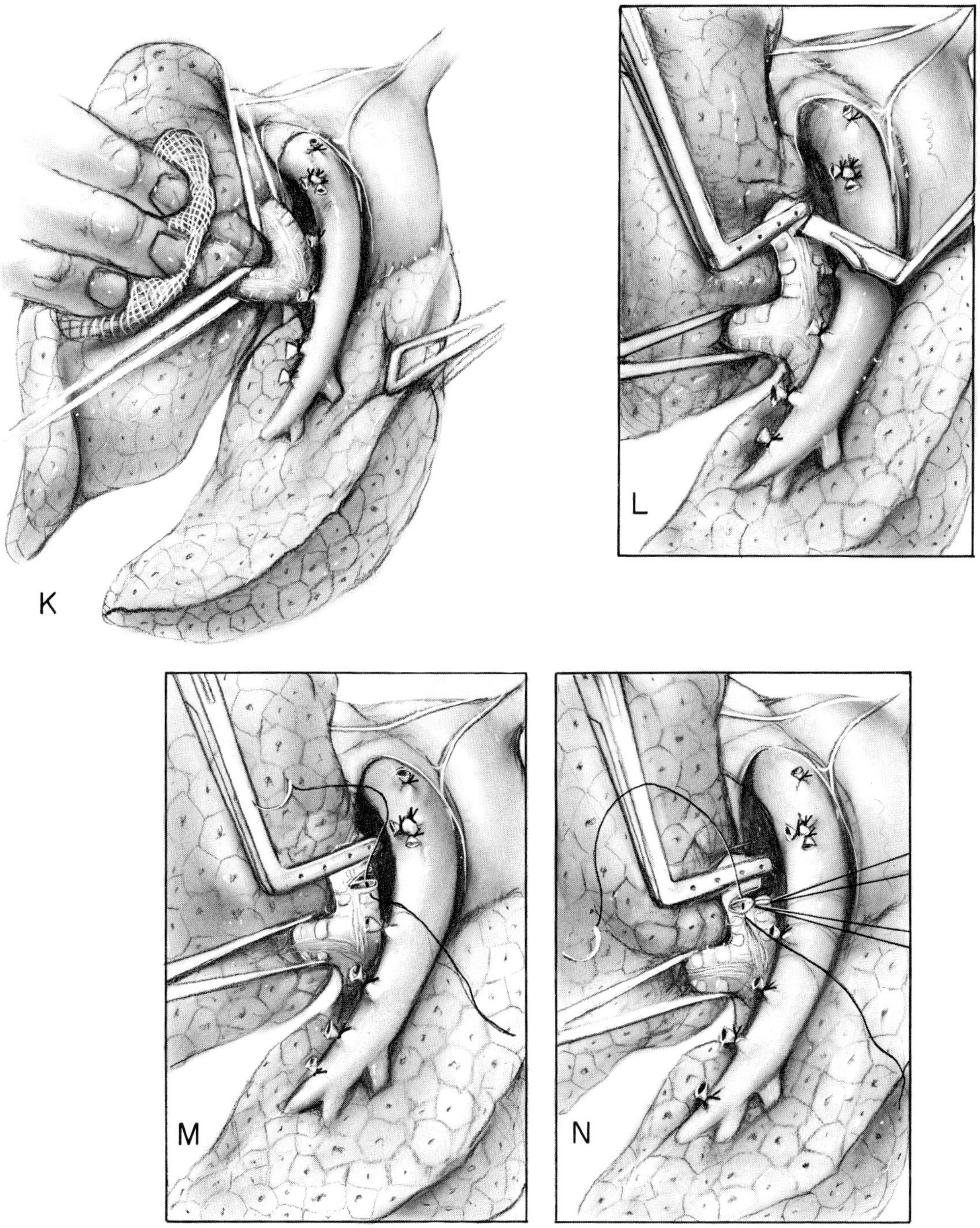
K
L
M
N

O. The closure of the superior stem bronchus is completed. The inferior or lingula branch bronchus will be occluded in like manner.

P. The closure of both stem bronchi is completed. They are held outward by traction on the angle closure sutures to show their relation to the surrounding structures.

Q. The sutures are cut, and the occluded branch bronchi are allowed to recede into their normal relation to the pulmonary artery and the ligated stump of the superior pulmonary vein.

R. A catheter (18 F.) is being anchored to the parietal pleura of the chest wall anteriorly to serve as an air vent.

S. The air vent catheter (18 F.) and a Foley (No. 18) catheter for underwater drainage of the pleural cavity are inserted, and closure of the costal cage is begun. Two double-strand pericostal sutures of No. 2 chromic catgut are inserted through periosteal "windows" underlying the sixth rib. The defect in the costal cage cephalad following segmental en bloc resection of the second, third, and fourth ribs is visible. The muscles of the posterolateral chest wall are closed in layers, using continuous double strand sutures of 00 chromic catgut.

T. The skin incision is closed with interrupted sutures of 000 silk to complete the operation. The exits of the catheters in relation to the incision are depicted.

Discussion—Dr. John C. Jones. An 80-year-old male complaining of constant pain in the axillary region for two months, having roentgenologic evidence of a peripheral lung lesion, must presumably have a lung malignancy of questionable resectability, regardless of normal bronchoscopic findings. The reasons for consideration of resectional surgery are (1) to relieve the pain, (2) to eradicate the source of hemoptysis, and (3) to prolong life by resecting the malignancy and its local extension. Certainly the source of hemoptysis may be eradicated by surgical excision of the lobe, but it is by no means certain that the patient will be free of pain following surgery, and debatable that an 80-year-old patient will live longer and as comfortably following radical resection of lung and chest wall as if he had been treated either by radiation and anticancer drugs or possibly radiation followed by excisional surgery.

The extent of the en bloc excision of chest wall is dictated by the lesion involving it after the pleural cavity is explored and found free of malignant implants.

The segment of chest wall is excised and dropped into the thorax along with its contiguous lobe before the hilar dissection is carried out. The technic may be modified, depending on the bulkiness of the tumor, the presence and status of the interlobar fissure, and the variations of the anatomy of the pulmonary artery branches. Not infrequently, it may be expedient because of difficult exposure to delay the sectioning of one or both lingular arteries until after the bronchus has been dissected and divided. Some surgeons prefer to divide the superior pulmonary vein before beginning the dissection of the branches of the artery, contending that the manipulation of the lobe during arterial dissection may be conducive to hematogenous metastasis. Only when the left upper lobe bronchus divides immediately near the main stem bronchus, or when carrying out segmental resection, do I employ the technic of a separate suture line for the superior and inferior segments of the left upper lobe. Peripheral malignancies confined to the left upper lobe that dictate lobectomy, and most of them do, should have the bronchus severed as close to the main bronchus (preferably one suture line) as possible. I am a confirmed advocate of a short bronchial stump under all resectional circumstances, malignancy or infection.

It is most important to utilize the two (anterior and posterolateral) drainage catheters loosely sutured to parietal pleura in most lobectomies, but particularly in upper lobectomy. They should be left in place until the remaining lobe, fully expanded, has obliterated the space defect at the apex. I prefer to have both tubes brought out through stab wounds (intercostal airtight drainage) rather than have either drainage tube emerge through the wound site. The bony defect resulting from the resection is well protected by the scapula and shoulder girdle musculature, so a prosthesis is not needed.

Prompt obliteration of the residual space left by lobectomy will prevent the incidence of complications of resection (residual air space, bronchopleural fistula, hematoma, and empyema). Suction drainage is frequently indicated. Phrenic crush at the diaphragm may be considered, but I prefer to institute immediate pneumoperitoneum to encourage early elevation of the diaphragm for space filling purposes. Air leaks from crossing incomplete fissures may require strong suction to encourage early and rapid lung expansion of the remaining segment of lung. Long suture lines of pleural edges to obliterate small bronchial leaks compromise the volume of the remaining lung, deform the lung's natural contours, and are to be avoided if possible by individual ligation of the air leak points.

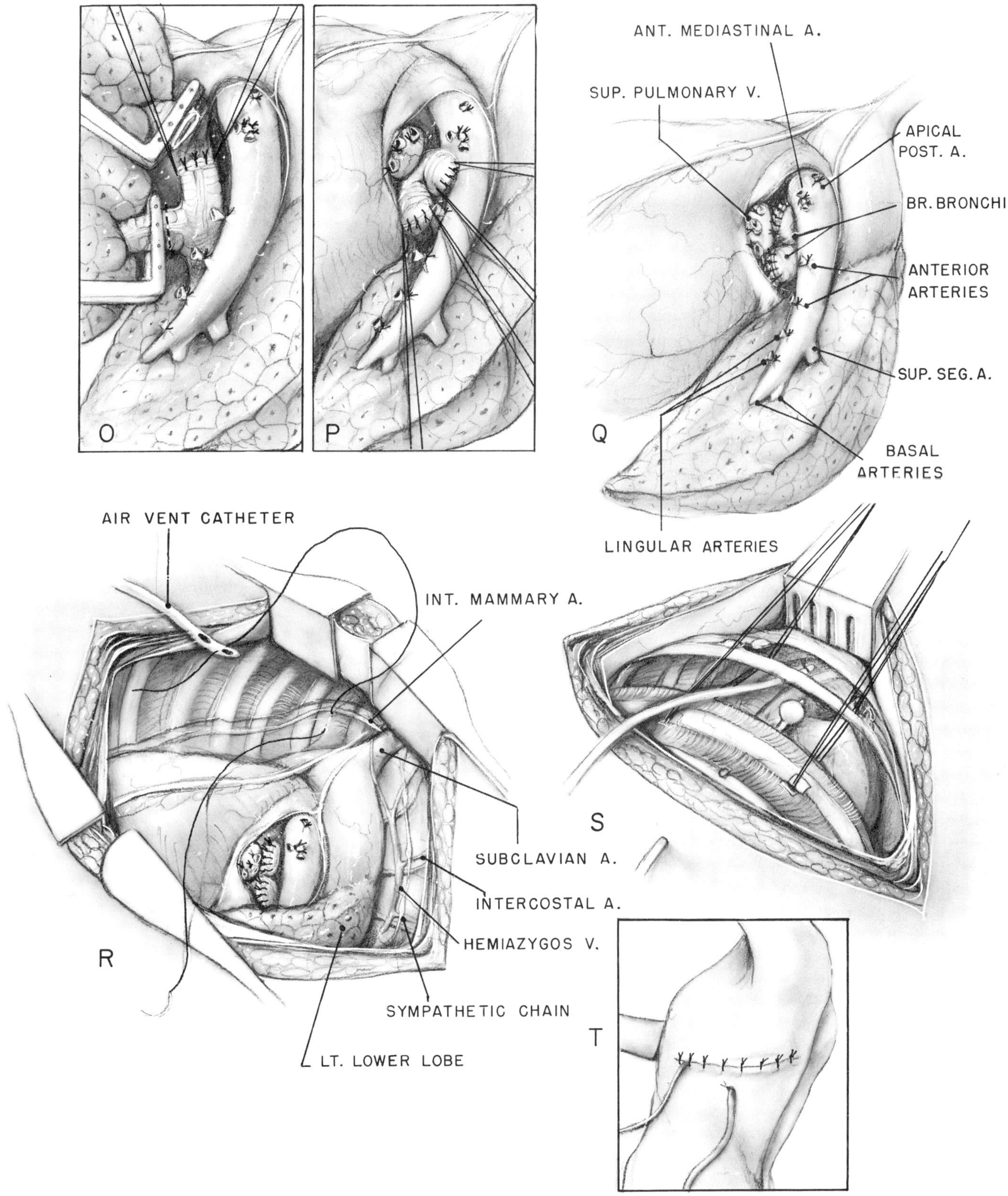
ANT. MEDIASTINAL A.
SUP. PULMONARY V.
APICAL POST. A.
BR. BRONCHI
ANTERIOR ARTERIES
SUP. SEG. A.
BASAL ARTERIES
LINGULAR ARTERIES
O
P
Q
AIR VENT CATHETER
INT. MAMMARY A.
SUBCLAVIAN A.
INTERCOSTAL A.
HEMIAZYGOS V.
SYMPATHETIC CHAIN
LT. LOWER LOBE
R
S
T

PULMONARY LOBECTOMY: LEFT LOWER LOBE

A. The patient is placed in the direct right lateral prone position, and the incision overlying the sixth intercostal space is outlined.

B. The left pleural cavity is entered, and the severance of the visceral pleura overlying the interlobar fissure for the exposure of the pulmonary artery and its branches is shown.

C, D. The left pulmonary artery and its branches to the upper and lower lobes are exposed. The artery to the superior segment of the lower lobe, which originates opposite the site of origin of the branch to the lingula segment of the upper lobe, is being encircled by a ligature of 00 silk (C) preliminary to its double ligation in continuity and severance (D).

DISCUSSION—DR. JOHN C. JONES. In women the anterior extremity of the posterolateral incision should be carried low enough so that it is not beyond the mammary fold or into the breast area; the incision should not cross above the angle of the scapula when the patient is in the normal upright position. In young patients I prefer the intercostal approach, incising the unresected rib bed of the sixth rib, but in older patients I usually resect the sixth rib. The latter are not infrequently plagued with postoperative thoracic pain, particularly if rib spreaders are spread too rapidly or too widely.

The dissection of the branches of the pulmonary artery will be guided by the completeness or incompleteness of the interlobar fissure, the extent and character of the lesion involving the lung, and the presence of hard fixed lymph nodes overlying the artery and its branches. Anticipating difficulties in the dissection, a tape passed about the main pulmonary artery or the main branch to the lower lobe will facilitate hemostasis and repair if branches of the artery are torn during the dissection. Usually the branch of the pulmonary artery to the superior segment must be divided first; the main branch to the lower lobe may then be divided some distance distal to it and below the lingular branch. Segmental resections require meticulous dissection of the various branches. However, most left lower lobectomies need only the ligation and division of the superior segment branch and the main branch to the lower lobe just distal to the lingular branch. I prefer to dissect the inferior pulmonary ligament up to the inferior vein and to clamp the mediastinal bleeders individually as they are encountered. Unless the superior segment is to be salvaged, the entire inferior pulmonary vein may be doubly ligated and divided. I place a suture ligature distal to the proximal tie.

The vast majority of lower lobe bronchi I have transected have been closed with one suture line. I believe this technic to be preferable to first individually dividing and suturing the superior segment branch bronchus. This I prefer to do without a bronchial clamp, using two stay sutures, one just below the upper lobe bronchus (anterior) and another just above the superior segmental bronchus (posterior). If necessary, I cut the bronchus on the bias, resulting in a short bronchial stump. Since 1942, I have employed 00000 (35 gauge) stainless steel sutures on swage needles for bronchus closure except in infants, when I use 00000 arterial silk. This technic eliminates two bothersome late complications: puddling of secretion in the long stump and bleeding from granulations at the sutured bronchial stump. I have not known of a patient who expectorated a wire suture.

After the major hilar structures have been dealt with, the lobe to be resected is carefully dissected from its contiguous lobe or lobes; gentle traction is applied to the bronchus clamp and the diseased lobe, and the smaller interlobar structures are divided individually as the dissection is carried along the interlobar fissure line, while the remaining lung is kept inflated with anesthesia positive pressure. It is much easier to dissect along the fissure line from the hilum outward to avoid tears and leaks in the lung tissue that is to remain.

Pleural grafts are not always feasible, but I would prefer to do without a graft cover than to transplant fat or tissue under tension and doomed to die. A bronchus not unduly denuded, with adequate bronchial blood supply to its stump end, properly sutured with stainless steel, and with the surrounding tissues dropping over it, is most unlikely to be complicated. The exceptions obviously are the resections in tuberculous patients whose organisms are resistant to antituberculosis drugs and patients in poor nutritional state.

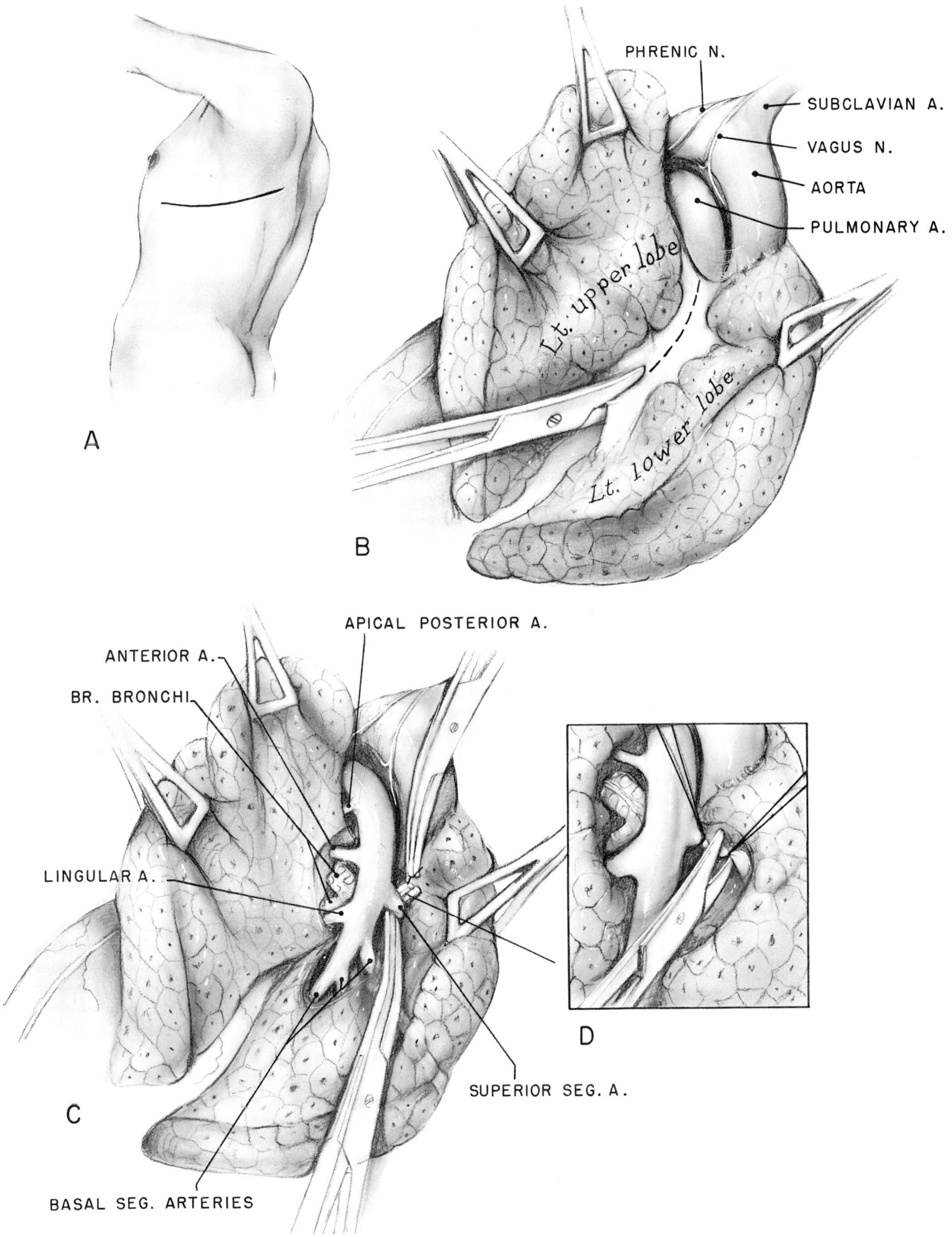
PHRENIC N.
SUBCLAVIAN A.
VAGUS N.
AORTA
PULMONARY A.
Lt. upper lobe
Lt. lower lobe
A
B
APICAL POSTERIOR A.
ANTERIOR A.
BR. BRONCHI
LINGULAR A.
SUPERIOR SEG. A.
BASAL SEG. ARTERIES
C
D

E. The remaining artery to the basal segment of the lower lobe is being doubly ligated in continuity.

F. A transfixion suture ligature of silk (000) is inserted just beneath the proximal ligature, and the artery is cut (broken line) between the transfixion and distal ligatures.

G. The inferior pulmonary ligament is doubly clamped and severed (broken line) by scissors.

H, I. The opening between the layers of the inferior pulmonary ligament is enlarged (H) to expose the inferior pulmonary vein, which is encircled by an untied ligature of 00 silk. (I)

J. The superior segmental tributary is doubly ligated in continuity (00 silk) and severed (broken line) between the ligatures.

K. The larger tributary from the basal segment is occluded in like manner, and the ligature (00 silk) that encircled the main trunk of the inferior pulmonary vein (I, J) is tied.

Discussion—Dr. Charles K. Kirby. The technic of left lower lobectomy has been very well described and illustrated. Many of the points which I made in my discussion of pulmonary lobectomy, left upper lobe, are also applicable here and are therefore not repeated.

The incision for left lower lobectomy may be made a little lower on the chest wall, and it may also be made shorter. Adequate exposure is provided by entering through either the sixth or seventh intercostal space, whereas the fourth intercostal space is preferable for left upper lobectomy. The reason why it is possible to make a shorter incision for left lower lobectomy is that it is not necessary to displace the scapula and shoulder upward for this procedure; nor is it necessary to open the rib spreader to such a great extent because dissection at the apex of the chest and at the superior and anterior aspects of the hilum are not necessary.

Mobilization of the left upper lobe is not necessary in most instances. It is chiefly for this reason that left lower lobectomy, in general, is a more benign procedure than left upper lobectomy. When dissection at the apex of the chest is not necessary, there is often considerably less blood loss and the patients seem to have less postoperative pain. In most instances of left lower lobectomy, the entire dissection is confined to the lower portion of the left hemithorax, and this is probably why this procedure seems less traumatic and stressful. One qualifying statement is advisable, however: in some instances the left upper lobe may have been trapped to some extent because of a previous inflammatory reaction and/or effusion; when this is the case and the total volume of the left upper lobe has been significantly decreased, decortication of the left upper lobe may become necessary. Under such circumstances, the magnitude of the entire operative procedure is increased to a considerable extent.

During the dissection of the segmental branches of the pulmonary artery in the depths of the fissure, it is necessary to retract the left upper and lower lobes in order to obtain adequate exposure, because inflation of these lobes by the anesthetist tends to interfere seriously with the clear visualization necessary for safe dissection. The application of lung clamps to the left upper lobe (B, C, F) has not in my experience been entirely safe. Potential injury to the pulmonary parenchyma, which is quite delicate, is more than a theoretical possibility, and I have observed such an injury with a troublesome air leak. A satisfactory method of obtaining adequate exposure is to use broad bladed malleable retractors, with moist sponges to protect the lobes at the tip of the blades. Sponge sticks, with loosely folded gauze inserted between the

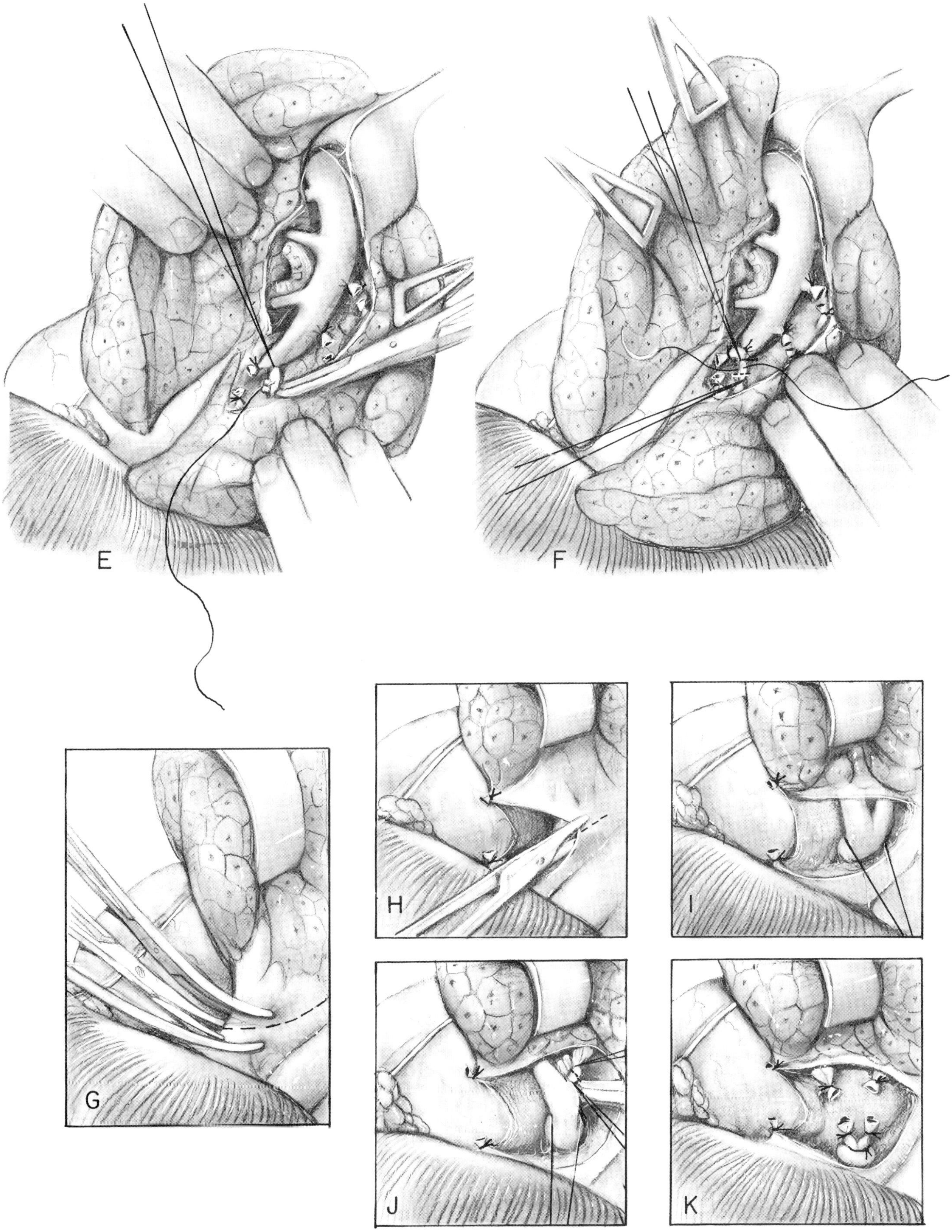
E
F
G
H
I
J
K

L. The ligation and severance of the blood vessels to the lower lobe is completed. The interlobar fissure is again exposed, and the branch bronchus to the superior segment of the lower lobe is clamped (Sarot clamp) distally preliminary to its transection proximally with scissors. Closure of the branch bronchi rather than the main stem bronchus prevents encroachment upon the lumen of the bronchus to the upper lobe.

M. The bronchus is serially severed with scissors and occluded with interrupted sutures of 000 silk swedged on a minimum trauma needle.

N. The lower lobe is removed, and the final suture to complete the closure of the bronchus to its basal segment is inserted.

O. The suture lines of the occluded branch bronchi are covered with free grafts of pleura to lessen the hazard of leakage.

Discussion—Dr. Kirby (cont.)

blades, also are very satisfactory for holding the fissure apart. It has seemed advantageous to have one person, such as the second assistant, hold the fissure open; he can control the inflation of both lobes to the extent desirable without risking injury. If two assistants are retracting the lobes, there is sometimes a tendency toward the application of excessive pressure on one side or the other.

Exposure of the main branch of the pulmonary artery and dissection of the segmental branches to the lower lobe are always somewhat hazardous. If there has been scar tissue formation in the depths of the fissure, the risk is somewhat greater. The key that opens the door to a safe dissection, in my opinion, is to enter the correct plane on the surface of the pulmonary artery. The precise location of this plane can only be learned by experience. In teaching younger men how to enter this plane, I have discovered that there is an understandable tendency to think that it lies somewhat more superficially than is actually the case. In order to find this plane, it is often helpful to pick up the adventitia with a forceps, cut it superficially with dissecting scissors, and then separate the tissues with a curved clamp. The surface of the pulmonary artery appears smooth and glistening when the proper plane has been entered. This plane can be safely followed up the entire length of the pulmonary artery and out on to the segmental branches by blunt dissection. It is essential to stay in this plane when going around the pulmonary artery. Injury posteriorly appears to be a common technical complication for the inexperienced when they are attempting to go around the main basal branch of the pulmonary artery.

It has been stated in some textbooks of anatomy that the pulmonary ligament is avascular. This is usually not the case. As a rule, the pulmonary ligament contains only three or four vessels that need to be clamped, however, so it is not necessary to clamp and ligate the entire ligament. There is nearly always a vessel at the diaphragmatic end of the pulmonary ligament, and it seems advisable to diivde 2 cm. of tissue in this area between clamps so that ligatures may be applied. The remainder of the pulmonary ligament can then be divided with scissors, bleeding points being clamped and ligated as they are encountered.

Whenever possible, the use of a free graft should be avoided in pleuralizing the bronchus (O). It is important to plan an adequate covering for the bronchial stump when beginning the posterior dissection of the hilum. Unless planning is begun at this time, all of the pleura and areolar tissue adjacent to the aorta may be shredded to such an extent that there will not be an adequate covering for the bronchial stump.

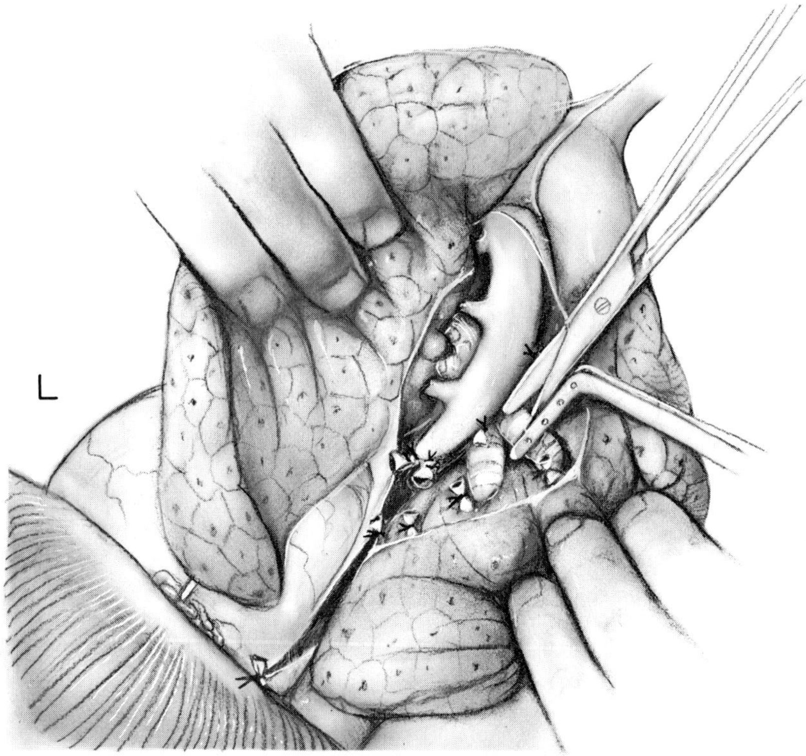

L

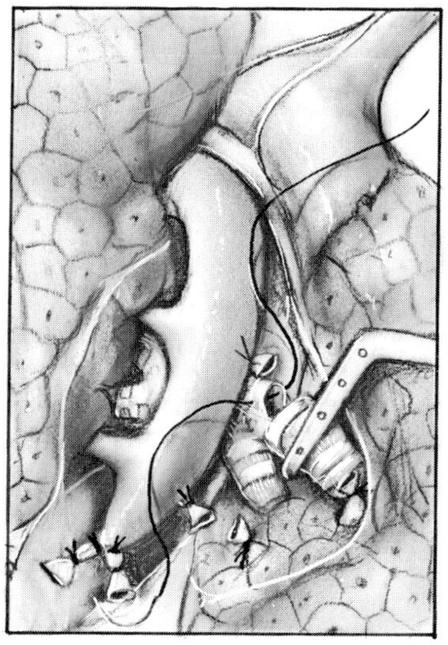

M

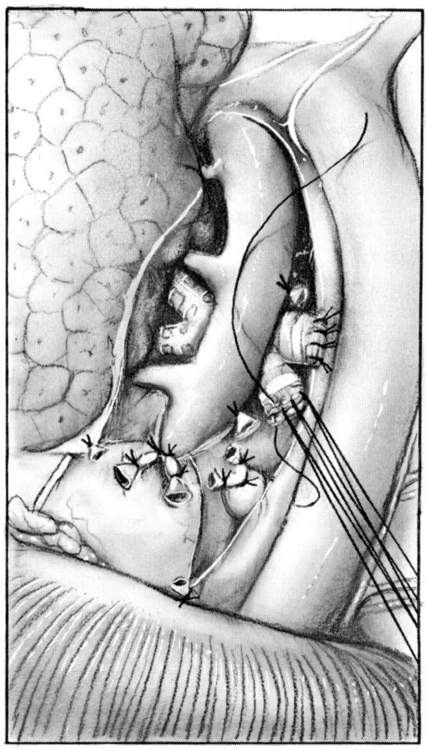

N

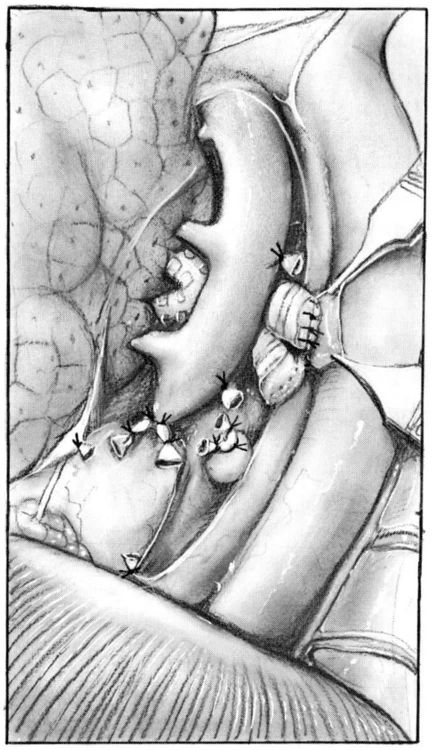

O

TOTAL PNEUMONECTOMY: LEFT

A. The patient is placed in the direct right lateral prone position and the left postero-lateral thoracotomy incision is outlined and cross hatched to facilitate later closure.

B. The left pleural cavity is entered through the fifth intercostal space (Brock technic), and the intrapleural viscera in relation to the surrounding viscera are depicted. The upper lobe of the left lung is manually retracted posteriorly, and the mediastinal pleura overlying the pulmonary hilum is severed (broken line) by scissor dissection.

C. The severance of the mediastinal pleura is completed to expose the left pulmonary artery and the left superior pulmonary vein. The apical posterior branch of the pulmonary artery is mobilized and elevated on a clamp preparatory to being encircled by a ligature of 000 silk.

D. The apical-posterior artery, doubly ligated (000 silk) in continuity, is being severed (scissors) between the ligatures.

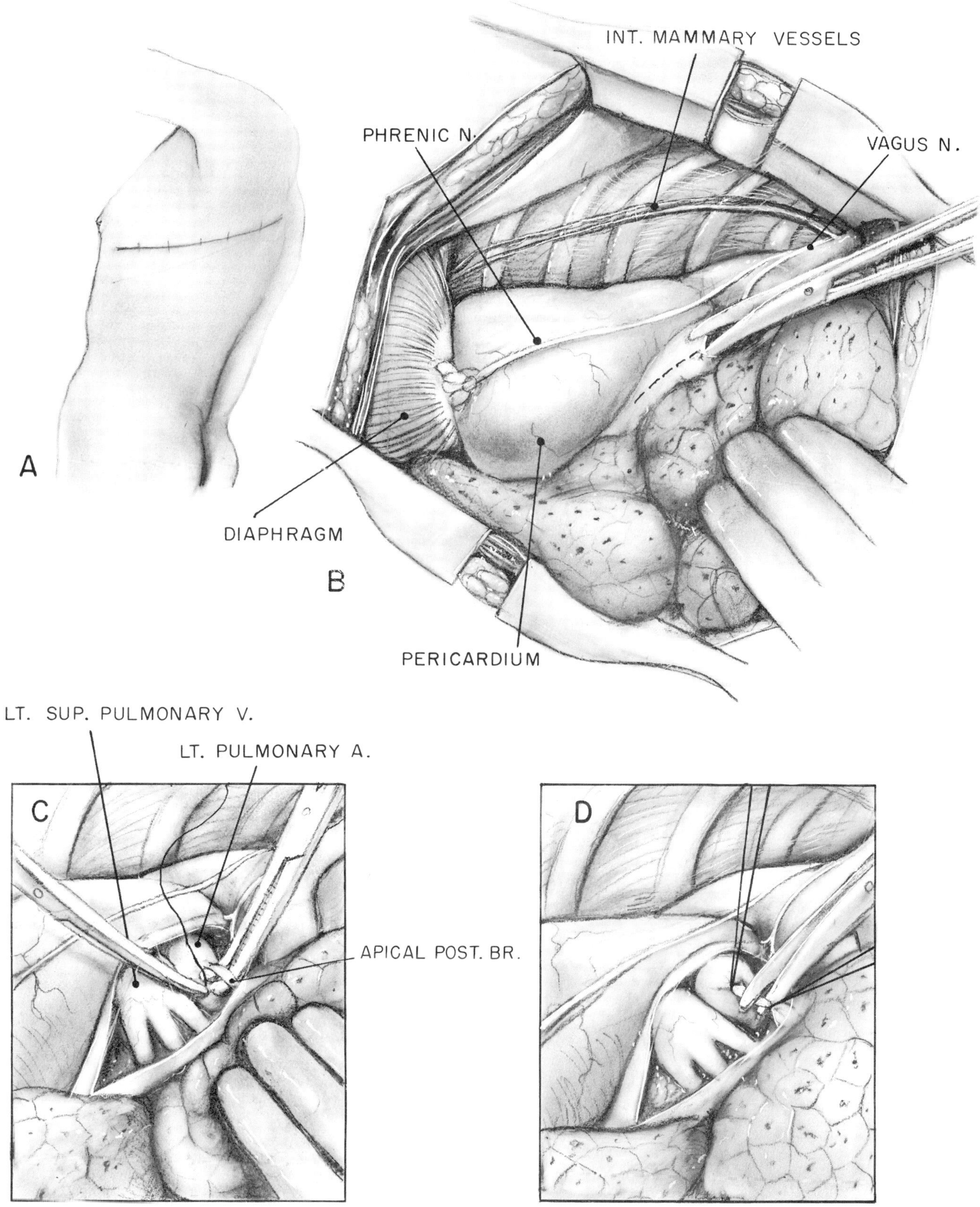
A
INT. MAMMARY VESSELS
PHRENIC N.
VAGUS N.
DIAPHRAGM
B
PERICARDIUM
LT. SUP. PULMONARY V.
LT. PULMONARY A.
C
APICAL POST. BR.
D

E, F, G. Pulmonary artery is being mobilized by combined digital and clamp dissection (E) and, finally, by digital dissection alone (F) before being encircled (G) by a ligature of 0 silk. The use of blunt digital dissection, particularly in the plane posteriorly, is a useful, safe, and efficient method for mobilizing the large vascular trunks in the pulmonary hilum.

H. The pulmonary artery is doubly ligated (0 silk) in continuity, and a transfixion suture (00 silk) is being inserted between the ligatures but closer to the proximal ligature.

I. The pulmonary artery is transected with scissors between the two proximal and single distal ligatures.

Discussion—Dr. Alton Ochsner. Whereas the anterior approach in the fourth interspace can often be used for pneumonectomy, the posterolateral incision is certainly preferable. I prefer an incision that extends farther anteriorly than illustrated in A, as it gives a little better exposure generally. The incision of the mediastinal pleura should be made in such a way as not to interfere with the phrenic nerve, which is easily identified (B). Generally, I think it is desirable to extend the incision up to the apex of the pleural cavity and begin the dissection above in order to remove any lymph nodes in the superior mediastinum, because on the left side a large involved node is often found about the arch of the aorta. It is important to examine this area early during the dissection in order to determine whether the lesion is resectable; even though involvement may be limited to the node, it can extend to the aorta, and if the aorta is actually involved, resection is not justified.

Although branches of the pulmonary artery can be individually ligated (C, D), it is generally my choice to isolate the pulmonary artery and ligate it as a common trunk. In every instance, however, I use transfixion in addition to ligation, which is particularly necessary in large vessels, such as the common trunk of the pulmonary artery.

Digital dissection is by far the most important and certainly the safest method. After complete isolation of the pulmonary artery from the superior pulmonary vein and the bronchus (G), a curved instrument is placed under the pulmonary artery, and the ligature is drawn around it. It is imperative to ligate on the cardiac side and on the pulmonary side with as much room between the ligatures as is possible. This is facilitated if the surgeon places his index finger behind the artery, "walks" the cardiac ligature into the mediastinum, and holds it in this position while the assistant ties the ligature. Transfixion both on the cardiac and pulmonary sides is important in addition to ligation. In fact, it is my custom to place two sutures proximally in such a way as to include four quadrants of the circumference of the vessel.

Generally, before ligating the superior pulmonary vein, it is desirable to mobilize the lower lobe of the lung by incising the inferior pulmonary ligament (M). This may facilitate isolation of the superior pulmonary vein. Again, the digital dissection is of importance here, as in the pulmonary artery, and ligation of the main trunk using the transfixion suture (K, L). Branches of the superior pulmonary vein can be ligated and transfixed separately, or, if there is sufficient room, ligation might be done as a trunk distally.

The inferior pulmonary vein is exposed by retracting the lower lobe anteriorly, and, again using digital dissection, the vein is completely isolated, after which ligation and transfixion ligation are done.

The bronchus is carefully dissected out, and all the nodes around the bronchi are removed together with the resected specimen. It is important that the bronchus be freed as far medially as possible up to the bifurcation because of the possibility of spread proximally. One can either utilize one bronchial clamp (P), or two, one placed proximally and the other distally. If the proximal clamp is used, it should not be applied tightly enough to crush the bronchus, however. The sutures introduced in the end of the bronchus (Q) should be tied only tightly enough to approximate the edges of the bronchus and not so tightly as to cut through the bronchus.

After removal of the lung and completion of the bronchial suture, it should be determined whether the suture is airtight. This is done by filling the thoracic cavity with saline solution and having the anesthetist increase the intrabronchial tension. If there is any leakage, bubbles will appear. Covering the bronchus with a flap of pleura is imperative in order to facilitate healing and prevent subsequent blowout of the bronchus. It is my policy, after completion of this phase of the procedure, to close the wound, leaving a catheter at the anterior end of the wound. The catheter is left in place until the wound has been completely closed and the patient placed back in a supine position. The anesthetist then inflates the opposite lung, which brings the mediastinum back into the midline position, during which time the catheter is kept open to permit egress of the trapped air. While the sound lung is maintained in the standard position, the catheter is withdrawn and the area sealed with vaseline gauze.

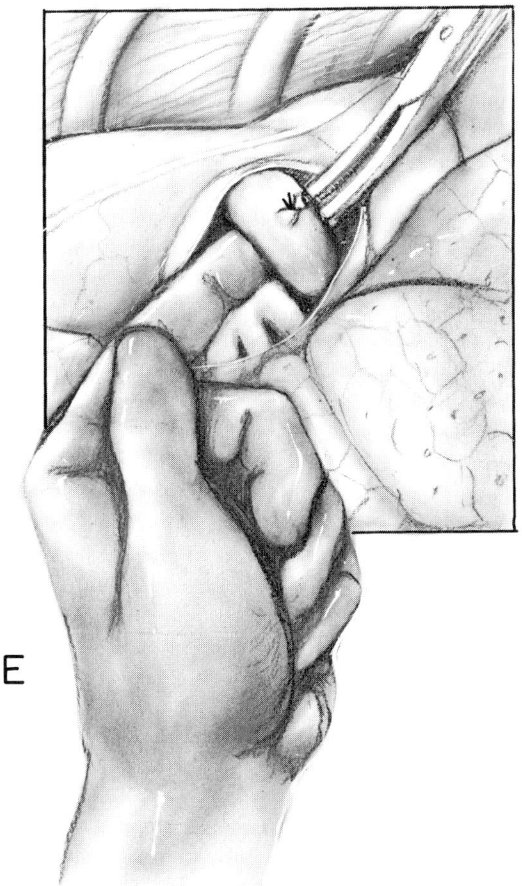

E

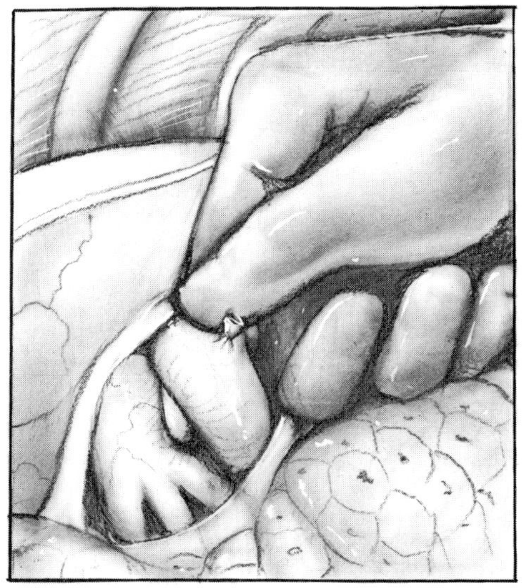

F

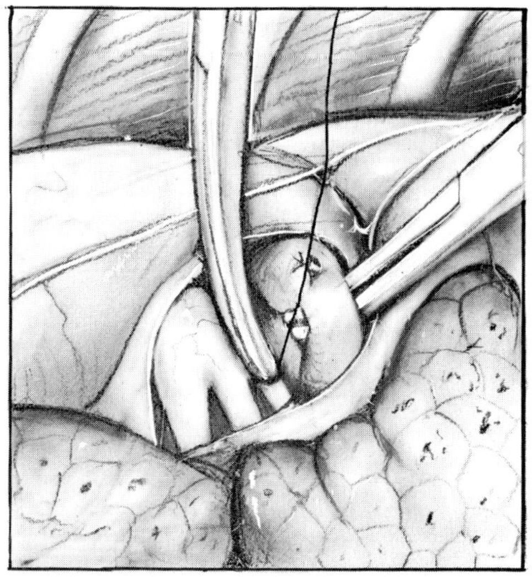

G

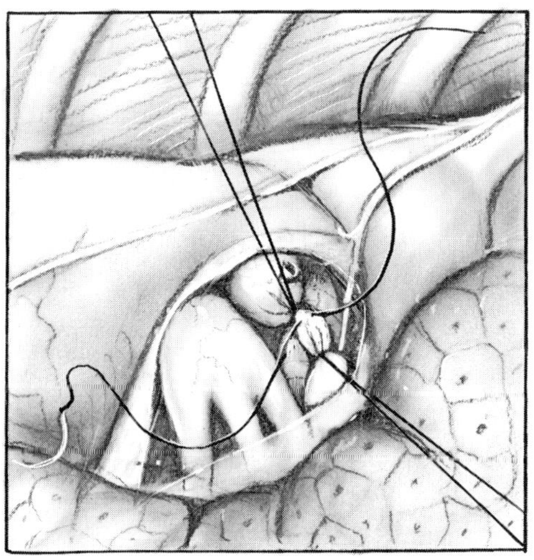

H

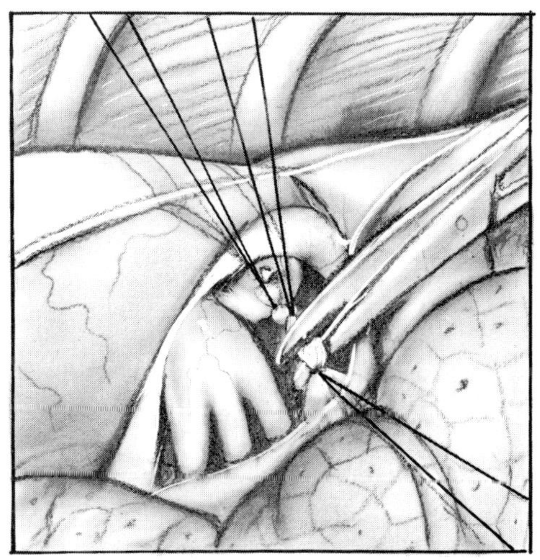

I

J, K. The superior pulmonary vein is mobilized posteriorly by blunt digital dissection (J) and then partially encircled by a clamp (K) for the withdrawal beneath it of a ligature of 0 silk.

L. The ligature (0 silk) about the superior pulmonary vein is tied, and its tributary veins are doubly ligated (000 silk) in continuity and severed (broken line) between the ligatures.

M, N. The lung is retracted medially and cephalad to make taut the inferior pulmonary ligament, which is doubly clamped and severed (M) to enter the posterior mediastinal space. The opening in this space is extended cephalad (N) to obtain exposure of the inferior pulmonary vein that forms the upper boundary of the inferior pulmonary ligament.

O. The inferior pulmonary vein is isolated, and its main trunk is occluded with a ligature of 00 silk. The tributary veins, superior (being severed with scissors) and basal, are doubly ligated (000 silk) in continuity and transected (scissors) between the ligatures.

Discussion—Sir Russell Brock. After identification of the vagus and dissection and clamping of the bronchus, the pleural incision is carried upward to the apex anterior to the vagus, the phrenic nerve and vessels are secured as on the right side, and the incision is then continued down in front of the phrenic nerve as far as the lower limit of the hilum, where the nerve and vessels are ligated and divided.

The pericardium is now opened and the veins dealt with as described for the right side, a common pulmonary venous trunk being easily displayed.

Once again it is preferable not to open the hilar areolar tissue to secure the upper lobe arteries as a preliminary to encircling the main left pulmonary artery. This is done more efficiently as far medially as possible. Indeed, this technic may make it possible to remove a cancerous lung that otherwise could not be resected.

The incision in the pericardium is carried high up into the concavity of the aortic arch, in front of the origin of the left pulmonary artery, so as to expose the ligamentum arteriosum. At this time it may be an advantage to clear the contents of the subaortic fossa, carefully identifying, freeing, and conserving the left recurrent laryngeal nerve. Occasionally heavy lymph node involvement may compel division of the nerve as well as the main vagus. Some surgeons prefer to free and to divide the ligamentum arteriosum in order to make a more radical clearance of the subaortic fossa. Usually an adequate clearance can be obtained without dividing the ligament, which is usefully preserved so that the most proximal ligature on the artery can be placed *medial* to it. There is little difficulty in defining the ligament by working from in front, from above and from behind. It will then be found that the left pulmonary artery is almost completely free, and a little more dissection enables it to be encircled and a transfixion ligature applied and the artery divided lateral to this.

It is always safer to apply *two* ligatures, one of which transfixes the vessel on the central end of the artery and of the veins.

The further steps of incision of the pericardium and clearance of the ligamentum latum and of the inferior tracheobronchial fossa are as described for the right side. The bronchus stump is similarly treated.

My own preference after pneumonectomy is to insert a drainage tube but *not* to leave it open all the time. If it is left, open air is expelled on coughing or straining and overdistention of the remaining lung occurs.

The tube should be clamped except for a few seconds every hour or so, when it is released to permit adjustment of pressure if there has been an increase from blood or serous collection. In other words, the drainage tube is used virtually as a manometer and safety-valve adjustment. It should be removed 18 to 24 hours after operation.

It is necessary to emphasize that, although the technic of dealing with the vessels may be thought to be too bold and too radical, it is in fact a simpler and safer method than dissecting within the hilum itself, especially when, as is often the case, this region is distorted and rendered rigid by adjacent growth. By working as near the origin of the vessels as possible, the tissues are less likely to be abnormal and are more easily dissected, and a much more radical clearance of diseased tissue is achieved.

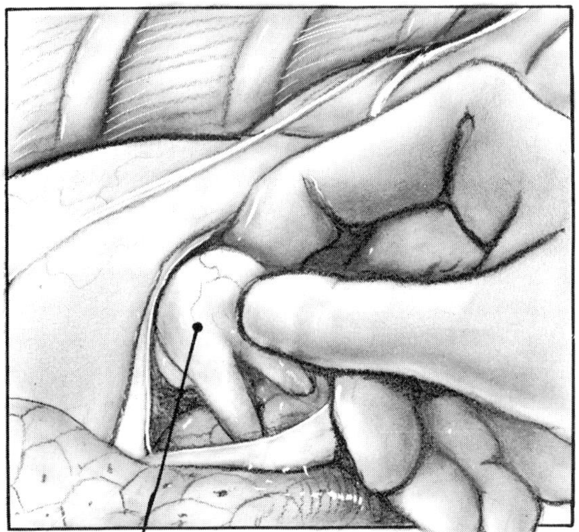
SUP. PULMONARY VEIN

J

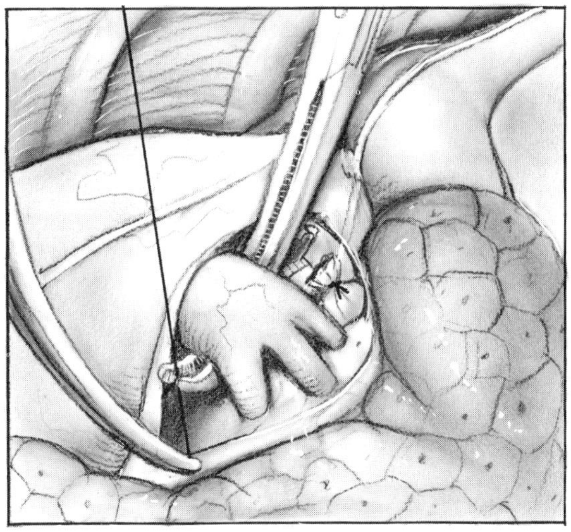

K

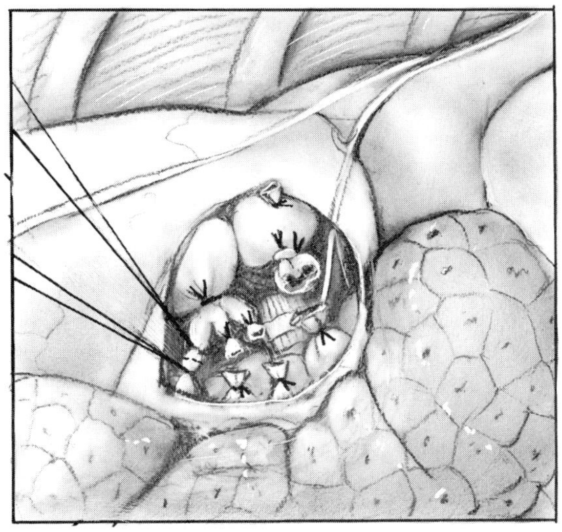

L

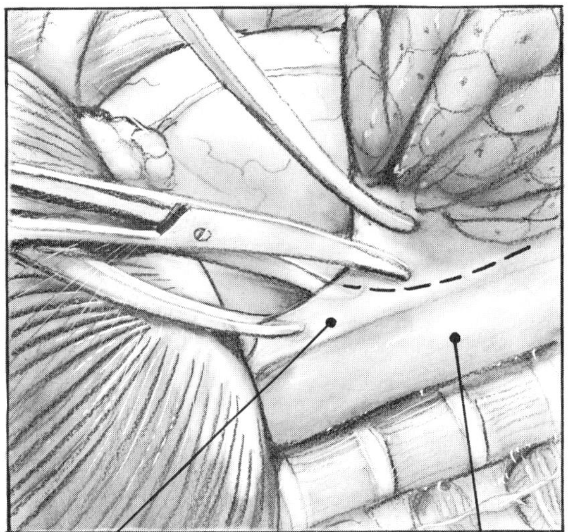
INF. PULMONARY LIG.
AORTA

M

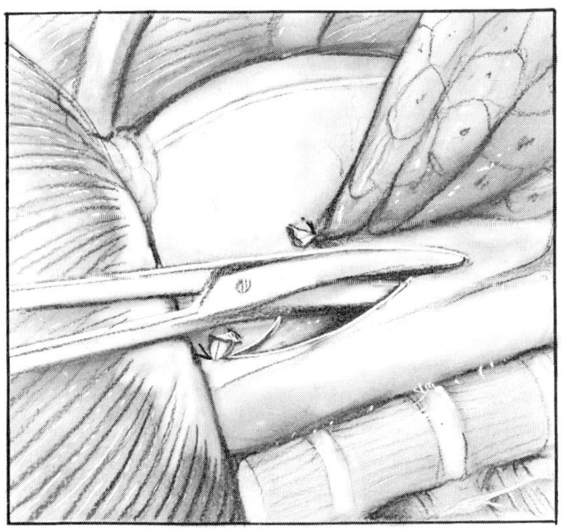

N

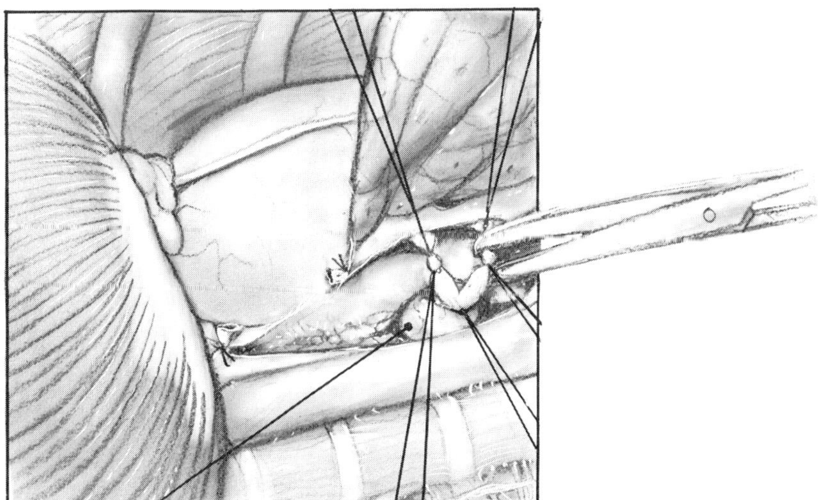
INF. PULMONARY VEIN

O

P, Q. The left lung, now attached by its bronchus only, is displaced posteriorly, and the main bronchus is occluded by a clamp (P). Proximal to the clamp, the bronchus is being severed and its open end serially occluded with interrupted sutures of 000 silk (P, Q) swedged on a minimum trauma needle.

R. The closure of the bronchus is completed, and traction is maintained on the angle sutures as a free graft of pleura is being applied over the suture line. The closure of the wound completes the operation. Water seal drainage of the pleural cavity is not employed. However, on completion of the wound closure, a negative pressure in the pleural cavity is established by aspiration with a syringe of the necessary quantity of air. This is indicated when the glass plunger is slowly drawn into the barrel of the syringe on inspiration.

DISCUSSION—DR. WILLIAM F. RIENHOFF, JR. In reference to left total pneumonectomy, the anterolateral incision is again preferred, and the same suggestions hold for the left side as for the right. Other than the exceptions stated, I greatly approve of the technic as illustrated.

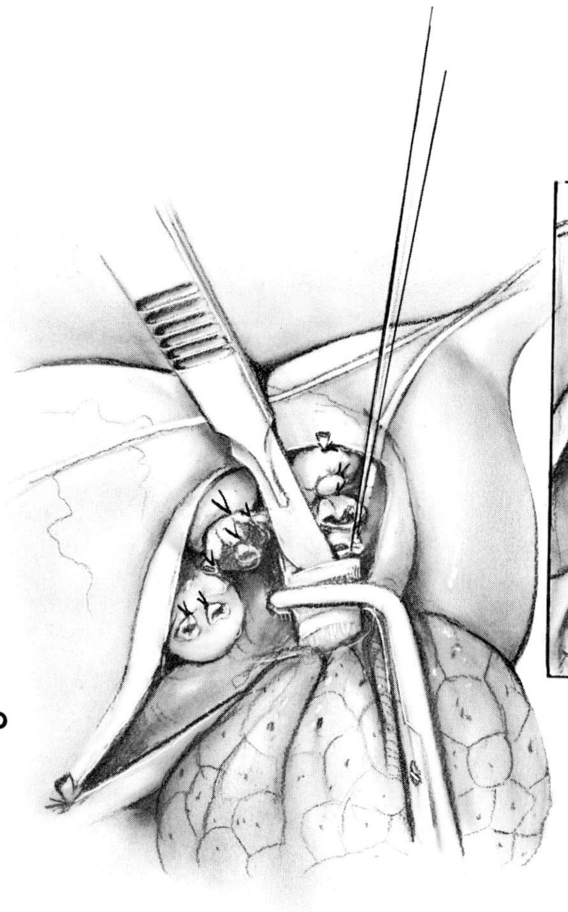

P

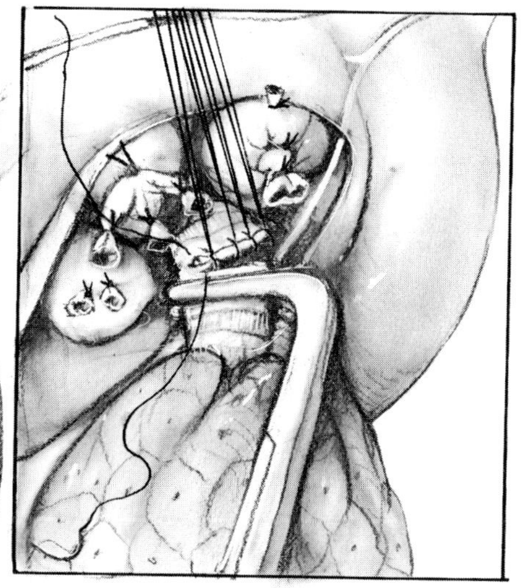

Q

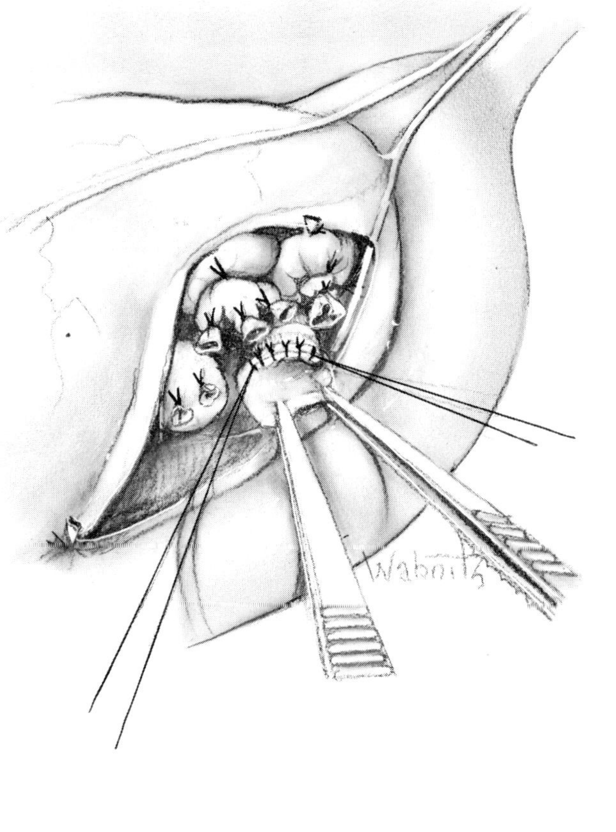

R

THYMECTOMY

The patient, a nine-year-old girl, had symptoms of myasthenia gravis of eight months' duration that were becoming progressively worse in severity. Because of the sex and age of the patient and the short duration and progressive character of the symptoms, thymectomy was advised. Prior to admission to the hospital, the patient was taking two tablets (120 mg.) of Mestinon (pyridostigmine bromide) three times daily. Two days subsequent to admission, Prostigmin (neostigmine bromide) one tablet (15 mg.) three times a day was substituted. The symptoms of dysphagia, dysarthria, and difficulty in breathing rapidly worsened. The Prostigmin (neostigmine methylsulfate) was then administered intramuscularly in the dose of 0.5 mg. every four hours; within 24 hours the dose was increased to 1.5 mg. every two hours. The difficulty in respiration persisted, and the use of an Emerson cuirass type of respirator was necessary. Accordingly, immediate thymectomy was done.

Admittedly, the performance of a thymectomy as an emergency operation may be questioned. However, the rapid deterioration in the general condition of the patient despite adequate medical treatment seemed to justify the surgical risk.

On the first postoperative day a tracheostomy was required because of the excessive bronchial secretions. It was originally planned to do a tracheostomy immediately upon completion of the thymectomy. However, the general condition of the patient appeared satisfactory, and it was not done. This proved an error in judgment. Whenever a thymectomy is performed for myasthenia gravis, in particular when respiratory difficulty is manifest, tracheostomy is believed mandatory.

On the second day after operation the patient was placed in a Drinker respirator and maintained therein for 12 days. Gavage feedings for 14 days were required. Prostigmin (neostigmine bromide) was administered in 1.5 mg. doses intramuscularly; first every two hours, then every three hours, for 12 days. It was then given by mouth, the dosage being two tablets (30 mg.) every two hours. Because of the excessive bronchial secretions, the medication was changed to Mytelase (abenonium chloride), and two tablets (20 mg.) every three hours were prescribed. The patient, now 18 months postoperatively, is very satisfactorily maintained on the oral ingestion of two tablets (20 mg.) of Mytelase (ambenonium chloride) four times a day.

A. The patient is placed in the supine position, and the midline sternal splitting incision (Duval-Barasty) is outlined. An alternate method for exposure of the thymus would be the use of a separate transverse "collar" incision and transection of the sternum in the fourth interspace, the level at which the midline sternal splitting incision would terminate.

B. The incision is deepened through the thin subcutaneous fatty tissue layer, and both the fascia and periosteum overlying the sternum are being incised.

C. The Stryker electric saw is used to split the sternum as sterile saline is being dripped to "lubricate" the cutting edge of the instrument.

D. Using a Lebsche knife, the initial split in the sternum is completed.

E. The cut margins of the sternum are separated with a self-retaining retractor (Finochietto), and the dissection of the mediastinal fat pad, which should not be mistaken for the thymus gland, is begun. An opening was inadvertently made in the right pleural cavity as depicted. Entrance into one or even both pleural cavities is not uncommon with this type of incision, which theoretically should preclude its occurrence.

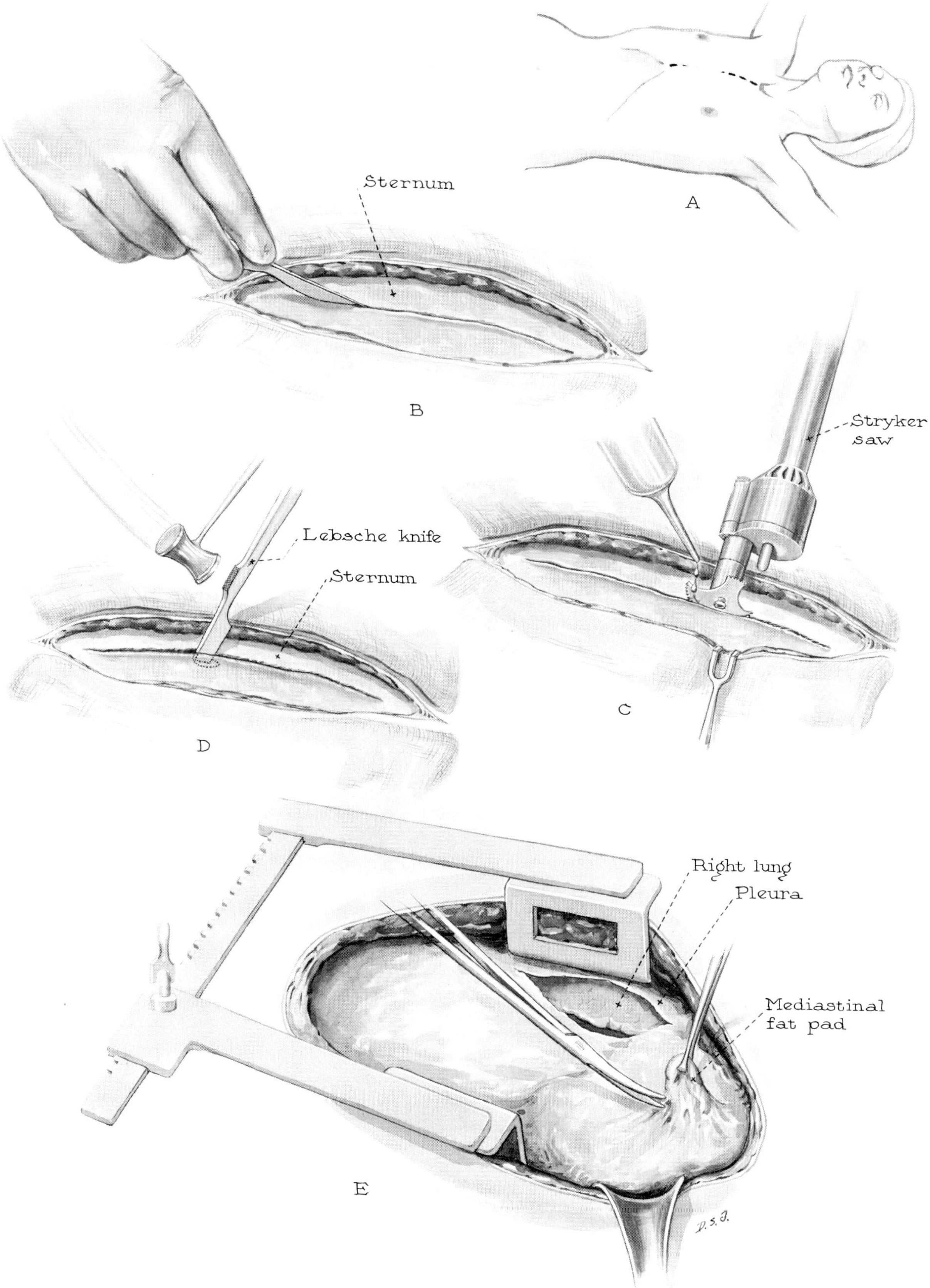
A
Sternum
B
Stryker saw
Lebsche knife
Sternum
C
D
Right lung
Pleura
Mediastinal fat pad
E
D.S.J.

F. The dissection of the fat pad is completed. The right lobe of the gland is grasped in a Potts type of Babcock clamp * and, as upward traction is maintained, it is mobilized from the adjacent tissues by scissor dissection.

G, H. A second "vascular" clamp is applied to the partially mobilized gland, and its dissection is completed.

I. The left lobe is similarly grasped in a "vascular" clamp, and its dissection is begun.

J. Traction is maintained cephalad on both lobes of the thymus gland, which are dissected from the underlying anterior surface of the pericardium. The pericardium is easily recognized by its bluish sheen and vascular pattern.

* Manufactured by Edward Weck & Co., Long Island City, N.Y.

Discussion—Dr. Merle M. Musselman. Thymectomy may be accomplished with facility, as illustrated so well by Dr. Madden. The operation itself poses little threat to the life of a patient. Patients die after the operation from pulmonary complications resulting directly or indirectly from the myasthenia. As suggested by Dr. Madden, operation should be planned when possible as an elective procedure during a remission. With proper preparation, technic of anesthesia, technic of operation, and postoperative care, the operation should carry little risk. A crisis either before or after operation is a grave complication in a patient with myasthenia gravis. Because of the weakness of the respiratory muscles, including the diaphragm, the patient cannot ventilate adequately and cannot clear secretions from the trachea and bronchi. Accordingly, atelectasis, pneumonitis, and asphyxia are associated complications.

It must be emphasized that a crisis may result from progress of the disease (*myasthenic crisis*) or from overtreatment with anticholinesterase drugs (*cholinergic crisis*). It is most important that a distinction be made between the two, which may be differentiated by the history and examination of the patient. However, both the symptoms and the physical findings are so similar that a correct diagnosis is difficult to make.

Fortunately, one can usually differentiate cholinergic from myasthenic crisis by the Tensilon * Test. One hour after the last dose of cholinergic drug, 0.2 mg. of Tensilon is given intravenously. If the patient has been overtreated, weakness will increase, muscle fasciculation will appear, and parasympathetic side reactions will occur. If the patient is undertreated, muscle strength will increase without fasciculation.

In the treatment of a crisis of either type, early tracheostomy as an elective procedure should be done as soon as the patient shows the first signs of respiratory difficulty. One should initiate positive pressure ventilation, using a cuffed tracheostomy

* Tensilon is the trade name of Roche Laboratories for edrophonium chloride.

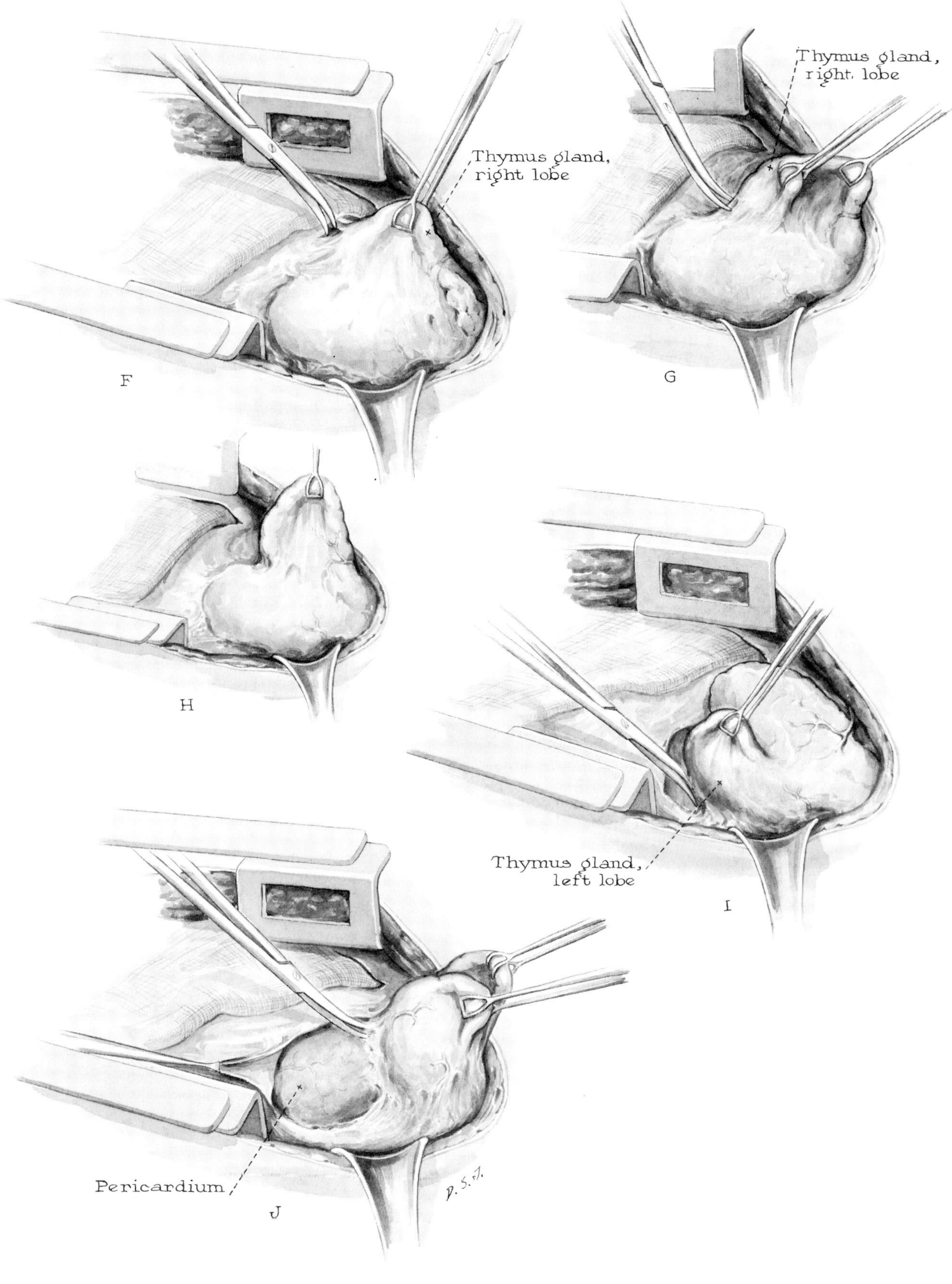
Thymus gland,
right lobe
F
Thymus gland,
right lobe
G
H
Thymus gland,
left lobe
I
Pericardium
J
D.S.J.

K. When the dissection posteriorly is completed, the lobes of the thymus are reposited to their normal position, and the artery to the right lobe is first doubly ligated in continuity (000 silk) and then severed between the ligatures.

L. The artery to the mid-portion and body of the thymus has been similarly ligated and severed, and the artery to the left lobe is being transected between ligatures of 000 silk. The arteries to the thymus gland are branches of the superior and inferior thyroid arteries and the internal mammary artery.

M. The mobilized gland is again retracted cephalad to expose its venous drainage, which in this patient was a solitary tributary vein of the left innominate vein.

N, O. The thymus vein is doubly ligated (000 silk) in continuity and severed between the ligatures.

Discussion—Dr. Musselman (cont.)

tube. If myasthenic crisis cannot be controlled by the use of Prostigmin Methylsulfate * intramuscularly or Mestinon Bromide † intravenously, it should be treated as a cholinergic crisis. In patients who have a cholinergic crisis, all medication should be stopped. After 72 hours the ventilatory assistance should be discontinued and the patient observed for his ability to get along without medication. If necessary, treatment with cholinergic drugs should be started again in low to moderate dosages, monitoring the results by the clinical response and by the Tensilon Test. The cholinergic drug should be given parenterally when necessary, but orally otherwise.

If thymectomy is to be done, on the morning of operation, the patient is given a cholinergic drug parenterally in a single dose that is calculated to maintain spontaneous respirations until the time of induction of anesthesia. Narcotics and barbiturates should be used, if at all, in small doses. Although belladonna-like drugs have the desirable effect of reducing the excess bronchial secretion produced by the cholinergic drugs, they should not be used, because they have the undesirable effect of thickening the bronchial secretions.

Cyclopropane has proved to be a good anesthetic, as it is easily administered, causes little irritation, and has little curare effect. Muscle relaxation is not necessary for thymectomy, and muscle-relaxing drugs of either the curare or succinyl choline types should not be used. In fact, their use is contraindicated.

In the postoperative care most patients do not require cholinergic medicine for 24 hours after operation because of the remission of symptoms. As the symptoms reappear, the parenteral use of cholinergic drugs is again started. One should undertreat the patient, giving only enough medicine to maintain respiration. Dosage should be checked repeatedly by the Tensilon Test. Myasthenic crises and cholinergic crises in association with inadequate ventilation, atelectasis, pneumonitis, and asphyxia are the greatest dangers after operation. They should be treated as previously described.

* Prostigmin Methylsulfate is the trade name of Roche Laboratories for neostigmine methylsulfate.

† Mestinon Bromide is the trade name of Roche Laboratories for pyridostigmine bromide.

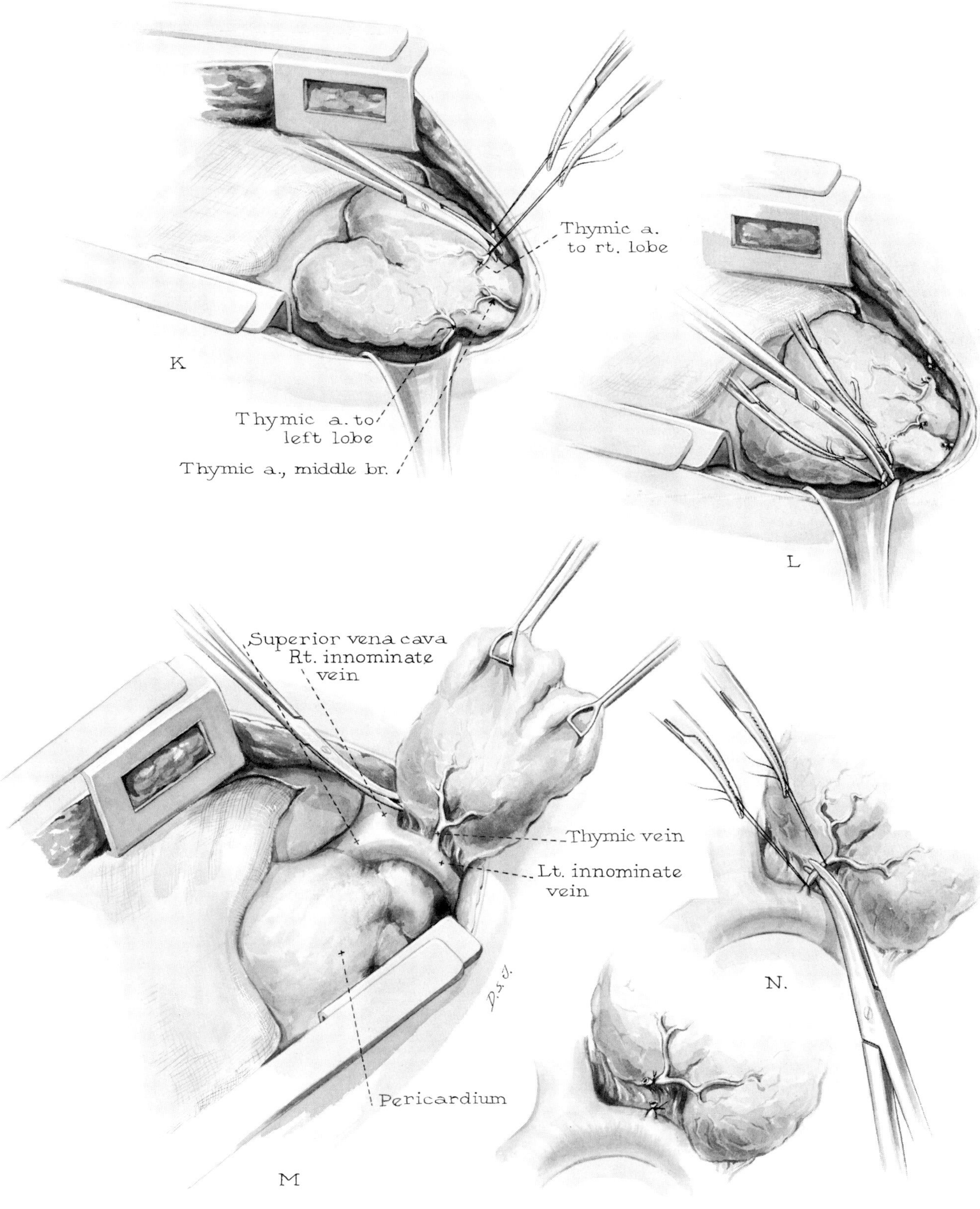
Thymic a.
to rt. lobe
K
Thymic a. to
left lobe
Thymic a., middle br.
L
Superior vena cava
Rt. innominate
vein
Thymic vein
Lt. innominate
vein
Pericardium
M
N.
O

P. Downward traction is made on the right lobe as the attachments (avascular) of its superior pole are being freed by scissor dissection. The thymus gland and also the parathyroid glands originate embryologically from the third branchial pouch. During fetal development the thymus descends downward behind the thyroid gland and terminates in the superior mediastinum. This explains the attachments of the superior poles of the gland, which extend cephalad on either side of the trachea to the level of the thyroid gland. The common site of origin of the thymus and parathyroid glands also explains the presence of parathyroid glandular tissue with the thymus in the superior mediastinum, which occurs in approximately 10 per cent of the patients.

Q. Similarly, the superior pole of the left lobe is mobilized and the gland is removed. Total removal of the gland is believed most important, both in the treatment of myasthenia gravis and thymomas.

R. Inset to show the resected gland, which weighed 25 g. This is in the range of the normal weight at puberty of 25-35 g. On histopathologic examination of the thymus, lymphoid hyperplasia, lymph follicle, and germinal center formations, the characteristic findings in myasthenia gravis were present.

S. The sternal incision is closed using peristernal sutures (double strands) of No. 2 chromic catgut. The age of the patient (nine years) and the corresponding pliability of the chest cage permitted approximation of the cut margins of the sternum without difficulty.

S′. An alternate method for the closure of the sternal incision using interrupted stainless steel wire (gauge 26) sutures.

T. The closure of the operative incision is completed. The pleural cavities, having been entered, are drained by water seal catheters. A subcutaneous rubber tissue drain has its exit in the cephalad angle of the incision.

Discussion—Dr. O. Theron Clagett. The development of myasthenia gravis in a nine-year-old child is relatively uncommon. However, this disease can occur at any age, even in newborn infants. While sudden worsening of the symptoms of myasthenia gravis can occur, one might suspect in this case that the sudden worsening might be related to the change in therapy from Mestinon to Prostigmine.

The wisdom of performing emergency thymectomy under the circumstances can be questioned. Patients with very severe myasthenia gravis can be carried along satisfactorily with assisted or controlled respiration for long periods of time, if necessary, and the operation can then be performed under more favorable circumstances, with the disease in remission or at least under better control. The effect of thymectomy on myasthenia gravis is so unpredictable and the time after operation when improvement appears varies so much that it would seem unlikely that thymectomy should be considered an emergency or life-saving procedure.

It would have seemed logical to perform tracheostomy at the time of thymectomy rather than on the following day. Tracheostomy is indicated in all instances of severe myasthenia gravis.

Postoperative management with controlled respiration, aspiration of tracheal secretions, and gavage feedings is highly appropriate. In patients with prolonged difficulty in swallowing, a small feeding gastrostomy has some advantages over the use of an indwelling nasogastric tube over many days.

Since this child requires approximately the same amount of Mestinon eighteen months after operation as before thymectomy, it does not appear that thymectomy has been effective in this patient. In my experience with this procedure, benefit has become apparent within six months of operation in the group that have been improved.

The technic of operation described is very appropriate and satisfactory. It must be appreciated that, regardless of the thoroughness of the surgical attempt to remove the entire thymus, some thymic tissue may be left behind. Thymic tumors occasionally develop out along the major bronchi or even in the lung parenchyma, so it seems inevitable that thymic tissue in ectopic sites may be left behind. Whether this may influence the effectiveness of thymectomy upon the course of myasthenia gravis is not known.

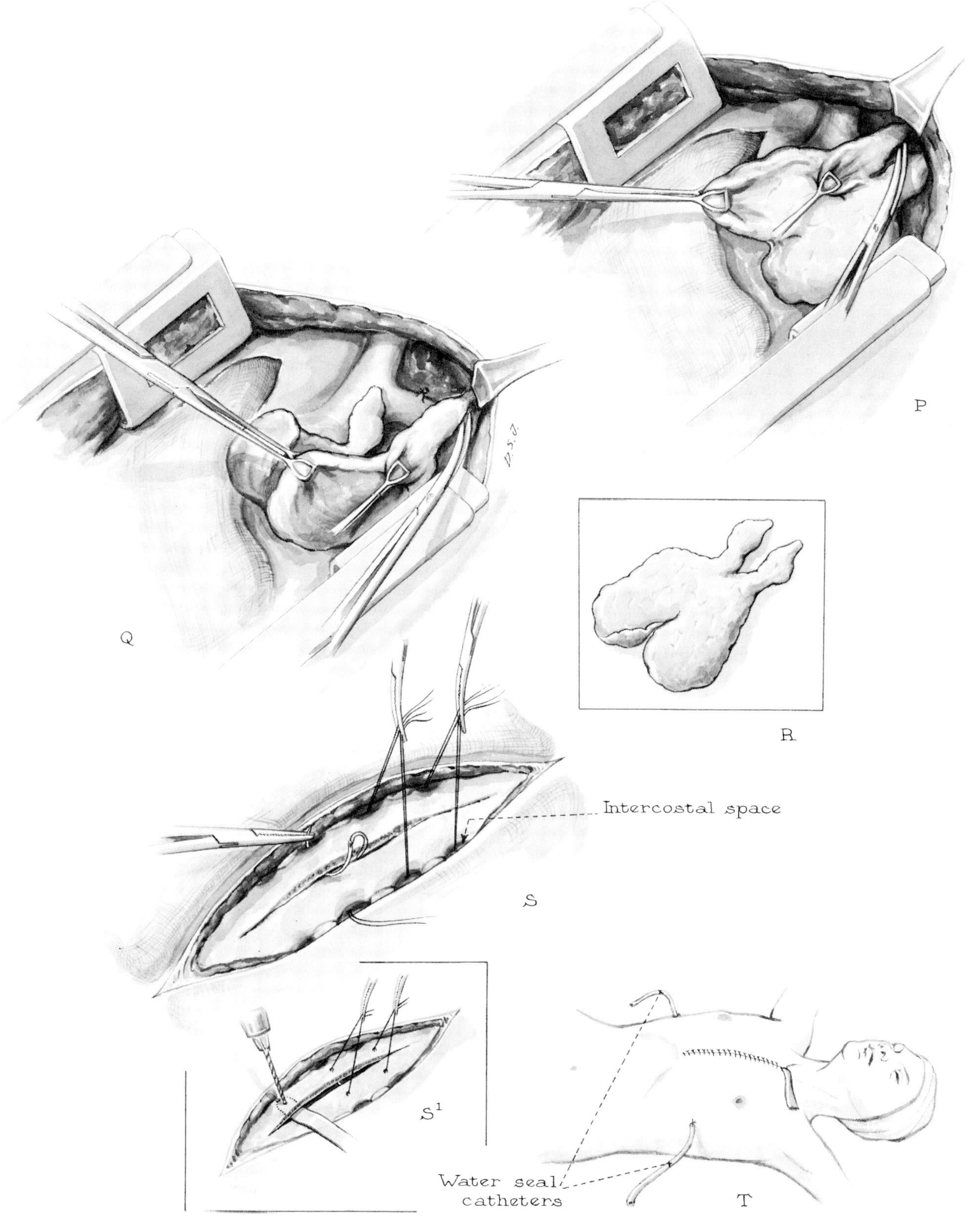
P
Q
R
Intercostal space
S
S1
Water seal
catheters
T

CONGENITAL ATRESIA OF THE ESOPHAGUS WITH TRACHEOESOPHAGEAL FISTULA

A. The patient is placed in the direct left lateral prone position, and the right thoracotomy incision is indicated by the solid line. A transpleural rather than an extrapleural approach is preferred.

B. The right pleural cavity is entered, and the azygos vein is severed between ligatures of silk (000). The site of the tracheoesophageal fistula and the adherence of the narrow proximal end of the lower portion of the esophagus to the widened cul-de-sac formed by the distal end of the proximal portion of the esophagus are shown.

B^{I}. Similar view as in B in a patient in whom the distance between the esophageal segment is greater. To bridge this distance the upper rather than the lower segment is extensively mobilized because otherwise there would be danger of compromise of the circulation to the lower segment.

C. The proximal end of the lower portion of the esophagus is severed in an oblique plane from its communication with the trachea, and the opening into the tracheal lumen is closed with interrupted sutures of silk (0000) which are swedged on minimum trauma needles. To obtain an adequate sized diameter of the lumen of the lower segment, a resection of a narrow portion of its proximal end, although not shown, is usually required.

D. The closure of the opening in the trachea is completed and traction guy sutures of silk (000) are inserted in the walls of the proximal and distal segments of the esophagus preliminary to the performance of the end-to-end anastomosis. The site of the incision to be made into the lumen of the proximal segment is indicated by the dotted line.

E, E^{I}, E^{II}, E^{III}. These close-up views depict the details of the end-to-end anastomosis of the esophagus. The first posterior layer consists of a series of interrupted mattress sutures which are all first inserted before being tied (E). These sutures produce an inversion of all of the layers of the esophagus into its lumen. The mattress sutures are tied, and interrupted sutures of silk (000) which include all the layers of the esophagus are inserted and tied. These sutures form the second posterior layer of the anastomosis (E^{I}) and are continued anteriorly as the first anterior layer. Although not shown in the illustrations, before inserting the first anterior layer of sutures, an intraluminal catheter (No. 8F) is inserted to facilitate the completion of the anastomosis anteriorly. When this is done, the catheter is removed. The sutures forming the first anterior layer are inserted from the "inside out" to the "outside in" so that when tied the knots are on the inside of the lumen (E^{I}). Each suture is inserted alternately from either end toward the center to avoid an angle closure of the anastomosis. When the last two sutures are tied in the midline anteriorly, they are encircled by a reinforcing figure of 8 mattress suture of silk (000) before being cut (E^{II}). The mattress suture is tied and the long ends are cut to complete the first layer of the anastomosis. For the second anterior layer interrupted horizontal mattress sutures of silk (000) are used (E^{III}). These sutures are inserted at right angles to the longitudinal layer of muscle fibers of the esophagus to obtain maximum holding power.

F, F^{I}, F^{II}, F^{III}, F^{IV}. This series of close-up views illustrates the "telescoping" technic described by Haight in the performance of an end-to-end anastomosis of the esophagus. Interrupted sutures of silk (000) are used for the first posterior layer. These sutures are all first inserted before being tied and include the mucosa layer only of the dilated proximal end of the esophagus and all of the layers of the narrow distal end of the esophagus (F). A catheter (No. 8F) is passed from the lumen of the upper segment of the esophagus into the lumen of the lower segment and a similar series of sutures is inserted anteriorly (F^{I}) to complete the first anterior layer of the anastomosis (F^{II}). The second layer of the anastomosis, both anteriorly and posteriorly, consists of a series of interrupted sutures which are inserted through the muscular layer only of the upper segment of the esophagus and through the whole thickness of the wall of the lower esophageal segment caudad to the level of the first layer of sutures (F^{II}, F^{III}). When tied, these sutures produce a "telescoping" of the narrow distal end of the esophagus into the wide proximal end which is best illustrated by a sagittal view of the completed anastomosis (F^{IV}).

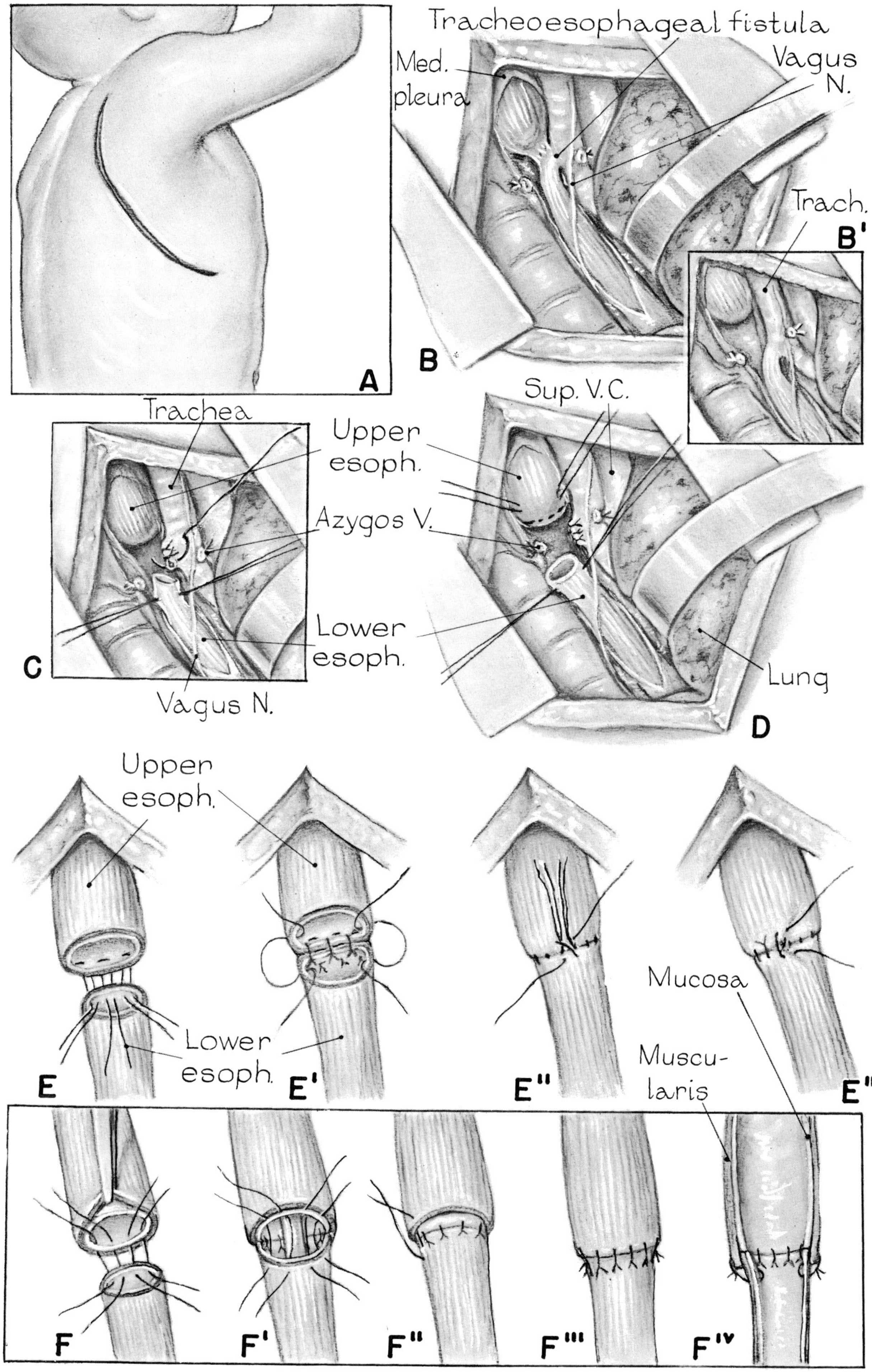
A
Tracheoesophageal fistula
Med. pleura
Vagus N.
Trach.
B'
B
Trachea
Upper esoph.
Azygos V.
Lower esoph.
Vagus N.
C
Sup. V.C.
Lung
D
Upper esoph.
Lower esoph.
E
E'
E''
E'''
Mucosa
Muscularis
F
F'
F''
F'''
F'v

In the surgical management of congenital atresia of the esophagus, the selection of the mode of surgical approach is determined mainly by the plain roentgenogram of the abdomen. In the absence of gas shadows in the gastrointestinal tract, a primary anastomosis of the esophagus is not considered. A primary esophagogastrostomy employing a right transpleural approach is preferred. In the presence of gas shadows in the gastrointestinal tract, an extrapleural thoracotomy on the right side may be employed, and, if possible, a primary anastomosis of the esophagus is performed. However, in a certain percentage of the patients in this group, a primary anastomosis of the esophagus may not be possible because of the wide separation of the esophageal segments. If this should obtain, a transpleural extension of the incision is recommended and the stomach mobilized into the right pleural cavity. If, following the mobilization of the stomach, the distal end of the esophagus is viable and the diameter of its lumen is adequate, a direct anastomosis of the esophagus may be performed. Otherwise, a primary intrapleural esophagogastrostomy is preferred. It is believed that every attempt possible should be made to reestablish continuity of the alimentary canal before resorting to a lifesaving multistage procedure.

Discussion—Drs. John M. Beal and Cranston W. Holman. Prematurity and aspiration pneumonia may present serious problems in the newborn infant who requires surgical correction of this congenital defect. For this reason, judicious preoperative preparation for 24 to 48 hours with antibiotics and parenteral fluids is usually indicated.

A right lateral transpleural approach through the fourth intercostal space gives the best exposure and requires less time. These are important considerations in operations upon small patients. To facilitate the anesthesia, the first step in the operation is to occlude the tracheoesophageal fistula which may easily be done by passing a small tape around the lower esophageal segment just below the tracheal communication. This prevents loss of the anesthetic agent, improves the respiratory exchange, and materially aids the anesthesiologist in the management of the patient.

The text has emphasized adequate mobilization of the esophagus. An anastomotic breakdown is more likely due to excessive tension than to the impairment of the blood supply resulting from mobilization of the esophageal segments. After the closure of the tracheal opening and completion of the esophageal anastomosis, it is desirable to place a flap of pleura between the esophageal suture line and the tracheal closure. This may be helpful in the prevention of a recurrence of the fistula.

A gastrostomy should be performed when the chest is closed. This permits early feedings which provide adequate nutrition until the oral intake is sufficient to satisfy the bodily needs. The operation is readily accomplished through a short left upper quadrant incision. A No. 12 F catheter is inserted through a small incision in the stomach wall which is encircled by a pursestring suture of 000 silk. The stomach should be attached to the peritoneum of the anterior abdominal wall with two or three sutures of the same material. The incision is closed about the gastrostomy catheter with 000 chromic catgut.

DISCUSSION—DR. CAMERON HAIGHT. The repair of congenital atresia of the esophagus with tracheoesophageal fistula can be performed readily through either a transpleural or extrapleural approach. The individual choice of the surgeon will usually dictate the type of exposure that is selected. My preference is for the extrapleural approach after the resection of the posterior half or two-thirds of the fourth rib, for the reasons that the exposure is entirely adequate, the anesthesia can be conducted more smoothly, and, most importantly, leakage of the anastomosis, should it occur postoperatively, can be dealt with more readily by simple drainage of the extrapleural wound and with a lower mortality than if a total empyema were to occur following the transpleural operation. The incision need not be started as high, as illustrated in A.

When a tracheoesophageal fistula is present, a primary esophageal anastomosis is almost always possible, providing adequate mobilization of the two portions of the esophagus is obtained, should it be necessary. A single-layer anastomosis (not illustrated) is used by some surgeons. Although it probably results in a lower incidence of stricture than does the two-layer anastomosis, it may result in a higher incidence of leakage. The thinness of the wall of the lower esophagus and the amount of tension on the anastomosis, should this be unavoidable, may govern the choice of the type of anastomosis that is used, and in these instances a single layer may be preferable. When there is adequate tissue for a two-layer anastomosis, the "telescoping" type illustrated in F-F^{iv} is preferable, although the suture material should not be larger than 000000 silk on the smallest available arterial needles. All knots of the inner layer should present within the esophageal lumen. The extrapleural wound is optimally drained with a No. 14 F. catheter and underwater suction for the first 24 to 36 hours.

CONGENITAL ATRESIA OF THE ESOPHAGUS WITH HYPOPLASIA OF THE LOWER ESOPHAGEAL SEGMENT

A. The incision for the extrapleural exposure of the mediastinum is depicted by the solid curvilinear line. For this exposure a segment of only one rib (fourth) is removed. The dotted line indicates the direction of the extension of the skin incision which was required in this patient when the extrapleural approach was converted into a transpleural one.

B. A self-retaining rib spreader (Tuffier) is inserted, and the extrapleural exposure of the mediastinum from the right side is shown. The dilated upper segment and the hypoplastic lower segment of the esophagus and their related structures are demonstrable. The azygos vein is doubly ligated and severed. The light and heavy dotted lines indicate the site of the incision through the parietal pleura and the line of extension of the skin incision respectively.

C. The right pleural cavity is entered, and the avulsion laceration of the hypoplastic lower segment of the esophagus at the cardia which occurred when clamp traction was applied to mobilize the stomach into the pleural cavity is visible.

D. The left gastric vessels are clamped, severed, and ligated, and the proximal portion of the stomach is mobilized with the aid of traction sutures of silk (000) into the right pleural cavity. During this mobilization the cardia and not the fundus was uppermost. Despite the extent of the intrathoracic mobilization of the stomach, the spleen was not seen. The dotted line in the upper segment of the esophagus indicates the site of the incision into its lumen for the anastomosis with the cardia of the stomach.

E. The cardia is mobilized into the apex of the right pleural cavity and the end-to-end esophagocardiostomy is completed. The area surrounding the anastomosis is enclosed by a rectangular shaped free graft of parietal pleura to lessen the incidence of leakage at the suture line. Closure of the chest wall and water-seal catheter (14F) drainage of the pleural cavity completes the operation.

Discussion—Drs. John M. Beal and Cranston W. Holman. The difficulties associated with this uncommon anomaly are much greater than with the type in which tracheoesophageal fistula is present. If a primary anastomosis is to be accomplished, as illustrated by the author, the stomach must be freely mobilized and brought into the chest. This procedure is followed by a higher mortality rate than that following an end-to-end anastomosis of the esophagus.

The postoperative course is complicated by frequent episodes of distention of the stomach transplanted into the right pleural cavity which causes compression of the lung and consequent pulmonary problems. Frequent regurgitation of gastric contents also complicates the postoperative management of the infant. These difficulties have influenced some surgeons to do a multistage operation consisting of a cervical esophagostomy and a gastrostomy with later restoration of gastrointestinal continuity by transplantation and interposition of the right colon. However, this particular type of anomaly is still a real challenge to the surgeon.

Discussion—Dr. Cameron Haight. Incomplete development of the lower segment of the esophagus occurs in slightly more than 10 per cent of infants with esophageal atresia. As there is no fistulous communication between the trachea and the lower portion of the esophagus, the diagnosis of this type of anomaly can be made by the absence of gas in the stomach and intestines.

Although the operations employing intrathoracic mobilization of the stomach, as recommended in the text, have been successfully performed in newborn infants, the mortality following these procedures is greater than that following the use of a multiple-stage plan. The generally accepted method of treating this anomaly, therefore, is by the use of a gastrostomy and cervical esophagostomy as the initial procedures. Later, after an interval of about two or more years, continuity is established, usually by the retrosternal interposition of a segment of colon between the cervical esophagus and stomach. With the use of the multiple-stage plan, the operative mortality is very low, and the late results to date have been excellent.

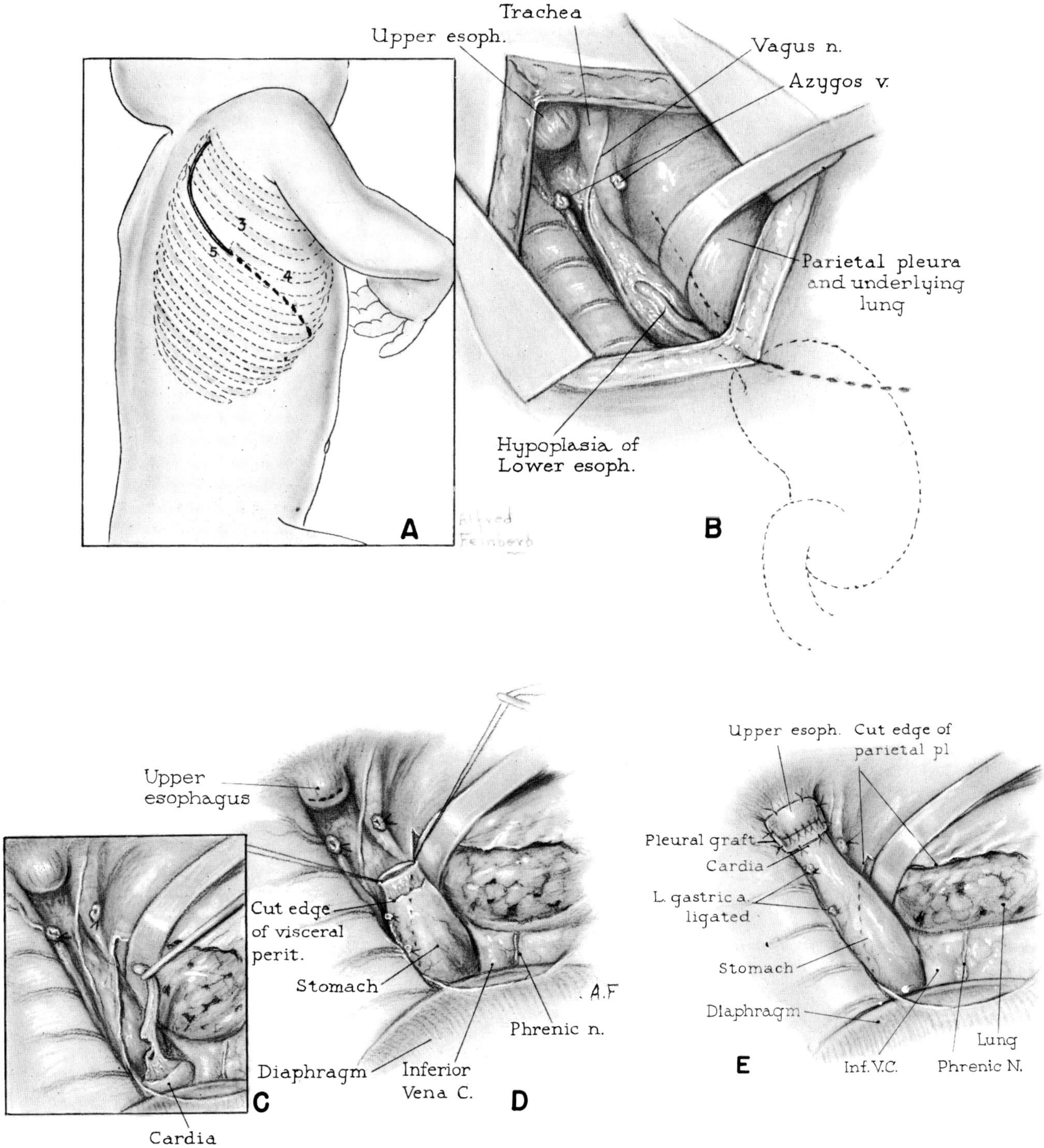

Trachea
Upper esoph.
Vagus n.
Azygos v.
Parietal pleura and underlying lung
Hypoplasia of Lower esoph.
3
4
5
A
Alfred Feinberg
B
Upper esophagus
Cut edge of visceral perit.
Stomach
A.F
Phrenic n.
Diaphragm
Inferior Vena C.
C
Cardia
D
Upper esoph.
Cut edge of parietal pl
Pleural graft
Cardia
L. gastric a. ligated
Stomach
Diaphragm
Lung
E
Inf.V.C.
Phrenic N.

RESECTION OF PHARYNGOESOPHAGEAL DIVERTICULUM

Diverticula of the esophagus are classified into two types: traction and pulsion. Traction diverticula most commonly occur on the anterior wall of the midportion of the thoracic esophagus in the region of the tracheal bifurcation. These diverticula are secondary manifestations of a surrounding inflammatory reaction and are true diverticula in that they contain all of the coats of the esophagus. However, this type of esophageal diverticulum is of little surgical significance.

The pulsion types of diverticula are most commonly found in the cervical region at the pharyngoesophageal level. They most commonly protrude on the left side, but they may be bilateral or protrude in the midline posteriorly. They may occur infrequently in the lower third of the esophagus just above the diaphragm, the so-called epiphrenic diverticula, and protrude either toward the right or the left side in the posterior mediastinum. The pulsion type of diverticulum is classified as false in that the mucosa of the esophagus herniates through the layers of overlying muscle fibers, and, accordingly, the diverticulum does not consist of the whole thickness of the wall of the esophagus. In the cervical region this protrusion usually occurs in the space between the lowermost fibers of the inferior constrictor muscle of the pharynx and the fibers of the cricopharyngeus muscle. Occasionally the protrusion may occur through the uppermost fibers of the cricopharyngeus muscle.

Pulsion diverticula are more commonly found in males (4:1) and occur most frequently in the sixth and seventh decades. However, in the illustrated technic the drawings were from sketches made by the artist while observing the operation performed in a 30-year-old man who had symptoms of progressive dysphagia of 14 months duration.

A. The patient is anesthetized, using intratracheal anesthesia. The oblique linear incision employed, paralleling the anterior border of the sternomastoid muscle, is depicted in dotted outline. Rarely, a right-side approach may be indicated for the exposure and the removal of a pharyngoesophageal diverticulum.

B. The incision is deepened through the platysma muscle and the anterior or investing layer of the deep cervical fascia to expose the fibers of the left sternomastoid muscle.

C. The anterior border of the sternomastoid muscle is mobilized and retracted laterally to expose the middle or pretracheal layer of the deep cervical fascia and its contained carotid sheath. The adjacent muscle structures are depicted.

D. The tendinous pulley, uniting the superior and inferior bellies of the omohyoid muscle, is elevated by a guy suture of silk (0) and retracted downward and medially. Severance of this tendon may be performed but this is generally not necessary. The retraction of the superior belly of the omohyoid muscle medially exposes the posterolateral portion of the left lobe of the thyroid gland and its overlying fascial (pretracheal) covering.

E. The middle or pretracheal fascial layer of the deep cervical fascia is incised to expose clearly the thyroid gland and the contents of the carotid sheath: the internal jugular vein, the vagus nerve, and the common carotid artery. In this patient there was an unusually large tributary vein as depicted which entered the internal jugular vein in the region conforming with the site of drainage of the common facial vein. Although it was in close approximation to the operative area, ligation and severance of this vein was not required.

F. The superior belly of the omohyoid muscle and the underlying sternothyroid muscle are retracted anteriorly and medially, and the sternomastoid muscle and the structures contained in the carotid sheath are retracted posteriorly and laterally to expose more clearly the posterolateral aspect of the left lobe of the thyroid gland. The inferior thyroid artery, a branch of the thyrocervical trunk of the subclavian artery, crosses horizontally beneath the carotid artery and divides into ascending and descending branches prior to its entrance into the gland structure. The inferior thyroid artery is a useful landmark for the identification of a pharyngoesophageal diverticulum which is usually located immediately subjacent to this vessel.

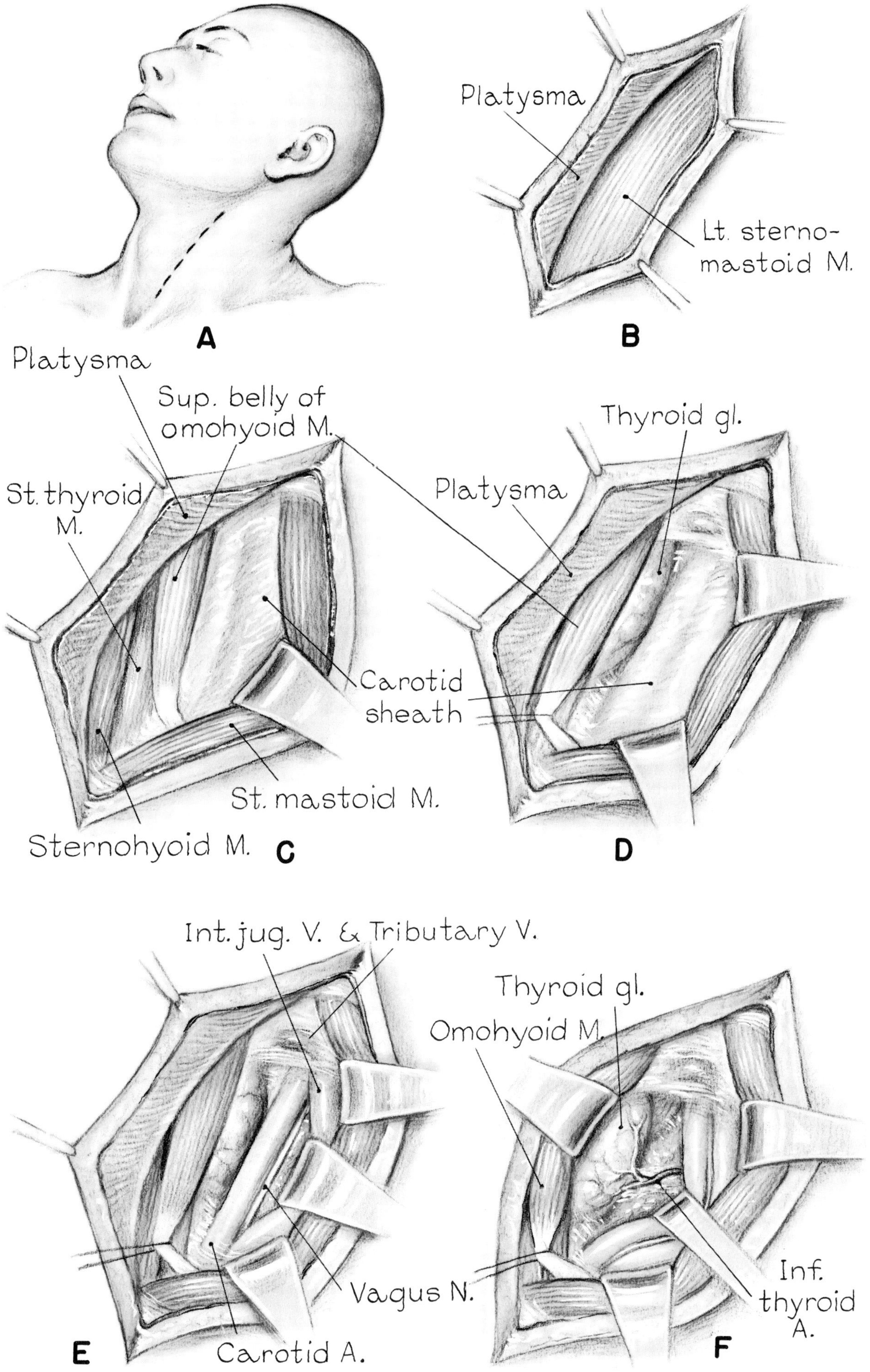
A
Platysma
Lt. sterno-
mastoid M.
B
Platysma
Sup. belly of
omohyoid M.
St. thyroid
M.
Carotid
sheath
St. mastoid M.
Sternohyoid M.
C
Thyroid gl.
Platysma
D
Int. jug. V. & Tributary V.
Vagus N.
Carotid A.
E
Thyroid gl.
Omohyoid M.
Inf.
thyroid
A.
F

G, H. The inferior thyroid artery is doubly ligated and severed (G) and the thyroid gland is retracted medially to expose the esophagus, the diverticulum, and the recurrent laryngeal nerve (H).

I. The recurrent laryngeal nerve, encircled by a guy suture of silk (000), bifurcated just prior to its passage beneath the lowermost fibers of the inferior constrictor muscle and its entrance into the larynx. The identification and isolation of this nerve is important in the prevention of injury to it during the operative procedure. The diverticulum, covered by fibroareolar tissue, may be seen to protrude through the space between the lower border of the inferior constrictor muscle of the pharynx above and the fibers of the cricopharyngeus muscle below. In some instances the protrusion may occur through the uppermost fibers of the cricopharyngeus muscle.

J, K. A Babcock clamp is applied to the fundus of the partially mobilized diverticulum (J), and, with traction maintained through the clamp, the mobilization of the diverticulum from the surrounding structures is completed by scissor dissection (K).

L. Inset showing a magnified view of the completely mobilized diverticulum and the demonstration of a technic for the determination of the level of the true neck of the diverticulum. In this particular patient the neck of the diverticulum appeared unduly wide in diameter. Accordingly, a catheter (16 F) was inserted through an opening in the fundus of the diverticulum and into the lumen of the distal portion of the esophagus where its tip could be readily palpated by the left index finger impinged against the outer wall of the esophagus. In this manner the true neck of the diverticulum was defined and the line for the resection indicated.

Discussion—Dr. Kenneth W. Warren. It has been an almost invariable practice at the Lahey Clinic to employ a long, oblique incision along the anterior border of the left sternomastoid muscle in approaching pharyngoesophageal diverticula. The choice of this type of incision is based upon the observation that one cannot prophesy preoperatively which diverticulum will be easily exposed, delivered, and dissected and which—because of its size, its adherence to the esophagus or related cervical structures—will prove to be difficult to manage. Until recently the majority of pharyngoesophageal diverticula treated at the Lahey Clinic were removed by the two stage operation. The long, oblique incision placed along the sternomastoid muscle afforded ample opportunity in this two stage procedure to permit fixation of the fundus of the diverticulum high in the cervical region so that the most dependent portion of the diverticulum would be at the junction of the sac with the longitudinal esophagus. Over 90 per cent of esophageal diverticula currently treated at the clinic are excised in a one stage maneuver. We still prefer this incision.

The skin and platysma are incised, and the anterior edge of the sternomastoid muscle on the left is reflected laterally, thus exposing the anterior belly of the omohyoid muscle. We have preferred to remove the anterior segment of this muscle completely rather than to retract it as is demonstrated in Plate 45 (D). The advantages of removing this segment of the omohyoid (while it is not necessary in every instance) are very great. This maneuver exposes the internal jugular vein with its branches running to the thyroid gland. After division of these lateral thyroid veins, the left lobe of the thyroid is elevated and rotated anteriorly and medially, thus exposing the common carotid artery which is then retracted laterally. Retraction of the carotid artery affords access to the inferior thyroid artery which is then divided between clamps and ligated. This division permits a greater degree of mobility of the left lobe of the thyroid. The left recurrent laryngeal nerve is then identified and its entire cervical course is exposed, but manipulation of this structure is avoided insofar as possible.

The preceding maneuvers expose the region of the pharyngoesophageal diverticulum which can now be identified. The fundus of the sac is grasped with Babcock forceps and the junction between the inner edge of the sac and the longitudinal esophagus is demonstrated. In some instances, the sac will be enveloped by a considerable thickness of fibers of the cricopharyngei which may make its identification difficult. In other instances, the sac may be extremely large and extend well down into the mediastinum. The delivery of such a large diverticulum from the mediastinum must be done with great care lest the diverticulum be perforated during this maneuver.

It should be borne in mind that the pharyngoesophageal diverticulum prior to its dissection lies

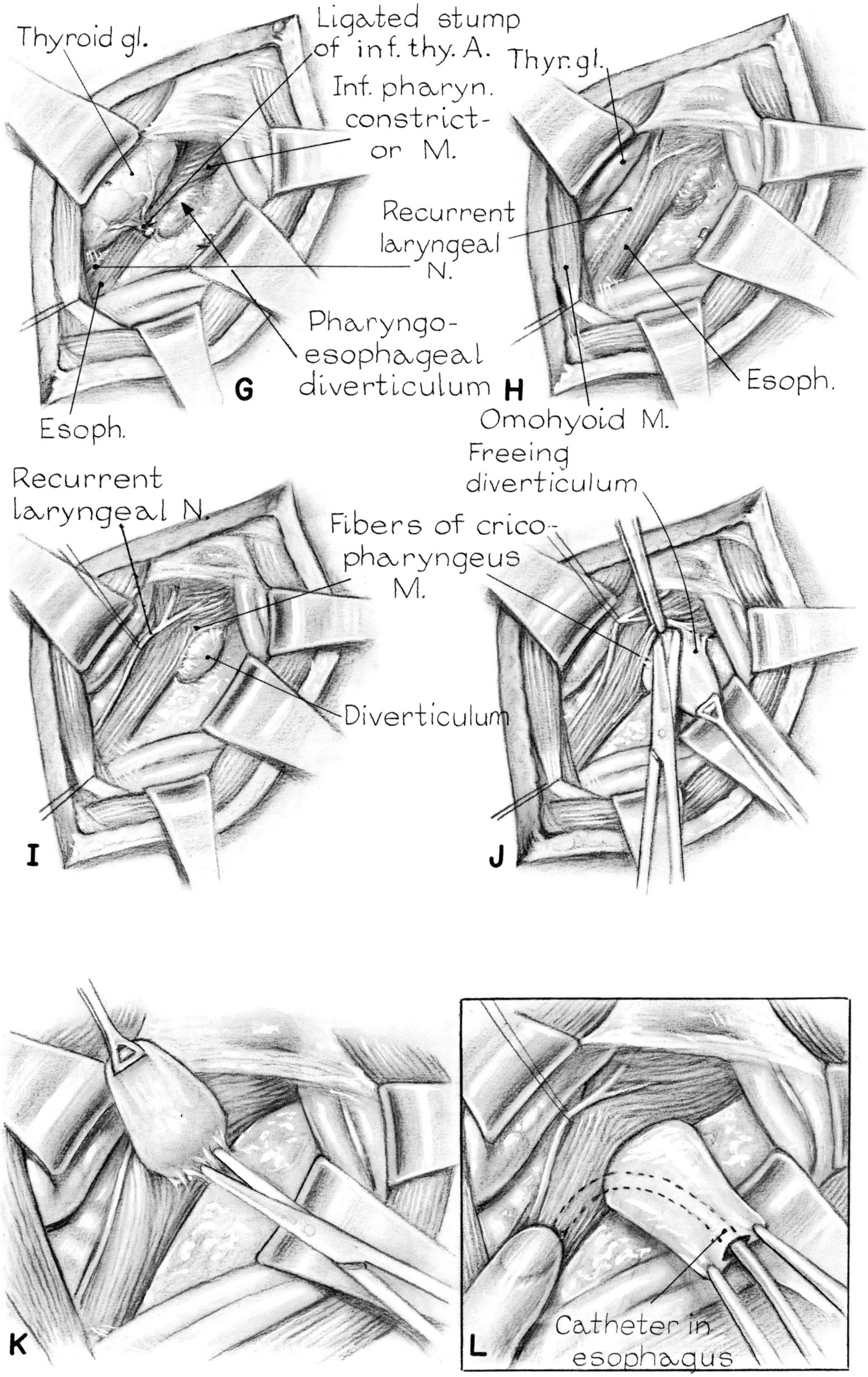
Thyroid gl.
Ligated stump of inf. thy. A.
Inf. pharyn. constrict- or M.
Recurrent laryngeal N.
Pharyngo- esophageal diverticulum
Esoph.
G
Thyr. gl.
Esoph.
Omohyoid M.
H
Recurrent laryngeal N.
Fibers of crico- pharyngeus M.
Diverticulum
I
Freeing diverticulum
J
K
Catheter in esophagus
L

M, N. Traction guy sutures of silk (000) are inserted through the neck of the diverticulum at its upper and lower borders, and the diverticulum is cross-clamped distally. The excision is begun by scissor dissection (M), and, following a partial resection, the cut margins of the mucosa and the submucosa layers of the esophagus are approximated with interrupted sutures of silk (000). In excising the diverticulum, excessive traction on its distal portion should be avoided. Otherwise, the walls of the esophagus may be tented into the line of resection with resulting constriction of the esophageal lumen.

O. The excision of the pharyngoesophageal diverticulum is completed, and the opening in the esophagus is closed with a series of interrupted sutures of silk (000).

O′. Inset to show an alternate method for the closure of the opening into the lumen of the esophagus. The interrupted sutures of silk (000) are inserted from the "inside out" to the "outside in" so that, when tied, the knots of the sutures are on the inside of the lumen.

P, Q. The defect in the musculature through which the diverticulum protruded is closed with interrupted sutures of 000 silk (P), and a Penrose (cigarette) drain is inserted into the cervical mediastinal space (Q).

R. The left sternomastoid muscle is gently retracted to show the relation of the surrounding muscles, previously labeled, to the carotid sheath and the site of drainage. The large tributary of the internal jugular vein previously mentioned is visible in the upper angle of the wound.

S. The operation is completed by closure of the skin incision about the drain, using interrupted sutures of silk (000).

Discussion—Dr. Warren (cont.)

parallel to the longitudinal esophagus and that as the dissection of the sac from the esophagus is carried out, an acute angle is made by the junction of the neck of the sac with the longitudinal esophagus. If recurrence of the diverticulum is to be avoided, it is extremely important to dissect the neck of the sac completely. It is easy to misjudge the degree of thoroughness of the dissection at this point, for the neck of the sac will be completely covered by an investment of the muscle fibers of the cricopharyngeus even though the sac has been liberated so that it hangs by its neck. We have always made it a point to dissect the neck of the sac until the pale white fibers of the submucosa of the sac are clearly visible. This dissection is relatively easily achieved in the inferior, superior, and left lateral positions. Unfortunately, dissection of the right side of the neck is more difficult since the fixed position of the cricoid cartilage and of the pharynx makes it impossible to rotate the posterior wall of the pharynx sufficiently to see the right lateral wall of the sac directly, except in those instances in which the diverticulum is very small and the neck quite narrow. If this phase of the dissection is done with care and with appreciation of the anatomic relationships and of the embryology of these diverticula, there will be no difficulty in determining the site of the junction of the diverticulum with the longitudinal esophagus.

When the sac has been thoroughly mobilized as previously described, one must decide how to deal with the neck of the sac. If the diverticulum is small or only moderately large and the neck is narrow, it is reasonable to ligate the neck of the sac flush with its junction with the longitudinal esophagus, using a 00 chromic catgut ligature. A clamp is then placed distal to this ligature and the sac is amputated, leaving an adequate amount of stump to insure that it will not retract through the previously placed ligature. When the neck of the sac is broad, it is best to divide its neck slightly distal to its precise junction with the longitudinal esophagus, and to close the defect with a continuous Connell inverting suture of fine catgut reinforced by a row of interrupted sutures of the same material. It is quite permissible to close this defect with interrupted sutures but we prefer to use inverting sutures, even though they be interrupted. After amputation of the sac and closure of the esophagus either by ligature or by the inversion suture method, it is important to approximate the cricopharyngei muscles over the closed neck of the sac. We usually employ a cigarette drain and bring it out in the lower angle of the incision.

This comment has been limited to the one stage procedure. However, it is well to remember that the two stage procedure still has merit in the presence of the large pulsion diverticulum of the pharyngoesophagus when the sac extends well down into the mediastinum and when diverticulitis and peridiverticulitis are prominent features. The two stage procedure should also have considerable appeal to those surgeons with a limited experience in esophageal surgery who, nevertheless, undertake to operate on pharyngoesophageal diverticula.

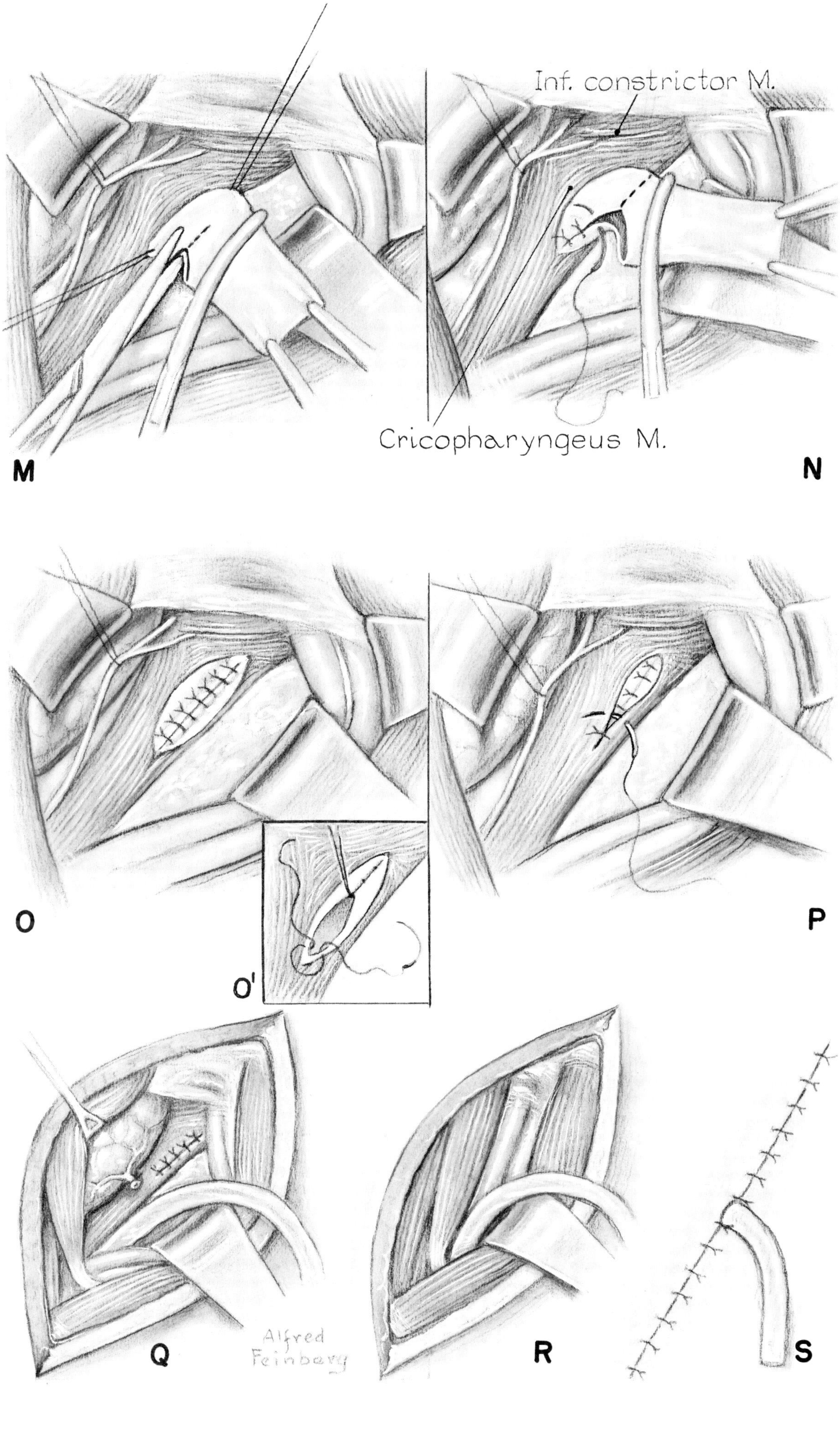
Inf. constrictor M.
Cricopharyngeus M.
M
N
O
O'
P
Q
R
S
Alfred Feinberg

ESOPHAGOCARDIOMYOTOMY—TRANSABDOMINAL APPROACH

A, B. The peritoneal cavity is entered through an upper left rectus muscle-splitting or muscle-retracting incision (A) and the underlying intraperitoneal viscera are demonstrable (B).

C. By manual retraction overlying a protective moist gauze pad the peritoneal attachment forming the left triangular ligament of the liver is made taut and severed as indicated by the dotted line.

D. The mobilized left lobe of the liver, covered by a moist gauze pad, is folded downward on itself and retracted medially to expose the opening in the peritoneal fascial layer overlying the esophagocardial junction. The lower end of the esophagus, the vagus nerves, and the esophageal hiatal ring formed by the superficial and deep muscle bundles of the right crus are visible. The tapered and thinned out terminal portion of the esophagus and the dilatation proximally, characteristic findings in achalasia, may also be seen.

E. By careful digital manipulation within the posterior mediastinum, the lower portion of the esophagus is mobilized and displaced downward into the peritoneal cavity.

F. The esophagus at the level of the esophagocardial junction is encircled by a tape of rubber tissue, and with downward traction maintained, a linear incision through the fibers of the longitudinal muscle layer of the esophagus and the adjoining segment of the stomach is begun.

Discussion—Dr. Richard H. Sweet. The operation of esophagomyotomy may be performed either through an abdominal incision, as originally advocated by Heller, or through a left thoracotomy incision. In my opinion the latter is preferable for the following reasons: (1) The incision through the left eighth intercostal space can be easily and quickly made and closed. (2) The exposure of the lower esophagus is more easily obtained, and access to the entire length of the lower segment is secured without dissection and mobilization which must always be employed when the abdominal approach is used. This makes it easier to avoid the vagus nerves and to minimize the amount of trauma in the lower esophageal region. (3) The fascial layers in the esophageal hiatus of the diaphragm are not greatly disturbed. (4) It is simple, using this approach, to repair a coexisting hiatus hernia with a minimum of dissection.

A technical matter which may make the difference between success and failure in the use of this operation for the treatment of megaesophagus is the length of the myotomy incision. As shown in Plate 48 (F), this incision must extend upward on the esophagus to a point where the diameter of the organ is large. It is not necessary, on the other hand, to extend the incision onto the wall of the stomach below the cardia. No hypertrophied circular muscle fibers are ever found distal to this point. It must be remembered that the abnormality is in the esophagus. The unnecessary extension of the incision into the stomach wall below the cardia usually is harmless, but because the muscular layers there are thin, it is easy to penetrate the mucosal layer. If this accident should occur, a careful closure of the opening should be made with sutures of fine silk.

The dissection between the circular muscle layer and the submucosa as shown in Plate 49 (H and I) is unnecessary and might even be harmful. It is much easier and safer merely to cut through the muscle layers with a sharp knife. It is absolutely essential, however, to divide every single circular muscle fiber in order to avoid leaving a stenotic point. Plate 49 (J) shows the appearance of the bulging mucosal layer when the division of the muscle has been completely accomplished, although in my opinion the incision as illustrated extends unnecessarily far into the wall of the stomach.

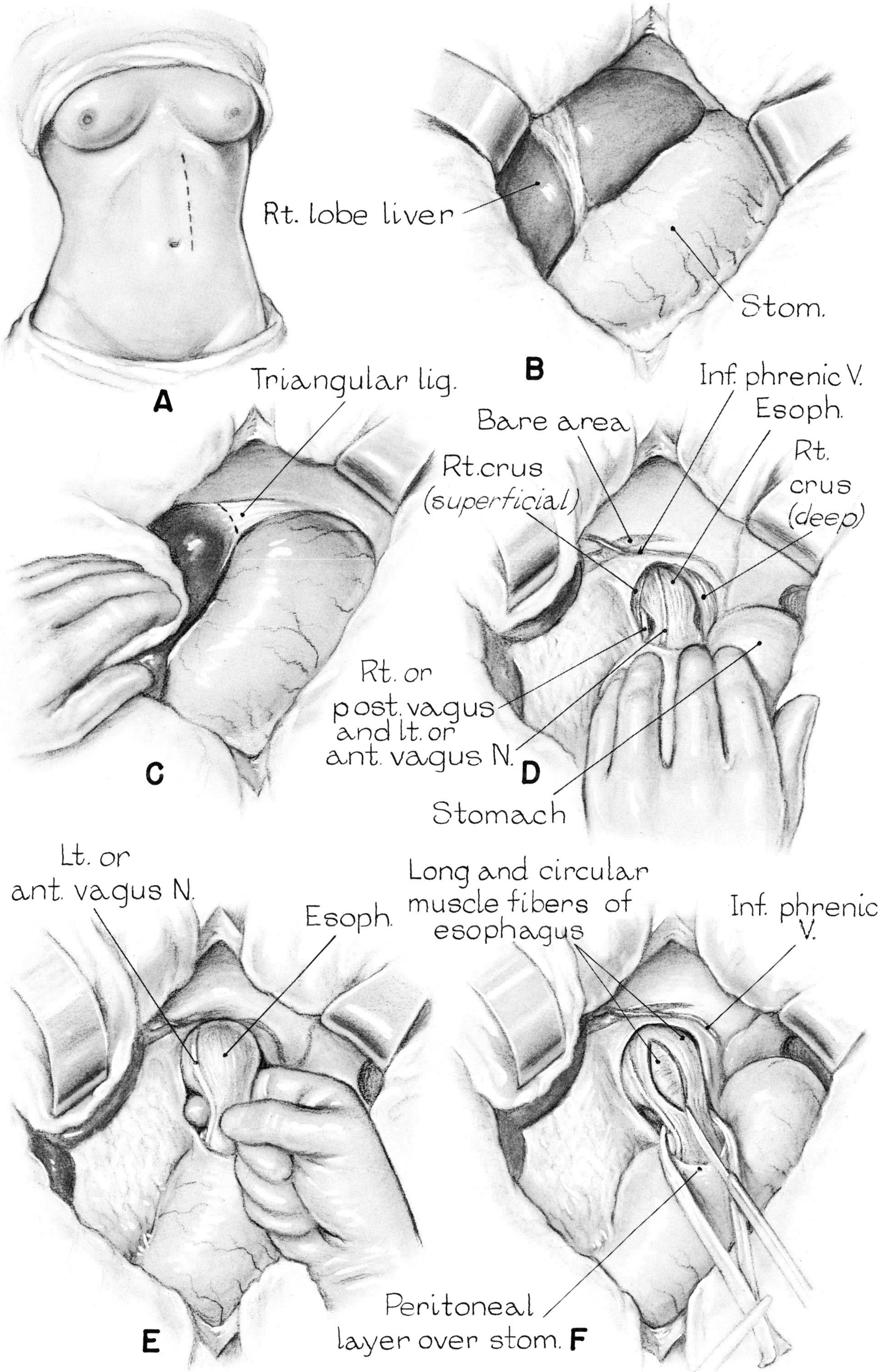
Rt. lobe liver
Stom.
A
B
Triangular lig.
Inf. phrenic V.
Esoph.
Bare area
Rt.crus
(superficial)
Rt.
crus
(deep)
Rt. or
post. vagus
and lt. or
ant. vagus N.
C
D
Stomach
Lt. or
ant. vagus N.
Esoph.
Long and circular
muscle fibers of
esophagus
Inf. phrenic
V.
Peritoneal
layer over stom.
E
F

G. The incision through the longitudinal muscle layer of the esophagus is completed, and the underlying layer of circular muscle fibers is visible. A vessel crossing transversely at the level of the cardia is shown elevated on a clamp prior to its double ligation and severance.

H, I. Following the completion of the incision in the longitudinal muscle layers of the esophagus, the cardia, and the segment of the gastric wall immediately below the cardia, the underlying circular layers of muscle fibers are elevated in segments and severed by scissor dissection.

J, K. The esophagocardiomyotomy is completed and the herniation of portions of the mucosa of the esophagus, the cardia, and the adjacent segment of the stomach respectively are depicted. The prominence of the vessels in the submucosal layer of the stomach may also be seen.

L, M, N. The wound is closed in layers using a double strand of a continuous interlocking suture of 00 chromic catgut for the peritoneum (L), interrupted sutures of 00 silk for the fascia (M), and 000 silk for the skin (N).

Discussion—Dr. Mark M. Ravitch. In many patients an oblique subcostal incision provides easy access to the esophageal hiatus. The rectus-splitting incision invariably paralyzes the portion of the rectus muscle medial to it and does not provide significantly better exposure than the rectus-retracting incision. For most gastric operations, unless the patient has a very flat costal arch, the midline incision, through the linea alba, is satisfactory and is technically the simplest. As emphasized in G through K, the esophagogastric incision is a long one, extending 5 cm. up on the esophagus and 5 cm. down on the stomach, through to the submucosa. Wangensteen suggested the passage of a balloon into the esophagus to distend it and to render this phase of the operation simpler.

It will be seen in D, E, and F that there is considerable dissection within the hiatus, and this may result in the appearance of a postoperative hiatus hernia. It is probable that a certain proportion of the unsatisfactory results following Heller's cardiomyotomy, are, in fact, due to the operative creation of a hiatus hernia. For this reason it is wise always to place one or two sutures behind the esophagus, approximating the fibers of the right crus, as in the repair of a hiatus hernia from the abdominal approach. In order further to prevent regurgitation into the esophagus and subsequent esophagitis, the bane of most other procedures for achalasia, Lortat-Jacob has emphasized the wisdom of tacking the gastric fundus up to the esophagus in order to re-create the angle of His and introduce what is almost a valvular mechanism at the esophagogastric junction, like the one produced by the normally acute angle of insertion of the esophagus into the stomach.

Discussion—Dr. C. Rollins Hanlon. I prefer an upper midline approach for this type of subdiaphragmatic exposure. A transverse epigastric incision dividing both rectus muscles may be adequate in patients with flaring costal margins.

Neither of these abdominal incisions provides full access to the esophagus for an upward extension of the myotomy, which is, at times, desirable. Conversely, it is easy to overextend the gastric portion of the muscle division, which may destroy the subdiaphragmatic portion of the esophageal sphincter. This destruction is conducive to reflux and, at times, to esophagitis.

The ability to explore the abdomen is an obvious advantage of the transabdominal approach but does not seem to be a dominant consideration.

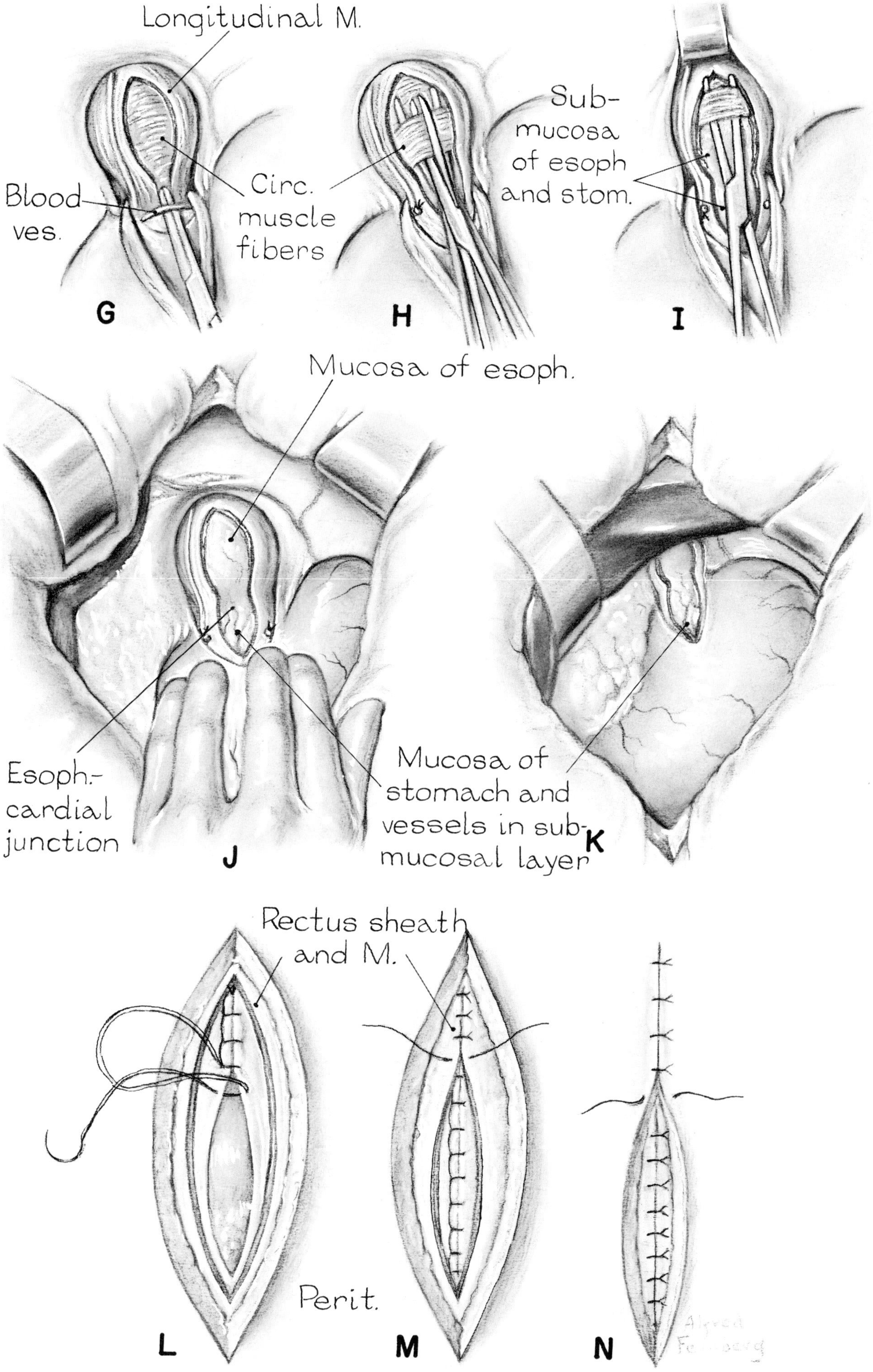
Longitudinal M.
Blood ves.
Circ. muscle fibers
Sub-mucosa of esoph and stom.
G
H
I
Mucosa of esoph.
Esoph.-cardial junction
Mucosa of stomach and vessels in sub-mucosal layer
J
K
Rectus sheath and M.
Perit.
L
M
N

ESOPHAGOCARDIOMYOTOMY—TRANSTHORACIC APPROACH

A. The patient is placed in the direct right lateral prone position. The incision overlying the eighth rib is indicated by the broken line.

B. The left pleural cavity is entered through the eighth intercostal space (Brock technic), and the related intrapleural structures are depicted. The lower lobe of the left lung, partly visible, is covered by a moist gauze pad and retracted cephalad. Sutures of 000 silk are inserted in the inferior pulmonary ligament, which is subsequently incised between the ligatures.

C. The incised margins of the inferior pulmonary ligament are retracted by sutures (000 silk), and the areolar tissue attachments about the esophagus are freed by scissor dissection.

D. The lower portion of the dilated esophagus is mobilized by blunt digital dissection from its "bed" in the posterior mediastinum.

DISCUSSION—DR. MARK M. RAVITCH. Ordinarily patients with achalasia who require operation have lost sufficient weight so that there is no difficulty in dissecting about the cardia through the transabdominal approach. It is easier, and does less violence to the hiatus, to bring the esophagus into the peritoneal cavity from below, than to bring the stomach up into the thoracic cavity from above. In either case, it is mandatory to make the esophagogastric incision a long one, and just as long (5 cm.) on the gastric side as on the esophageal side of the esophagogastric junction.

Heller originally advised two incisions, one anterior and one posterior. This would make assurance doubly sure but does not appear to be necessary. Whether the operation is done from above or from below, the hiatus should be reinforced at the conclusion of the esophagocardiomyotomy. Tacking the fundus to the side of the esophagus is as feasible in the transthoracic as in the transabdominal approach.

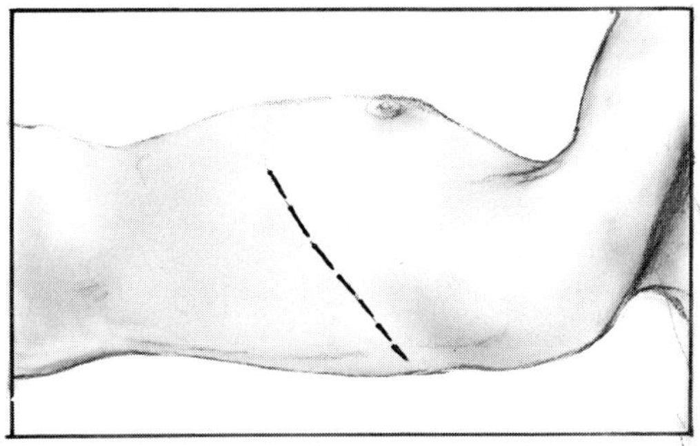

A

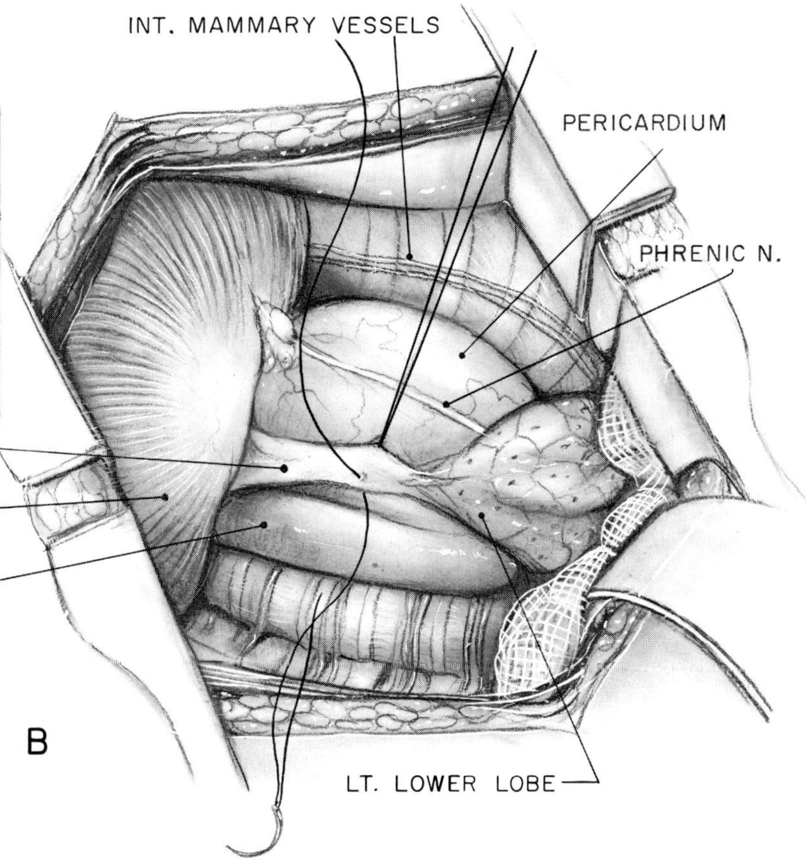
INT. MAMMARY VESSELS
PERICARDIUM
PHRENIC N.
INF. PUL. LIG.
DIAPHRAGM
AORTA
LT. LOWER LOBE

B

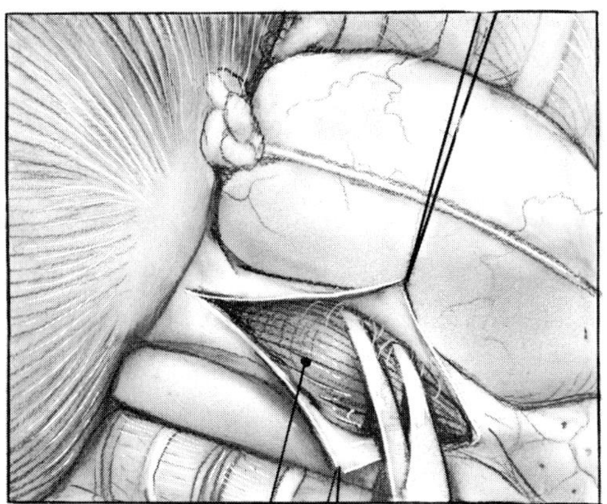
ESOPHAGUS

C

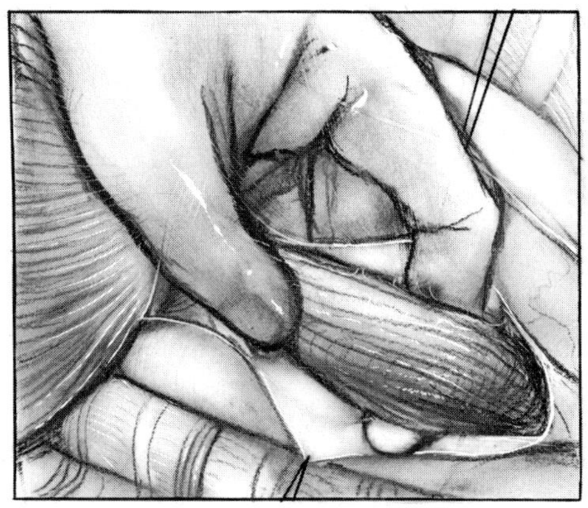

D

E, F, G. A rubber-tissue tape is inserted beneath the esophagus (E) to encircle it (F), and as traction on the tape is maintained, the esophagus is mobilized by scissor dissection of its areolar tissue attachments (G). The right or posterior vagus nerve in relation to the partly mobilized esophagus is visible (G).

H. A second rubber-tissue tape encircles the esophagus caudad, and as traction is maintained on the tapes, the longitudinal or outer layer of muscle fibers in the lower portion of the esophagus is incised. Through the incision some of the fibers of the underlying circular muscle layers may be seen.

I. The incision in the outer (longitudinal) muscle layer is completed, and the inner (circular) muscle layer, elevated on a curved (Kelly) clamp, is incised.

J. The circular muscle layer cephalad is similarly elevated on a Mixter clamp, and the severance of its fibers is completed (broken line).

Discussion—Dr. C. Rollins Hanlon. It seems clear that esophagocardiomyotomy, omitting the posterior of the two incisions advocated by Heller, is the best treatment for achalasia of the esophagus. I prefer a transthoracic approach, despite the occasional occurrence of annoying intercostal neuralgia after this procedure. Satisfactory access may be obtained by excision of the seventh, eighth, or ninth rib; entry through the eighth intercostal space gives adequate exposure.

The technic portrayed in illustrations B through G is quite satisfactory. Particular care should be taken not to damage either vagus nerve, because vagotomy tends to aggravate the dysfunction. In contrast to use of the knife in H, I use Metzenbaum scissors to divide both layers of muscle, thus minimizing the likelihood of mucosal perforation, especially at the important lower end of the dissection. The incision is usually 10 cm. long and extends over the stomach only far enough to insure complete division of all circular esophageal muscle fibers. Excessive prolongation of the incision on the stomach or damage to the right crus may explain some cases of late, regurgitant esopha-

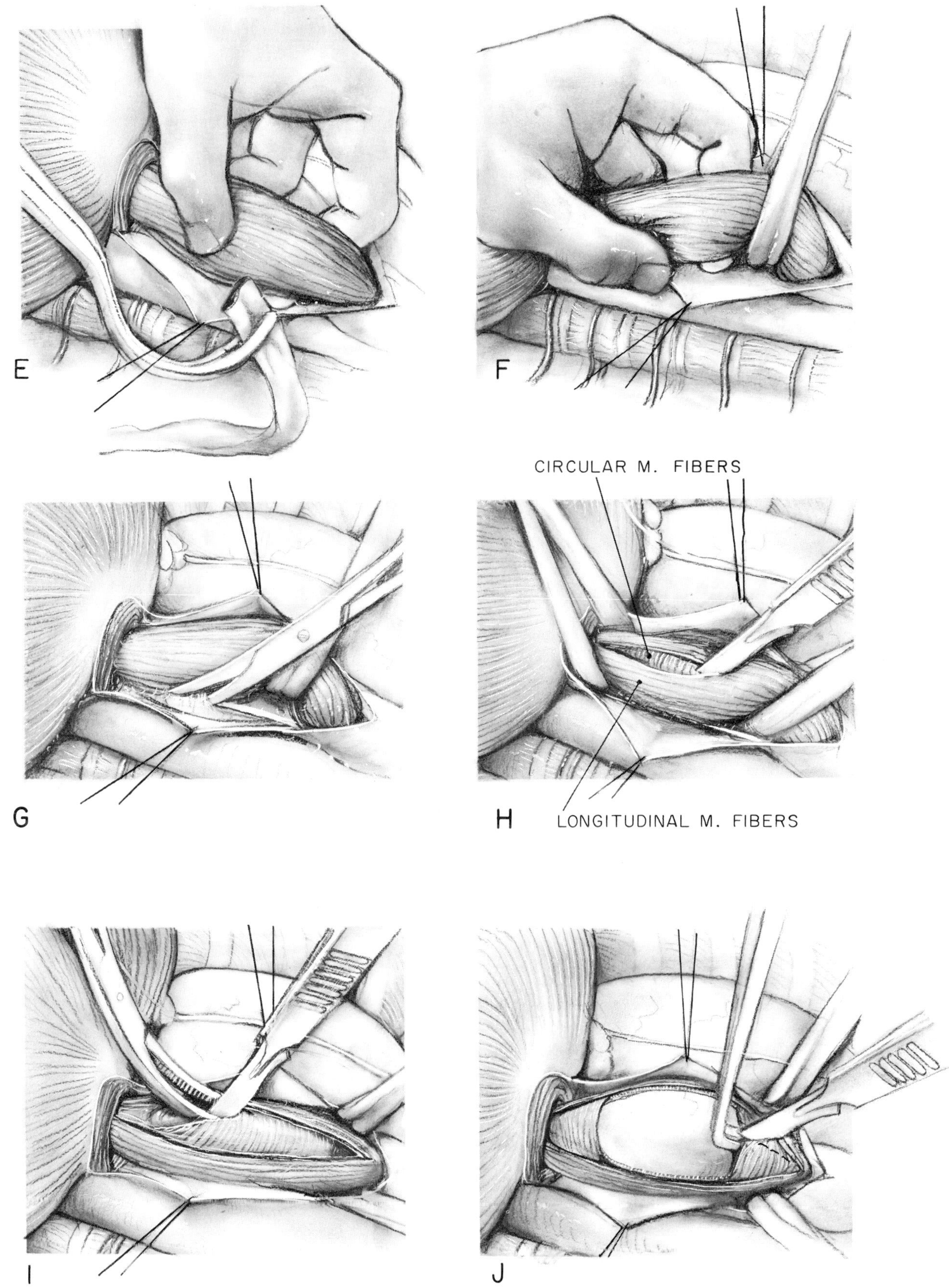
E
F
CIRCULAR M. FIBERS
G
H
LONGITUDINAL M. FIBERS
I
J

K. The fibers of the remaining and caudad segment of the circular muscle layer are transected as indicated (broken line).

L. The esophagocardiomyotomy is completed, and the herniation of the mucosal layer of the esophagus is visible. The relation of the incised margins of the muscle layers of the esophagus to the muscle fibers of the right crus of the diaphragm which form the esophageal hiatal ring is also visible.

M. A close-up view shows more clearly the relation of the lower portion of the esophagus to its hiatal ring. A segment of the right (posterior) vagus nerve is also seen.

N, O. The operative field before (N) and after (O) approximation of the pleural leaflets overlying the diaphragm is shown. The mediastinal pleural leaflets are not sutured. Expansion of the lung and closure of the thoracic incision complete the operation. A waterseal drainage catheter (18 F) is used during the closure of the wound and may be removed as the final skin suture is being tied about it.

Discussion—Dr. Hanlon (cont.)

gitis. If hiatus hernia is present or is rendered likely by the dissection, a few sutures may be placed for approximation of the fibers of the right crus posteriorly.

The mucosa should bulge over a wide area, as shown in L. Passage of a sound or easy inflation of a pneumatic dilator (60 F) by the anesthesiologist assures one that the size of the cardia is adequate. In addition, it may demonstrate persistent circular muscle fibers requiring division. Though some have advocated retrograde passage of the fingers or a balloon dilator through a gastrotomy, this seems unnecessarily complex and increases the risk of infection in the pleural space. With an incidence of mucosal perforation in the vicinity of 10 per cent, it seems safer to leave an intercostal waterseal drainage catheter in place for a day or two, especially if a recognized perforation has been sutured.

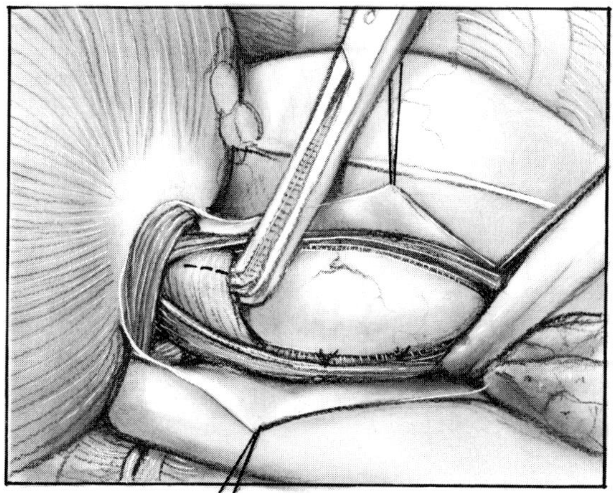

K

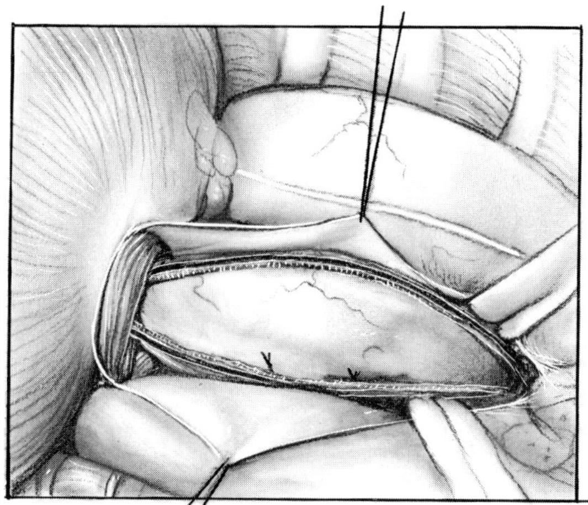

L

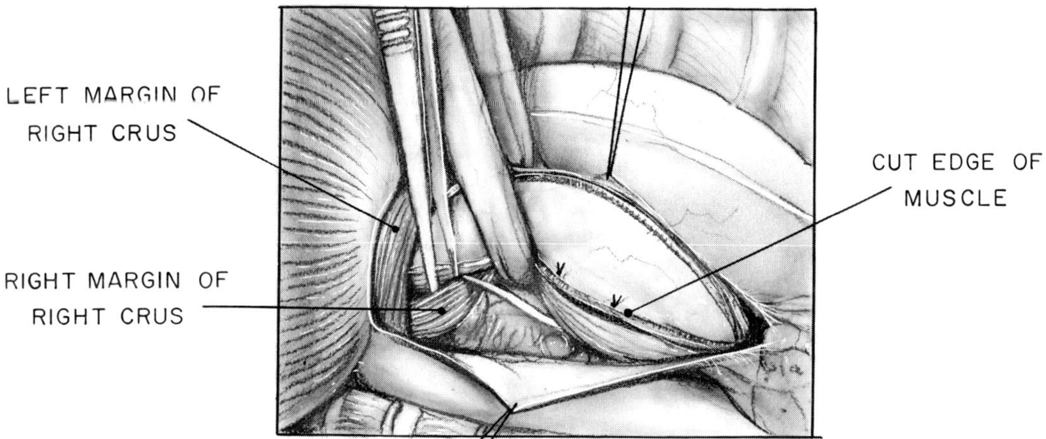
LEFT MARGIN OF
RIGHT CRUS
RIGHT MARGIN OF
RIGHT CRUS
CUT EDGE OF
MUSCLE

M

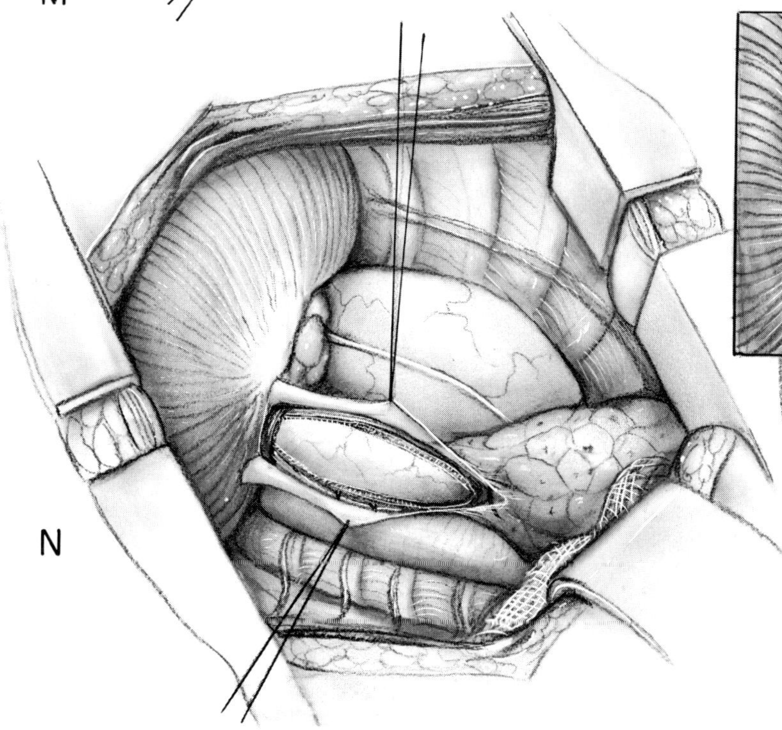

N

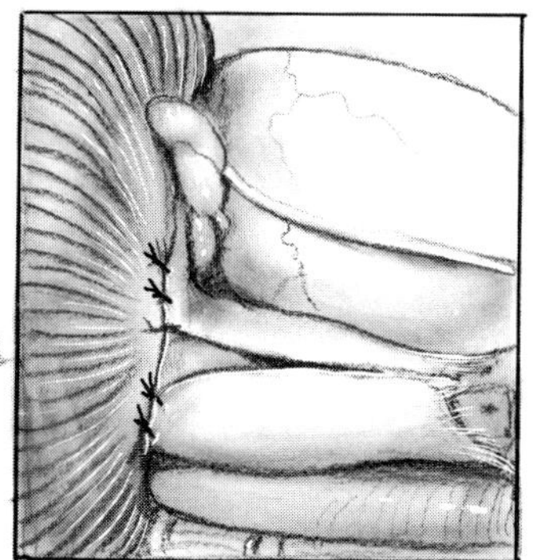

O

ESOPHAGECTOMY. LEFT TRANSPLEURAL, TRANSDIAPHRAGMATIC APPROACH WITH SUPRAAORTIC AND INFRAAORTIC ESOPHAGOGASTROSTOMY

A. The patient is placed in the direct right lateral prone position, and the left thoracotomy incision is shown in dotted outline. Although not shown, the seventh rib is partially resected and segments (2 cm.) of the vertebral ends of the sixth and eighth ribs are also removed. The related intercostal neurovascular muscle bundles are clamped, severed, and ligated with suture ligatures of silk (00).

B. The left pleural cavity is entered, and the rib cage is separated over protective moist towels with a self-retaining retractor (Finochietto). The incision in the posterior mediastinal pleura is depicted by the dotted line.

C. The cut margins of the mediastinal pleura are retracted with guy sutures (0000 silk) and the tumor of the esophagus is exposed. The lower portion of the esophagus, previously mobilized by blunt digital dissection, is encircled by a cotton tape for traction. With traction maintained anteriorly and toward the midline, the esophageal branches of the thoracic aorta are isolated, doubly ligated in continuity, and then severed between the ligatures. Usually two and at the most three arterial branches are ligated in the area between the arch of the aorta and the diaphragm.

D, E. Dissection with scissors is continued in the fibroareolar tissue layer surrounding the tumor until it is completely mobilized from the surrounding structures. In the dissection at this level there is danger of injury to the azygos vein which is not visible and which may be adherent to the right side of the tumor bearing area of the esophagus.

F. The mediastinal pleura above the aortic arch and lateral to the subclavian artery is incised and the cut margins are secured with guy sutures of silk (0000).

G, G′. The supraaortic segment of the esophagus is encircled by a cotton tape and retracted in various planes as the surrounding fibroareolar tissue is severed (dotted lines) by scissor dissection. In performing the dissection in this area the surgeon should be cognizant of the proximity of the lymphatic duct and the increased likelihood of its injury.

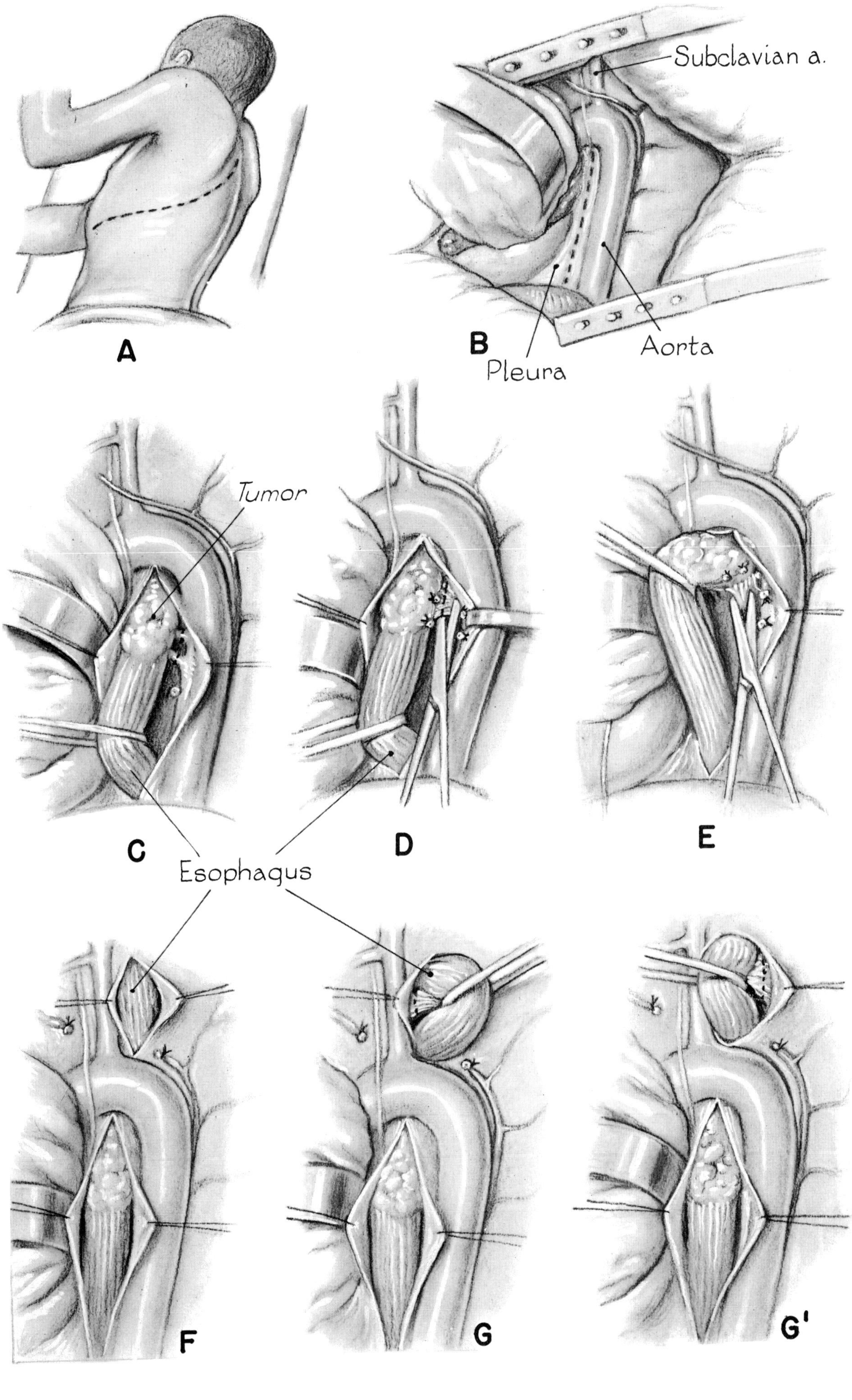
Subclavian a.
Pleura
Aorta
Tumor
Esophagus
A
B
C
D
E
F
G
G'

H. The supraaortic and infraaortic segments of the esophagus are encircled by cotton tapes through which traction is applied to elevate the esophagus and the tumor mass from the depths of the mediastinum. Traction guy sutures of silk (00) are used to tent a portion of the left leaflet of the diaphragm which is incised in the direction indicated by the dotted line. This radial incision extends through the esophageal hiatal ring preparatory to the mobilization of the esophagocardial junction.

I. The transdiaphragmatic incision is completed and the subjacent intraperitoneal viscera are demonstrated. This incision converts the left pleural and the subjacent peritoneal cavity into one common cavity.

J. The anterior wall of the stomach is grasped in a Babcock clamp through which traction is applied to displace the stomach upward into the left pleural cavity. The severance of the gastrocolic ligament below the gastroepiploic arch is indicated in dotted outline.

K. The mobilization of the greater curvature of the stomach is continued by doubly clamping and severing (dotted line) the gastrosplenic ligament and its contained vasa brevia.

L. The completely mobilized greater curvature of the stomach is grasped in Babcock clamps and retracted anteriorly and cephalad to show the left gastric vessels, contained in the gastropancreatic fold of peritoneum, triply clamped prior to their severance between the two distal clamps.

L′. The clamped and severed left gastric vessels are occluded proximally with a ligature of silk (00) and the lowermost clamp is removed. A second suture, a suture ligature of 00 silk, is inserted distally beneath the uppermost clamp which is removed as the suture is tied.

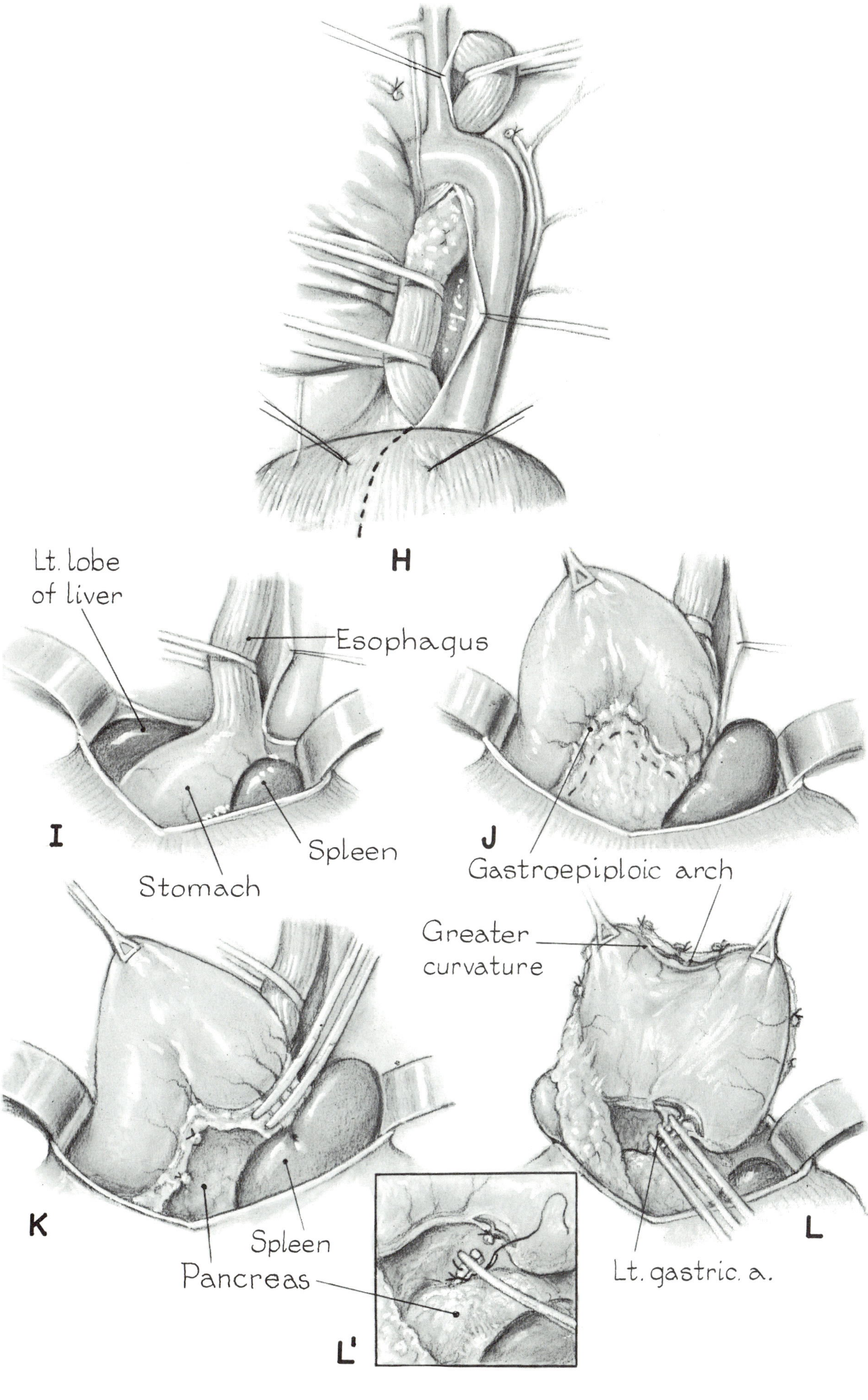
H
Lt. lobe of liver
Esophagus
I
Stomach
Spleen
J
Gastroepiploic arch
K
Spleen
Pancreas
Greater curvature
L
Lt. gastric. a.
L'

M. The completely mobilized stomach, anchored only by its esophageal and duodenal attachments, is secured proximally with Babcock clamps, and the line of transection of the stomach below the clamp-occluded esophagocardial junction is shown in dotted outline.

N, O. The oblique opening in the proximal segment of the stomach is closed with interrupted sutures of silk (000). The sutures are inserted from the "inside out" and from the "outside in" so that when tied the knots are on the inside of the lumen. The reinforcing second layer of interrupted horizontal seromuscular mattress sutures (Cushing) are inserted to complete the closure of the transected stomach. The esophagogastric stump proximally (O) is covered by a piece of rubber dam and occluded with two ligatures of No. 1 silk.

P, Q. The long strands of the proximal ligature which occludes the distal end of the esophagus are passed upward behind the aortic arch, and, by traction through these strands from above and digital manipulation from below (P), the tumor mass and the distal segment of the esophagus are displaced upward behind the arch of the aorta to a position anterior to the aortic arch (Q).

R. Traction sutures (000 silk) are inserted in the fundus of the stomach, and, immediately subjacent, a horizontal incision is made through the seromuscular layer of the stomach at the site of election for anastomosis to the esophagus. The vessels in the submucosal layer are undersewn with hemostatic suture ligatures of silk (0000). The performance, at this time, of this particular step in technic obviates troublesome bleeding when the opening into the lumen of the stomach is subsequently made (R′). The excision of a circular area of stomach wall is neither practiced nor recommended. A careful mucosa to mucosa approximation is considered the best prophylaxis for stenosis at the stomal site.

R′. The first posterior layer of interrupted sutures are being inserted. On the esophageal side the sutures are inserted at right angles to the fibers of the longitudinal muscle layer to increase the holding power of the tissues. The dotted line on the posterior wall of the esophagus indicates its site of transection. The opening into the lumen of the stomach is being enlarged by scissor dissection between the two rows of the previously inserted hemostatic ligatures which have been tied and cut.

R″, R‴. A second posterior layer of interrupted and untied mattress sutures of silk (000) is inserted (R″); these, when tied (R‴), effect an inversion of the tissue layers into the lumen of the anastomosis. A third posterior layer of interrupted sutures (000 silk) is inserted (R‴) through the whole thickness of the inverted layers of the stomach and the esophagus.

Discussion—Dr. John H. Garlock. For adequate exposure, I have found it necessary to remove only one rib, usually the seventh, in most instances. By opening the rib spreader slowly and in stages, it is possible to obtain adequate room without cracking, accidentally or purposely, the ribs above or below. In heavy chested men, it may be necessary to divide the sixth or eighth ribs or both, and this is done without disturbing the intercostal neurovascular bundles.

I would suggest using soft Penrose tubing instead of cotton tape when mobilizing the esophagus. Many patients with cancer of this organ exhibit friable musculature, and, unless the traction tape has considerable resiliency and "give," the organ may be torn at a site which is not to be excised. If the surgeon limits his dissection close to the esophagus in the supra-aortic area, he need have little fear of injuring the thoracic duct.

The use of grasping clamps, as depicted (Plate 54, K and L) is to be avoided for reasons stated previously. The stomach can be easily and gently displaced above the opening in the diaphragm by the gloved hand.

When ligating the left gastric vessels, the surgeon should make every effort to clear this vascular pedicle of all lymph nodes. In more than 50 per cent of our cases, squamous cell cancers of the thoracic esophagus have metastasized retrogradely to the nodes along the left gastric artery.

As stated before, I would suggest a wider excision

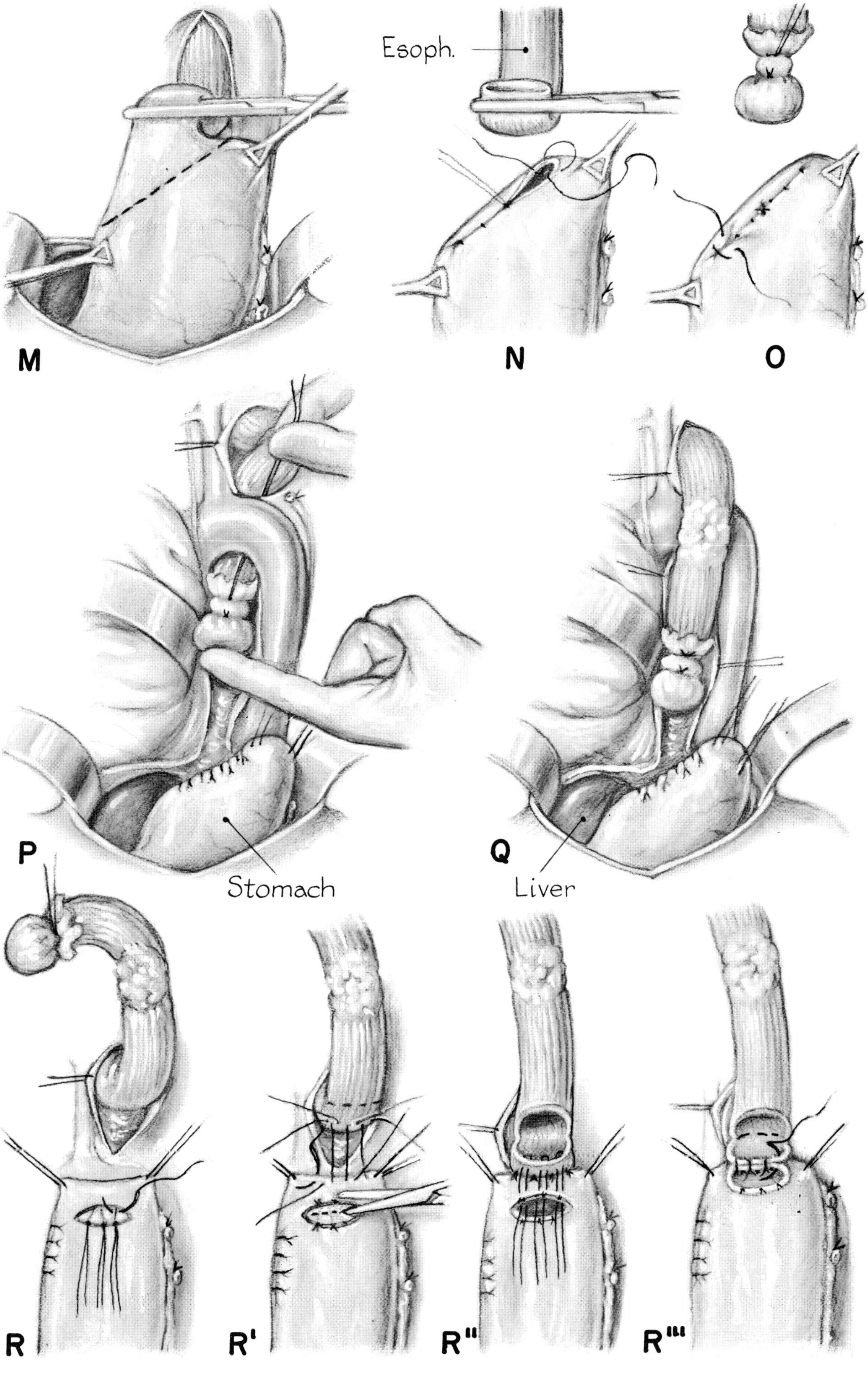
Esoph.
M
N
O
P
Stomach
Q
Liver
R
R'
R''
R'''

S. The first anterior layer of the anastomosis is begun by inserting the angle sutures which are inserted from the "inside out" on one side and from the "outside in" on the other side, so that when tied the knots are on the inside of the lumen. Traction on the long strands of the angle sutures posteriorly facilitates the inversion of the first anterior layer.

S′. The interrupted inversion sutures are inserted alternately from either end toward the center at which juncture the first two sutures are encircled by a figure of 8 mattress suture before being cut.

S″. The mattress suture is tied and cut and the second anterior layer of the anastomosis, a series of interrupted horizontal mattress sutures (Cushing), is begun.

T. The left supraaortic esophagogastrostomy is completed. The intrathoracic portion of the stomach is anchored with interrupted silk (000) sutures to the mediastinal pleura, and the incision in the diaphragm is closed snugly about the transplanted stomach with interrupted silk (00) sutures.

U, U′. Inset to show the extent of resection (U) and the completed infraaortic esophagogastrostomy (U′) for the surgical removal of a carcinoma in the region of the esophagocardial junction.

V, V′, V″. Inset to show an alternate method, used in one patient in the treatment of a carcinoma of the midthoracic segment of the esophagus (V). The thoracic aorta is completely mobilized by ligation and severance of the paired intercostal arteries and rotated anteriorly (V′). This permits the transplantation of the mobilized stomach into the esophageal bed within the mediastinum and the establishment of the esophagogastric anastomosis posterior and superior rather than anterior and superior to the arch of the aorta (V′, V″).

W. A Foley catheter (18 F) is partially withdrawn through a stab wound drainage site in the eighth intercostal space and connected to a water-seal drainage bottle. Periosteal "windows" are made in the eighth rib and two pericostal sutures of double strands of No. 2 chromatic catgut are inserted to encircle the eighth and sixth ribs. When tied these sutures will approximate the rib cage about the partially resected seventh rib. The partially resected segments (2 cm.) at the vertebral ends of the sixth and eighth ribs are also visible. The formation of periosteal "windows" is believed to lessen the incidence of postthoracotomy pain.

X. The completed closure of the skin incision with interrupted silk (000) sutures and the relation of the water-seal drainage catheter to the anterior rather than the middle or posterior portions of the incision is depicted.

Discussion—Dr. Garlock (cont.)

of the beginning of the greater curvature of the stomach than is depicted in Plate 55, M. The step of mobilization of the duodenum is always carried out in left sided esophagectomy for the reasons previously stated.

I believe there is an easier method of making the anastomosis in the supraaortic area than that depicted in Plate 55, R, R′, R″, R‴. Before placing the first posterior row of sutures, a button of stomach wall is excised from the upper anterior wall of the stomach. All vessels are carefully ligated with very fine silk. After aspiration of stomach contents (blood and mucus), the opening is approximated to the esophagus at a site proximal to the area of subsequent transection. The first posterior layer of sutures is now placed in a dry field, the esophagus is transected and the anastomosis is completed. Trying to ligate vessels in the stomach wall at the site of anastomosis while the stomach is located high in the chest greatly complicates the details of an already difficult procedure.

Finally, I have abandoned the operation of infraaortic anastomosis for squamous cell tumors of the distal esophagus because it is important to excise as much esophagus as possible proximal to the growth in order to get well beyond the submucosal spread so frequently seen in this location.

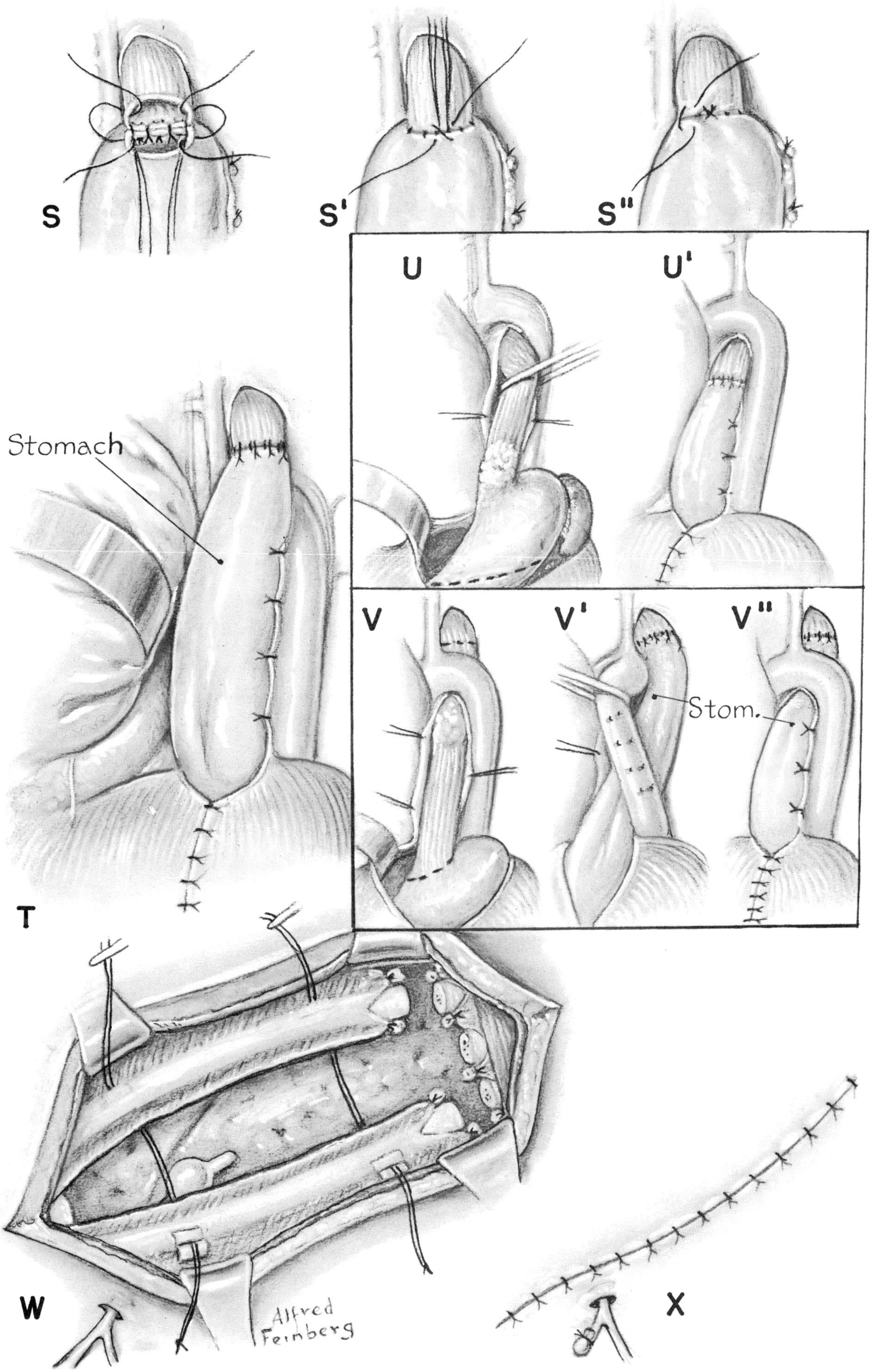
S
S'
S"
U
U'
Stomach
V
V'
V"
Stom.
T
W
Alfred Feinberg
X

ESOPHAGECTOMY. COMBINED RIGHT CERVICAL, RIGHT THORACIC, AND LEFT ABDOMINAL APPROACH, WITH CERVICAL ESOPHAGOGASTROSTOMY

A. The patient is placed in the supine position and the head is rotated to the left. The cervical incision, the first to be made, is demonstrated by the solid line. The right anterior thoracotomy and the left upper paramedian abdominal incisions, which are made in the order mentioned, are indicated in dotted outline.

B. The cervical incision is deepened through the subcutaneous fatty tissue and the platysma muscle layers to expose the sternomastoid muscle, the anterior border of which is being mobilized by scalpel dissection.

C. The mobilized anterior border of the sternomastoid muscle is retracted posteriorly, and the underlying anatomic structures are exposed.

C¹, D, D¹. The middle thyroid vein is firstly doubly ligated (000 silk) in continuity and then severed between the ligatures (C¹). This permits retraction of the right lobe of the thyroid gland anteriorly toward the midline and exposure of portions of the recurrent laryngeal nerve, the trachea, and the esophagus (D). The cervical portion of the esophagus, mobilized by finger dissection, is encircled by a traction tape of rubber tissue. The left index finger of the surgeon is inserted along the outside of the esophagus into the superior mediastinum and the tumor, located in this segment of the esophagus, is palpated (D¹). The use of this maneuver at this time may frequently indicate whether or not the lesion is locally resectable and thereby avoid the necessity of making either a thoracotomy or abdominal incision.

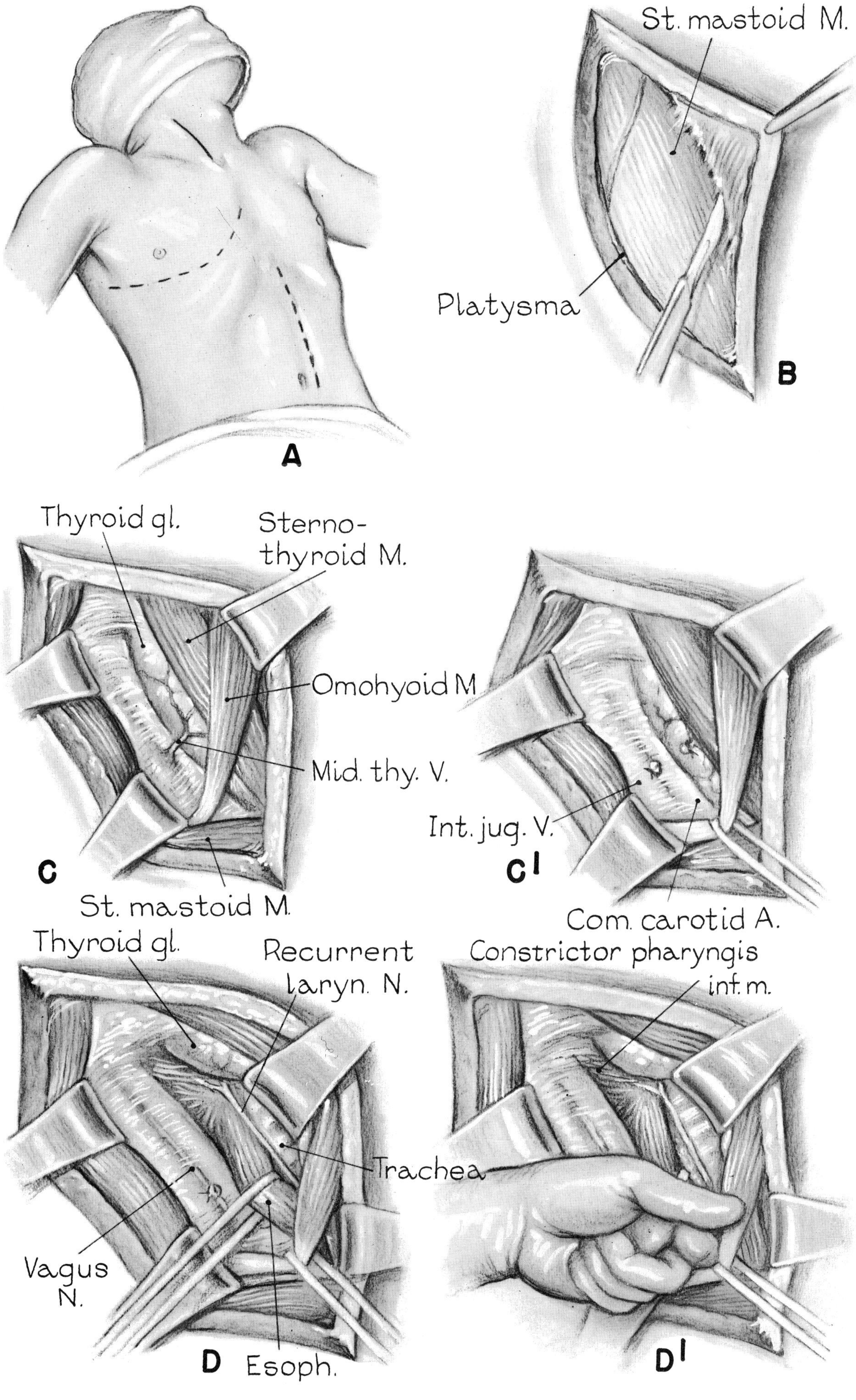
St. mastoid M.
Platysma
A
B
Thyroid gl.
Sterno-
thyroid M.
Omohyoid M
Mid. thy. V.
Int. jug. V.
C
C'
St. mastoid M.
Com. carotid A.
Thyroid gl.
Recurrent
laryn. N.
Constrictor pharyngis
inf. m.
Trachea
Vagus
N.
D
Esoph.
D'

E. The cervical mediastinotomy and the digital exploration of the superior mediastinum is completed. The second incision to be made, a right anterolateral thoracic incision, is indicated in dotted outline.

F, F¹. The incision is deepened through the underlying pectoralis major and the latissimus dorsi muscles, the superficial muscle layers (F), and then through the pectoralis minor and serratus anterior (magnus) muscles, the deep muscle layers, to expose the rib cage and one of the related intercostal muscle layers (F¹).

G. The wound margins are retracted and portions of the second, third, and fourth ribs are exposed. An incision is made in the periosteum throughout the length of the exposed portion of the fourth rib and with a periosteal elevator the periosteum is removed from the lower half of the rib.

G¹. The dissection of the periosteum from the fourth rib posteriorly is completed, and, by blunt digital dissection, a plane of cleavage is obtained between the endothoracic fascia and the posterior aspects of the second and third ribs respectively after the manner of Sir R. C. Brock. The adjacent intercostal muscle bundles are doubly clamped, severed, and ligated with suture ligatures of 000 silk. The incision in the endothoracic fascia and the parietal pleura behind the fourth rib is shown in dotted outline.

H. The right pleural cavity is entered and the wound margins are retracted over protective moist towels with a self-retaining retractor (Finochietto) to expose portions of the lobes of the lung.

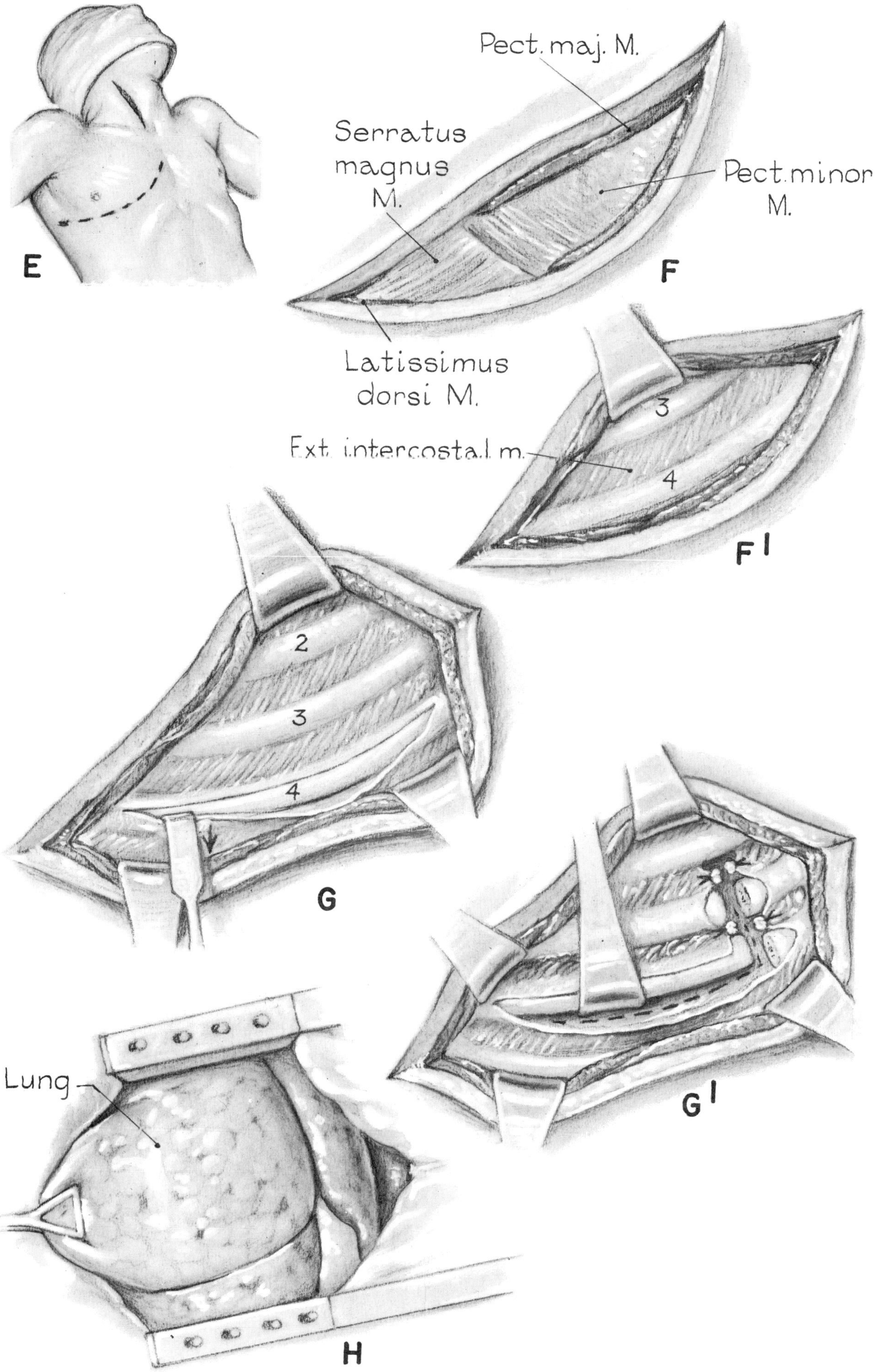
E
Pect. maj. M.
Serratus
magnus
M.
Pect. minor
M.
F
Latissimus
dorsi M.
3
Ext. intercostal m.
4
F'
2
3
4
G
G'
Lung
H

I, J. The right lung is retracted anteriorly and toward the midline to expose the related structures posteriorly. The azygos vein is mobilized on a curved clamp preparatory to withdrawing the first of two silk (00) ligatures for ligation of the vein in continuity (I). Subsequently the azygos vein is doubly clamped between the two ligatures and severed. Each clamp is then replaced by a suture ligature of 00 silk (J).

K, K¹. The severance and ligation of the azygos vein is completed (K), and the mediastinal pleura is incised to expose the thoracic segment of the esophagus and the tumor located in its proximal portion above the aortic arch (K¹).

L. The caudad end of the thoracic esophagus is encircled by a cotton tape for traction as mobilization of the esophagus is continued by blunt digital dissection.

L¹. The partially mobilized thoracic esophagus is retracted laterally and posteriorly and the second of two of the esophageal arterial branches from the thoracic aorta is doubly clamped prior to its severance. One of the ligated stumps of the esophageal artery previously ligated and severed is also visible.

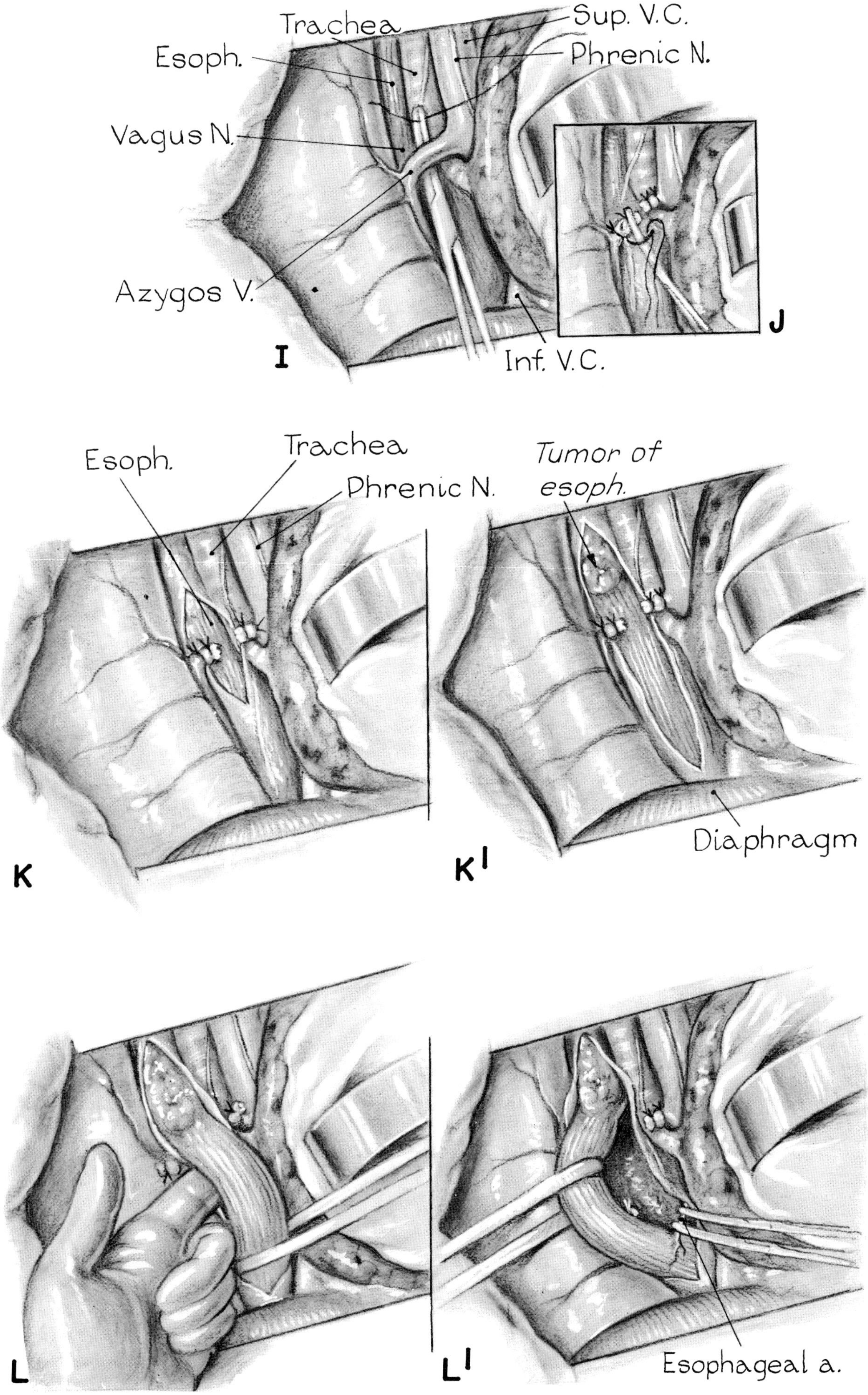
Trachea
Sup. V.C.
Esoph.
Phrenic N.
Vagus N.
Azygos V.
Inf. V.C.
I
J
Esoph.
Trachea
Phrenic N.
Tumor of esoph.
Diaphragm
K
K'
L
L'
Esophageal a.

M, M¹, M². The third incision, an upper left paramedian muscle-retracting (lateral) abdominal incision is depicted in dotted outline (M). This incision is deepened through the anterior rectus sheath, and the underlying left rectus muscle is mobilized from its midline attachment (M¹). An incision is made in the posterior rectus sheath and anterior parietal peritoneum, and the incised margins are grasped in clamps (M¹) preparatory to extension of the incision both cephalad and caudad to expose the underlying intraperitoneal viscera (M²).

N. The left lobe of the liver, mobilized by severance of the avascular left triangular ligament, is turned downward on itself and retracted toward the midline. By manual traction the stomach is displaced downward, and by scissor dissection an opening is made through the musculofascial fibers of the diaphragm overlying the lower end of the esophagus immediately cephalad to the esophagocardial junction.

N¹. By digital dissection within the posterior mediastinum the lower end of the esophagus is mobilized on the index finger. The anterior (left) vagus nerve is severed and a silver brain (Cushing) clip is applied to its proximal cut end. The posterior (right) vagus nerve is mobilized on a nerve hook prior to its severance. The transection of the vagus nerves is a technical aid in the freeing of the esophagus from its surrounding attachments.

O, O¹. The completely freed lower end of the esophagus is encircled by a tape of rubber tissue for both future identification and traction (O). Mobilization of the greater curvature of the stomach below the gastroepiploic arch is begun by serially clamping and severing the gastrocolic ligament (O¹). The maintenance of continuity of the gastroepiploic arch is important in assuring an adequate blood supply to the stomach when its mobilization is completed.

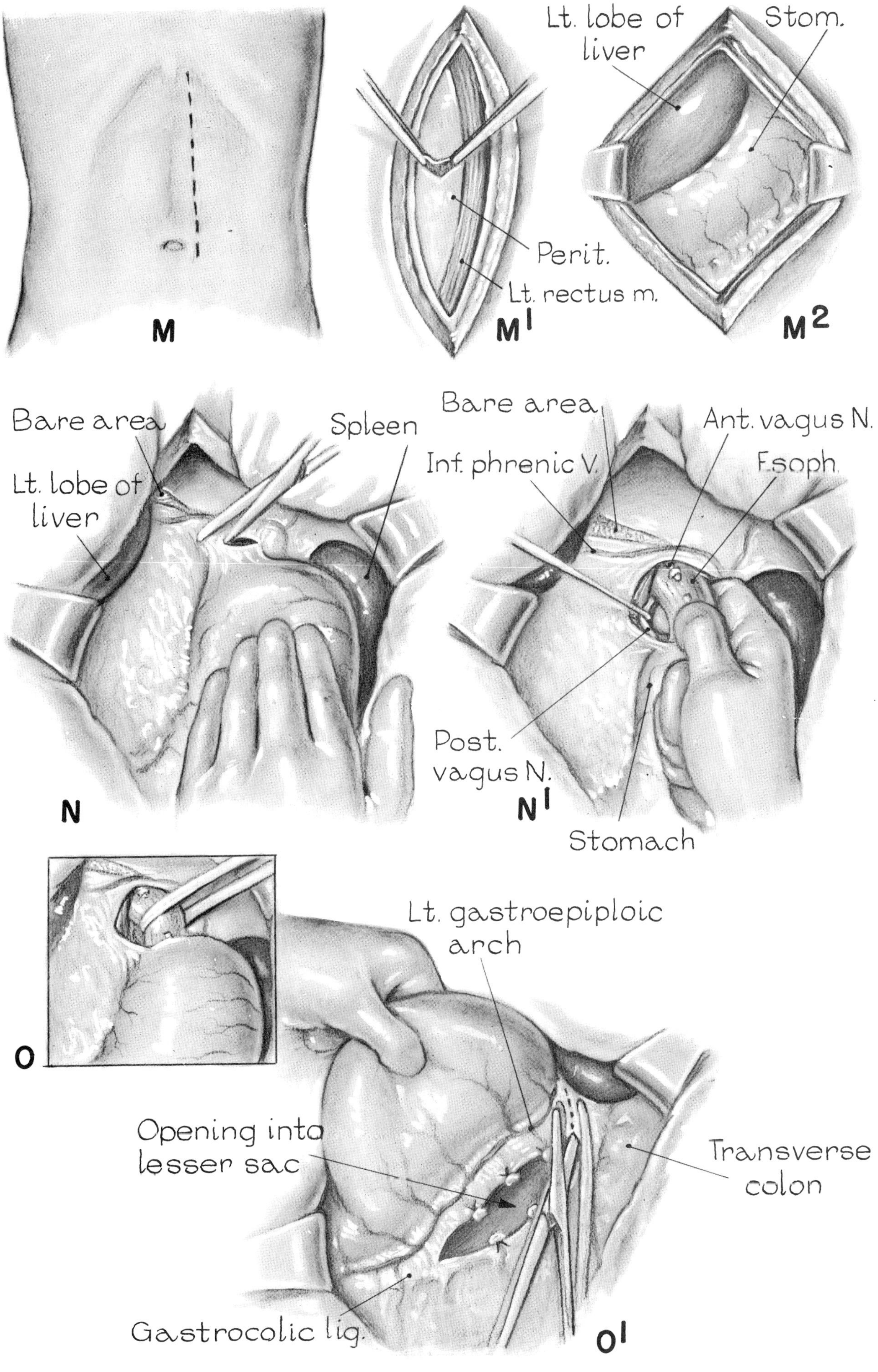
Lt. lobe of liver
Stom.
Perit.
Lt. rectus m.
M
M1
M2
Bare area
Spleen
Lt. lobe of liver
N
Bare area
Ant. vagus N.
Inf. phrenic V.
Esoph.
Post. vagus N.
N1
Stomach
O
Lt. gastroepiploic arch
Opening into lesser sac
Transverse colon
Gastrocolic lig.
O1

P. Mobilization of the greater curvature and fundus of the stomach is continued by serially clamping and severing the gastrosplenic ligament and its contained vasa brevia.

Q. Upon completion of the mobilization of the fundus of the greater curvature of the stomach, an incision, indicated by the dotted line, is made in the posterior parietal peritoneum lateral and inferior to the descending (second part) and horizontal (third part) portions of the duodenum before freeing it by blunt digital dissection posteriorly.

Q¹. The duodenal loop and the head of the pancreas are mobilized by blunt digital dissection in the relatively avascular areolar tissue plane posteriorly, and the related anatomic structures are depicted. The dissection of the horizontal portion of the duodenum is continued medially until the superior mesenteric vascular stalk and the uncinate process of the pancreas are identified. In this dissection caution must be observed to avoid making a rent in the base of the mesentery of the colon through which the small bowel may herniate.

Q². The finger of the right hand of the surgeon is inserted behind the mobilized greater curvature of the stomach, and after transgressing the lesser sac, an opening is made in the velumous gastrohepatic ligament from behind by blunt digital dissection. The transection of this ligament to mobilize the whole of the lesser curvature of the stomach is indicated by the dotted line. The continuity of the right gastric artery on the lesser curvature similar to the continuity of the right gastroepiploic artery on the greater curvature is preserved.

Discussion—Dr. John H. Garlock. It has been and still is my practice to use the right sided approach for cancers of the esophagus located behind the aortic arch or more proximally up to the general level of the suprasternal notch. The technic of Ivor Lewis, requiring three separate incisions, as depicted in A, Plate 57, has been replaced by a right thoracoabdominal incision, traversing the sixth or seventh interspace with division of the cartilaginous costal arch and extension downward along the upper midabdomen. Of course, the final esophagogastric anastomosis in the neck requires a cervical incision either on the right or left side, depending on how easily the cervical esophagus swings to one or the other side. To accomplish this operative approach, the thoracic portion of the operation can be more expeditiously carried out if the patient is tilted forward about 45 degrees. When mobilization of the stomach becomes indicated, the table may be tilted backwards so that the patient assumes the straight supine position. This makes it much easier to separate the stomach from its vascular attachments and permits the surgeon to handle the stomach with a minimum of trauma, an important feature in the prevention of thrombosis in the stomach wall. The cervical incision is, therefore, the last one made, after it has been determined that one is dealing with a resectable tumor. It is usually not possible to determine operability of an esophageal cancer located in the superior mediastinum by finger exploration through the cervical incision.

With the use of the thoracoabdominal incision, it is unnecessary to remove ribs, thereby eliminating all possibility of subsequent intercostal neuralgia, a disabling aftermath which frequently follows the maneuvers depicted (Plate 58, E through H).

Dissection of the esophagus from the mediastinum should include all removable areolar tissue and careful ligation of the segmental esophageal arteries arising from the descending aorta. Fatal postoperative

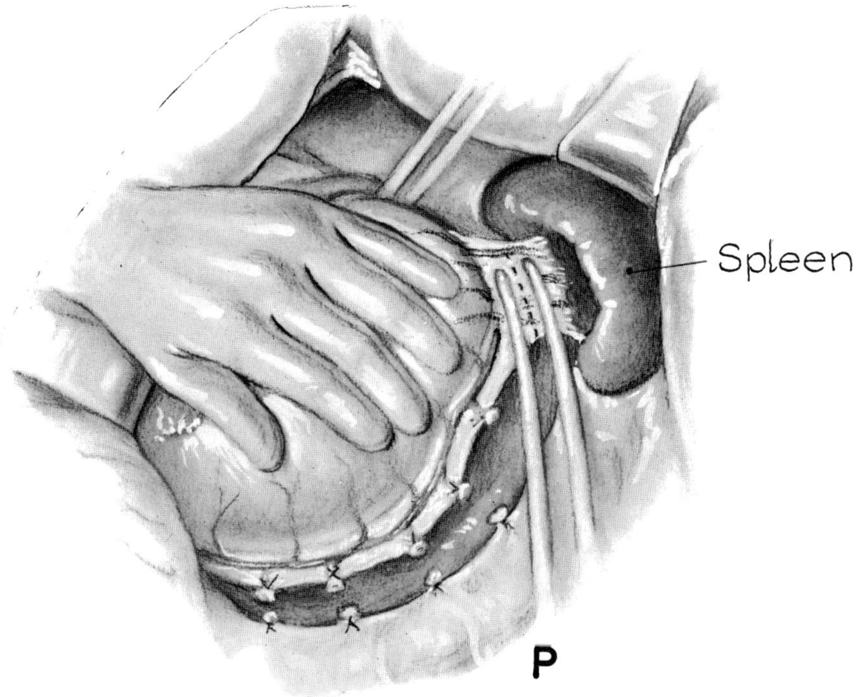
Spleen

P

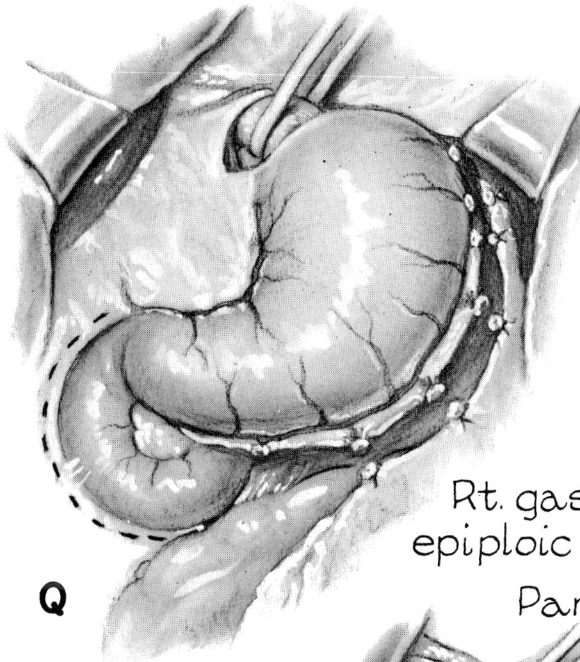

Q

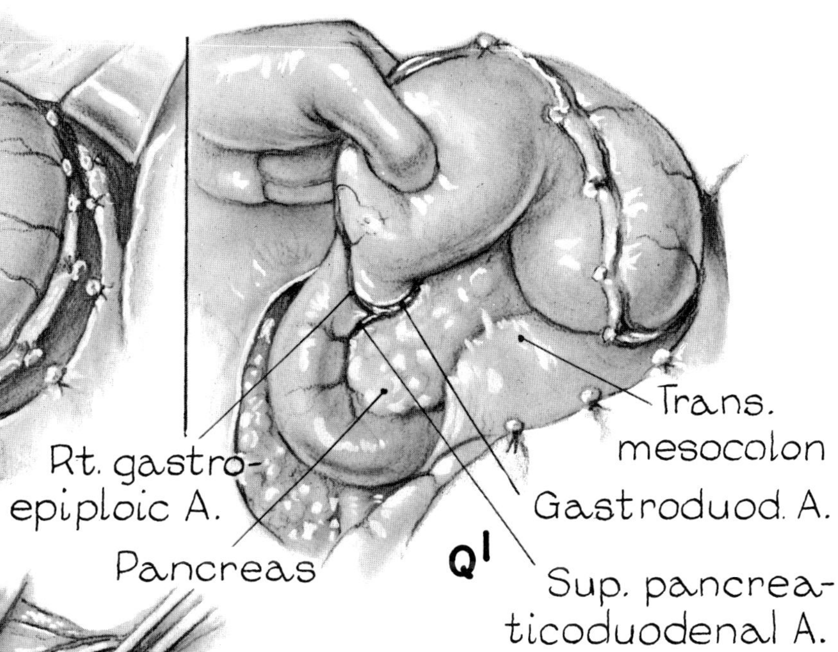
Trans. mesocolon
Rt. gastro-epiploic A.
Gastroduod. A.
Pancreas
Sup. pancreaticoduodenal A.

Q¹

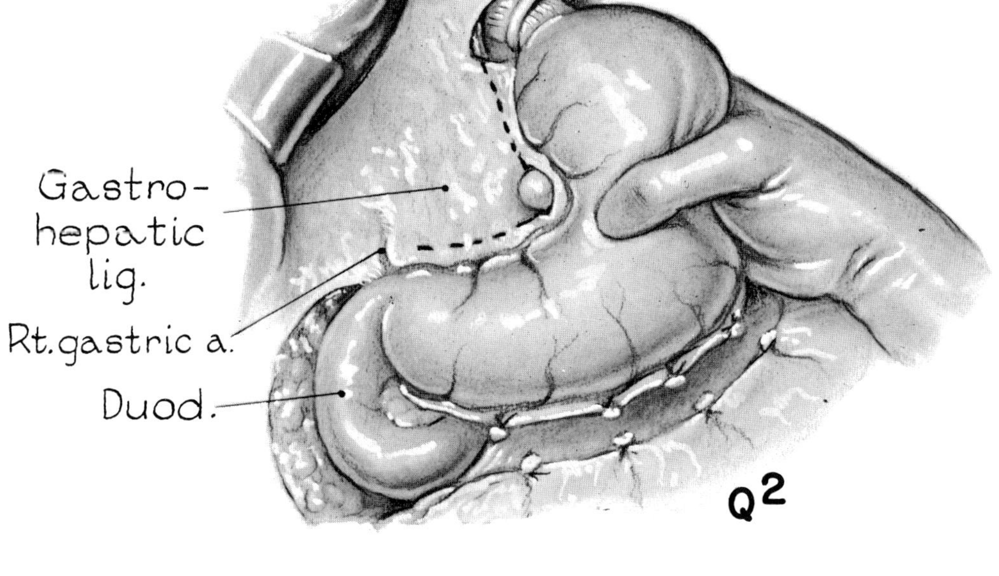
Gastro-hepatic lig.
Rt. gastric a.
Duod.

Q²

Q[3]. The mobilized greater curvature of the stomach is rotated anteriorly and retracted cephalad to demonstrate the left gastric vessels contained within the gastropancreatic fold of peritoneum, triply clamped prior to severance between the two distal clamps.

Q[4]. The stomach is replaced in its normal position and the remaining intact segment of the gastrohepatic ligament is serially clamped and severed as indicated.

R. The mobilization of the lesser and the greater curvatures of the stomach is completed and the lower portion of the esophagus and proximal portion of the stomach are retracted to expose the hiatal ring which is formed by the separation of the muscle fibers of the right crus into superficial and deep muscle layers.

R[1]. The cardioesophageal region, encircled by a cotton tape for traction, is displaced downward and laterally to demonstrate the transection of the superficial layer of muscle fibers of the right crus which forms the right margin of the hiatal ring. This maneuver enlarges the hiatal ring and facilitates the transplantation of the mobilized stomach from the peritoneal cavity into the right pleural cavity.

S. By manual manipulation from below and upward traction from within the thoracic incision above, the stomach is displaced through the enlarged esophageal hiatus into the right pleural cavity.

S[1]. The transplantation of all but the distal segment of the pyloric portion of the stomach into the right pleural cavity is completed, and the change in position of the related viscera within the peritoneal cavity is illustrated.

Discussion—Dr. Garlock (cont.)

hemorrhage has been known to occur from one of these vessels ligated too close to the aorta.

The importance of gentle handling of the stomach through all phases of its mobilization and subsequent transplantation in the chest cannot be overemphasized. There is every reason to believe that local trauma may produce thrombosis and localized necrosis with perforation in the early postoperative period. Another important feature in the adequate mobilization, depicted in Plate 61, Q and Q[1], is concerned with the freeing of the second and third parts of the duodenum. This maneuver prevents axial rotation of the duodenum when the stomach is transplanted into the chest and also provides increased length to the stomach in its new position.

In Plate 63, T, the line of transection of the stomach is indicated by a dotted line. I would suggest removal of at least two more inches of the beginning of the greater curvature so that the line of transection is more oblique than depicted. The reason for this is that the most precarious area from the standpoint of adequate blood supply is located here. Almost all postoperative leakages have occurred in this region. This usually fatal complication has been obviated in recent years by removal of the potentially dangerous area.

The importance of not inserting too many sutures at the anastomosis is clearly shown in V through V[7], Plate 64. Oversuturing this area may lead to obliteration of the tenuous blood supply of the esophageal stump which receives its nourishment here from small branches of the inferior thyroid arteries.

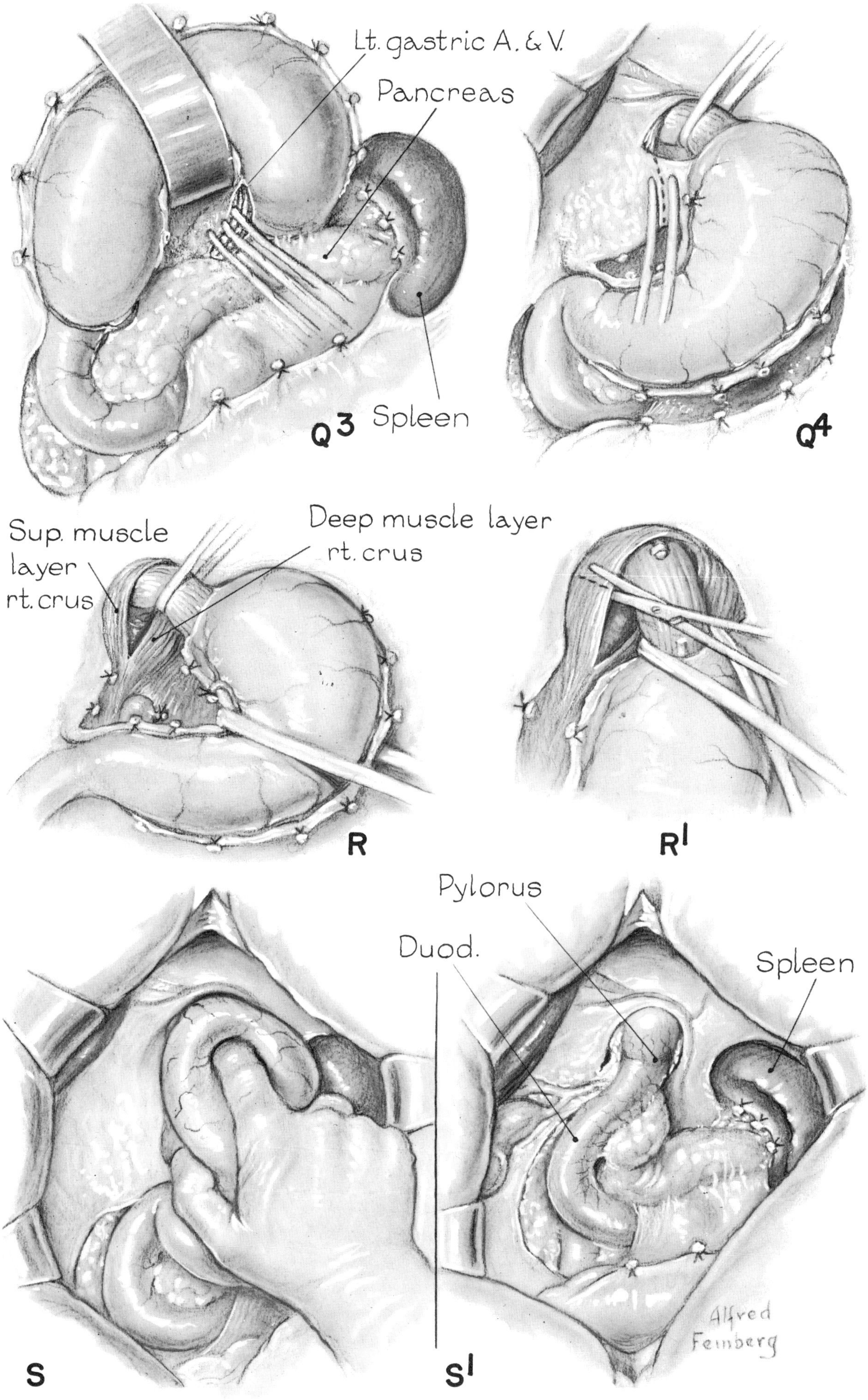
Lt. gastric A. & V.
Pancreas
Spleen
Q3
Q4
Sup. muscle layer rt. crus
Deep muscle layer rt. crus
R
R1
Pylorus
Duod.
Spleen
S
S1
Alfred Feinberg

T, T[1]. The completion of the transplantation of the stomach into the right pleural cavity is shown. The lower end of the esophagus is occluded by a clamp preparatory to the resection of a subjacent segment of the stomach which is indicated by the dotted line. Accordingly, resection of the whole of the caudad portion of the esophagus is assured. The transected esophagogastric stump is occluded with a piece of rubber dam and the opening in the gastric lumen is closed in two layers using interrupted sutures of 000 silk (T^1).

U, U[1]. By a combination of digital traction through the cervical incision and manual manipulation from within the thoracic incision (U), the mobilized thoracic and abdominal segments of the esophagus are displaced upward into and out through the right cervical incision (U^1). In like manner the fundus of the transplanted stomach, secured by traction guy sutures of silk (00), is mobilized into the cervical mediastinum (U^1).

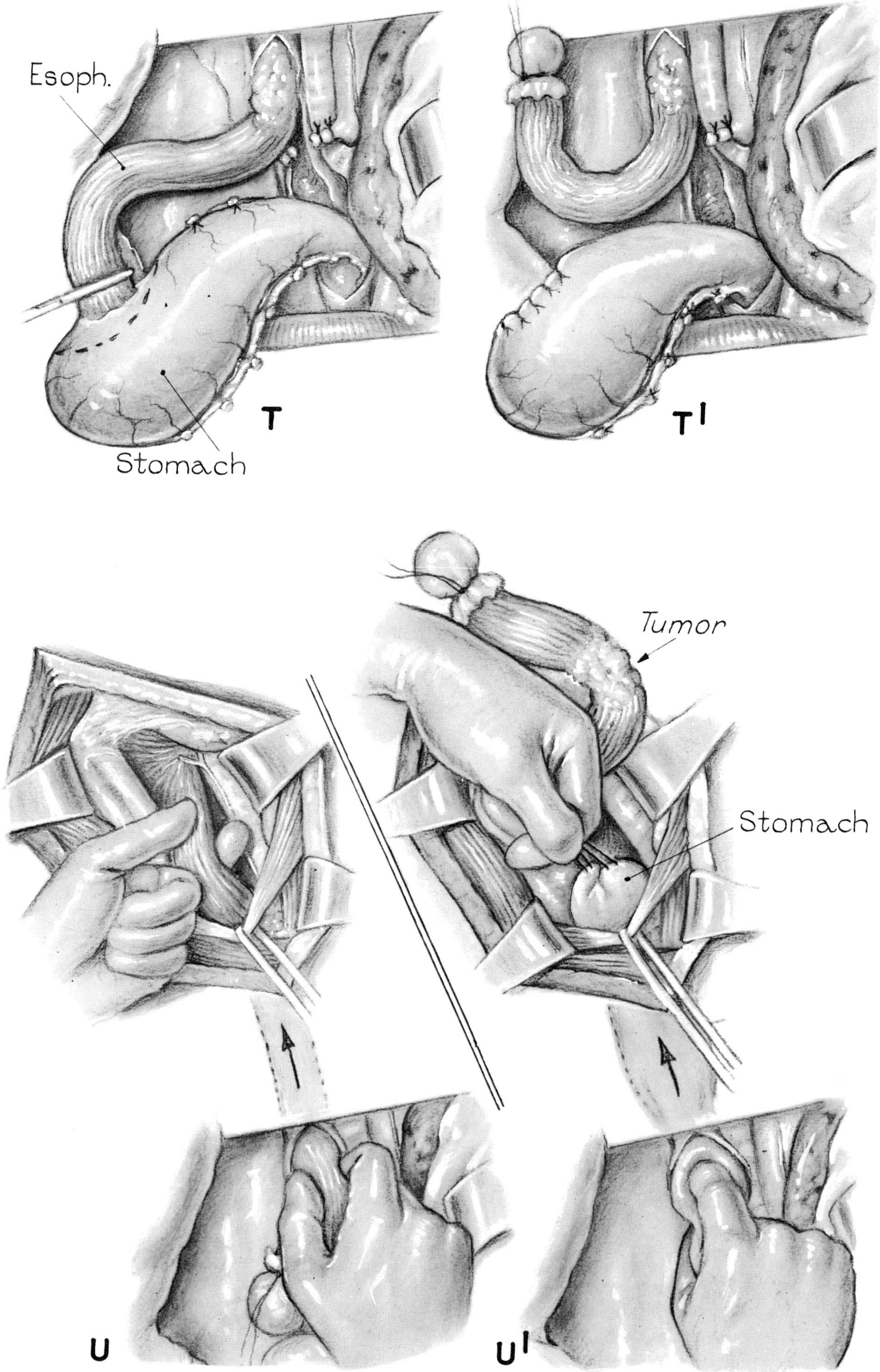
Esoph.
Stomach
T
T'
Tumor
Stomach
U
U'

V. For technical expediency an opening is made in the fundic portion of the stomach before the insertion of the interrupted silk sutures (000) which form the first posterior layer of the esophagogastric anastomosis. To increase the holding power of the tissues of the esophagus these sutures are inserted in the wall of the esophagus at right angles to its longitudinal layer of muscle fibers.

V^1. The first posterior layer of sutures is tied to approximate the posterior wall of the stomach and the fundus of the esophagus. Two of the series of through and through interrupted sutures which will comprise the second posterior layer are inserted at either angle of the anastomosis but are not tied.

V^2. The insertion of the second layer of sutures posteriorly is completed, and the transection of the esophagus anteriorly is being completed by scissor dissection.

V^3. The first anterior layer of the anastomosis consists of a series of interrupted silk (000) sutures which are inserted from the "inside out" to the "outside in" so that, when tied, the knots are on the inside of the lumen. The first angle suture anteriorly is inserted but not tied. Traction in the long axis of the anastomosis is applied to the strands of the angle suture posteriorly as the anterior angle suture is tied. This facilitates the inversion of the first layer of the anastomosis anteriorly.

V^4. V^5. V^6, V^7. The interrupted sutures are inserted alternately from either end toward the center (V^4) where the first layer anteriorly terminates (V^5). The site of termination of these sutures is encircled by a figure of 8 mattress suture (V^5) which, when tied (V^6), lessens the likelihood of an anastomotic leakage. For the second layer anteriorly a series of interrupted mattress sutures (000 silk) is used (V^6). These sutures are inserted at right angles to the layer of longitudinal muscle fibers of the esophagus (V^6) and when tied (V^7) a telescoping of the esophagus into the serosal lined wall of the stomach is effected.

W. This is a view through the cervical incision showing the completed esophagogastrostomy and its relation to the surrounding structures.

X. This is a view from within the right pleural cavity showing the right lung retracted anteriorly toward the midline and the transplanted stomach attached to the cut margins of the mediastinal pleura with a series of interrupted silk (000) sutures.

Y. The operation is completed and the cervical, thoracic, and abdominal incisions are closed. The relation of the transplanted stomach to these incisions is depicted in transparent outline.

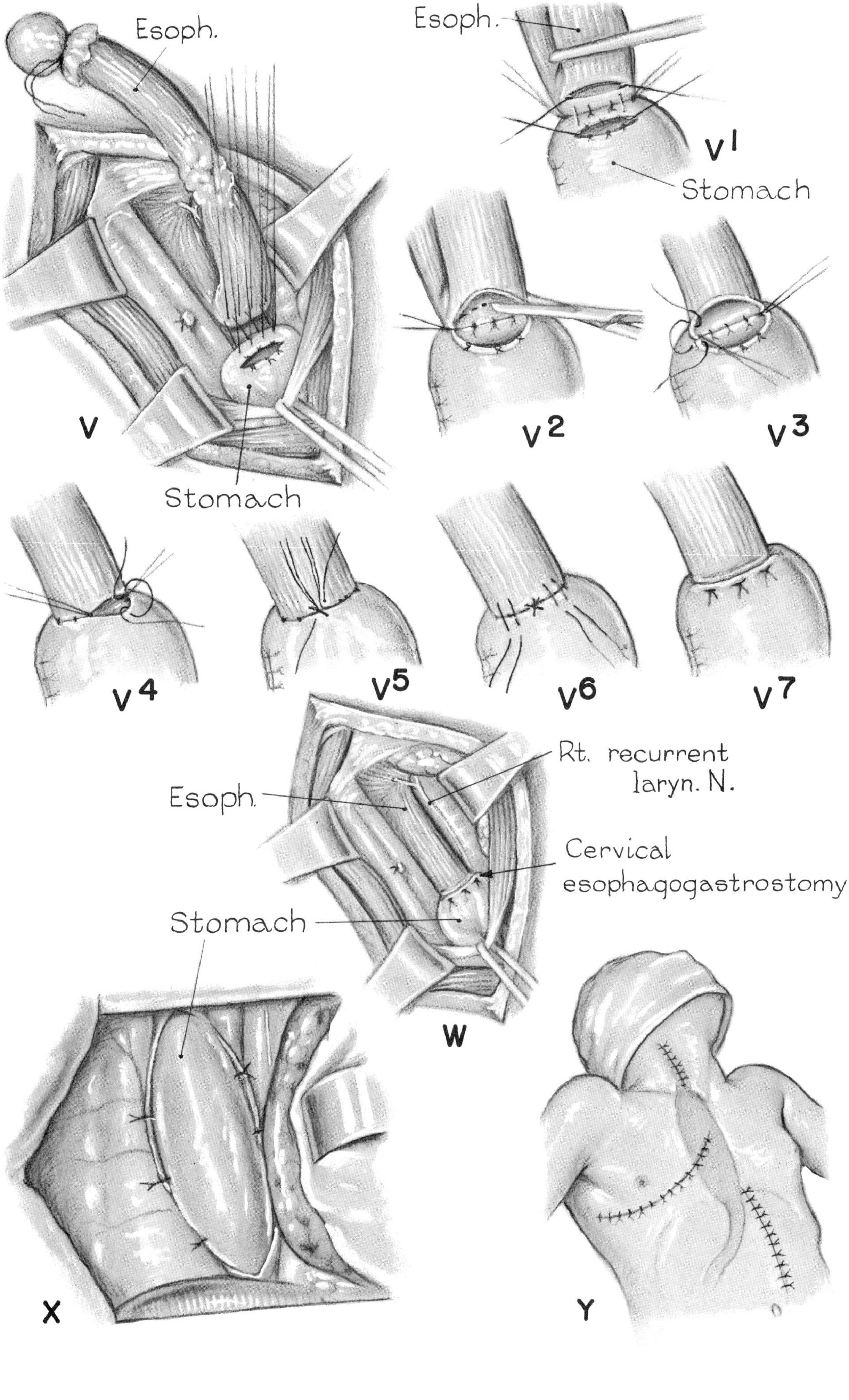
Esoph.
Stomach
V
Esoph.
Stomach
V1
V2
V3
V4
V5
V6
V7
Rt. recurrent
laryn. N.
Esoph.
Cervical
esophagogastrostomy
Stomach
W
X
Y

ESOPHAGECTOMY—RIGHT TRANSPLEURAL APPROACH

A. The patient is placed in the direct left lateral prone position with the left side elevated on a pillow support. The oblique posterolateral incision is shown by the solid line and its subsequent anterior extension by the broken line.

B. The sixth rib is partially resected, as is a segment of the fifth rib posteriorly. This additional segmental resection posteriorly is usually unnecessary. The severed and ligated ends of the fifth intercostal muscle bundle are visible.

C. The pleural cavity is entered through an incision in the bed of the sixth rib, and the rib margins are retracted. Filmy adhesions between the lung and the underlying esophagus are separated by blunt dissection with a gauze pledget.

D. The tumor of the esophagus is now exposed, and its relation to the remaining adherent segment of the right lung is visible.

E. The dissection of the adherent lung is completed, and the mobilized tumor bearing segment of the middle and lower thirds of the esophagus is encircled by cotton tapes and elevated from its "bed" in the posterior mediastinum. The relation of the tumor to the surrounding structures is depicted.

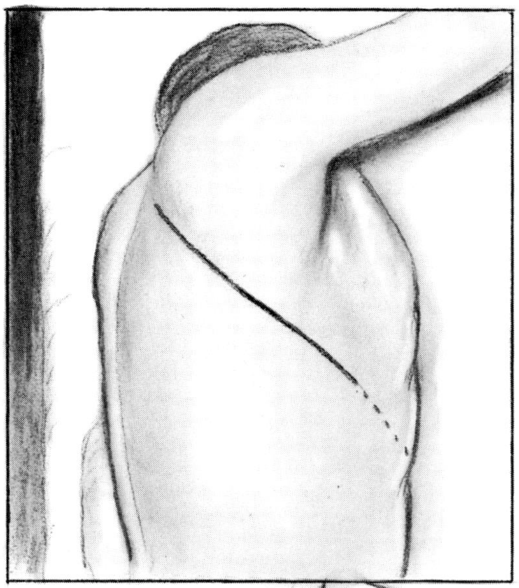

A

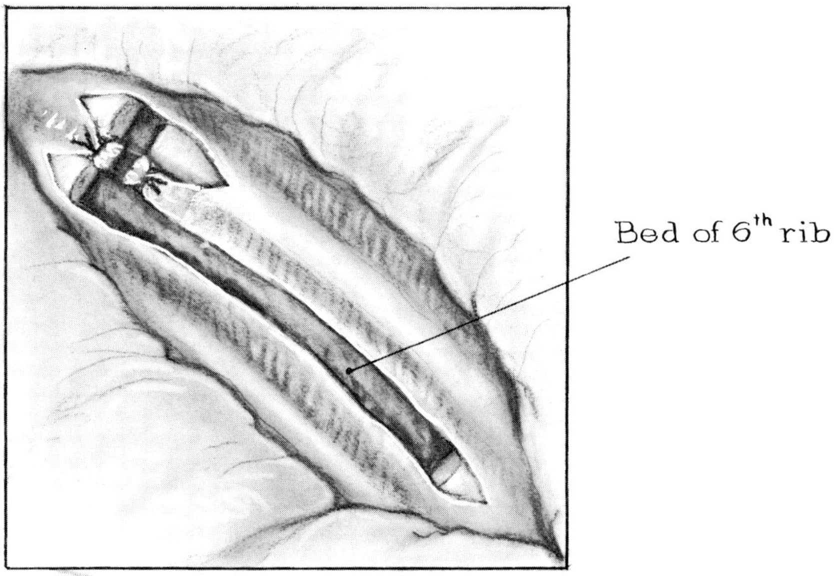
Bed of 6th rib

B

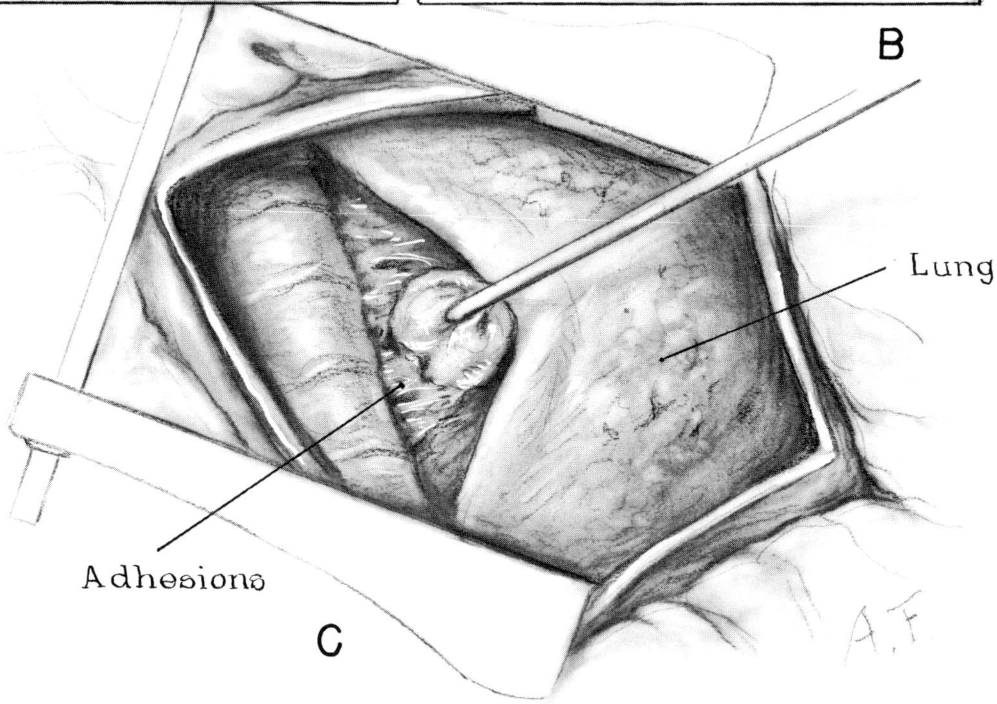
Lung
Adhesions
A.F.

C

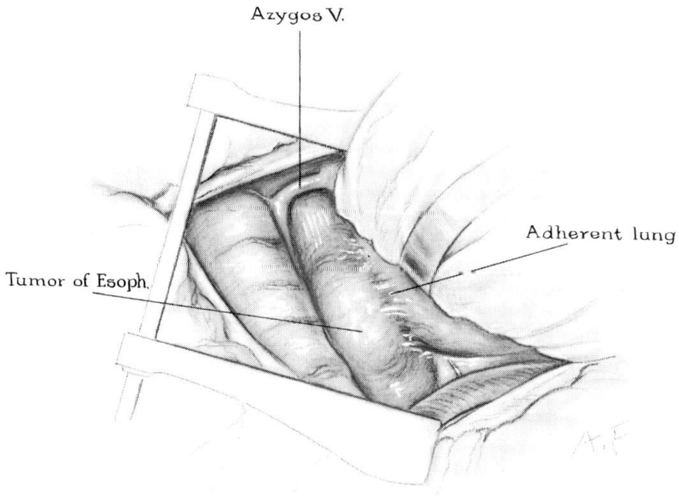
Azygos V.
Adherent lung
Tumor of Esoph.

D

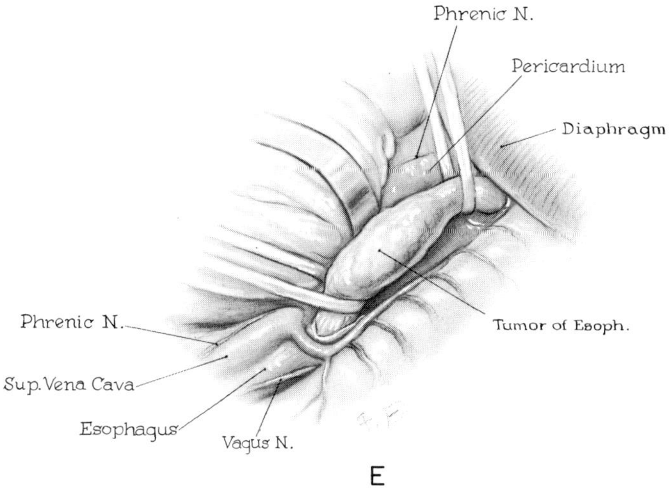
Phrenic N.
Pericardium
Diaphragm
Tumor of Esoph.
Phrenic N.
Sup. Vena Cava
Esophagus
Vagus N.

E

F. The stomach is mobilized upward through the esophageal hiatus into the right pleural cavity. During the transplantation from the peritoneal to the pleural cavity, branches of the left gastric artery were clamped, severed, and ligated to free the lesser curvature of the stomach. The esophagus at the esophagocardial junction is doubly clamped with right-angled clamps and transected between the clamps as indicated by the broken line.

G. The cardiac orifice of the stomach is closed in two layers using interrupted sutures of 000 silk. The fundus of the stomach is elevated with forceps, and the site of the anastomotic incision is indicated (broken line). The proximal transected end of the esophagus is retracted cephalad, and the opening to be made into its lumen for anastomosis with the fundus of the stomach is represented by the broken line.

H. The two-layer anastomosis posteriorly is completed, interrupted sutures of 000 silk being used. The first layer is an approximation of the serosa of the stomach to the muscle wall of the esophagus. The second layer is comprised of a series of through-and-through sutures that include all the layers of the cut margins of the esophagus and stomach. The Levin tube is inserted beyond the anastomosis into the lumen of the stomach.

I. The first suture layer anteriorly is begun. Each suture is inserted from the inside-out on the esophagus and from the outside-in on the stomach, so that when tied the knot is on the inside of the lumen. Medial traction on the suture previously inserted facilitates the inversion of the cut margins. The sutures are inserted alternately from either end and terminate in the center of the anastomosis, where they are encircled by a figure-of-8 mattress suture to complete the first anterior layer of sutures.

J. The second anterior layer of the anastomosis is comprised of a series of interrupted mattress (Lembert-Cushing) sutures that are inserted at right angles to the longitudinal muscle fibers of the esophagus to reinforce the holding power of the tissue.

K. The mattress sutures are all first inserted and tied individually and then cut to complete the esophagogastrostomy. When tied, the sutures forming the second anterior layer effect a cap-like covering of serosa on the esophagus.

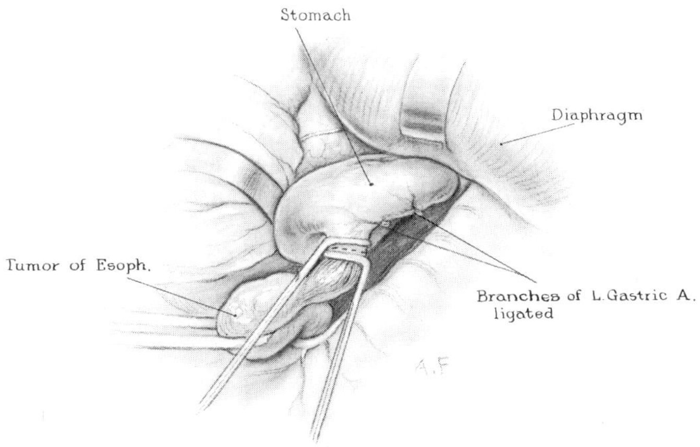
Stomach
Diaphragm
Tumor of Esoph.
Branches of L.Gastric A. ligated

F

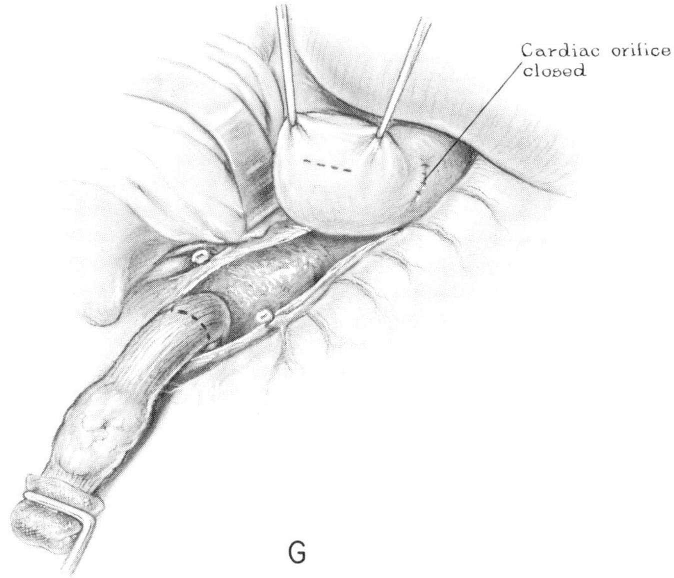
Cardiac orifice closed

G

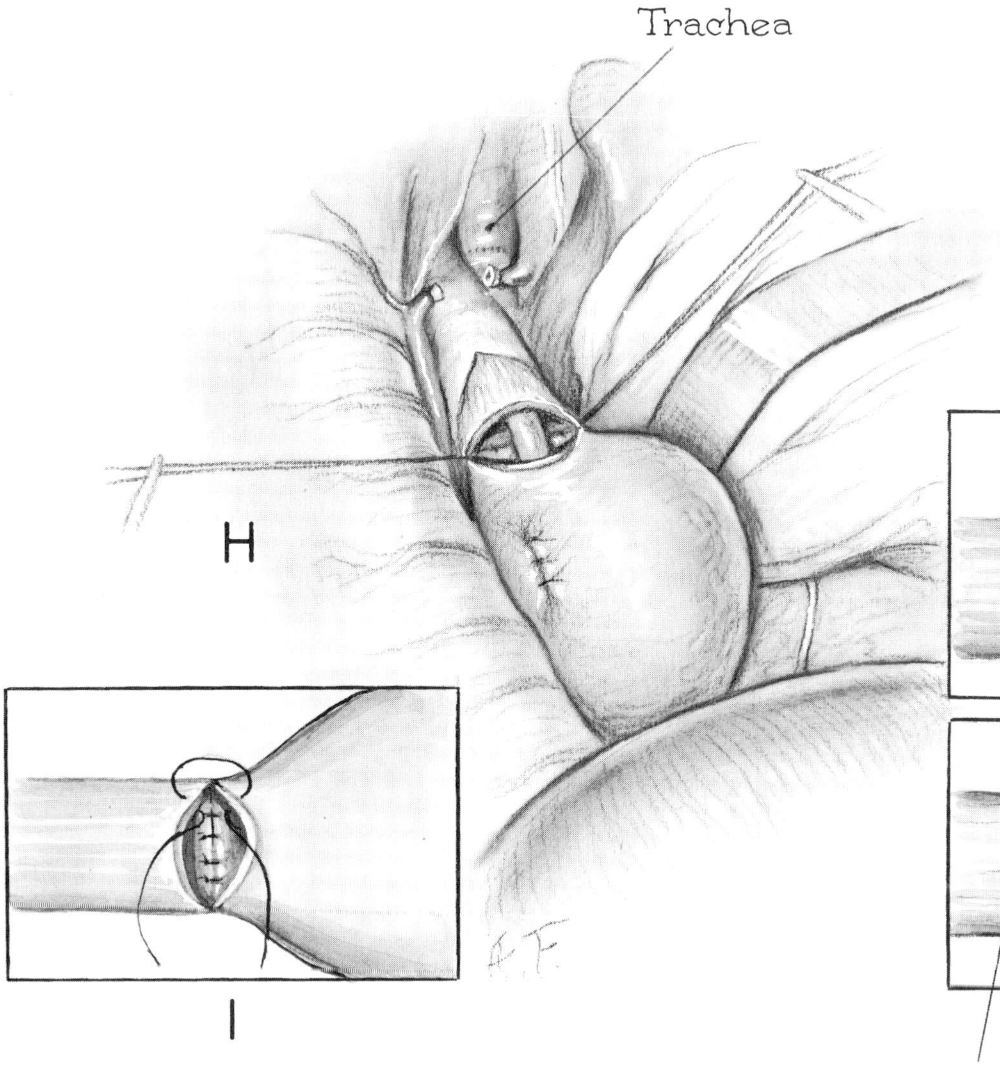
Trachea

H

I

J

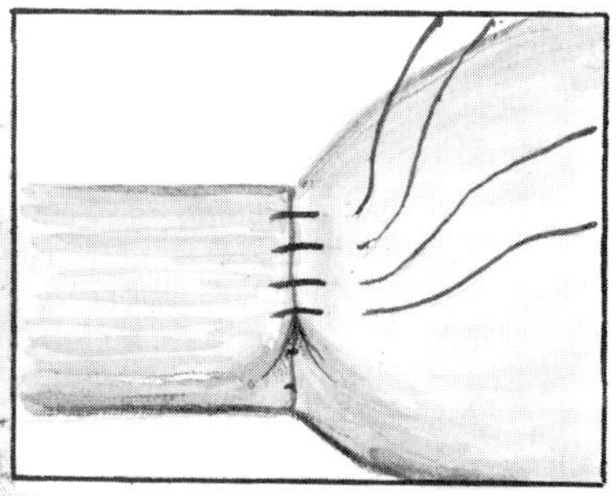

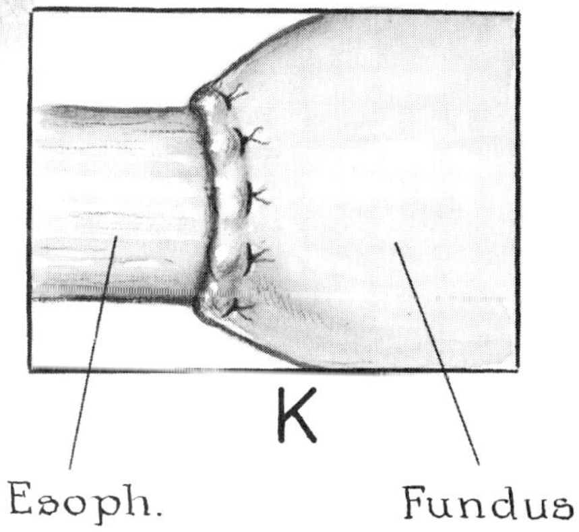
Esoph.
Fundus

K

ESOPHAGECTOMY AND COLON TRANSPLANT

A. The patient is placed in the supine position, and the right side is elevated to a 20°-25° angle with the horizontal. The right paramedian abdominal incision and the right anterolateral thoracic incision are indicated by solid and broken lines, respectively.

B. The peritoneal cavity is entered, and the right side of the colon is mobilized by severance of the fascia fusion layer Toldt ("white line") and the right phrenocolic ligament as indicated by the broken line. The transverse colon is subsequently mobilized by dissection of the relatively avascular attachments of the greater omentum.

C, C′. The superior mesenteric artery and its branches in relation to the small and large bowel are depicted (C). The mobilization of the ileocolic segment for esophageal bypass is begun by the transection of the branches of the ileocolic artery proximal to the marginal colic artery (C, C′).

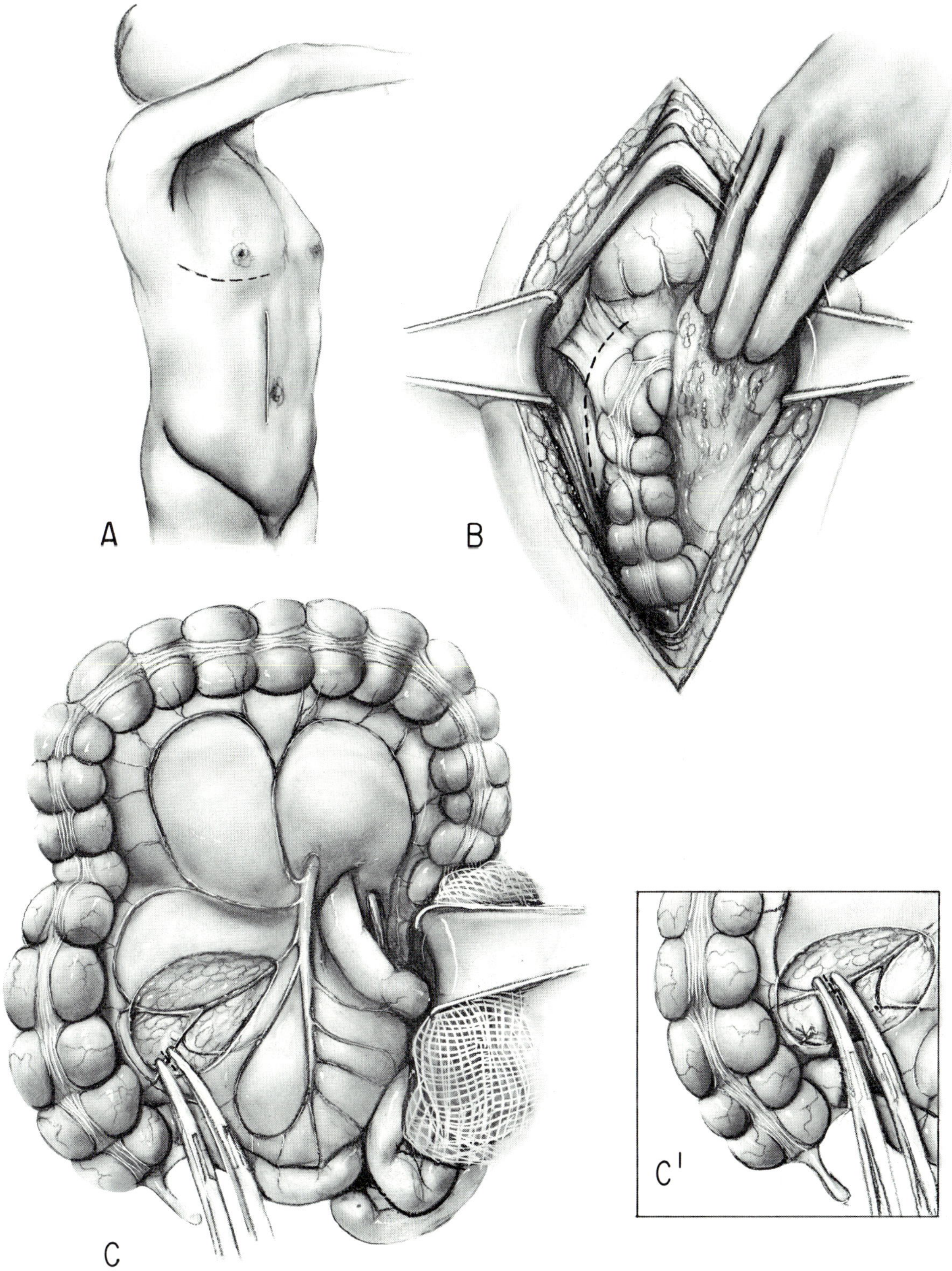
A
B
C
C'

D. The mobilized segment of cecoascending colon and its intact marginal artery are visible. The terminal ileum is severed (broken line) between clamps, the jaws of which are held firmly together but not locked.

D_1, D_2, D_3, D_4. The distal end of the terminal ileum is inverted in two layers, using interrupted sutures of 000 silk as indicated. The first layer of sutures is inserted from the inside-out to the outside-in (D_2) so that, when tied, the knots are on the inside of the lumen. For the second layer of closure interrupted seroserosal or Lembert sutures are employed (D_3). The appendix is then removed and its stump inverted with a pursestring suture of 000 silk (D_4).

DISCUSSION—DR. EARLE B. MAHONEY. The use of colon transplant in esophageal surgery, which has become a commonly accepted procedure during recent years, may be used in a rather wide variety of conditions. The right or the left colon may be used to reconstitute the gastrointestinal tract following total esophagectomy for carcinoma or for replacement when benign lesions, such as intractable strictures, may require esophagectomy. The colon may be used as a bypass for intractable strictures or as a palliative bypass around an inoperable carcinoma. The choice of whether the right or left colon is used depends on a surgeon's experience, but I prefer the right colon and frequently use the distal right colon with terminal ileum. The technic of the operation is very demanding, and extreme care must be used in handling tissue. Failure to observe the minute details of careful surgical technic will lead to necrosis of the transplant and failure of the operative procedure.

The technic of esophagocoloplasty for bypass of a lesion in the lower esophagus is very well illustrated and accurately described. This technic may be used when a benign or malignant lesion is encountered, usually one causing obstruction and in the presence of a normal proximal esophagus. There are, however, several alternate minor details of technic that may at times be very helpful. In the procedure illustrated the terminal ileum is not used in the transplant but is turned in and closed, as indicated in illustrations D-D_4. The vascular arcades of the terminal ileum and of the cecum vary in individuals, and I have found that frequently a much longer segment of the terminal ileum may be saved with very adequate blood supply and this can be used for the proximal anastomosis to the esophagus. In this technic it may be necessary to use only a portion of the ascending colon in addition to the terminal ileum. This involves, of course, conserving a longer segment of the ileo-colic vessels and utilizing the anastomotic arcades to the terminal ileum.

E shows division of the ileocolic artery and of

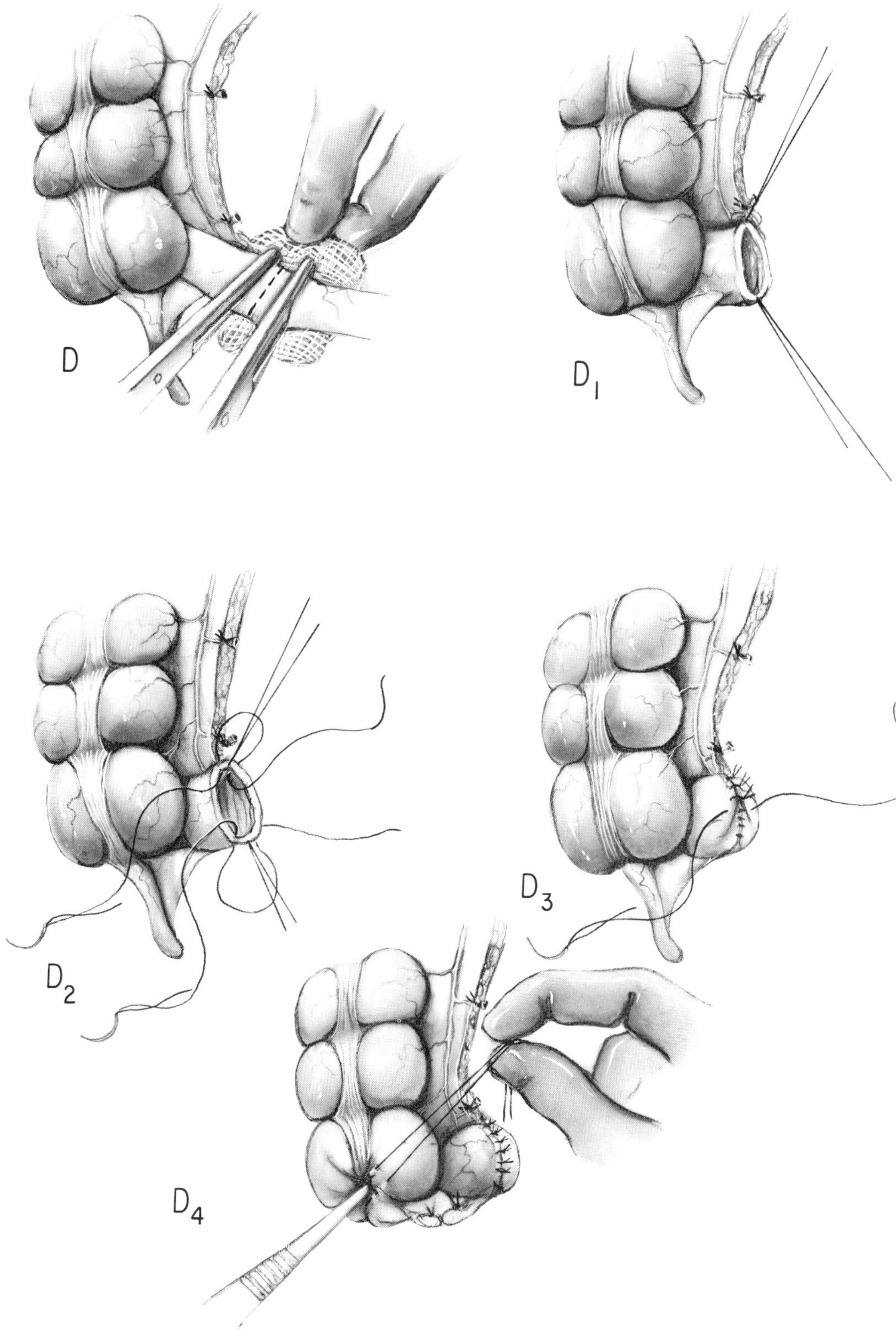
D
D_1
D_2
D_3
D_4

E. The ileocecal segment is mobilized, and its relation to the retroperitoneal structures—viz., the ureter, the spermatic vessels and the psoas muscle—is visible. The right colic artery in juxtaposition to the marginal colic artery is transected and ligated, and the left branch of the middle colic artery is being transected between ligatures by a scalpel.

E_1. The transverse colon is compressed between fingers rather than clamps as it is transected at the site of election in the mid-transverse colon.

F. The mobilization of the ileocolic segment is completed, and its relation to the surrounding structures is visible. The viability of the mobilized bowel segment is maintained through the marginal artery by the middle colic artery and its intact right branch.

Discussion—Dr. Mahoney (cont.)

the right colic artery. I prefer to temporarily occlude these vessels at the point where division is anticipated and observe the circulation in the colon segment for fifteen or twenty minutes before making the decision as to the points of ligation. During this time, if the circulation to the transplant is to be adequate, one can see pulsations in the marginal arteries. This time need not be wasted, because the appendix may be removed and the ileum divided at the appropriate level while the vessels are temporarily occluded. In addition, it has been my custom to divide the right colic artery immediately adjacent to its origin from the superior mesenteric, since this gives a larger number of vessels feeding the marginal artery. By appropriate incisions in the mesentery, adequate length may be obtained even though numerous branches of the artery have been left. Also, E indicates that the left branch of the middle colic artery is being ligated and divided. In my experience the middle colic usually bifurcates sufficiently low that it is not necessary to divide its left branch. The colon is divided and the mesentery split down to the division of the middle colic artery and the left branch may be preserved. If this artery is divided, one depends on the left colic artery entirely for the viability of the splenic flexure of the colon.

G shows the manner in which the terminal

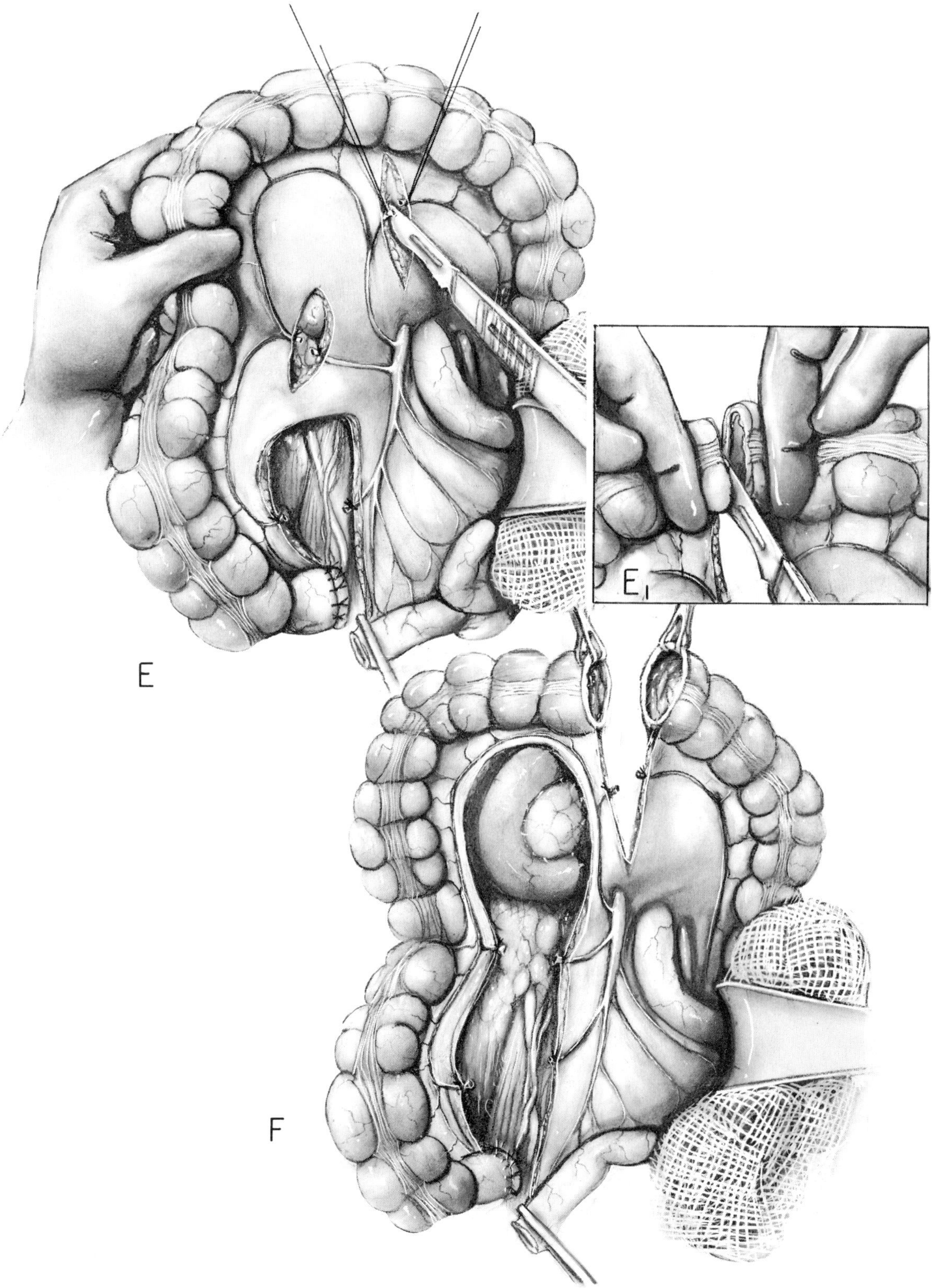
E₁
E
F

G. The open end-to-end ileocolostomy is begun by the insertion of the mesenteric coapting suture (Lee), which, when tied, closes the mesenteric angles of each intestinal segment. The mesenteric vascular stalk (middle colic artery) and marginal artery of the excluded ileocolic segment are depicted.

G_1, G_2. The insertion of the last of a series of horizontal mattress sutures (000 silk) comprising the first posterior layer of the anastomosis is completed (G_1). When tied, these sutures evert the cut margins of the intestines and facilitate the insertion of the interrupted through-and-through (all layers) sutures that comprise the second suture layer posteriorly (G_2).

G_3, G_4. The sutures (000 silk) at each angle of the anastomosis are inserted from the inside-out on the ileal side and from the outside-in on the colon side, so that when tied the knots are on the inside of the lumen (G_3). These sutures are inserted alternately from either angle to terminate in the center, where they are encircled by a "figure of 8" suture to complete the first anterior layer of the anastomosis (G_4).

G_5, G_6. The insertion of a series of interrupted seroserosal (Lembert) sutures (G_5, G_6) completes the second layer anteriorly, subsequent to which the opening in the mesentery is occluded with interrupted sutures of 000 silk (G_6).

Discussion—Dr. Mahoney (cont.)

ileum is brought up anterior to the vascular pedicle of the transplant, but it should be emphasized that the vascular pedicle of the transplant is also passed behind the stomach. If this is not done, compression of the pyloric end of the stomach by the middle colic artery and pyloric obstruction may result. The transplant in the illustrated procedure is brought up through an incision in the diaphragm anterior to the liver. It may also be brought up through a substernal tunnel or if the esophagus has been removed, it may be brought up through the esophageal bed. Two types of anastomoses are shown between the transplant and the esophagus: one a side-to-side and the other an end-to-end anastomosis. If circumstances permit, I would certainly favor the end-to-end anastomosis with division of the esophagus and, if esophagectomy is not to be performed, closure of the distal esophagus. The distal end of the transplant may be anastomosed to the stomach on either the posterior or anterior surface, depending upon the position which seems to give the least tendency toward kinking. At this stage a pyloroplasty probably should be added to give adequate drainage to the stomach.

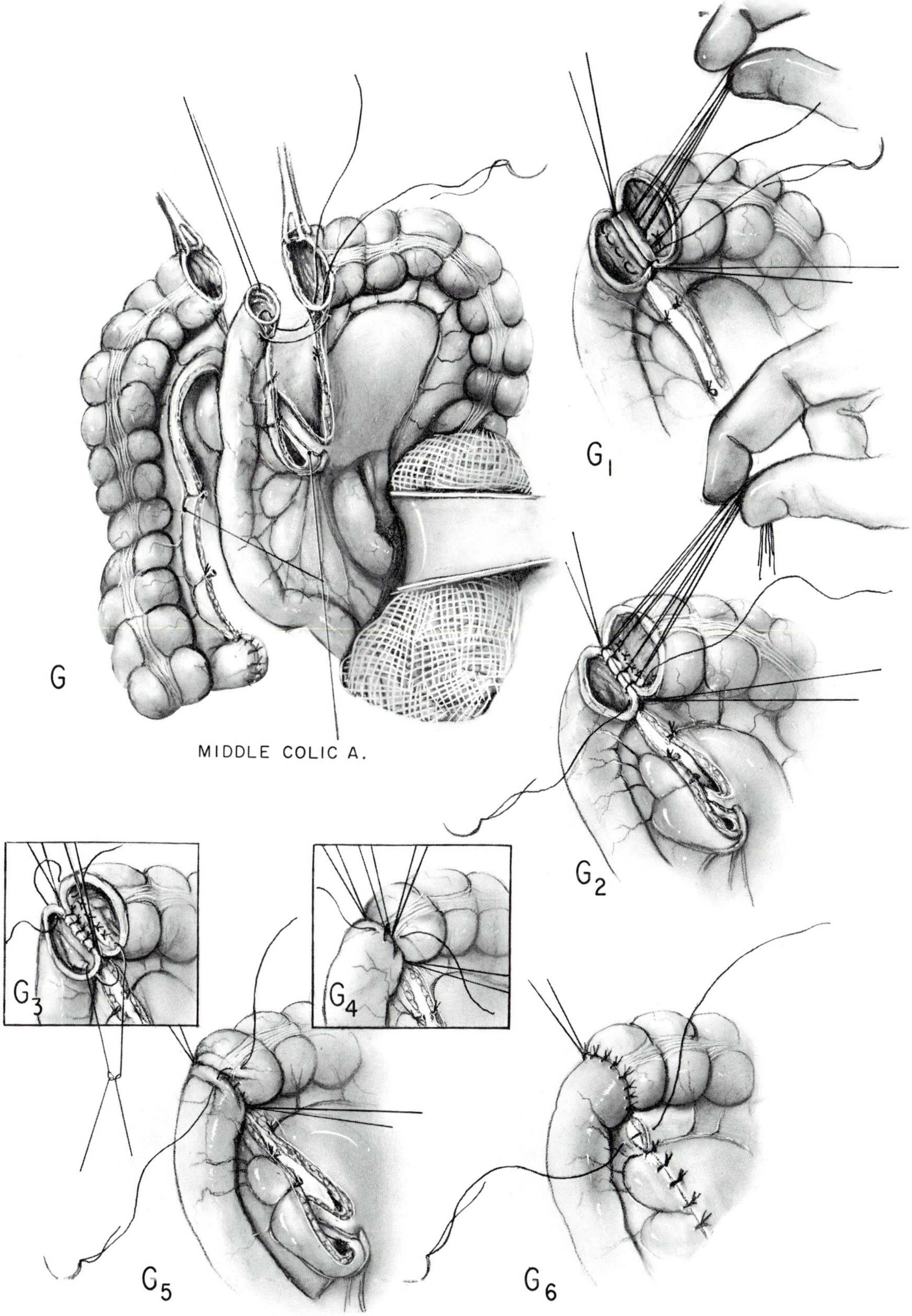
G
MIDDLE COLIC A.
G_1
G_2
G_3
G_4
G_5
G_6

H. On completion of the ileotransverse colon colostomy, a moist pad is placed in the abdominal wound, and the right anterolateral thoracic incision is shown.

I. The right pleural cavity is entered, and the azygos vein, doubly ligated in continuity, is being transected with scissors.

J, J_1. The ileocecal end of the ileocolic segment is transplanted from the peritoneal cavity through an opening in the diaphragm (J_1) into the apex of the right pleural cavity, where it is approximated to the side of the supra-aortic segment of the esophagus using interrupted sutures of 000 silk (J).

K, L. The first posterior layer of the esophagocolostomy is completed, and an incision is made into the lumen of the esophagus (K) and extended by scissor dissection (L).

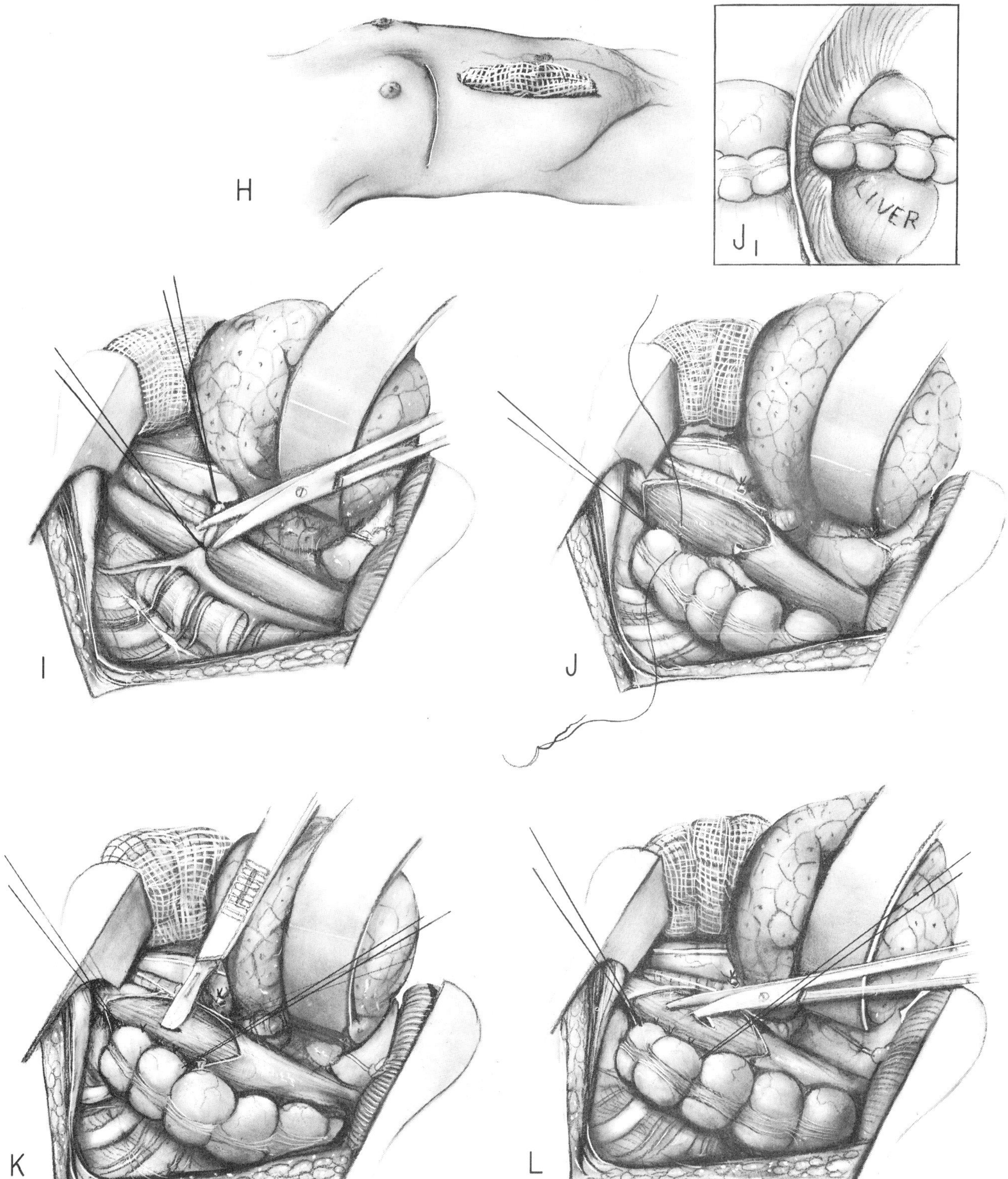
H
LIVER
J1
I
J
K
L

M, N. The stab wound incision in the cecoascending colon is enlarged by scissor dissection (M) preparatory to the start of the second posterior suture layer (N).

O, P. The first of the angle sutures is inserted cephalad and passes from the inside-out on the esophageal side and from the outside-in on the colon side so that, when tied, the knot is on the inside of the lumen (O). The sutures (000 silk) are inserted alternately from either angle and terminate in the center anteriorly, where a "figure of 8" suture is inserted to complete the first anterior layer of the anastomosis (P).

Q. The last of a series of Halsted mattress sutures are inserted to complete the second layer anteriorly of the side-to-side esophagocolostomy.

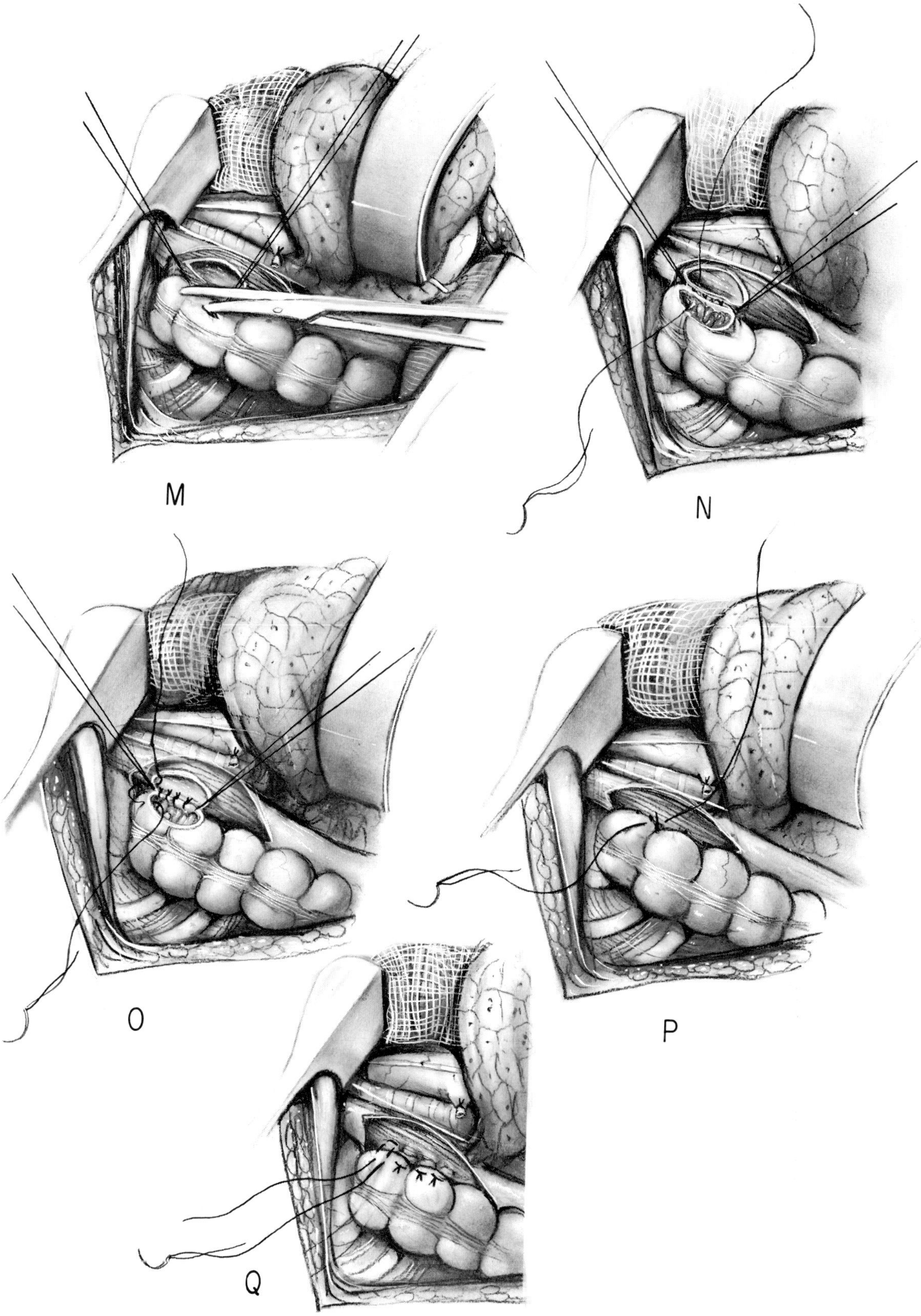

M N O P Q

R. In some patients the location of the lesion may necessitate the transplantation of the colon into the cervical region. Accordingly, the cervical esophagus is exposed through an oblique cervical incision that parallels the anterior border of the sternomastoid muscle. The esophagus is shown elevated on the left index finger just cephalad to the superior belly of the omohyoid muscle. The site of transection of the esophagus is indicated by the broken line. The vagus nerve, visible between the trachea and esophagus, bifurcates just before passing beneath the lowermost fibers of the inferior constrictor muscle of the pharynx to enter the larynx.

S. The proximal segment of the esophagus is secured by guy sutures of 000 silk, and its distal turned-in segment is gently displaced downward into the superior mediastinum by a clamp, the tip of which is covered by a gauze sponge. The tendinous union between the inferior and superior bellies of the omohyoid muscle is encircled by a cotton tape for traction as indicated.

T. The long strands of the ligature (No. 1 silk) about the gauze covered end of the colon are used for upward traction to facilitate the transplantation of the colon from the right pleural cavity into the cervical incision.

T_1. The interrupted mattress sutures of 000 silk that form the first posterior layer of the esophagocolostomy are all first inserted, and as traction is being maintained on the suture strands, the colon is approximated to the esophagus by gentle manipulation with anatomic tissue forceps.

T_2. The suture strands of the first posterior layer are tied and cut, and the last of the interrupted sutures that form the second posterior layer are inserted through the everted cut margins of the esophagus and colon.

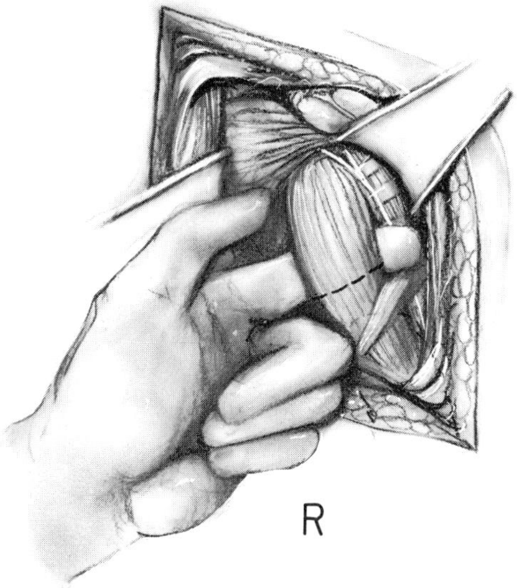

R

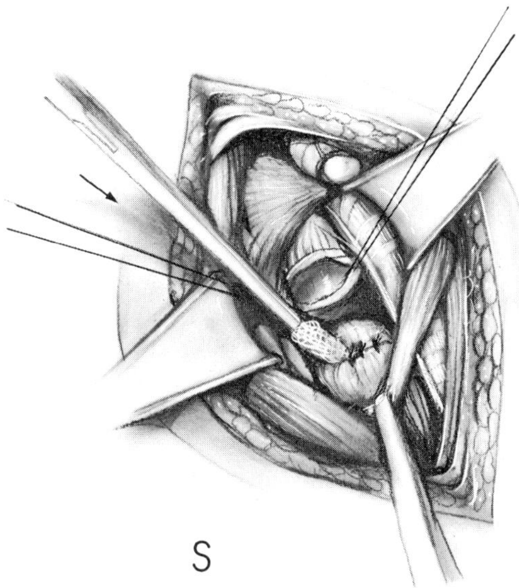

S

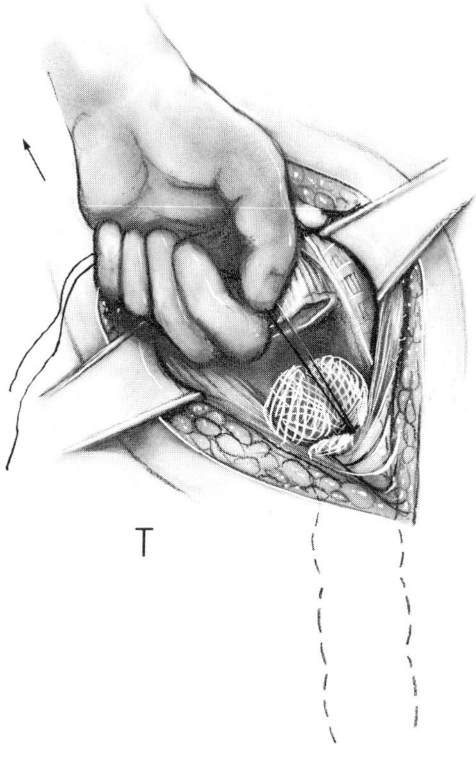

T

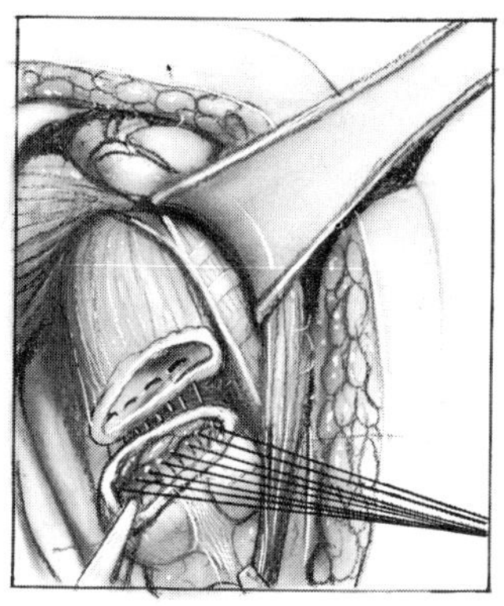

T_1

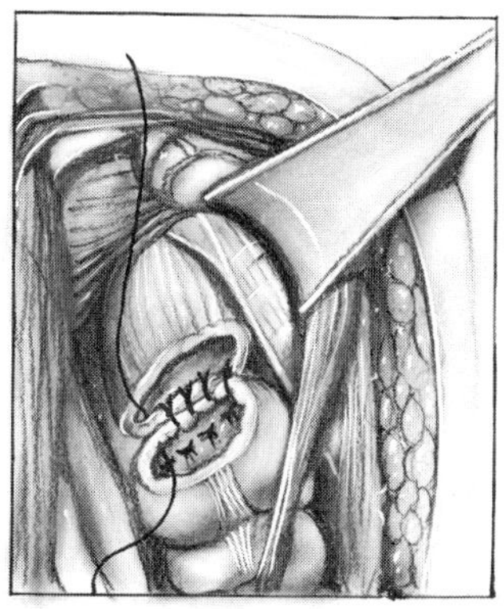

T_2

U, U_1, U_2. Interrupted sutures (000 silk) are inserted at each angle (U), and proceed from the inside-out on the esophageal side and the outside-in on the colon side so that, when tied, the knots of the sutures are on the inside of the lumen. Sutures are inserted alternately from either angle (U_1), and as each suture is being tied, medial traction on the previously inserted suture facilitates the inversion of the tissue margins. The sutures terminate in the center anteriorly, where they are encircled by a "figure of 8" suture (U_2) that, when tied, completes the first anterior layer of the anastomosis.

U_3, U_4. The second anterior layer is comprised of a series of interrupted mattress sutures (Lembert-Cushing) in which the sutures are inserted at right angles to the longitudinal muscle fibers of the esophagus to enhance the holding power of the tissue (U_3). When tied, these sutures effect a serosal cap-like covering of the suture line (U_4).

U_5, U_6. On completion of the esophagocolostomy a Penrose "cigarette" drain is inserted in juxtaposition to the anastomosis (U_5) and has its exit through the mid-portion of the cervical incision, which is closed with interrupted sutures of 000 silk (U_6).

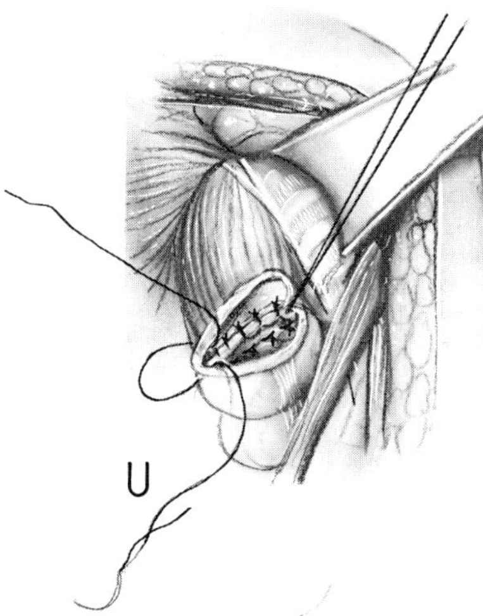

U

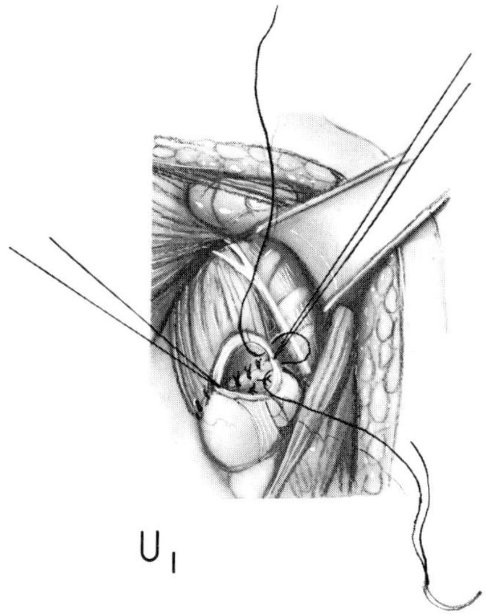

U_1

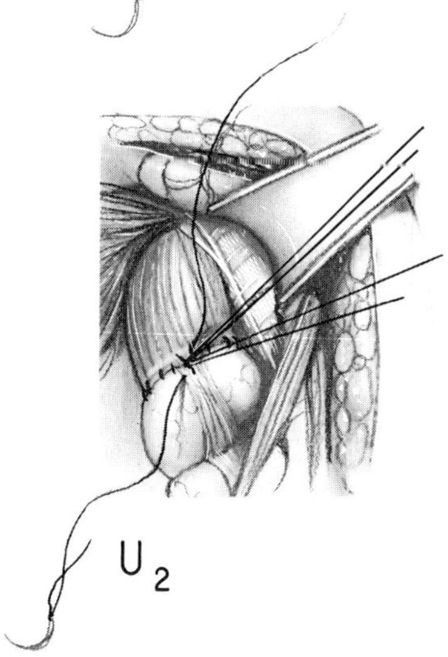

U_2

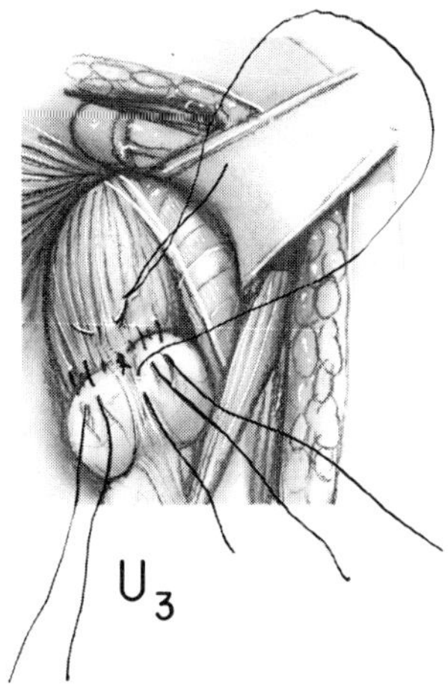

U_3

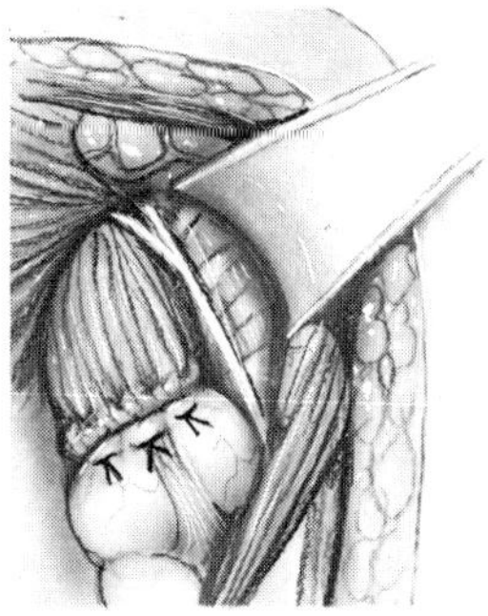

U_4

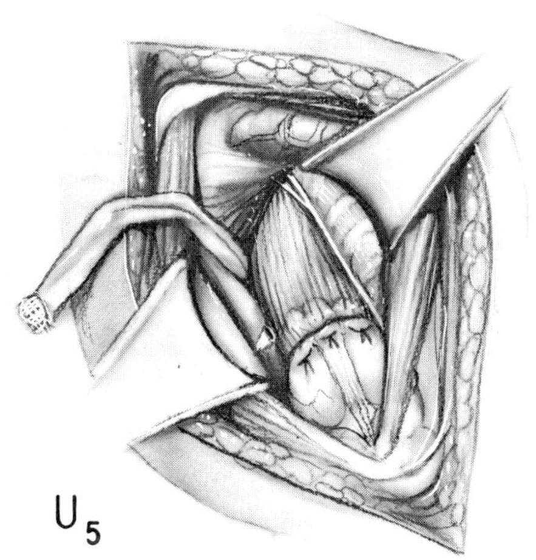

U_5

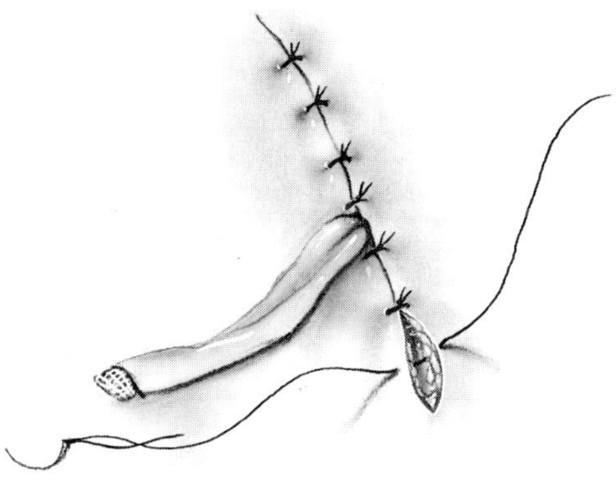

U_6

V, V_1. On completion of the esophagocolostomy, the peritoneal cavity is again entered for the performance of the cologastrostomy. A longitudinal opening is made in the anterior wall of the stomach, preferably much closer to the fundus than depicted. Interrupted mattress sutures are used for the first posterior layer (V) and interrupted through-and-through sutures for the second layer posteriorly (V_1).

V_2, V_3, V_4. The sutures that comprise the first anterior layer (V_2, V_3) are inserted as previously described and terminate in the center of the anastomosis (V_3). A series of Halsted mattress sutures is used to complete the serosal layer anteriorly (V_4).

W. This view of the peritoneal cavity shows the completed abdominal portion of the operation and the relation between the end-to-side cologastrostomy and the end-to-end ileotransverse colon colostomy.

X. This inset shows the completed esophagocoloplasty. The abdominal, thoracic, and cervical incisions are depicted, and the esophagocolic, the cologastric, and ileocolic anastomoses are illustrated in broken outline.

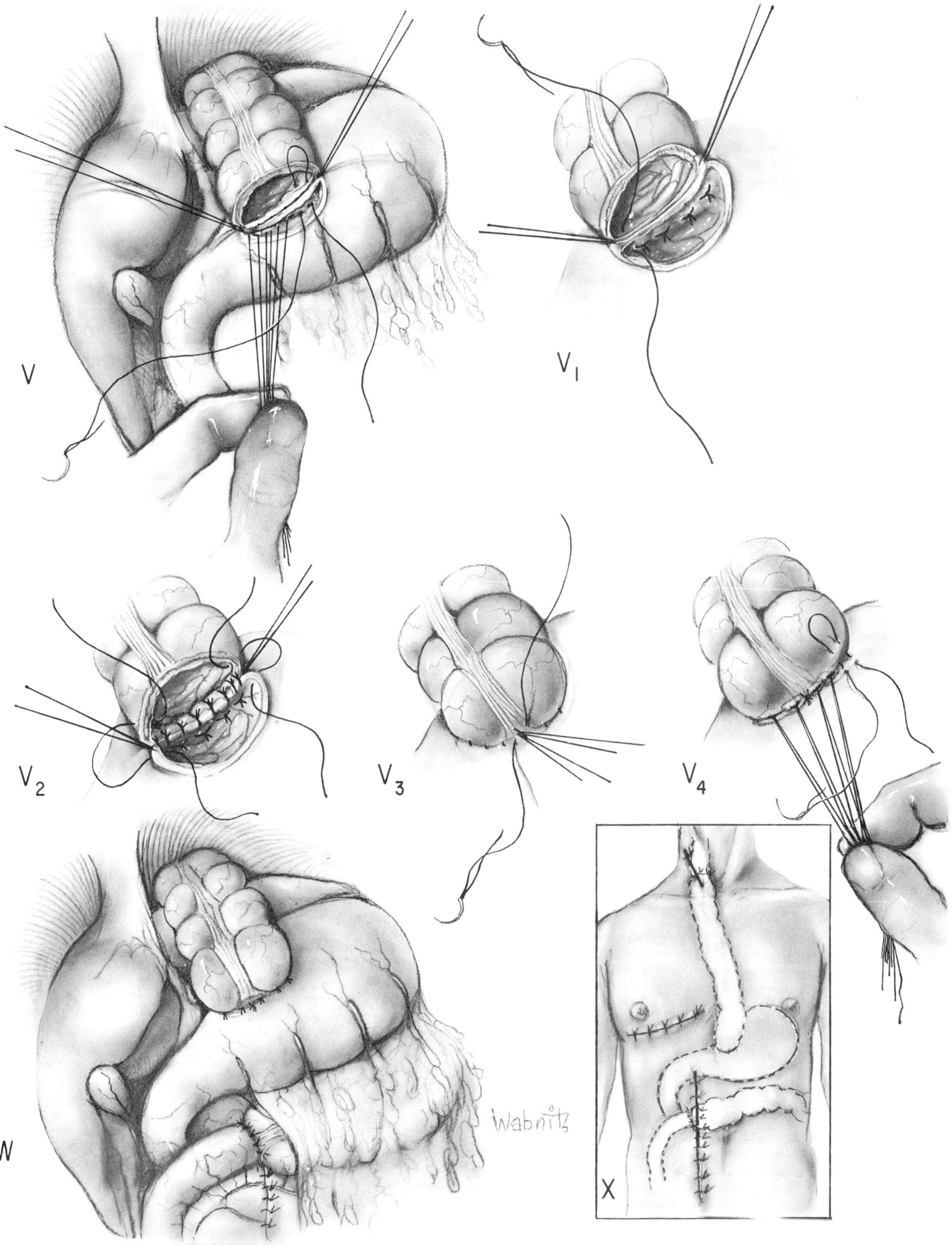
V
V_1
V_2
V_3
V_4
W
Wabnitz
X

In the transplantation of the colon to the cervical region, the substernal extrapleural route is preferred by many. This route is shorter than the transpleural, and in the event of infection secondary to leakage of the anastomosis, the morbidity and mortality are lessened.

Y. By concomitant blunt digital dissection through the cervical and abdominal incisions a tunnel is initiated in the substernal tissue plane.

Y_1. The dissection is continued with moist gauze sponges held in sponge stick forceps to complete the substernal tunnel.

Y_2. The colon is transplanted from the peritoneal cavity into the substernal tunnel and cervical region by gentle taxis from below and traction from above as illustrated.

Z. This inset shows the fixation of the mesentery of the transplanted colon to the mediastinal pleura in those patients in whom the transpleural route is used to transplant the colon into the cervical incision.

Discussion—Dr. Mahoney (cont.)

Y and Z show anastomosis of the transplant to the esophagus above the clavicle. It has been my experience that frequently the proximal end of the transplant, at this stage, will show some edema and duskiness. If this occurs, the anastomosis is not performed at this stage. The proximal end of the esophagus and the transplant are brought out through the incision in the neck, and the procedure is terminated. Usually the edema of the transplant subsides after four to seven days, and at this time normal color has returned and the anastomosis is performed as a secondary procedure. Particular care must be taken with this anastomosis, and I prefer interrupted fine silk throughout.

The second operation illustrated depicts utilization of the transverse colon with the splenic and hepatic flexures as a transplant. I have used the transverse colon for short bypass procedures, particularly in those situations where only the terminal esophagus is to be resected. If the left colon is to be utilized for a long transplant, we prefer the descending colon and sigmoid brought up as an antiperistaltic loop.

It should be emphasized that the anatomy varies considerably with each individual and that the surgeon must approach this procedure with an open mind as to the type of technic which shall be used. No hard and fast rules can be laid down as to the exact procedures to be followed, and frequently the surgeon must tailor the operation to meet the individual situation.

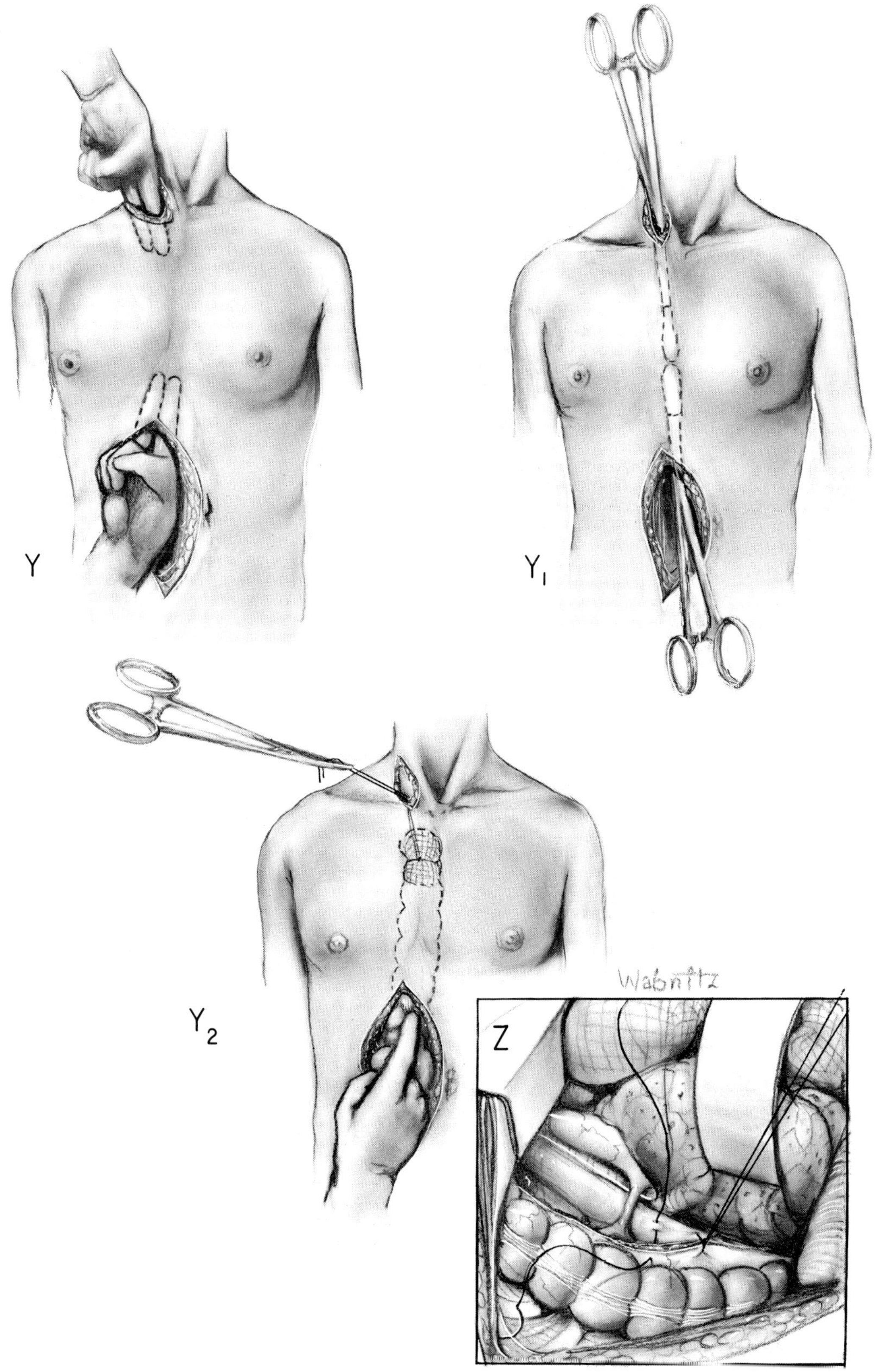
Y
Y1
Y2
Wabnitz
Z

A. In some patients, particularly those in whom extra length of colon is required, the use of the left colon is frequently preferred. Mobilization of the left colon is begun by scissor dissection along the fascia fusion layer of Toldt and is indicated by the broken line (A). Next the lesser sac is entered cephalad to the transverse colon, serially clamping and severing the gastrocolic ligament (broken line).

B. The entrance into the lesser sac permits the approximation of the transverse and descending colons, which facilitates the application of manual traction downward as the phrenocolic and splenocolic ligaments are severed with scissors.

C. The blood supply to the right side of the colon, the transverse colon, and splenic flexure is depicted. The broken lines indicate the sites of severance of the middle colic and right colic arteries and the ascending colon. In this specimen the viability of the excluded colon segment will be maintained by the left colic artery through the marginal artery.

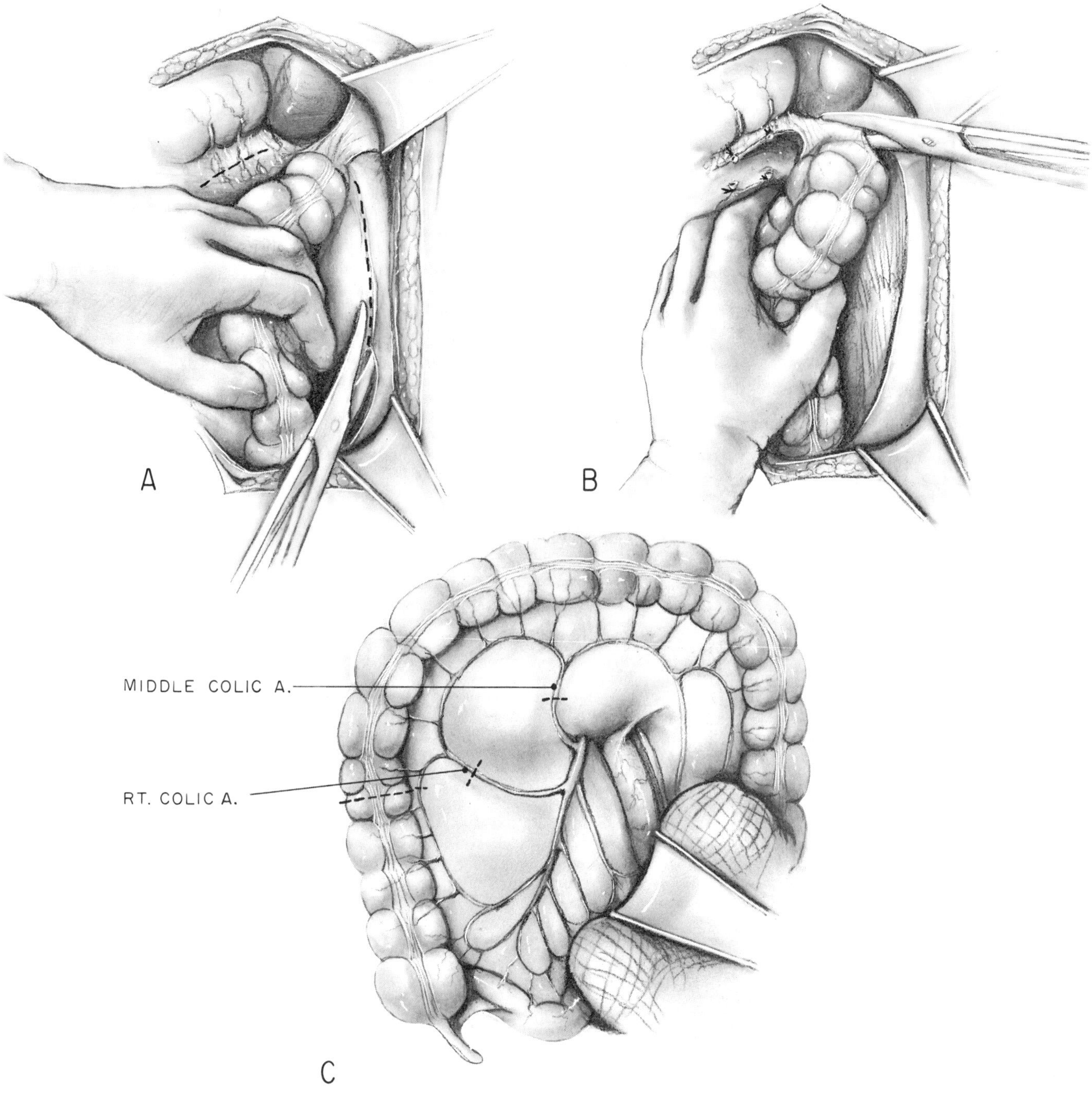
A
B
MIDDLE COLIC A.
RT. COLIC A.
C

D. The right colic and middle colic arteries are severed, and the transected ends of the ascending colon are occluded by Babcock clamps modified on the Potts principle.* The broken lines indicate the sites for transection of the remaining blood vessels and bowel to complete the mobilization of the left colon for transplantation.

E. The excluded colon segment and its blood supply maintained through the marginal artery by the left colic artery are depicted. The intact inferior mesenteric vein is also visible.

* Manufactured by Edward Weck & Co., Long Island City, N.Y.

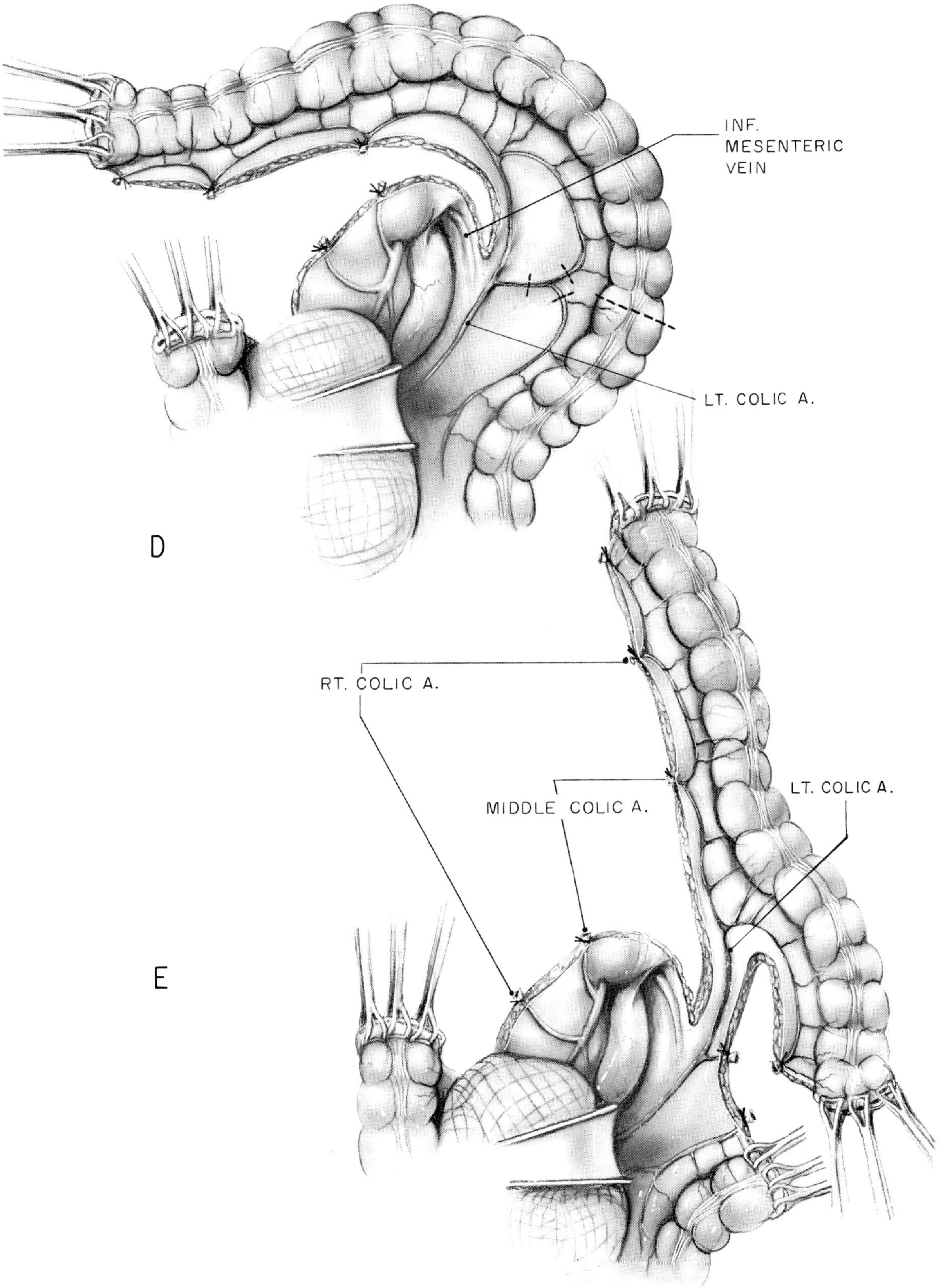
INF.
MESENTERIC
VEIN
LT. COLIC A.
D
RT. COLIC A.
MIDDLE COLIC A.
LT. COLIC A.
E

THE TRANSTHORACIC REPAIR OF AN ESOPHAGEAL HIATUS HERNIA

TOP

Artist's illustrations of the inferior or abdominal aspect of the diaphragm drawn from a fresh cadaver specimen. The right crus, longer, thicker, and more tendinous than the left, separates into superficial and deep muscle bundles to form completely the esophageal hiatus. The superficial layer forms the right margin and the deep layer the left margin of the hiatal ring, effecting a slinglike arrangement of the fibers of the right crus. The close relation of the tendinous portion of the diaphragm and the inferior phrenic vein to the anterior angle of the hiatal ring is depicted.

MIDDLE

A. Artist's interpretation of the anatomy of the esophageal hiatus drawn from a fresh cadaver specimen showing the esophageal hiatus from the abdominal view. The formation of the hiatal ring or sling by the muscle fibers of the right crus is depicted. The greater length and width of the right crus compared to the left are demonstrated.

B. The esophageal hiatus as it appears looking obliquely downward from the head of the cadaver specimen. The thick or deep layer of muscle fibers of the right crus which forms the left margin of the hiatal ring lies superficial to and crosses the superficial or thin layer of muscle fibers of the right crus which forms the right margin of the hiatal ring.

C. Diagrammatic representation of the slinglike arrangement of the muscle fibers of the right crus of the diaphragm in the formation of the esophageal hiatal ring.

BOTTOM

These two artist's illustrations were drawn from fresh cadaver specimens and show the variations in the anatomy of the esophageal hiatus from that previously described.

Left. The muscle fibers of the left crus are separated into superficial and deep layers. The fibers of the superficial layer cross over the deep layer of muscle fibers of the right crus, and join with the fibers of the superficial layer of the right crus to form the right margin of the esophageal hiatal ring.

Right. In this specimen a thick bundle of muscle fibers from the left crus crosses beneath the deep layer of fibers of the right crus and ultimately blends with the superior or thoracic surface of the superficial layer of muscle fibers of the right crus. This particular anatomic configuration was originally described by Low and the crossing bundle of fibers of the left crus is commonly called the band of Low.

DISCUSSION—DR. PAUL C. SAMSON. The first plate illustrates two facts of great importance: (1) the esophageal hiatus nearly always comprises muscles fibers from the *right* crus of the diaphragm; (2) the hiatus is oval, with the long axis in a generally anteroposterior direction. The anterior "angle" is rounded and firm; the posterior angle is usually the "weak spot" and is formed by the crossing or decussation of muscle fibers from the right (or medial) and left (or lateral) margins of the hiatus.

Illustrations A through U depict a method of transthoracic repair that differs in several details from the one I usually employ. In D, resection of the eighth rib is acceptable and may give more room without undue spreading of the ribs. In E, there is no point in injecting the left phrenic nerve. In fact, I think it is contraindicated. The anesthesiologist can easily control diaphragmatic motion during operation. In addition, I have seen hours and days of phrenic paralysis from injection alone. In F, the label should read simply *"pulmonary ligament,"* since there is no *inferior* pulmonary ligament. Regarding H and I, careful dissection of the esophagus is necessary, but the vagi should *not* be separated from the esophagus and should not be put on great tension. A drain passed around the esophagus should include both vagus nerves. Also, I carefully free the muscle fibers of the right crus circumferentially from the hernial sac for a distance of 6 or 7 mm., which prevents a "rolling in" of the muscle when the hernia is reduced. In J, my counterincision is longer and roughly parallels the curve of the left (lateral) margin of the hiatus. This is because I believe strongly in Allison's method of tacking remnants of the sac, phrenoesophageal ligament and peritoneum to the undersurface of the diaphragm (see B). Regarding K, L, and M, I do not *excise* any portion of the sac, but with a wide horizontal (anteroposterior) incision a generous cuff is left attached to the region of the esophagogastric junction. From four to six, spaced, 000 silk sutures taken in the cuff at this stage are later passed through the counterincision, reneedled, and sewn to the undersurface of the diaphragm approximately 7 to 10 mm. from the left margin of the hiatus. In passing, I must confess that most illustrators make the phrenoesophageal ligament much more easy to identify than I am frequently able to do at the operating table. In O, since the anterior rounded "angle" of the hiatus usually is firm, I doubt if I employ sutures at the anterior angle in more than 10 per cent of cases. In P and Q, the essence of repair is the

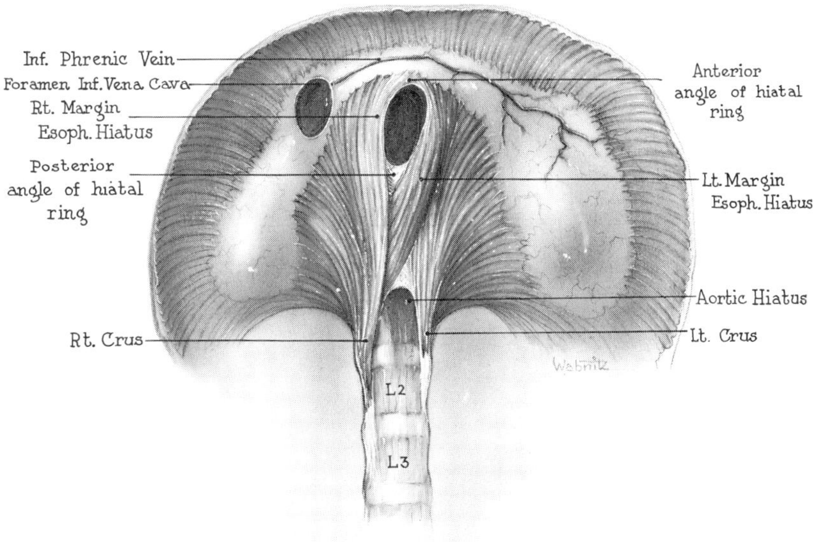
Inf. Phrenic Vein
Foramen Inf. Vena Cava
Rt. Margin Esoph. Hiatus
Posterior angle of hiatal ring
Anterior angle of hiatal ring
Lt. Margin Esoph. Hiatus
Aortic Hiatus
Rt. Crus
Lt. Crus
L2
L3

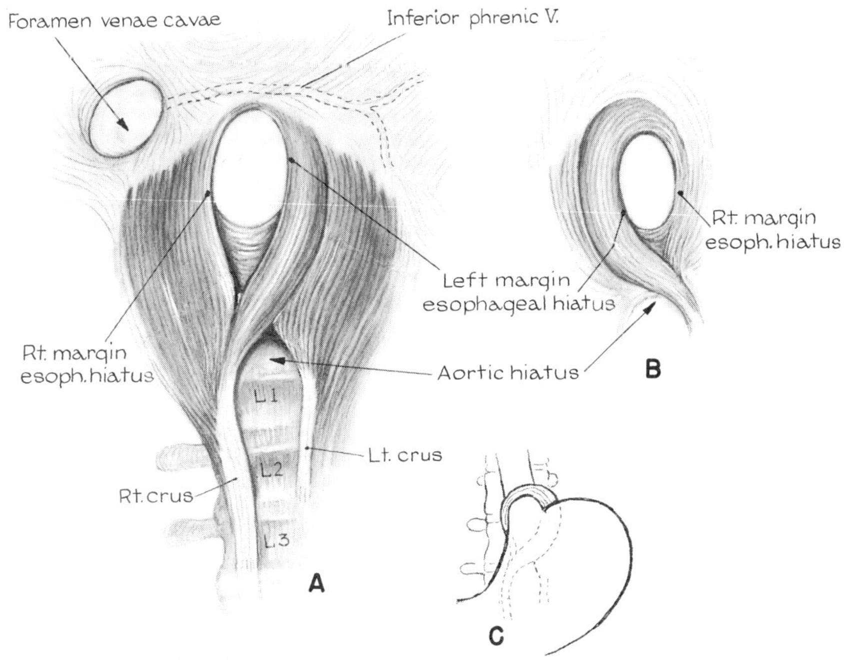
Foramen venae cavae
Inferior phrenic V.
Left margin esophageal hiatus
Rt. margin esoph. hiatus
Aortic hiatus
Rt. margin esoph. hiatus
L1
L2
L3
Lt. crus
Rt. crus
A
B
C

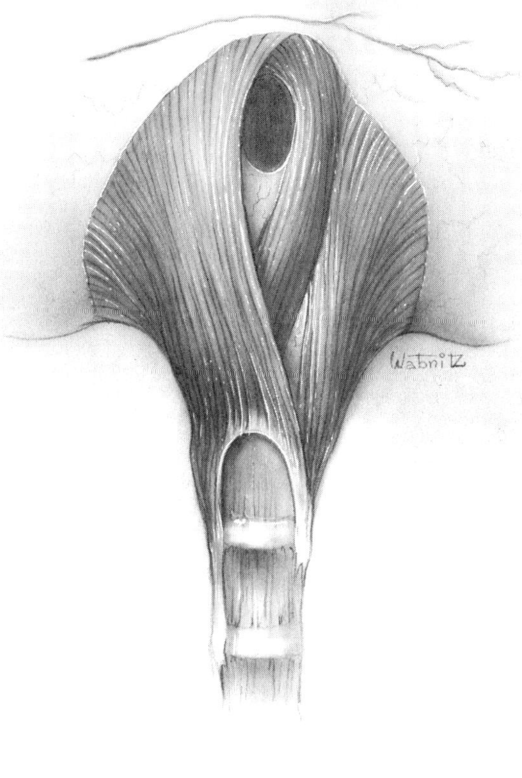

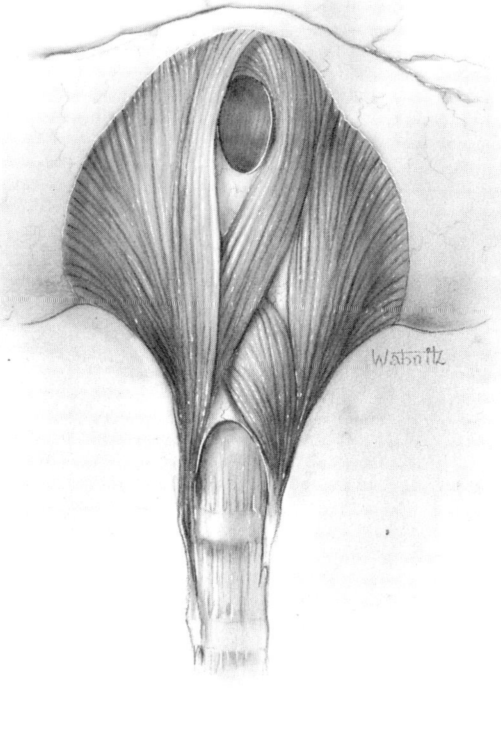

A. The patient is placed in the right lateral prone position, and the incision overlying the eighth interspace is outlined.

B, C, D. The incision is deepened through the underlying muscle layers to expose the line of incision in the eighth interspace.

E. The left pleural cavity is entered, and the wound margins are retracted with two self-retaining rib retractors of the Tuffier type. The resection of a rib is not required. The phrenic nerve is not crushed by clamping, but temporary paralysis of the diaphragm is obtained by injection of the nerve with 6 to 8 ml. of procaine solution (one per cent). Paralysis of the phrenic nerve by crushing destroys the bellowslike action of the diaphragm which is believed to predispose to postoperative pulmonary complications.

F. The deflated left lung is displaced upward and maintained in position by retraction over a moist gauze pad. This exposes the characteristic protrusion of the sliding hernia in the esophageal triangle. This triangle is bounded medially (anteriorly) by the pericardium and laterally (posteriorly) by the aorta. The base is formed by the diaphragm and the apex by the proximal portion of the inferior pulmonary ligament. The inverted T-shaped incision in the mediastinal and diaphragmatic pleura is depicted by the dotted lines. The horizontal portion of this incision extends medially (anteriorly) to the base of the pericardium and laterally (posteriorly) to a point just beyond the thoracic aorta.

G. The flaps of mediastinal pleura are retracted by guy sutures of silk (000), and the extension of the underlying muscle fibers of the diaphragm onto the base of the hernial protrusion may be seen.

Discussion—Dr. Samson (cont.)

posterior closure, where the fibers from the left (lateral) and right (medial) margins of the hiatus frequently appear to decussate. I think medium heavy silk (0 or 1), is better than fine silk. Dr. Madden rightly points out that the right marginal fibers are thin, and heavier silk will not cut. In this connection, I always seek to buttress any muscle sutures by passing the needle through pleura, peritoneum, or an available portion of the sac, which frequently I can pull up from below. The silk is tied with four throws of the knot. I am sure there have been some recurrences simply because the silk came untied early in the postoperative period. The closure usually needs only two to four sutures. With a Levin tube in the esophagus, the closure should be snug to the passage of the tip of the index finger.

In R, the closure of the counterincision must be in two layers, with interrupted silk. In all of the hernias occurring through the counterincision that I personally have seen, either single-layer silk or catgut closures had been employed. R, S, and U show a typical closure for an intercostal incision. When a rib is removed, subperiosteally, interrupted silk is used to close the pleural cavity. By taking generous bites of intercostal muscle, the intercostal nerve is protected and pain is less. No pericostal sutures are then employed.

I, II, and III illustrate well the modification described. As I have stated, I prefer to suture the cuff beneath the diaphragm. This technic is not difficult or time-consuming particularly if the counterincision is a little longer and parallels the left margin of the hiatus. It does mean that there will be several millimeters further reduction of the hernia.

The last two plates nicely illustrate an unusual problem and its solution. I think they emphasize the necessity of accurate anatomic delineation of the entire situation before repair has commenced.

The plates show clearly the steps in the transabdominal repair of an esophageal hiatus hernia. The end result of the repair should be the same as with the transthoracic approach. I may say that there is no uniformity of opinion regarding the method of approach. Some general surgeons believe the transthoracic approach is superior, while, conversely, some thoracic surgeons, particularly those who now perform a more complicated operation as a routine, have switched to the abdominal route. In a given case, complete familiarity with one or the other approaches should be the guiding factor. The operation from either aspect is not one of critical proportions, but there are a number of important technical details which must be remembered, and I think it is fair to say that the occasional operator will not have as high a percentage of success, as the surgeon who does the operation frequently.

If other abdominal pathologic lesions (possibly requiring surgery) are uncovered during the preoperative workup, then the operation should be peformed from below. If, however, the gall bladder and stomach are not implicated, if the patient is quite fat (as many are), or if other abdominal surgery has preceded the prospective repair, then I think there is fairly general agreement that the transthoracic approach is superior.

Finally, I have encountered a rare situation when with a transthoracic approach, vagotomy and pyloroplasty seem called for. In such an instance, I have not hesitated to do the vagotomy through the chest, repair the hernia (if possible), and after closing the thoracic incision, turn the patient supine and perform a pyloroplasty through a separate small abdominal incision.

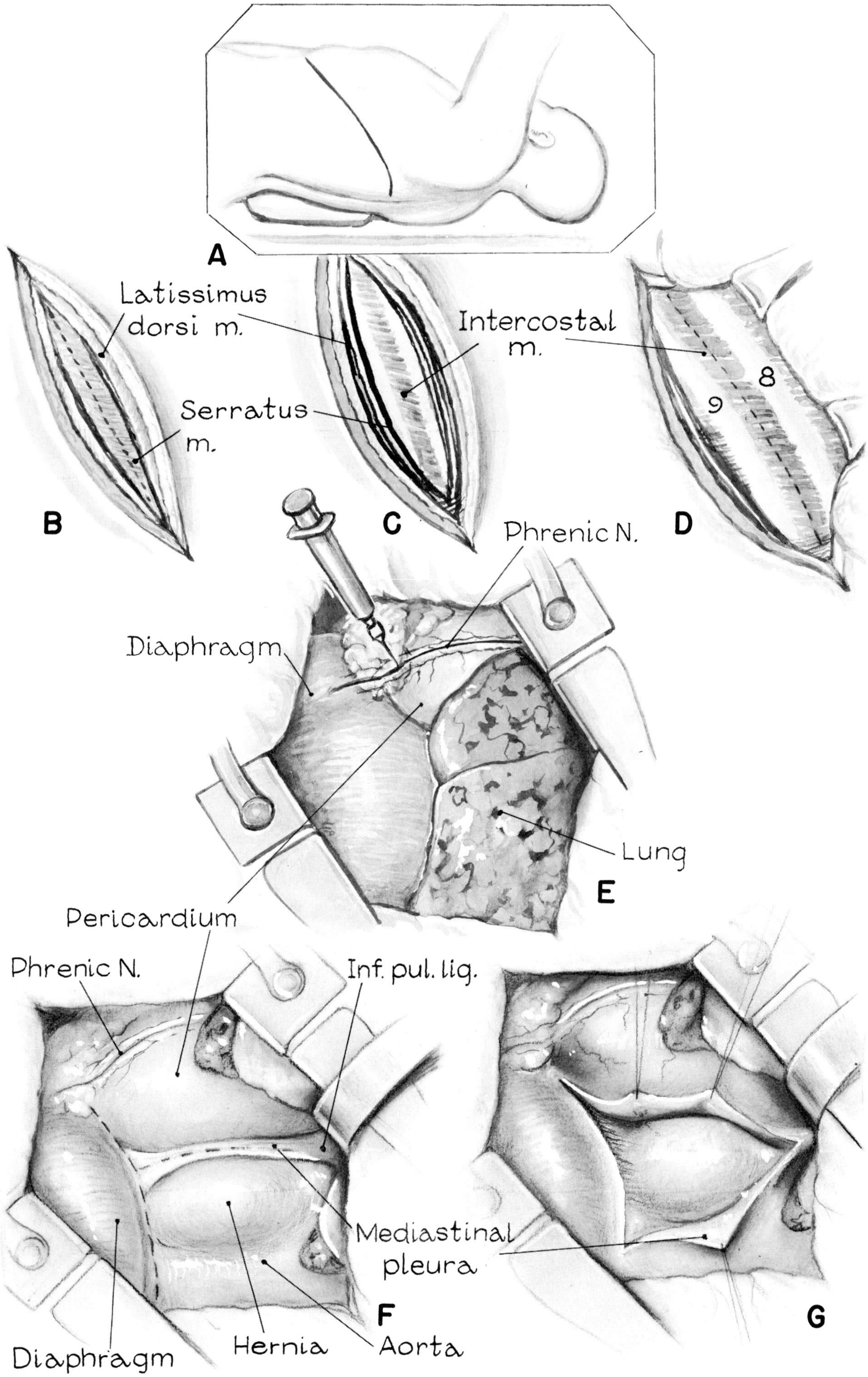
A
Latissimus dorsi m.
Serratus m.
Intercostal m.
8
9
B
C
D
Phrenic N.
Diaphragm
Lung
E
Pericardium
Phrenic N.
Inf. pul. lig.
Mediastinal pleura
F
G
Diaphragm
Hernia
Aorta

H, I. The distal portion of the esophagus is first mobilized by blunt digital dissection and then encircled by a rubber tissue drain. Traction upward on the esophagus is maintained and the hernia is mobilized by scissor dissection to expose the whole of the hiatal muscle ring which is formed completely by the muscle fibers of the right crus of the diaphragm (I). This step is considered an essential part of the operative technic. The thick layer of muscle fibers of the right crus which forms the left margin of the esophageal hiatal ring is anterior (lateral) and crosses superficial to the thin layer of muscle fibers of the right crus which is posterior (medial) and which forms the right margin of the esophageal hiatal ring.

J. A segment of the diaphragm in juxtaposition to the esophageal hiatus is tented by Babcock clamps and incised as indicated by the dotted line.

K. The left index finger of the surgeon is inserted through the incision in the diaphragm into the peritoneal cavity and then upward through the esophageal hiatus into the herneal sac. The overlying structures are tented on the index finger, and the phrenoesophageal ligament is incised to expose the underlying layer of the parietal peritoneum which forms the anterior wall of the sliding hernial sac. The area of the phrenoesophageal ligament to be excised is depicted in dotted outline. This ligament is a definite anatomic structure, possessed of good holding power and best demonstrated by elevation on the index finger as indicated.

L, M. Similarly, as in K, the peritoneum is incised and the lumen of the hernial sac is entered. This exposes the posterior wall of the hernial protrusion which is formed by the anterior wall of the stomach and thereby conforming to the definition of a sliding hernia. A sliding hernia defined is an irreducible hernia in which a portion of the wall of the sac is formed by the protruding or herniated viscus.

Discussion—Dr. Richard H. Sweet. A knowledge of the anatomy of the diaphragm and particularly of the structures in and about the esophageal hiatus is essential to an understanding of the principles involved in the successful repair of a hiatus hernia. Plate 79 (Top) shows the configuration of the muscle bundles of the right crus and the relations of the right and left crura. It should be emphasized, however, that this is a view of the inferior surface of the diaphragm. When viewed from above on the mediastinal surface, the right margin of the hiatus becomes the deep layer and the left margin is the superficial layer. This distinction is important for those who use the thoracic approach. The view in Plate 79, Top, is that of the surgeon who uses the abdominal approach. This is true also of Plate 79, Middle, A. Plate 79, Middle, B, shows the relations of these bundles as seen when the thoracic approach, which is preferred, is employed.

These relations of the muscle fibers which constitute the margin of the hiatus are of interest to the surgeon, but of even greater importance is an understanding of the disposition of the fascial layers and of the peritoneum in both the normal condition and in the presence of an esophageal hiatus hernia. One must realize that the pouch of peritoneum which comprises the hernial sac in the sliding variety in hernia pushes up in front of and to the right of the anterior surface of the herniated portion of stomach. Because of its anatomic relations it is impossible for the sac to envelop the entire circumference of the stomach, the anterior wall of which always makes up the posterior wall of the sac. Thus the term "sliding type" is the technically correct designation for this kind of herniation.

The fascial layer called by Allison the "phrenoesophageal ligament" is often so stretched out over the herniated stomach and the sac that it may not be recognized unless the surgeon realizes that this layer is always present. It is made up of a reflection of the transversalis fascia below and of the mediastinal fascia above which fuse at the margins of the hiatus to provide a loose tissue attachment for the esophagus. It is difficult to demonstrate this layer in a drawing, but it is important to place sutures in it at the operation. An impression of the relations of this layer may be gained from Plate 81, K, L, and M.

The impression is gained from Plates 81 and 82 that the cardia must always be pulled down below the hiatus by means of a sling inserted through a counter incision in the diaphragm. Although this maneuver is helpful, it is by no means always necessary. Actually the majority of hernias, excepting those which are unusually large or when the patient is excessively fat, can be handled without opening the diaphragm. This is done either by plication of the sac when it is small or by incision of the sac in the larger hernias. In the latter, additional sutures placed in the fascial layer are often needed to maintain a complete reduction of the hernia.

Plates 81 and 82 demonstrate clearly all of the steps in the repair of the hernia. The placing of sutures across the hiatus in front of the esophagus as shown in Plate 82, O, P, and Q, is essential when the shape of the hiatus is that of an ellipse, thus leaving a triangular defect in front. In the majority of instances, however, the hiatus is U or horseshoe shaped with a rounded contour in front. In these it is necessary merely to place a few sutures behind the esophagus.

The situation illustrated in Plates 85 and 86 appears to be somewhat theoretical. I have never encountered it. With any anomaly of the diaphragm at the esophageal hiatus, a thorough knowledge of the normal anatomy should make it possible to improvise a satisfactory technic for closure.

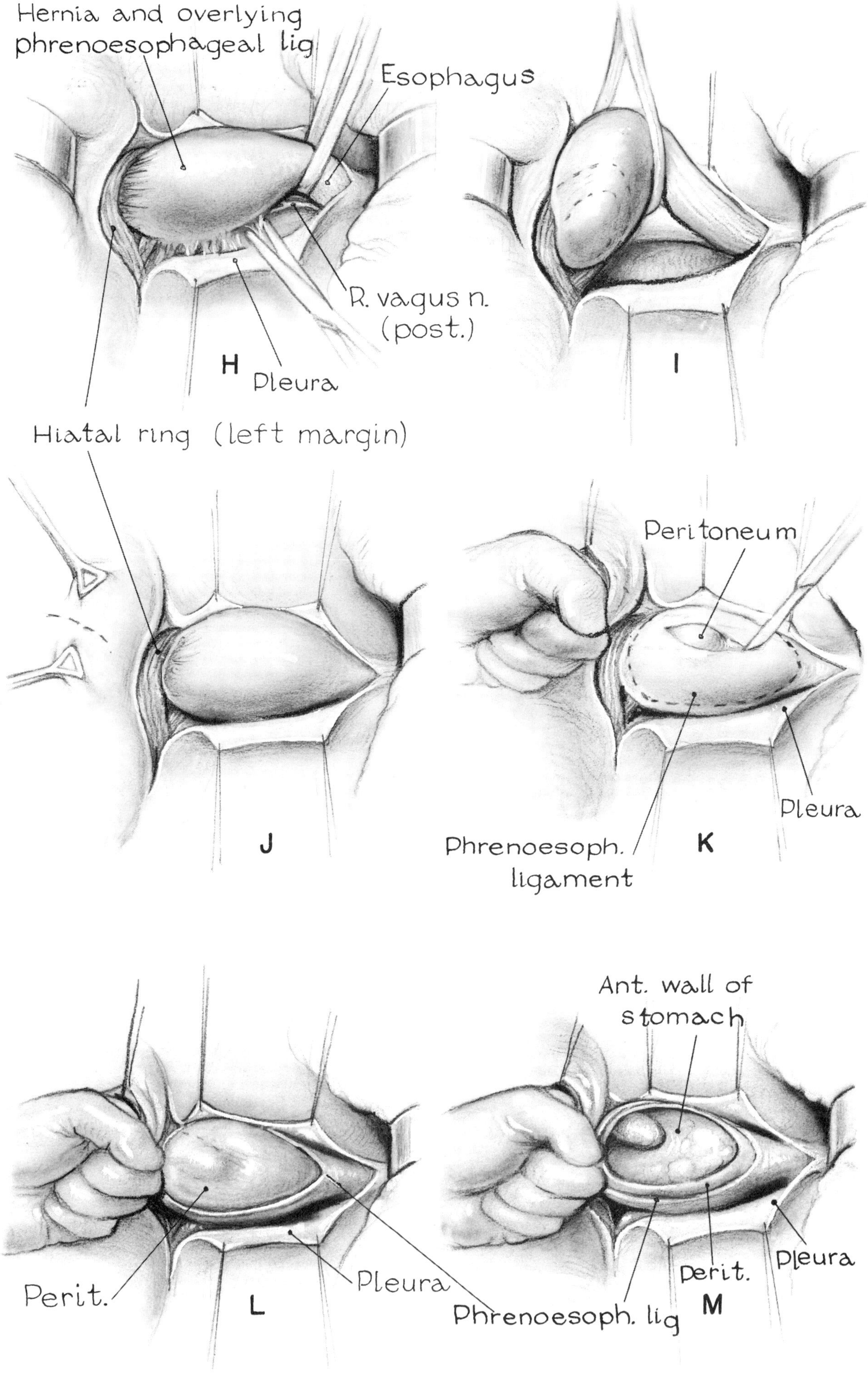
Hernia and overlying phrenoesophageal lig
Esophagus
R. vagus n. (post.)
H
Pleura
I
Hiatal ring (left margin)
Peritoneum
J
Pleura
Phrenoesoph. ligament
K
Ant. wall of stomach
Perit.
Pleura
L
Phrenoesoph. lig
Perit.
M
Pleura

N. The hernia is reduced either by traction through the diaphragm as shown or by downward displacement with the aid of a pledget of gauze held in a ring clamp (P). If desired a combination of both maneuvers may be used.

O. After reduction of the hernia, the esophagus is retracted laterally (posteriorly) and the innermost or "crown" suture is inserted. This suture approximates the muscle fibers of the right crus which forms the medial (anterior) angle of the hiatal ring. This angle is in juxtaposition to both the tendinous portion of the diaphragm and the inferior phrenic vein. Accordingly, caution should be observed in the placement of sutures to avoid injury to the inferior phrenic vein. A second suture in this area may or may not be required.

P, Q. The esophagus is displaced medially (anteriorly) and the lateral (posterior) sutures (No. 1 silk) are inserted. These sutures approximate not the right and left crura as so commonly thought but the superficial and deep muscle layers of the right crus of the diaphragm which form the right and left margins respectively of the esophageal hiatal ring. The muscle fibers of the superficial layer (right margin of the esophageal hiatus) are frequently thinned out and have a poor holding power. Accordingly, in the suture approximation of the superficial and deep layers of the muscle fibers of the right crus, tension on the suture line should be avoided. When completed, the closure of the hiatal ring is snug but not too tight.

R. The incision in the diaphragm is closed (00 silk) and the flaps of diaphragmatic pleura are approximated with sutures of fine silk (0000). The posterior mediastinal pleura is not sutured because, in the event of an infection, the more readily treated complication, a pleural empyema, rather than a mediastinal abscess would then occur.

S, T, U. Two pericostal sutures of silk (No. 3) or, if preferred, double strands of chromic catgut (No. 2), are used to approximate the rib cage, and the muscle layers of the wound are closed with interrupted sutures of silk (000). Periosteal "windows" are formed along the inferior border of the lower rib to prevent impingement upon either the intercostal nerve or the sensitive periosteum. A water-seal catheter drainage of the pleural cavity is routinely employed. This catheter is withdrawn approximately 36 hours postoperatively.

Discussion—Dr. Denton A. Cooley. In regard to the technic described by the author for transthoracic repair of the hernia a larger secondary incision in the diaphragm should be used so the esophagus can be anchored with sutures below the diaphragm. The phrenicoesophageal ligament can be used for this purpose. Overcorrecting the hernia into the abdomen is important, since roentgenographic studies after operation may otherwise suggest an incomplete repair.

Discussion—Dr. John Robinson Brooks. In recent years at the Peter Bent Brigham Hospital, increasing use of the abdominal approach for repair of esophageal hiatus hernia has been prompted by a number of factors. It has been shown that approximately 40 per cent of patients coming to operation for esophageal hiatus hernia have some concomitant process within the abdomen, such as peptic ulcer or biliary tract disease, which may be treated at the same sitting. When gastrointestinal bleeding becomes a problem with site unknown and with both peptic ulcer and esophageal hernia present, it is almost mandatory to explore the abdomen in order to evaluate properly and correct the source of blood loss. Moreover, the abdominal approach may be said to compromise less the pulmonary reserve of patients with hiatus hernia, many of whom are elderly and have chronic lung disease. Although the pulmonary complications following subdiaphragmatic surgery do exist, there is, nevertheless, no question that pulmonary reserve is more compromised intraoperatively during a chest procedure than during an abdominal procedure. The abdominal approach confines the surgeon to one cavity. The transthoracic approach involves an incision through the diaphragm (with possible interference of the phrenic nerve in the course of this procedure), thereby opening both the pulmonary and abdominal cavities simultaneously.

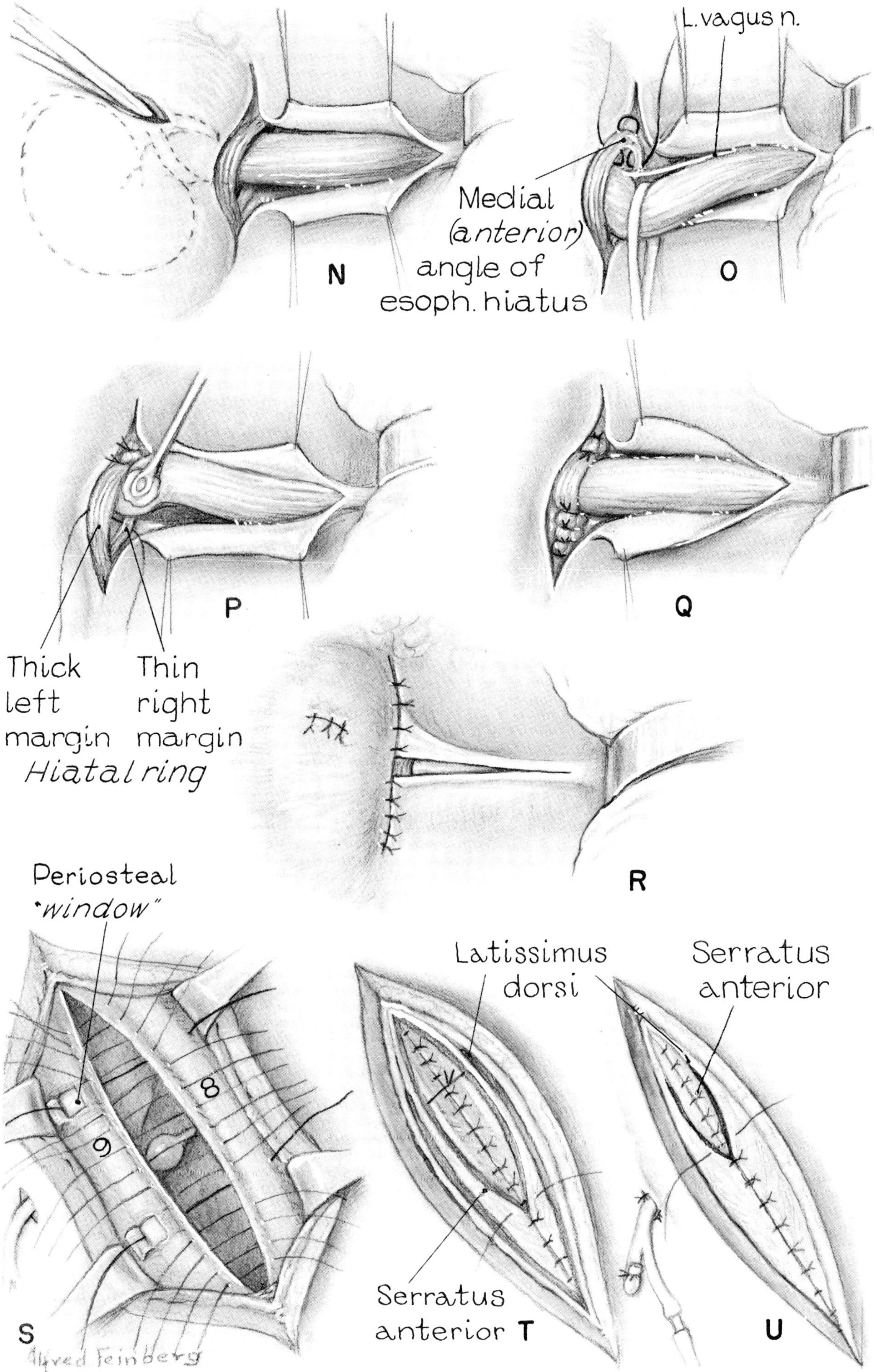
L. vagus n.
Medial (anterior) angle of esoph. hiatus
N
O
P
Q
Thick left margin
Thin right margin
Hiatal ring
R
Periosteal "window"
8
9
S
Latissimus dorsi
Serratus anterior
Serratus anterior
T
U
Alfred Feinberg

These illustrations depict diagrammatically the three most commonly used methods in the repair of a hernia through the esophageal hiatus of the diaphragm.

I. *a.* The anatomic pathologic findings in a sliding hernia through the esophageal hiatus are shown. The posterior wall of the sac is formed by the protruding viscus, the stomach, and thereby conforms to the definition of a sliding hernia.

b. The posterior mediastinal pleura, the phrenoesophageal ligament, and the peritoneum are incised to enter the lumen of the hernial sac. The extent of the resection of the phrenoesophageal ligament and the peritoneum is indicated by the small solid black lines.

c. The herniated segment of the stomach into the posterior mediastinum is reduced, and the superficial and deep muscle layers of the right crus of the diaphragm are approximated around the esophagus just above the cardia. The diaphragmatic pleura, but not the opening in the posterior mediastinal pleura, is sutured. This method of repair of a sliding hernia is the same as shown in the preceding artist's illustrations.

II. *a, b.* These sketches demonstrate an essential step in the Allison method of repair. Following the excision of segments of the phrenoesophageal ligament and the peritoneum (anterior wall of the sac), the cuff formed by the proximal cut margins of the phrenoesophageal ligament and peritoneum is sutured to the under surface of the diaphragm. Another important step in the Allison method, although not illustrated in the sketches, is the closure of the muscular hiatal ring in a vertical plane, "with the grain," posterior to the esophagus.

III. *a, b, c.* These sketches outline the essential steps in the technic advocated by Sweet for the repair of small and medium sized hernias. A series of circumferential or longitudinal plication sutures are inserted in the overlying phrenoesophageal ligament and peritoneum to obliterate the sac. The closure of the lax muscle ring of the hiatus about the esophagus completes the repair of the hernia.

Discussion—Dr. Brooks (cont.)

In preparation for hiatus herniorrhaphy, an evaluation of gastric secretion is mandatory. A high acid level in the face of coexisting esophagitis may indicate the need for concomitant vagotomy. Esophagoscopy is performed if possible to evaluate more accurately the lower esophagus and rule in or out ulceration, esophageal ring, or tumor. Finally, the presence of ulcer disease with or without pyloric stenosis may indicate the need for pyloroplasty or vagotomy and pyloroplasty at the time of hernia repair. Careful roentgenographic examination of the esophagus to rule out a diverticulum, an esophageal web, or ring is important and may be clarified by cineradiography.

The incision for the abdominal approach to hiatus herniorrhaphy can be adapted to the patient at hand. If herniorrhaphy alone is to be performed, a left rectus muscle-retracting incision is preferable and should be extended up lateral to the xiphoid, which may be removed if indicated. A right rectus "hockey stick" incision carried across the midline up to the left of the xiphoid is used if concomitant biliary tract disease is present and is to be treated.

It is characteristic of the abdominal approach that exposure becomes easier as the operation proceeds. Frequently, the most difficult aspect of the operation is with mobilization and retraction of the left lobe of the liver. In instances where that lobe is small, severance of the triangular ligament may not be necessary. In most cases, however, this must be done and may be difficult to perform in patients with a high-riding diaphragm and an overhanging costal margin. Once the triangular ligament is severed and the left lobe of the liver is retracted to the right, exposure rapidly becomes easier, and reduction of the hernia can then be carried out with ease. It is only the extremely rare, longstanding hernia with periesophageal inflammatory changes that is difficult to reduce below the diaphragm. Dissection is carried around the esophagus. The sac is excised, and an incision is made in the attenuated phrenoesophageal ligament, the proximal portion of which will later be sutured to the undersurface of the diaphragm. Approximately 2 in. of esophagus is thereby mobilized, and the vagus nerves can then be severed if indicated.

The esophagogastric junction is retracted to the left, and the two limbs of the right crus of the diaphragm located posteriorly are cleared of overlying tissue and peritoneum. The more posterior

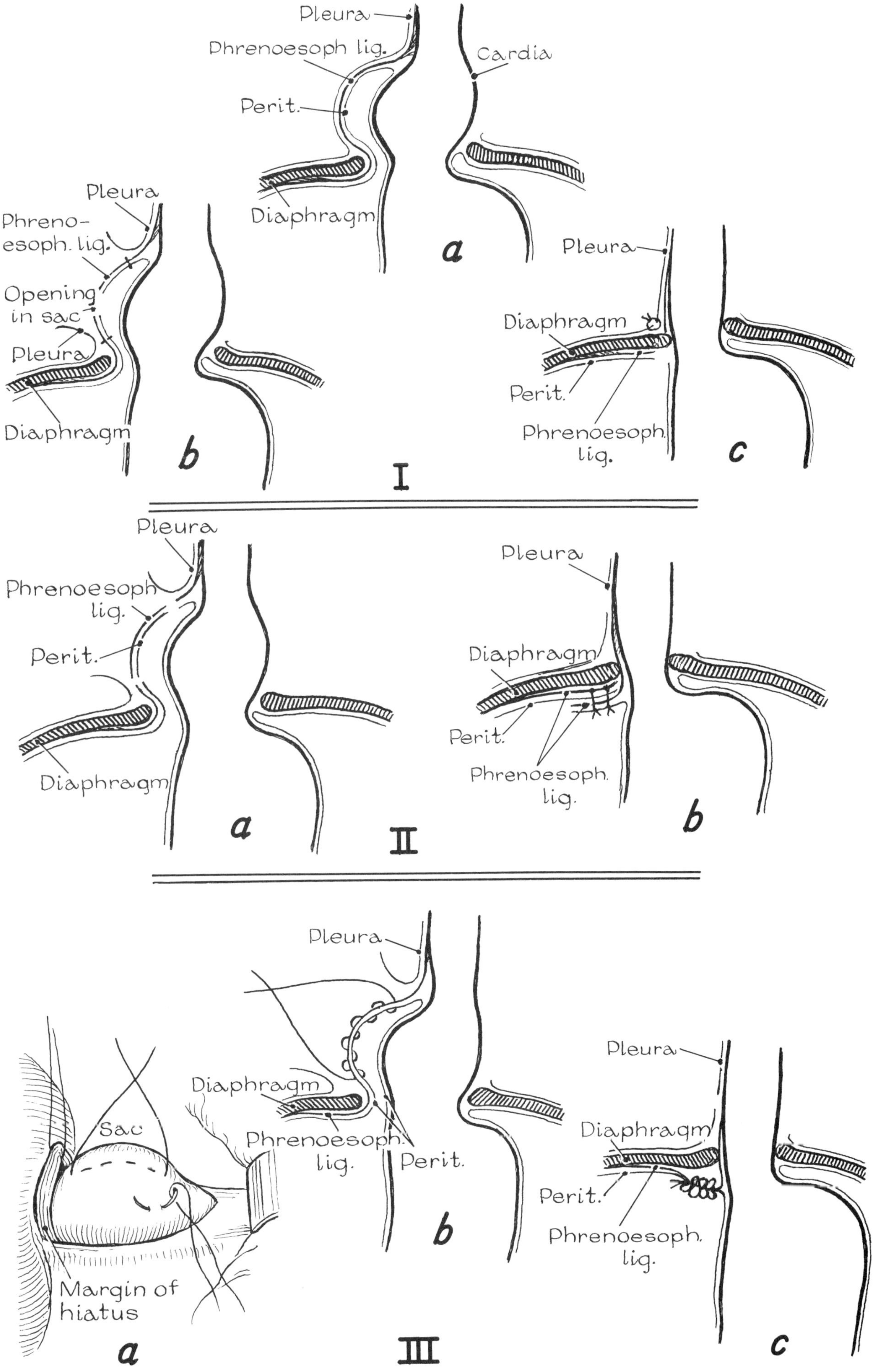
Pleura
Phrenoesoph lig.
Cardia
Perit.
Diaphragm
a
Pleura
Phreno-
esoph. lig.
Opening
in sac
Pleura
Diaphragm
b
Pleura
Diaphragm
Perit.
Phrenoesoph.
lig.
c
I
Pleura
Phrenoesoph
lig.
Perit.
Diaphragm
a
Pleura
Diaphragm
Perit.
Phrenoesoph.
lig.
b
II
Pleura
Diaphragm
Phrenoesoph.
lig.
Perit.
Sac
Margin of
hiatus
a
b
Pleura
Diaphragm
Perit.
Phrenoesoph.
lig.
c
III

The modification of the Allison method which is now used routinely as the preferred technic in the repair of an esophageal hiatus hernia is illustrated. The main modification is that the proximal cuff formed by the phrenoesophageal ligament and the peritoneum is sutured to the upper rather than the under surface of the diaphragm. Technically this is simpler, and it is believed not to lessen the anchorage effect on the esophagus.

The modification of Allison's method, recently suggested by Johnsrud, has much to recommend it. In this technic the phrenoesophageal ligament and the peritoneum forming the anterior wall of the hernial sac is not incised but instead inverted through the esophageal hiatus into the peritoneal cavity. The double thickness of the wall of the inverted hernial sac is then sutured to the under surface of the diaphragm with a series of interrupted silk sutures.

A. Through an incision in the diaphragm, the index finger is inserted into the peritoneal cavity and then through the esophageal hiatus into the lumen of the sac. The phrenoesophageal ligament is incised, and the underlying peritoneal layer is tented on the tip of the index finger.

B. The peritoneal layer which forms the anterior wall of the sac is incised, and the lumen of the hernial sac is entered. The anterior wall of the stomach which forms the posterior wall of the sac is visible. A cuff of the phrenoesophageal ligament and peritoneum is formed proximally by making the incisions indicated by the dotted lines.

C, D. The ends of the traction tape of rubber tissue which encircles the esophagus are withdrawn through the esophageal hiatus into the peritoneal cavity and then through the opening in the diaphragm into the pleural cavity. By traction on this tape the hernia is reduced into the peritoneal cavity and the muscle bundles of the right crus which form the boundaries of the esophageal hiatus are approximated both medial (anterior) and lateral (posterior) to the esophagus.

E. The proximal cuff formed by the phrenoesophageal ligament and peritoneal layers is sutured to the upper or pleural surface of the diaphragm for anchorage of the esophagus. The incision in the diaphragm is closed and the flap of diaphragmatic pleura, but not the mediastinal pleura, is sutured.

F. A diagrammatic illustration of the completed operation is shown in profile.

DISCUSSION—DR. BROOKS (cont.)

portion of these two can be felt rising up to the left of the aorta and is usually bulkier than the more anteriorly located right portion. In mobilizing these muscle bundles, care must be taken not to damage the inferior phrenic artery or the inferior vena cava. An appropriate number of braided silk interrupted sutures are taken so that the esophageal hiatus is snug. If the esophageal hiatus is made too snug, dysphagia may occur and require postoperative esophageal dilatation. As a general rule, however, most patients have some transient symptoms of esophageal hold-up for several weeks following an "adequate" repair.

Following suture of the hiatus, the phrenoesophageal ligament is sutured to the undersurface of the diaphragm if it can be obtained as a significant structure. If not, small fine silk stitches of 0000 silk are taken between the esophageal wall and the undersurface of the ring of the hiatus to secure the esophagogastric junction at this point and prevent retraction up into the mediastinum. The usual anchoring stitches of silk are then taken between the lower esophagus and the undersurface of the diaphragm and between the cardia of the stomach and the undersurface of the diaphragm. No attempt is made to reperitonize these surfaces.

A concomitant vagotomy and pyloroplasty is done if severe duodenal ulcer disease exists or if there is esophagitis with ulceration and beginning stenosis of the lower end of the esophagus. Under these circumstances, an inlying gastrostomy tube is placed, using a No. 16 Foley with a 5 cc. bag. This is brought out to the left of the incision and remains in place until the patient is eating well. In the usual patient with esophagitis without fibrosis, no vagotomy is performed.

The repair of an hiatus hernia from below the diaphragm is easily performed and can be carried out in elderly people with relatively little risk. There is less chance of impairing pulmonary reserve. A statistical evaluation of the end results shows no higher recurrence rate following repair from below than that from above, and when done from below, coexisting intra-abdominal disease can be handled at the same time.

Complicated lower esophageal strictures and problems of esophageal shortening or hernia fixation above the diaphragm can be readily handled by extending the abdominal incision across the costal margin into the left side of the chest if indicated. In my experience this is rarely required.

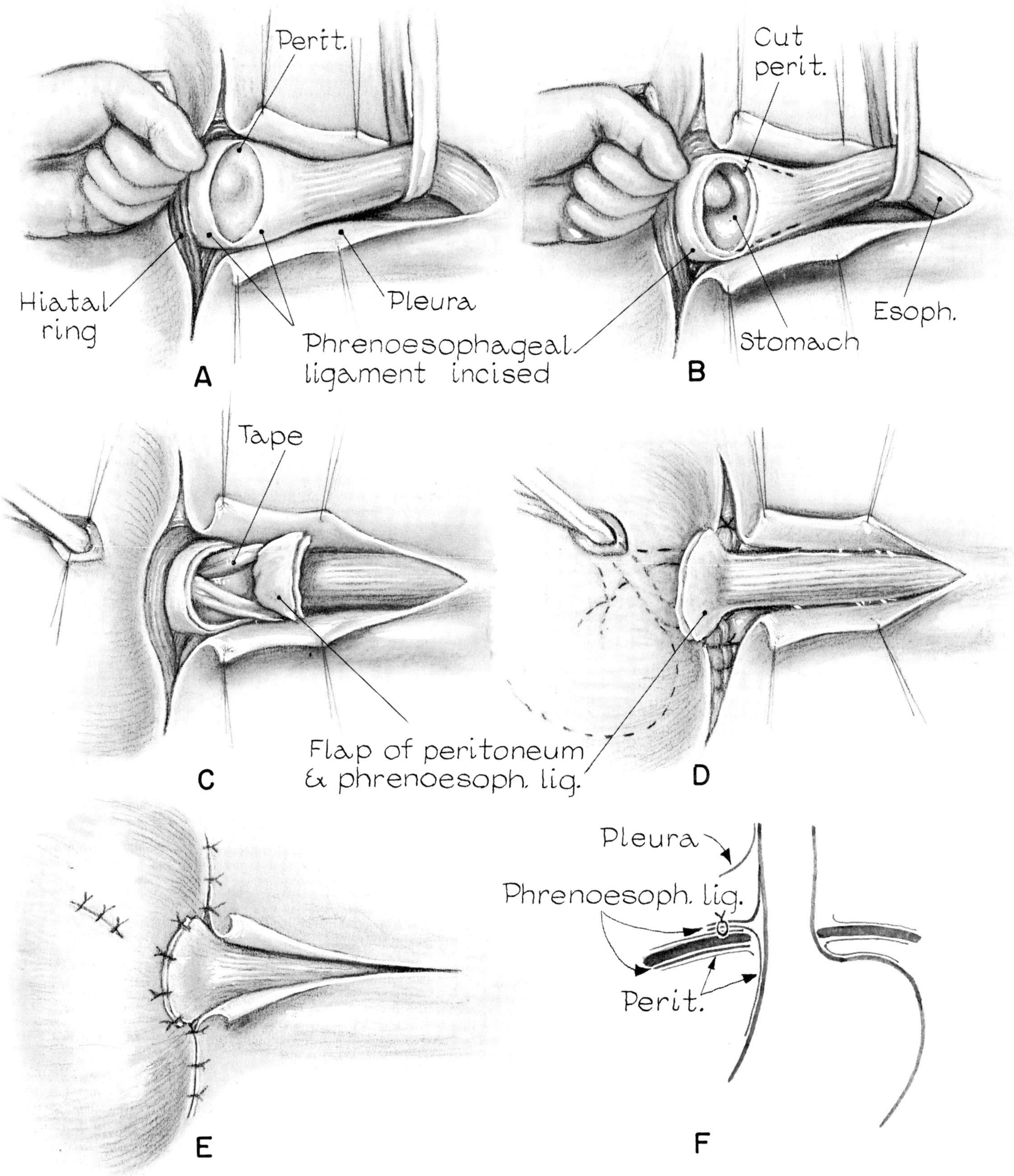
Perit.
Hiatal ring
Pleura
Phrenoesophageal ligament incised
A
Cut perit.
Esoph.
Stomach
B
Tape
C
Flap of peritoneum & phrenoesoph. lig.
D
E
Pleura
Phrenoesoph. lig.
Perit.
F

Allison emphasized the importance of closure of the hiatal ring in a vertical plane posterior to the esophagus. In the succeeding illustrations the difficulty in performing this method of closure when the long axis of the hiatus is in the transverse or horizontal plane is shown.

A. The esophageal hiatus viewed from the lower or abdominal surface of the diaphragm. The dilated hiatal ring prior to closure is demonstrated. The long axis of the ring is in a horizontal plane.

B. The excessive angulation and tension on the suture line and the inadequacy of the closure on attempted approximation of the muscle layers of the right crus in a vertical plane posterior to the esophagus are shown.

C, D. The muscle fibers of the right crus are approximated in a horizontal plane to the left of the esophagus. The closure is adequate and there is a minimum of tension on the suture line.

Although in many instances the illustrated technic has proved satisfactory, it is believed anatomically unsound. The inherent weakness in the method is the suturing of the muscle fibers of the right crus in the reconstruction of the esophageal hiatus.

Muscle tissue has a minimal "holding" power for sutures, and, as a consequence, when the muscle contracts, the sutures tear through, even though the tension on the suture line is not excessive. This occurrence has been observed repeatedly during operations, and on several occasions it was necessary to abandon the method.

The rationale of attempting to decrease the size of the hiatus is questioned. Frequently in the performance of abdominal operations the hiatus is explored digitally to estimate its size. Often it will admit three to four fingers, yet no hernia is demonstrable surgically, radiographically, or by clinical manifestations. On the contrary, a hernia may be present in a patient with a relatively small esophageal hiatus. Accordingly, the size of the hiatus is not the basic factor in the presence or absence of an esophageal hiatus hernia.

If these tenets are accepted—viz., (1) the muscle fibers of the hiatal ring should not be sutured and (2) the presence of esophageal hiatal hernia is not dependent upon the size of the hiatus—the logical question is, What operation should be performed? Admittedly, I do not know. However, it is believed that the sac should always be opened and a flap formed cephalad of peritoneum (sac) and phrenoesophageal ligament (transversalis fascia). The hernia is next reduced, and the flap previously formed is sutured to the pleural surface and tendinous portion of the diaphragm. In this manner a firm serosa-to-serosa apposition of tissues possessed of good "holding" power is obtained. Since the principle of the method is believed of basic importance, anchorage of the flap to the under or peritoneal surface of the diaphragm is not considered necessary. In fact, this procedure not only is technically more difficult but also necessitates the apposition of fascia (phrenoesophageal ligament) to serosa rather than the preferred serosa-to-serosa union that is obtained with the technic previously described. The union of serosa to serosa is a time-honored principle in intestinal surgery.

In some instances the ends of the peritoneal-fascia flaps are sutured together behind the esophagus to form a circular cuff about the esophagocardial junction. The lower margin of the cuff is then sutured in a circular manner to the adjacent cut margins of the diaphragmatic pleura and the underlying tendinous portion of the diaphragm. Again, serosa-to-serosa apposition is obtained with concomitant fascia reinforcement on each side of the suture line. This technic, from theoretical as well as practical considerations, is preferred.

In each of the technics described the transthoracic route is required. Accordingly, this route is of necessity preferred. Many surgeons elect the abdominal route so that an artificial angle of His may be more easily established by suture of the fundus of the stomach to the undersurface of the diaphragm in juxtaposition to the hiatus. The basis for this maneuver is more theoretical than real. What is more important is the reduction of the hernia and the maintenance of its reduction, which may be more ably accomplished by use of the transthoracic approach.

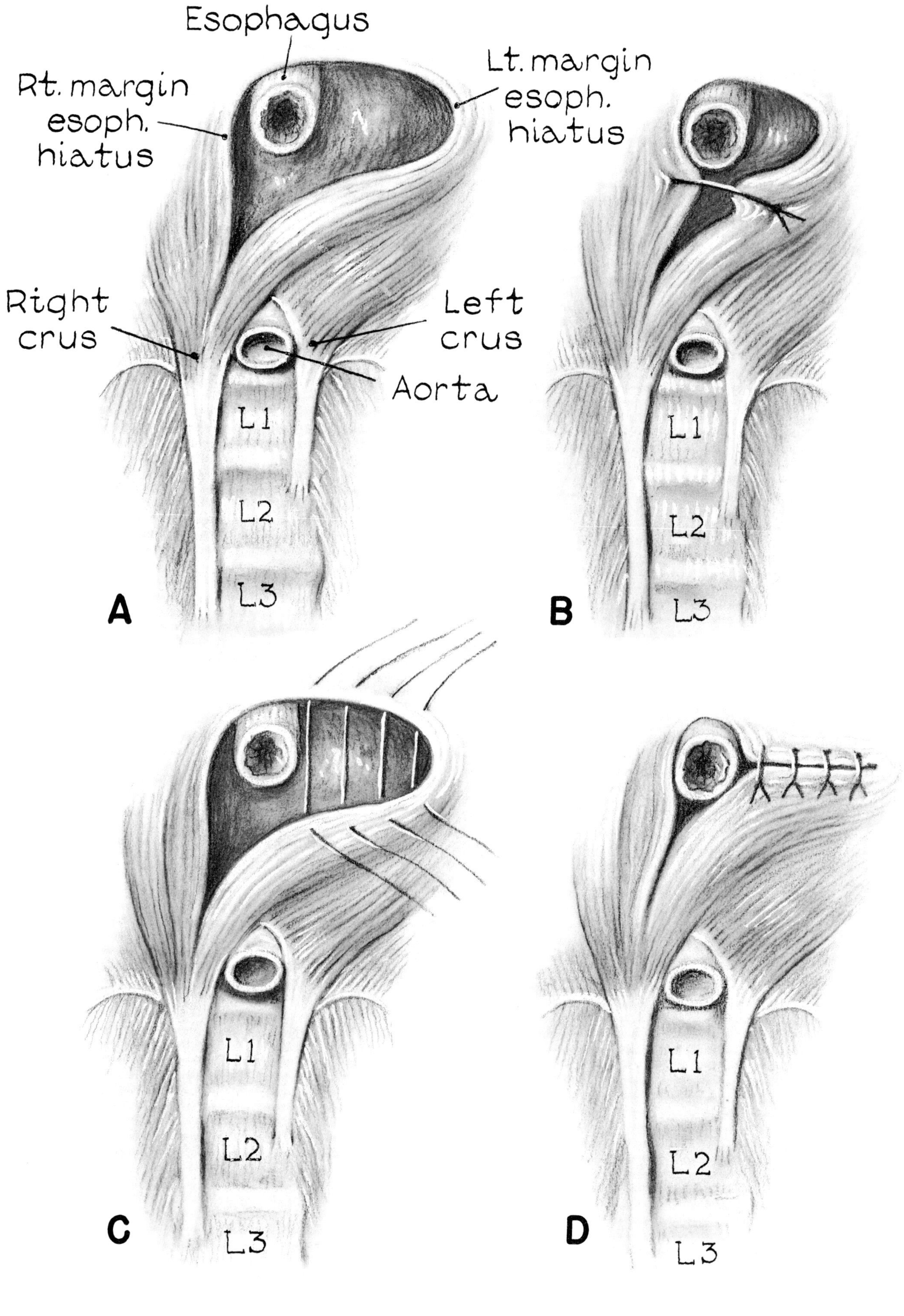
Esophagus
Rt. margin esoph. hiatus
Lt. margin esoph. hiatus
Right crus
Left crus
Aorta
L1
L2
L3
A
B
C
D

The same illustrations as in Plate 85 when viewed from the upper or thoracic surface of the diaphragm with the patient in the direct right lateral prone position.

A. The thick layer of muscle fibers of the right crus, the left margin of the hiatal ring, crossing superficial to the thin layer of muscle fibers of the right crus, the right margin of the hiatal ring, is shown. The long axis of the hiatus is in the left lateral or horizontal plane.

B. The excessive angulation and tension on the suture line and the inadequate closure on attempted approximation of the muscle fibers of the right crus in a vertical plane posterior to the esophagus is demonstrated.

All too frequently artist's illustrations depicting the transthoracic approach for the repair of an esophageal hiatus hernia will show the thoracic incision being properly made with the patient in the right lateral prone position. But when the left pleural cavity is entered, the anatomic relations of the hiatal ring and the method for its closure are illustrated as if the patient were supine. It is believed that such illustrations are perpetuations of error which have led to needless confusion and misunderstanding of both the anatomy of the hiatal ring and the methods of surgical repair. The surgeon should remember that in the transthoracic approach, with the patient in the right lateral prone position, the posterior angle of the hiatal ring is always facing toward him. Furthermore, it is at this angle that the crossing of the fibers of the right crus occurs (A).

Commonly in the transthoracic approach, closure of the hiatal ring in the lateral plane to the left of the esophagus (C) is described as anterior to the esophagus. Similarly, closure in the opposite or right lateral plane (D) is described as posterior to the esophagus. However, a careful study of the comparative relation of the hiatal ring to the esophagus in the supine (Plate 85) and in the right lateral prone positions (Plate 86) should aid in the correction of these anatomic misinterpretations.

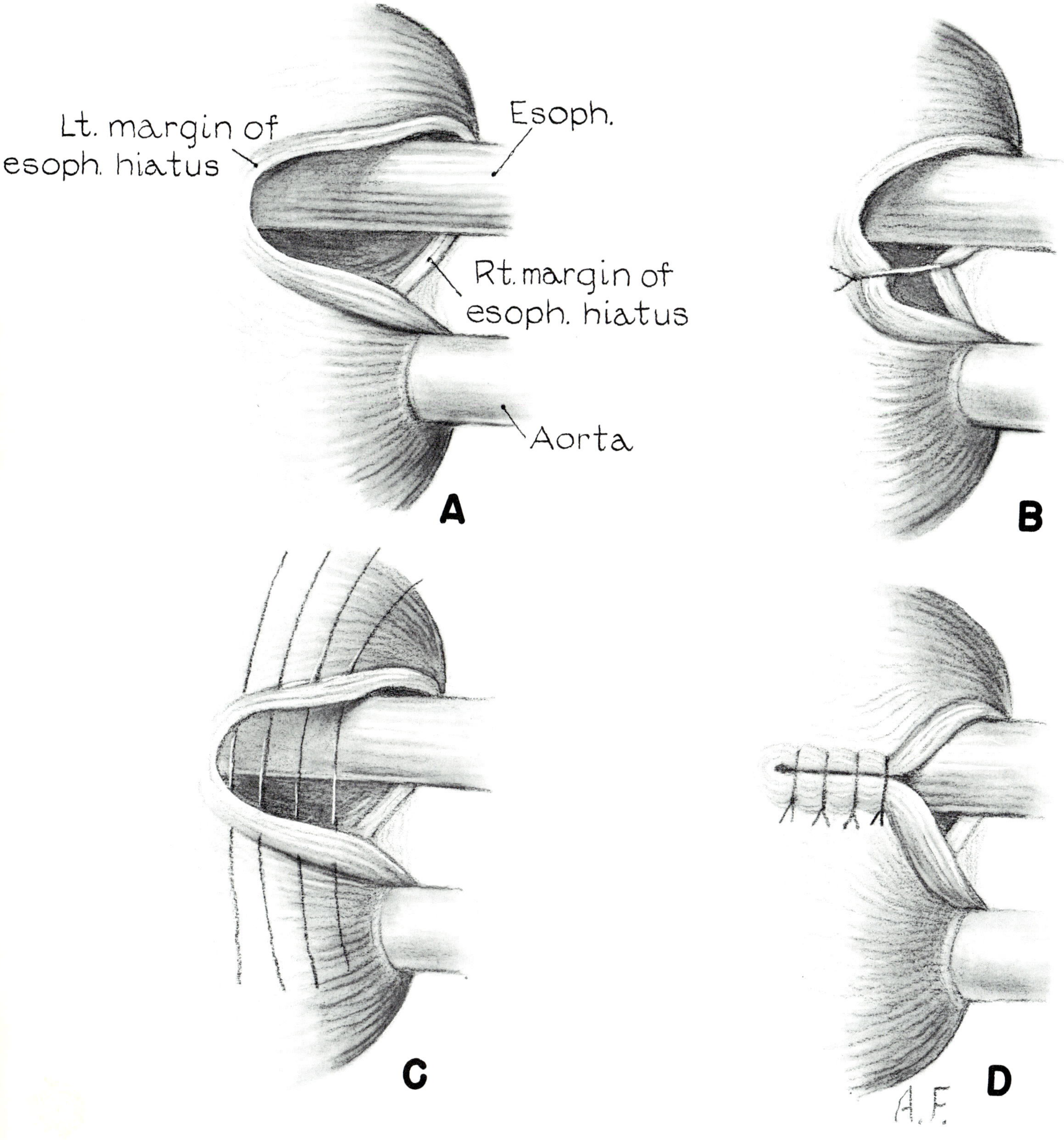
Lt. margin of esoph. hiatus
Esoph.
Rt. margin of esoph. hiatus
Aorta
A
B
C
D
A.F.

THE TRANSABDOMINAL APPROACH FOR THE REPAIR OF AN ESOPHAGEAL HIATUS HERNIA

A. The patient is placed in the supine position, and the incision of choice, a long left paramedian muscle-retracting (lateral) incision, is outlined.

B. The peritoneal cavity is entered, and the related intraperitoneal viscera are demonstrable. By manual retraction the left lobe of the liver is displaced downward toward the midline, and its mobilization is commenced by the severance of the avascular left triangular ligament. In some instances the left lobe of the liver is elongated and the left triangular ligament is markedly foreshortened. Under such circumstances the esophagocardial region is exposed by the retraction upward of the left lobe of the liver, the surface of which is protected by a moist gauze pad.

C. The mobilized left lobe of the liver is turned downward and inward on itself, and, after being covered with a moist gauze pad, it is retracted medialward. By manual traction the herniated segment of the stomach into the posterior mediastinum through the esophageal hiatus is reduced, and the layer of peritoneum overlying the esophagocardial junction is severed by scissor dissection.

D. The posterior mediastinal space is entered and the terminal portion of the esophagus, mobilized previously by digital dissection, is encircled by a rubber tissue drain for the purpose of traction.

E. The reduction of the hernia is maintained by downward traction. The terminal 4 cm. of the esophagus is exposed, and its relation to the vagus nerves and the right and left margins of the esophageal hiatus formed by the superficial and deep muscle layers respectively of the right crus of the diaphragm are demonstrated.

F. The esophagus is displaced to the left to show the enlarged esophageal hiatus and its formation by the separation of the fibers of the right crus into thin superficial (right margin) and thick deep (left margin) muscle layers.

G. The superficial and deep muscle layers of the right crus of the diaphragm, the right and left margins respectively of the hiatal ring, are approximated in a slightly oblique plane posterior to the esophagus, using two or three interrupted sutures of silk (No. 1). In this approximation, tension on the suture line should be avoided.

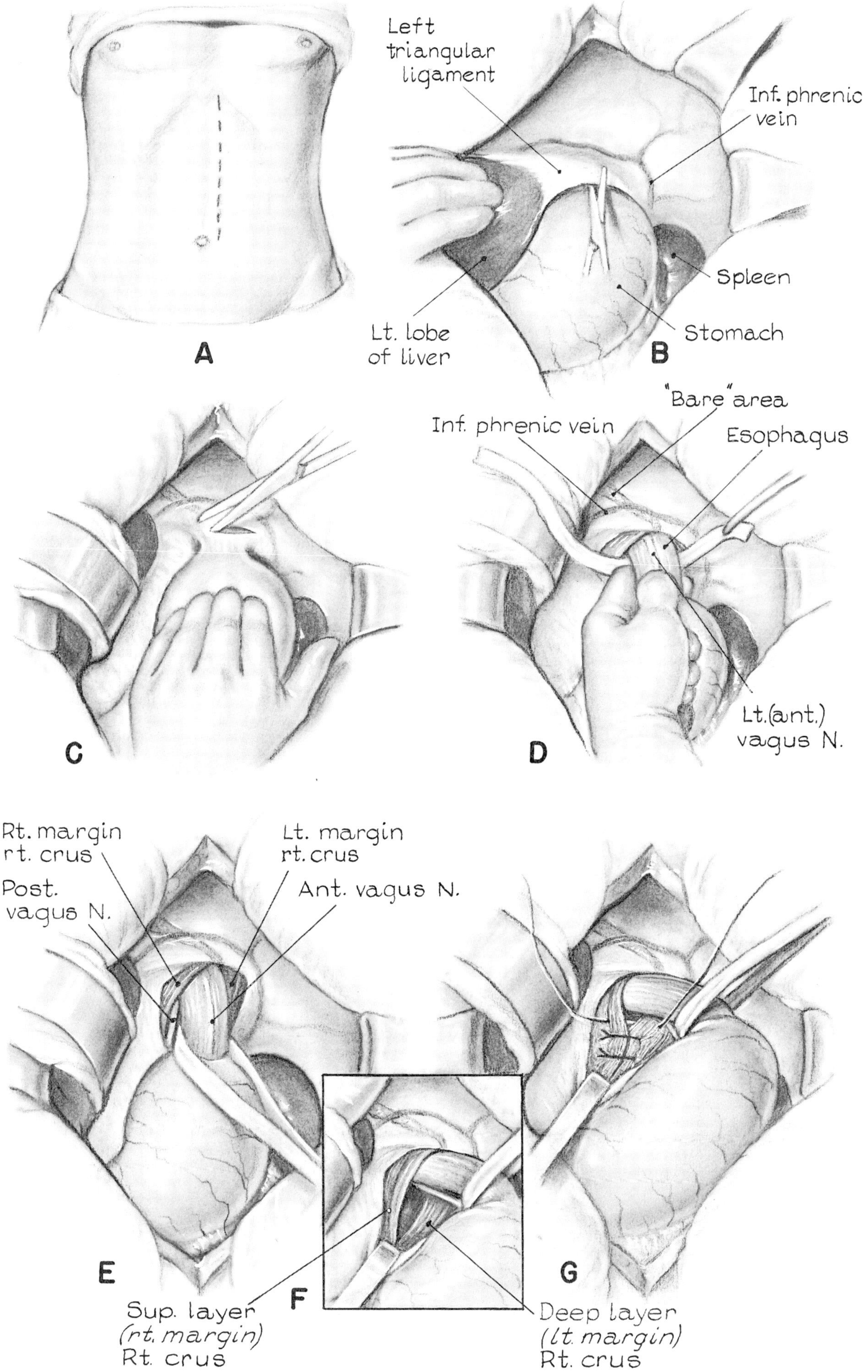
A
Left triangular ligament
Inf. phrenic vein
Spleen
Stomach
Lt. lobe of liver
B
C
"Bare" area
Inf. phrenic vein
Esophagus
Lt. (ant.) vagus N.
D
Rt. margin rt. crus
Lt. margin rt. crus
Post. vagus N.
Ant. vagus N.
E
F
G
Sup. layer (rt. margin) Rt. crus
Deep layer (lt. margin) Rt. crus

Discussion—Dr. Denton A. Cooley. Indications for the transthoracic or transabdominal approach in the repair of an esophageal hiatal hernia were not part of this presentation, yet this aspect of the technical problem is important and deserves careful consideration. After an experience with a sizable series of patients operated upon by both technics, I have concluded that the transabdominal approach should be the procedure of choice. Two exceptions to this policy would be, first, the extremely obese patient in whom surgical exposure in the upper abdomen would be difficult and, second, the patient with a recurrent hernia. Recurrence of an esophageal hiatal hernia is difficult to repair from the abdominal route, since adhesions about the hiatus and herniated stomach located in the mediastinum or pleural space are difficult to divide transabdominally. In some of the more complicated recurrences with a history of more than one attempted repair, consideration should even be given to a combined thoraco-abdominal incision so the repair can be accomplished from above and below the hiatus.

Selection of the transabdominal approach for all other elective situations depends upon a number of factors. Exposure of the anatomy about the hiatus is best demonstrated from below. Anatomists and artists support this viewpoint, since their descriptions and drawings usually emphasize this surface of the diaphragm. Avoiding the thoracotomy incision also eliminates the intercostal nerve pain or troublesome neuralgia, which may simulate the symptoms caused by the hernia. Efforts to eliminate this postoperative chest pain by technics of reapproximating the ribs, as described by Dr. Madden, are helpful but by no means completely effective. Moreover, pericostal sutures of heavy silk should probably be replaced by absorbable chromic catgut. The midline abdominal incision is less difficult than a paramedian and is easier to repair. Nonabsorbable Dacron or Mersilene sutures in the linea alba give a firm repair with a low incidence of incisional hernia.

An important step in repair of the lesion is complete reduction of the hernia and withdrawal of the esophagus well down into the subdiaphragmatic position. This can best be accomplished by the vertical downward traction from the upper abdomen with the patient lying supine. Since the muscle fibers of the crus are usually attenuated and friable, interrupted sutures have a tendency to cut through the fibers. Thus, from the transabdominal approach these sutures should be placed through the covering peritoneum for additional support. Repair of the hiatus, in my opinion, should always be done by approximating the fibers of the crus posterior and inferior to the hiatus, leaving the anterior sling unrestricted by plicating sutures. The size of the hiatus should be carefully controlled and should not be too tight because edema may cause dysphagia after operation. After the repair, the opening should accommodate an index finger easily alongside the esophagus.

When the hernia is completely reduced, a portion of 2 to 3 cm. of longitudinal muscle fibers of esophagus above the esophagogastric junction is visible below the newly repaired hiatus. Usually the phrenicoesophageal ligament, which in my opinion is overrated as a useful structure in the repair of the hernia, is located well down in the abdominal cavity. An important part of the repair is placement of a circle of interrupted 000 nonabsorbable sutures, about six or eight in number, to anchor the esophagus to the hiatal fibers. Another technical point that may be important is to place a row of interrupted sutures between the gastric cardia and the adjacent esophagus. The maneuver maintains the acute esophagogastric angle that is important to prevent esophageal reflux. The vagus nerves should not be divided or sutured into the repair unless the patient requires additional surgery for peptic ulcer or reflux esophagitis.

Perhaps the strongest argument in favor of the transabdominal approach is the opportunity afforded for exploration of the peritoneal cavity for additional pathologic lesions. Among the more common associated lesions in my experience were chronic cholecystitis with cholelithiasis and duodenal ulcer. Occasionally unsuspected retroperitoneal or intraperitoneal neoplasms have also been discovered: they were the actual cause for the patient's symptoms. Routine appendectomy was also employed in our patients.

Discussion—Dr. Richard H. Sweet. The *abdominal approach* for the repair of a hiatus hernia is well illustrated in Plate 87. Here also precise knowledge of the anatomy is absolutely essential. In fact, the failures which result from the use of this approach are undoubtedly due to inaccuracy in dealing with the structures involved. As with all surgery, a wide exposure of the operative field must be obtained. It is this aspect of the employment of the abdominal approach which creates the greatest technical problem.

The incision must be long and must reach upward to the costoxiphoid angle (Plate 87, A). So also the left lobe of the liver must be retracted away from the operative field. This step requires the division of the left triangular ligament and the folding under of the liver edge as shown in Plate 87 (B and C).

It should be stressed also that, with the abdominal approach as with the thoracic, the margins of the hiatus must be exposed to view so that sutures can be inserted in the muscle bundles. This is best accomplished by retracting the esophagus to the left (Plate 87, F and G).

Little remains of the peritoneal sac after the dissection necessary to expose the lower esophagus and the muscle bundles of the right crus has been completed, but nothing much need be done about it. Any redundant edges of peritoneum, however, can be trimmed away and the peritoneal layer closed with sutures which attach it to the undersurface of the diaphragm as an additional safeguard against recurrence.

EVENTRATION OF THE DIAPHRAGM

A. The patient is placed in the direct right lateral prone position, and the incision overlying the eighth rib is indicated by the solid line.

B. The elevated left leaflet of the diaphragm which caused a compression atelectasis of the lower lobe of the left lung is shown. Despite the high elevation of the diaphragmatic leaflet, its muscle tone was surprisingly good. No tendinous portion was visible.

C. The diaphragm is retracted downward, and the flaps of the posterior mediastinal and diaphragmatic pleura are raised to expose the lower portion of the esophagus and the muscular esophageal hiatal ring. This ring is formed by a separation of the muscle fibers of the right crus into two layers, superficial and deep. The superficial layer forms the right margin and the deep layer the left margin of the esophageal hiatus. From the thoracic approach as illustrated, the thick layer of fibers which forms the left margin crosses superficial to the thin layer of fibers which forms the right margin of the hiatus. The reverse is true when the hiatus is viewed from the abdominal side with the patient supine. It should also be observed that with the patient in the right lateral prone position, the posterior angle of the esophageal ring is directed toward the surgeon. This anatomic point is stressed because it is so frequently misrepresented in artist's illustrations. In this patient a concomitant finding was a small sliding hiatus hernia.

D. The lower portion of the esophagus is encircled by a cotton tape for traction, and the left leaflet of the diaphragm, tented by guy sutures of silk (000), is incised. The incision is subsequently extended by scissor dissection as indicated by the dotted line.

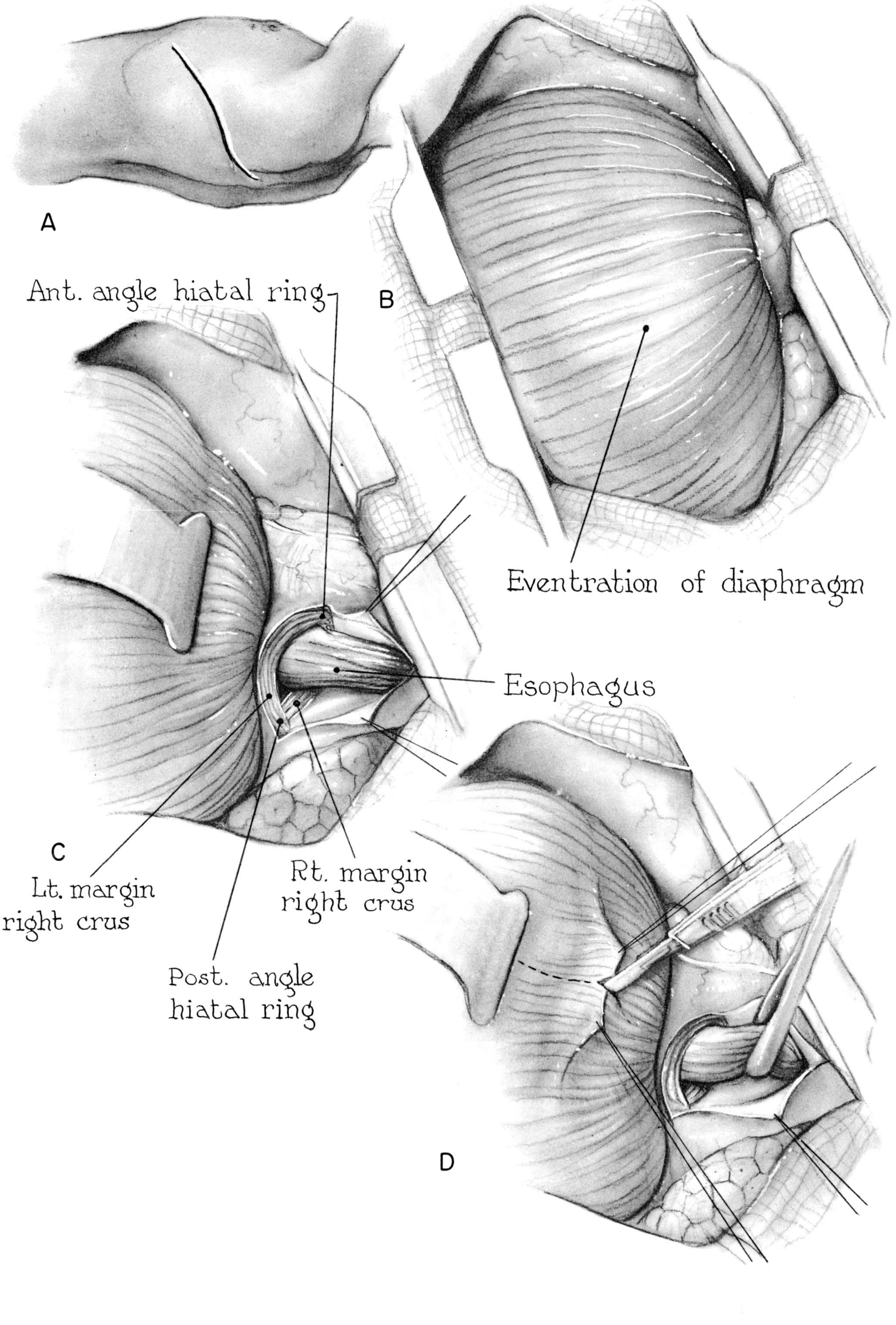

A
B
Ant. angle hiatal ring
Eventration of diaphragm
Esophagus
C
Lt. margin right crus
Rt. margin right crus
Post. angle hiatal ring
D

E. The incised margins of the diaphragm are grasped in Babcock clamps and the scissor dissection is continued. Underlying portions of the stomach and the left lobe of the liver are visible.

F. The long ends of the cotton tape which encircle the lower portion of the esophagus are passed through the hiatus into the peritoneal cavity and then through the opening in the diaphragm into the left pleural cavity. By traction on the tape the small herniated segment of the stomach is reduced, and the closure of the hiatal ring posteriorly is begun by the insertion of a suture of No. 1 silk. In this illustration the anterior border of the spleen is visible.

G. The closure of the hiatal ring posteriorly using two interrupted sutures of silk (No. 1) is completed, and the insertion of the imbricating mattress sutures of silk (0) for the repair of the eventration of the diaphragm is begun.

H. All but one of the imbricating mattress sutures are inserted. The insertion of these sutures is begun farther from the incised margin of the diaphragm anteriorly than posteriorly so that, when they are tied, an overlap (imbrication) of the cut margins of the diaphragm is obtained.

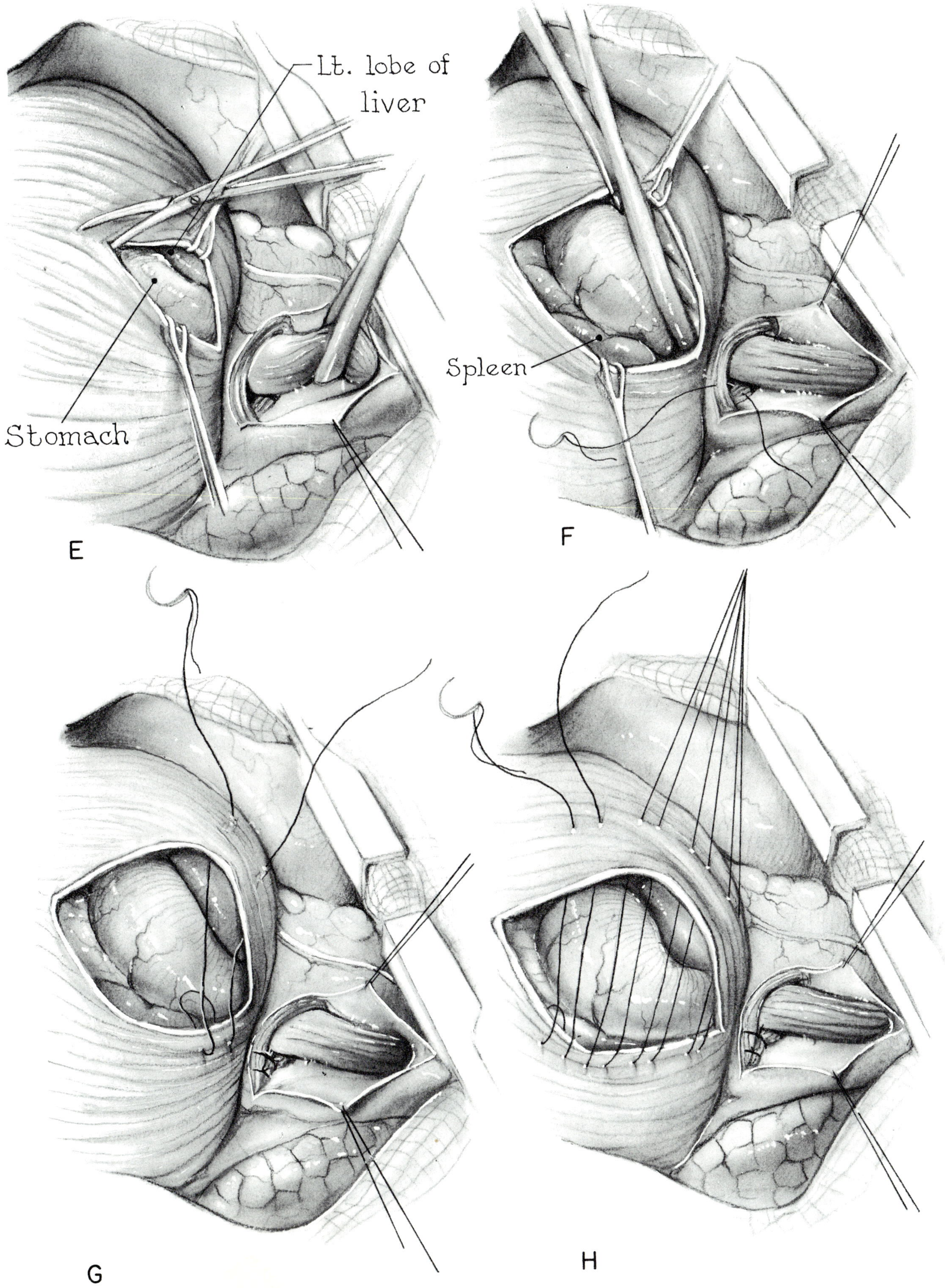
Lt. lobe of liver
Stomach
E
Spleen
F
G
H

I. The imbricating mattress sutures of silk are tied, and the excess of the overlapping portion of the diaphragm is excised as indicated by the dotted line.

J. The free cut margin of the overlapping portion of the left leaflet of the diaphragm is sutured to its subjacent portion with interrupted sutures of 0 silk.

K, L. In this patient some laxity of the diaphragm persisted following the repair as depicted. Accordingly, a secondary inversion layer of interrupted sutures of 0 silk was first inserted (K) and the sutures then were tied (L). Following the completion of this procedure, the relation of the left leaflet of the diaphragm to its opposite side and to the adjacent intrapleural structures appeared normal. The lower lobe of the left lung was easily expanded to its full capacity, and the flaps of diaphragmatic pleura were approximated with interrupted sutures of silk (000). The flaps of posterior mediastinal pleura were not sutured. Accordingly, in the event of an infection, a complicating pleural empyema which is easily drained rather than a mediastinal abscess which is difficult to drain would most likely occur.

This patient, a 63-year-old obese white man, was admitted to the hospital because of massive gastrointestinal bleeding. A gastrointestinal series revealed a true "upside-down" stomach associated with a high elevation of the left leaflet of the diaphragm as depicted in the illustrations. The summit of the elevation was at the level of the third rib anteriorly. Because of the severity of the hemorrhage and the previous history of symptoms consistent with the diagnosis of a duodenal ulcer, operation was advised. Although the relation of the esophagocardial junction to the hiatal ring appeared normal in the roentgenograms, at operation there was an associated small esophageal hiatal hernia of the sliding variety. In addition to the surgical correction of the eventration of the diaphragm as illustrated, a transdiaphragmatic antecolic gastrojejunostomy, in conjunction with a transthoracic partial resection of the vagus nerves, was done. Postoperative roentgenograms of the chest revealed normal position and mobility of the left leaflet of the diaphragm.

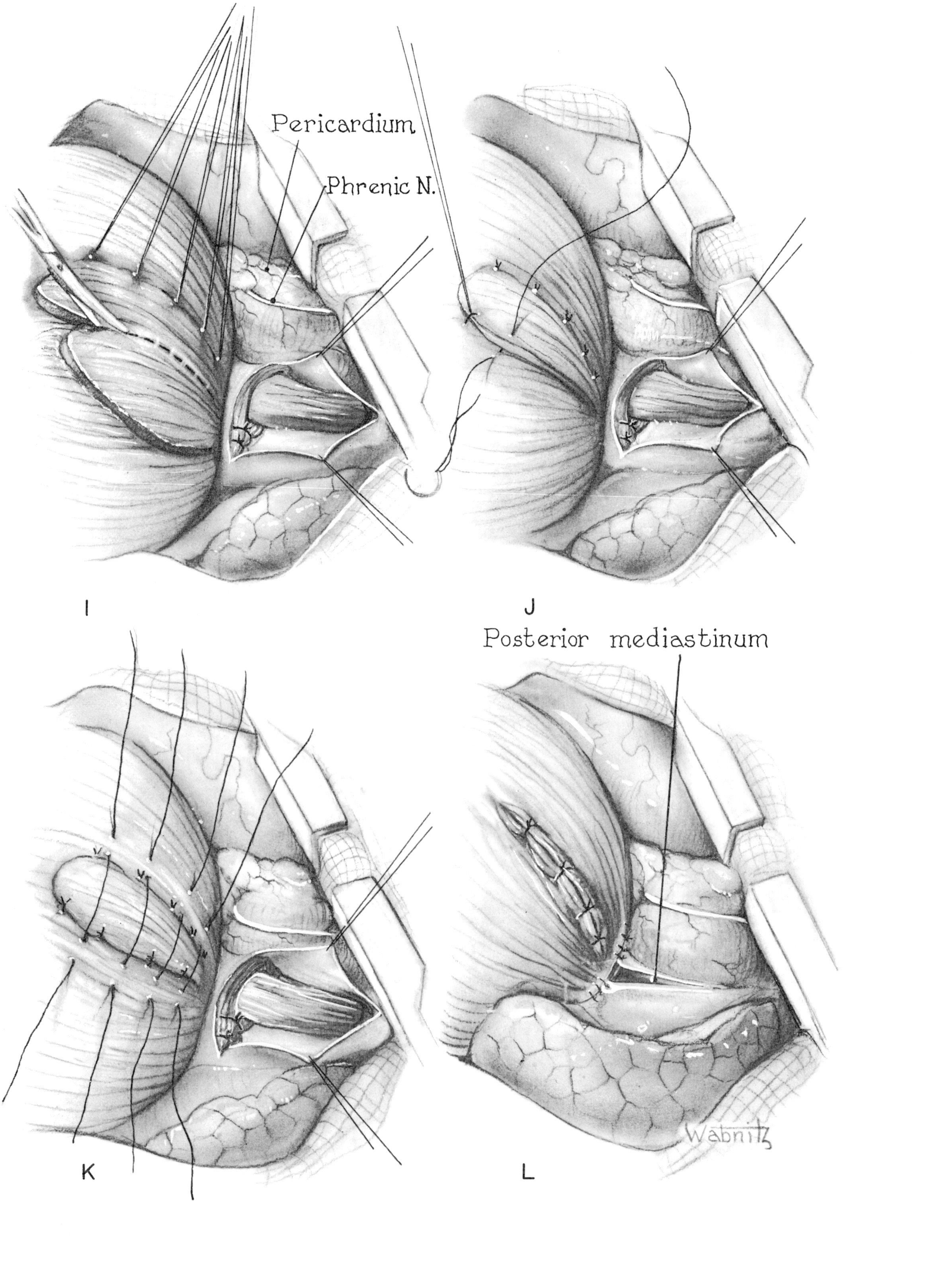
Pericardium
Phrenic N.
I
J
Posterior mediastinum
K
L
Wabnitz

INFRADIAPHRAGMATIC RESECTION OF THE VAGUS NERVES AND ANTECOLIC GASTROJEJUNOSTOMY

A, B, C. The peritoneal cavity is entered through a left paramedian muscle-retracting (lateral) incision.

D. The wound margins are retracted, and the structures in the region of the esophago-cardial junction are shown. The site of severance of the avascular left triangular ligament is shown in dotted outline. In some instances this ligament may be too short to sever. Under such circumstances, a moist protective pad is placed beneath the left lobe of the liver which is gently retracted upward.

E, F. An incision is made through the peritoneal and fascia layers overlying the lowermost portion of the esophagus, and the posterior mediastinal space is entered. The relation of the esophagus to the margins of the right crus of the diaphragm which form completely the esophageal hiatal ring is shown.

Discussion—Dr. Lester R. Dragstedt. In the transabdominal approach for resection of the vagus nerves, it has been my usual practice to divide the triangular ligament to the left lobe of the liver, as illustrated in D, Plate 91. I believe that this gives better access to the lower portion of the esophagus. However, some surgeons of experience, including Dr. Joseph Weinberg of Los Angeles, omit this step and retract the left lobe of the liver upward with a large broad blade retractor. In entering the mediastinum, I have found it wise to make the opening midway between the esophageal hiatus and the large inferior phrenic vein, as demonstrated in the illustrations E and F, Plate 91. I customarily do this by picking up the diaphragm with forceps with protruding teeth, making a small nick with a pair of scissors, and

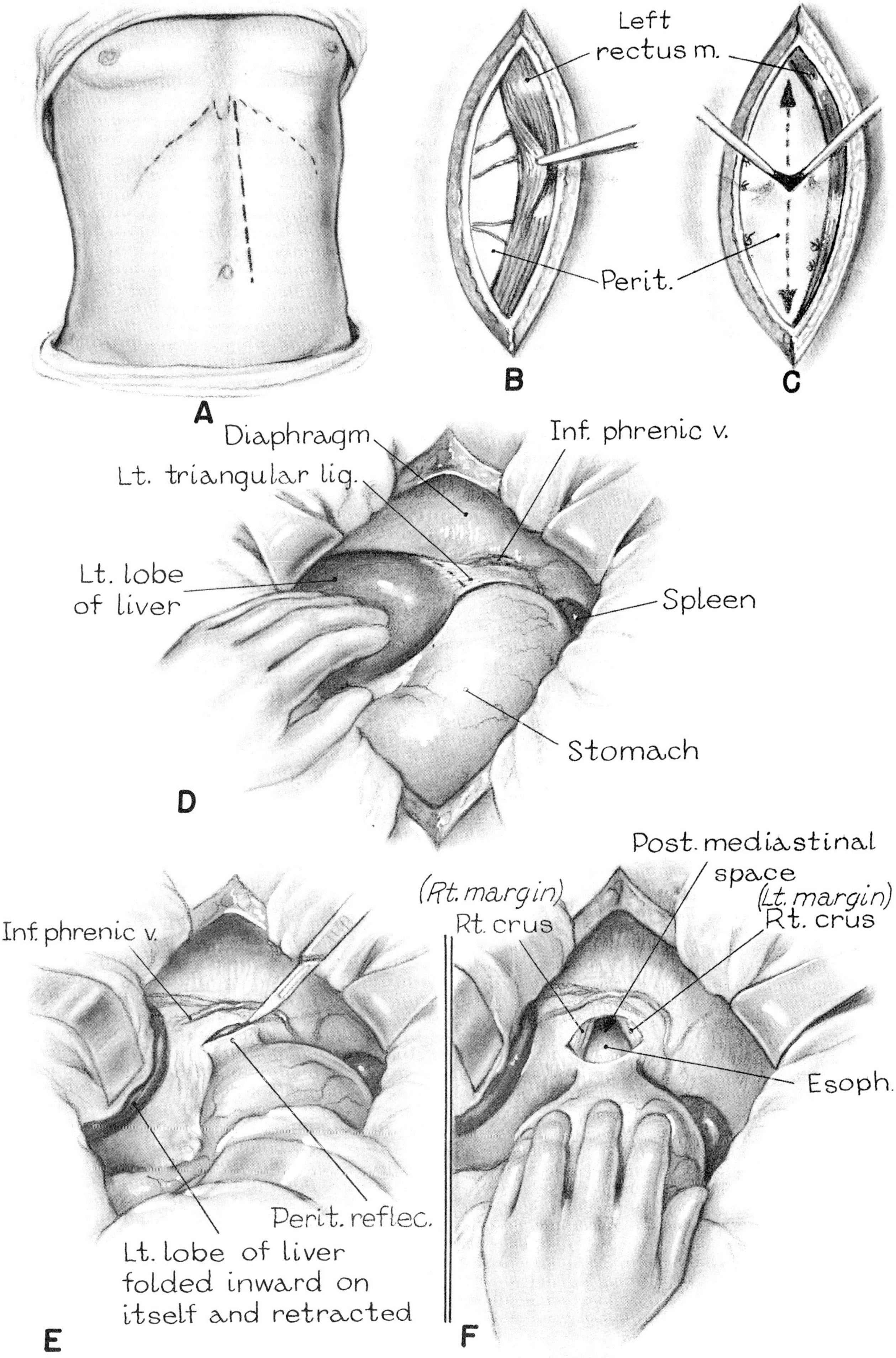
A
Left
rectus m.
Perit.
B
C
Diaphragm
Lt. triangular lig.
Inf. phrenic v.
Lt. lobe
of liver
Spleen
Stomach
D
Inf. phrenic v.
Perit. reflec.
Lt. lobe of liver
folded inward on
itself and retracted
E
Post. mediastinal
space
(Rt. margin)
Rt. crus
(Lt. margin)
Rt. crus
Esoph.
F

G. The lower end of the esophagus is mobilized by blunt digital dissection and encircled by a rubber tissue traction tape. The left anterior vagus nerve which is always in close relation to the anterior surface of the esophagus is visible.

H, I. The esophagus is displaced to the left by traction, and the right or posterior vagus nerve located in the fibroareolar tissue posterior and medial to the esophagus is mobilized on the right index finger and secured on a nerve hook.

J. The right (posterior) vagus nerve is divided with scissors between a silver clip marker above and a clamp below.

K. The left (anterior) vagus nerve is similarly divided, and careful digital exploration of the periesophageal region for additional nerve fibers is being performed. This is considered a most important part of the operation. A minimum of 3 and a maximum of 13 additional nerve fibers have been identified by this maneuver.

L. The duodenojejunal junction at the base of the transverse mesocolon, as indicated by the ligament of Treitz, is visualized, and a segment of jejunum, 9 to 12 inches distally, is isolated by two guy sutures of silk.

Discussion—Dr. Dragstedt (cont.)

then thrusting the scissors into the mediastinum, thus enlarging the opening. Sometimes I think this may avoid troublesome hemorrhage.

In mobilizing the esophagus by blunt finger dissection it is important to emphasize that this be done gently. Several cases have been reported where the esophagus has been opened with rough handling. Upon mobilization of the esophagus it is my practice to sweep the fingers of the right hand around the esophagus in an effort to include all of the vagus fibers within their grasp. The esophagus and vagus nerves are then pulled downward into the abdomen whereupon the posterior vagus nerve, which is felt against the yielding esophagus, is pulled over to the left and a segment excised between ligatures of nonabsorbable suture material. The use of silver clips is equally satisfactory.

If a gastrojejunostomy rather than pyloroplasty is selected as a drainage procedure, I believe it is wise to place the gastroenterostomy stoma within five or six cm. of the pylorus. We have encountered a number of patients where a high-lying gastrojejunostomy failed to drain adequately the antrum of the stomach, and the stasis of food in this area caused an excessive secretion of gastric juice of humoral or hormonal origin. It has also been my practice to make a small gastroenterostomy opening so that when the operation is completed the stoma is approximately one-and-one-half cm. in diameter. It is my conviction that such a small stoma decreases the incidence and severity of the dumping syndrome.

The transthoracic approach for division of the vagus nerves, such as indicated in the illustrations of this operation, was the method that I first employed. However, this operation has been very largely abandoned by me because it does not provide an opportunity to add a drainage procedure to the vagotomy, it does not permit inspection of the ulcer and possible associated pathology, and because of the frequency of postoperative intercostal pain. This approach, however, may be used for the treatment of recurrent gastrojejunal ulcers after repeated gastric resection and possibly in some other special situation.

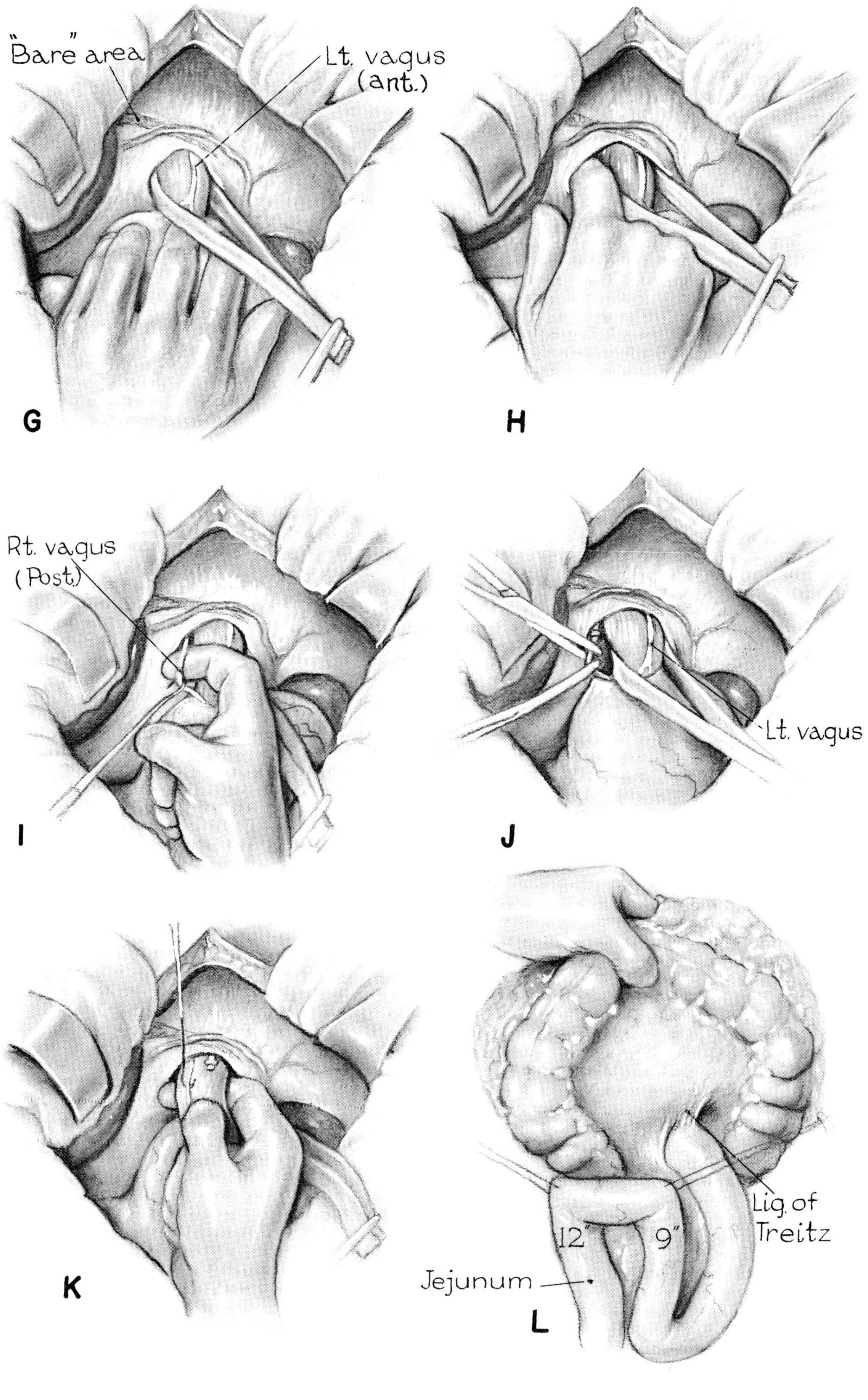
"Bare" area
Lt. vagus (ant.)
G
H
Rt. vagus (Post.)
I
Lt. vagus
J
K
Lig. of Treitz
12"
9"
Jejunum
L

M, N. A segment of the anterior wall of the stomach in juxtaposition to the most dependent portion of the greater curvature is mobilized by Babcock clamps, and the anterior gastric branches of the gastroepiploic arch are serially clamped, severed, and ligated.

O. The anterior, and all but one of the posterior, gastric branches of the gastroepiploic arch have been severed and ligated, and the lesser sac is entered.

P. The segment of jejunum previously isolated is brought anterior to the transverse colon and approximated to the posterior wall of the greater curvature of the stomach by a series of interrupted silk (000) sutures. If preferred, the jejunum may be brought through an opening in an avascular portion of the transverse mesocolon and a "short loop" retrocolic gastrojejunostomy performed. The sites of incision in the jejunum and in the avascular plane of the greater curvature of the stomach are indicated in dotted outline. No clamps are used in the performance of the anastomosis. This is the preferred technic.

p′. Inset to show the relation of the first posterior layer of sutures to the mesenteric border of the jejunum.

Q. Incisions are made through the seromuscular layers of the jejunum and the greater curvature of the stomach, and the vessels in the submucosal layers are undersewn with hemostatic suture ligatures of silk (0000).

R. The lumen of the stomach is first entered by an incision with a scalpel, and the opening is extended by scissor dissection. The opening, similarly made previously into the lumen of the jejunum, is visible. Soiling of the operative field with either gastric or jejunal contents is minimized by aspiration with the suction tube.

Discussion—Dr. Stanley O. Hoerr. I prefer a midline incision that will extend to the left of the xiphoid and, if necessary, to the left of the umbilicus (A, B, C). It is very important for ease of exposure to go as high as possible. A self-retaining retractor of the Balfour type may be used instead of hand-held retractors (D). Exposure of the diaphragmatic reflection at the cardioesophageal may be obtained by a ribbon or malleable retractor elevating the left lobe of the liver; in my experience, division of the left triangular ligament is rarely necessary.

Instead of tugging on the esophagus with an encircling rubber tape or catheter (G, H, J), I employ traction on the stomach to make the nerve stand out like a bowstring. The first assistant is instructed to pull the stomach (grasped through a gauze pad) toward the left great toe of the patient. The surgeon may wish to do this first himself, using his right hand, while with his left forefinger he palpates the nerve. While palpating the nerve, he transfers the stomach to his assistant, who maintains the same degree of traction. A long nerve hook with a right-angle tip (rather than a curved one as shown in I and K) may be used to break through the overlying thin layer of peritoneum, thus omitting the stages shown in E and F. A second nerve hook may be used to free up a segment of nerve for easy division and removal of a segment for the pathologist. Sometimes the nerve trunk, particularly the posterior trunk, is accompanied by a small blood vessel; both cut ends should then be clipped or ligated (J). After division of the main trunks, the operator standing on the right side of the patient may encircle the esophagus with his *left* forefinger, permitting the surface to be inspected for additional fibers. The posterior (right) vagus nerve at the level of the cardioesophageal junction may lie a centimeter or more posterior to the esophagus, and characteristically overlies the aorta, coursing slightly to the left as it descends. Sometimes elevating the stomach slightly (toward the ceiling) while maintaining traction toward the feet will facilitate exposure of this trunk. Inexperienced surgeons may easily overlook even a sizable posterior vagus nerve. Reconstruction of the hiatus may be done after severance of the nerves but is rarely indicated. An exception may be the coexistence of an hiatus hernia believed to be symptomatic.

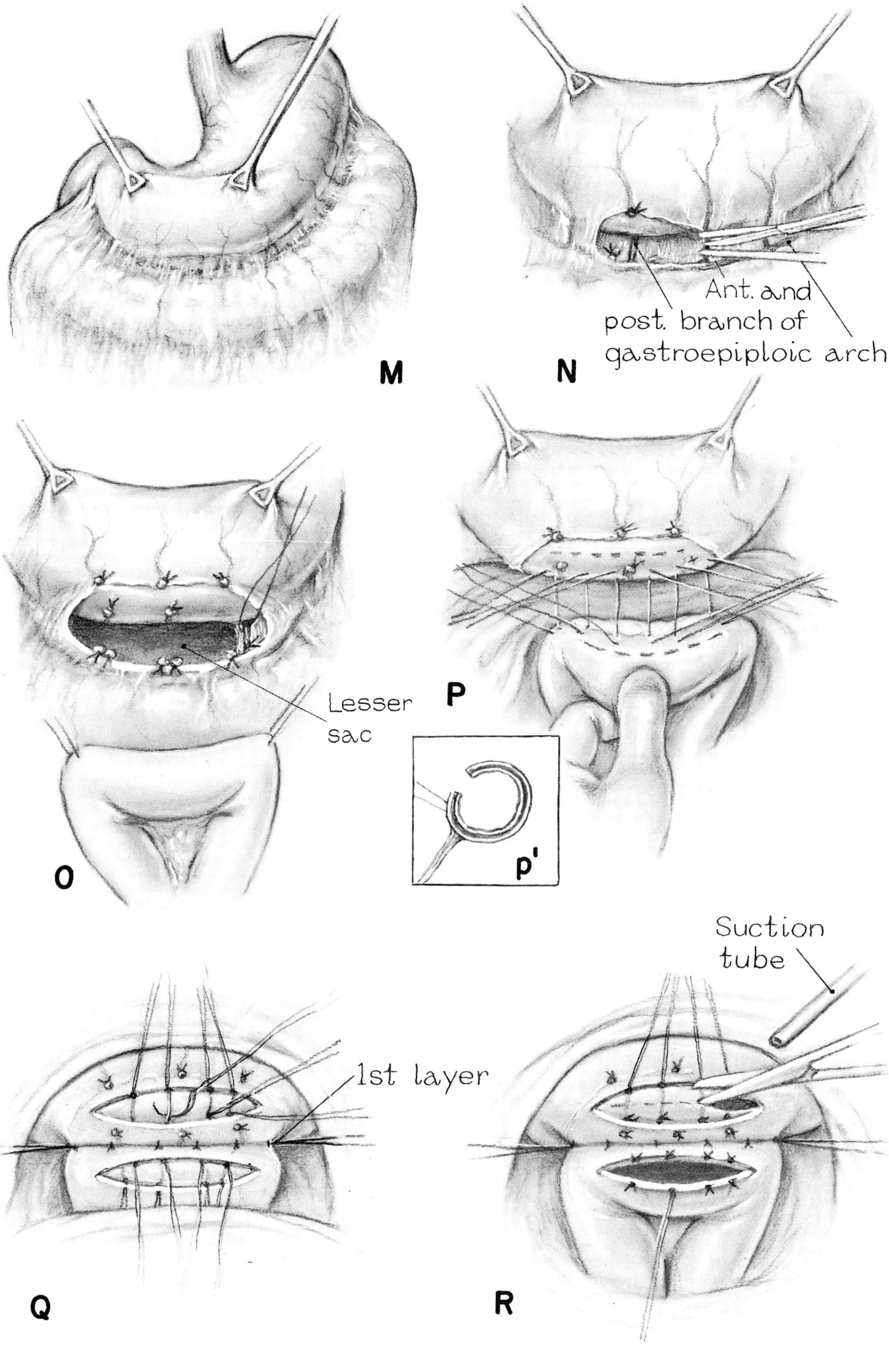
M
Ant. and
post. branch of
gastroepiploic arch
N
Lesser
sac
O
P
p'
Suction
tube
1st layer
Q
R

S. The middle hemostatic sutures on the anterior cut margins of the jejunum and stomach respectively are left long for traction, and the second posterior layer of interrupted sutures of silk (0000) are inserted. No complications have ensued from the use of silk sutures for the mucosal layer. In fact, this method of suture is preferred to the use of a continuous interlocking suture of fine chromic (00) catgut.

T. The closure of the second posterior layer is completed with a wide approximation of the adjacent posterior serosal surfaces.

U. The first anterior layer of silk sutures (0000) are inserted. The sutures at either angle are inserted from the "inside out" to the "outside in" and are tied as oblique traction is maintained on the angle sutures of the second posterior layer. This type of suture produces an inversion of the serosal surfaces with the suture knot on the inside of the lumen.

U′. Inset to show the use of interrupted inversion sutures throughout for the closure of the first anterior layer.

V. The closure of the first anterior layer with single through and through interrupted silk sutures is completed and the insertion of the second anterior layer of interrupted seromuscular sutures (Lembert) of fine silk (0000) is begun.

W. The antecolic, isoperistaltic gastrojejunostomy along the most dependent portion of the greater curvature of the stomach is completed.

X, Y. The commencement of the wound closure, using interrupted sutures of silk (00) for the peritoneum is shown. If preferred, interrupted silk sutures of the mattress variety, or a continuous chromic catgut (00) suture that is doubled, may be used. The fascia and skin layers are closed with interrupted sutures of 00 and 000 silk respectively.

Discussion—Dr. Hoerr (cont.)

The ligament of Treitz should invariably be identified directly (L). After selecting a suitable segment of jejunum—as close as possible to the ligament of Treitz without creating tension at the proposed site of the anastomosis—the proximal end of the segment may be grasped with a "soft" Allis clamp (teeth filed off to avoid injury to the bowel), and the distal end of the segment may be grasped by a Babcock clamp. Since A comes before B in the alphabet, the mnemonic 'A' for Allis and 'B' for Babcock will identify the proximal and distal jejunum and may help avoid confusion once the ligament of Treitz is no longer in view.

The use of the greater curvature for the gastric stoma (M, N, O) is very sound practice and permits accurate placement at the most dependent portion of the stomach. I refer to this as an "antecolic dependent gastrojejunostomy" rather than as an anterior gastrojejunostomy, which may be interpreted as being to the anterior surface of the stomach.

The figures show proximal jejunum to the left of the anastomosis. Ordinarily this will be the more "comfortable" from a mechanical standpoint. The surgeon should not hesitate, however, to turn the jejunum in the opposite direction if this would seem to be more free of undesirable kinks or twists.

Interrupted silk sutures for both layers make an excellent anastomosis. I personally employ two layers of continuous 00 chromic catgut on an atraumatic needle, with emphasis on the bites being sufficiently deep into muscularis but creating minimal inversion with the outer layer. The end result with either suture material seems to be the same, but a continuous suture is a little faster. Nonabsorbable materials such as silk and cotton are not suitable for continuous sutures.

If a midline incision has been used, interrupted No. 30 stainless steel wire is a convenient mass suture for the deep layers.

The surgeon should utilize antecolic dependent gastrojejunostomy as shown in these figures when feasible, but in an occasional patient with a long transverse mesocolon and a heavy omentum, a posterior gastrojejunostomy may be simpler. It is best to remain openminded as to the type of gastrojejunostomy until the exact situation in the given patient has been assessed.

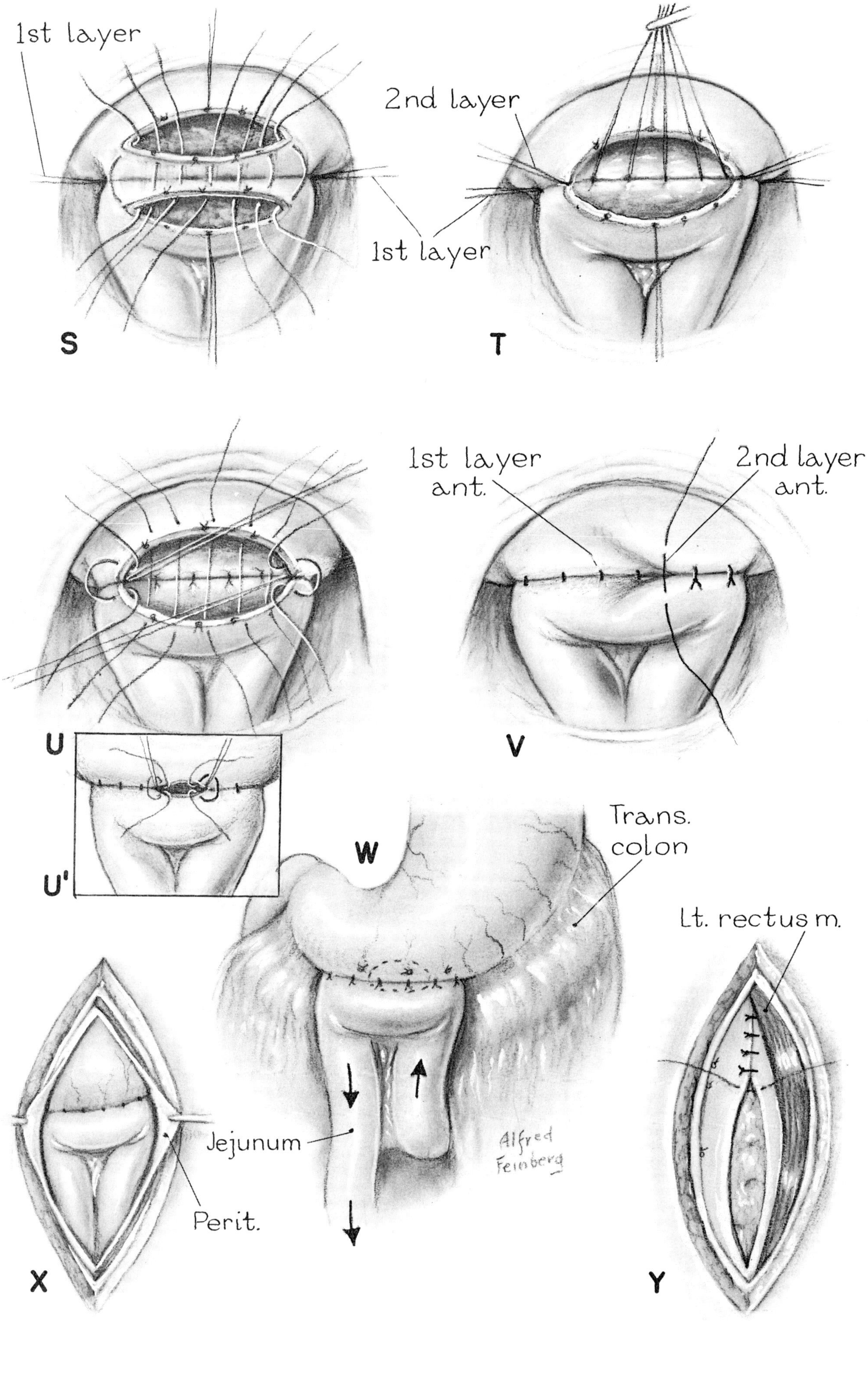
1st layer
S
2nd layer
1st layer
T
1st layer ant.
2nd layer ant.
U
U'
V
W
Trans. colon
Lt. rectus m.
Jejunum
Perit.
Alfred Feinberg
X
Y

PATENT DUCTUS ARTERIOSUS

A. The surgical approach for the ligation or severance of the patent ductus arteriosus may be through either an anterolateral or a direct lateroposterior incision as demonstrated. Although both have been used, the lateroposterior, originally suggested by Harrington for operations upon the patent ductus, is preferred.

B. The pleural cavity is entered through either the fourth or fifth interspace, preferably the fourth. The visible structures are depicted. The inverted Y-incision in the mediastinal pleura, midway between the phrenic nerve anteriorly and the vagus nerve posteriorly, is shown in dotted outline.

C. The mediastinal pleural flaps are retracted by guy sutures of silk (000) to expose the underlying fibroareolar tissue layer and the vagus nerve, which is retracted by an encircling ligature of silk (000). In some instances, although not necessary in this particular patient, ligation and severance of the highest intercostal vein may be required.

D. The lappet of pericardium overlying the region of the patent ductus is held taut by a traction suture of silk (000), preliminary to its dissection from the anteromedial surface of the aorta as indicated by the curvilinear dotted line.

E. The dissection of the pericardial lappet is completed, and the anterior, superior, and inferior surfaces of the patent ductus are clearly exposed. In this dissection the important landmark for the identification of the ductus is the recurrent laryngeal branch of the vagus nerve, which courses beneath the inferior border of the ductus at its aortic end and then continues upward behind the arch of the aorta into the neck.

Discussion—Dr. Herbert C. Maier. In our opinion, the posterolateral incision is preferable because of the better exposure it affords should any difficulty arise during the intrathoracic manipulations. The upper posterior end of the incision can be kept surprisingly low in children and yet permit ready access to the fourth or fifth interspace; in females, this lower scar may be of considerable cosmetic importance in later life. The midportion of the incision should be below the tip of the scapula. An interspace incision without any rib section is adequate in children provided the incision is carried anteriorly to a sufficient extent. The incision in the mediastinal pleura should be made sufficiently posterior to the phrenic nerve with its vessels in order to avoid the risk of injury to these structures when the mediastinal pleura is later sutured. Care must be taken that only gentle traction is applied on any temporary encircling thread placed around the vagus nerve. Dissection is best begun over the aorta, as it is easier to identify the proper cleavage plane here. Some surgeons recommend that the aorta be freed in its entire circumference, both above and below the ductus, before dissection of the ductus itself is begun. They advise this so as to permit quick clamping of the aorta if the ductus should inadvertently be torn. This maneuver is not without its own risks; an intercostal or bronchial branch of the aorta may be injured in such a dissection. We only employ this technic in special situations where more than the usual risk of ductal injury is anticipated. Patience and gentleness on the part of the surgeon are among the most important factors in avoiding ductal injury during its dissection.

If umbilical tape is employed to obliterate the ductus, it is mandatory that the tape be thoroughly vaselinized so that some vaseline will actually exude as the knot is firmly tied. Otherwise, it is difficult to tell when a tape has been tied sufficiently tight. If this point is carefully observed, tying with umbilical tape can be very satisfactory because two such tapes (one at the aortic and the other at the pulmonary end of the ductus) will give a broad area of ductal occlusion. The ends of each of the tapes are transfixed and tied together with a silk suture. No metal clips are employed. Thorough closure of the mediastinal pleura is mandatory if umbilical tape is employed; otherwise, erosion of the projecting knot into the adjacent lung is a possibility. We have not seen this occur when the mediastinal pleura is closed. The pleural cavity is routinely drained with a rubber tube which is inserted through a stab wound. The tube is connected for underwater closed drainage.

In cases of patent ductus arteriosus with sufficient pulmonary hypertension to cause possible reversal of flow through the ductus during at least a part of the cardiac cycle, the ductus should at first be clamped with a Potts ductus clamp in order to de-

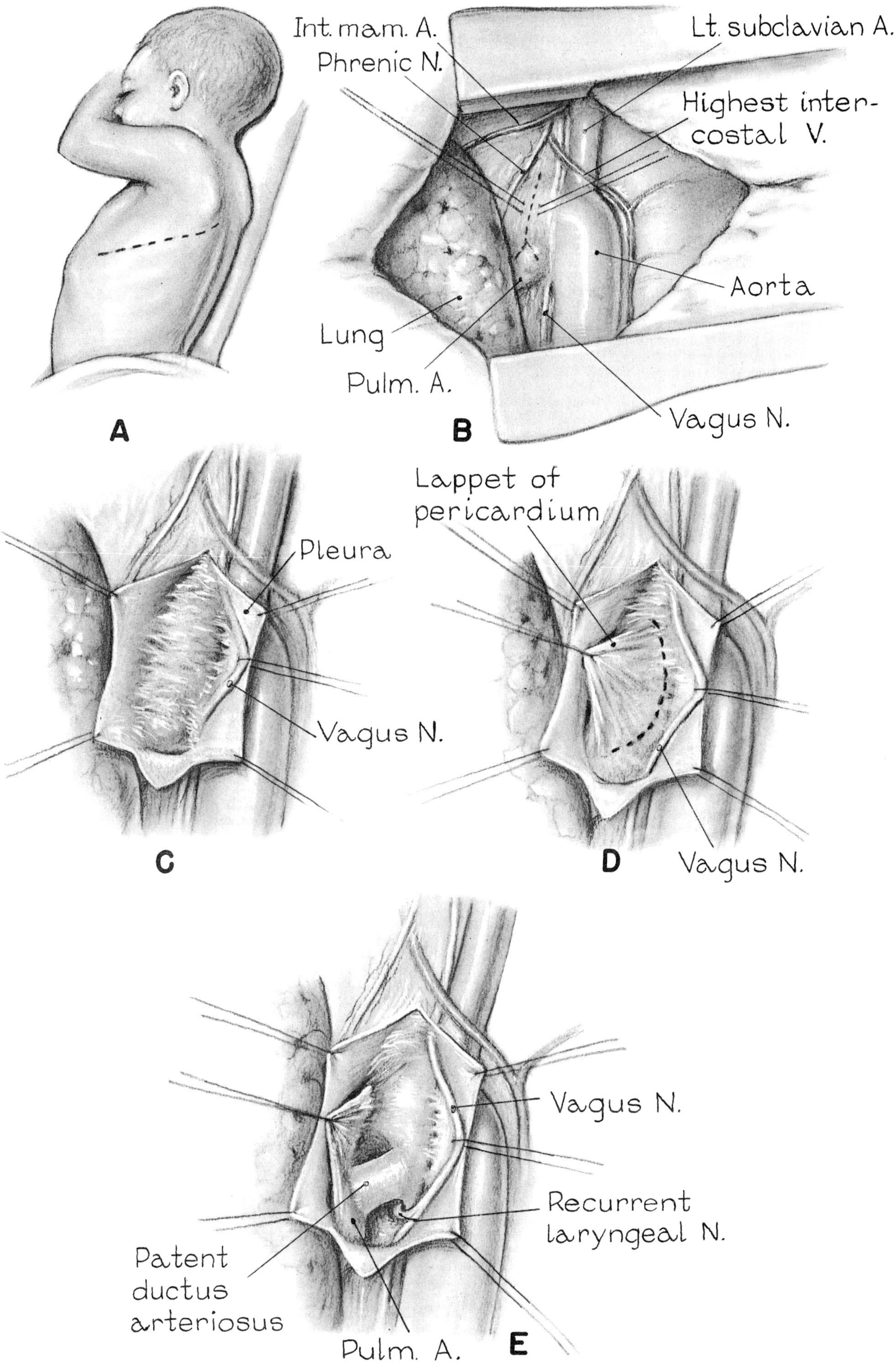
Int. mam. A.
Phrenic N.
Lt. subclavian A.
Highest inter-
costal V.
Aorta
Lung
Pulm. A.
Vagus N.
A
B
Pleura
Vagus N.
Lappet of
pericardium
Vagus N.
C
D
Vagus N.
Recurrent
laryngeal N.
Patent
ductus
arteriosus
Pulm. A.
E

F. The ductus is freed posteriorly by blunt dissection with a Mixter type clamp. This dissection is facilitated if the index finger of the left hand of the surgeon is inserted above the ductus in the sulcus between the aortic arch and the pulmonary artery. In freeing the ductus posteriorly, the blunt dissection is maintained toward its aortic end where the tissues are thicker and, accordingly, the danger of producing a tear in the ductus is lessened. This complication is most likely to occur during the posterior dissection and usually at the line of junction of the ductus and the pulmonary artery.

G. The Mixter type clamp is inserted from above the ductus down into the dissected space posteriorly to confirm the completeness of the dissection.

H. A clamp is inserted behind the mobilized ductus preparatory to withdrawing an encircling ligature of No. 1 braided silk.

H_1. Inset to show an alternate method of placing the encircling ligature using a malleable ligature carrier with a ball-point protective tip. This instrument was originally designed for use in operations upon the patent ductus.

I. The ductus arteriosus is occluded with two ligatures of No. 1 braided silk, and Cushing silver brain clips are placed on the ends of the ligatures just distal to the knots. These clips serve as a roentgenographic landmark and also prevent the knots of the ligatures from slipping. The use of umbilical tape as a ligature has been discontinued because of the inability to set the knots sufficiently tight to obtain satisfactory obliteration of the ductus.

J. If preferred the mobilized ductus may be doubly clamped (Potts multitoothed clamps) and severed as indicated. This method, practiced routinely by Gross and Potts, is admittedly the best technic to assure complete and permanent obliteration of the ductus. However, with the use of this method, the possibility of technical errors is increased. Accordingly, double ligation in continuity is preferred as the routine method. However, in selective cases, particularly when the ductus is wide in diameter, severance of the ductus and suture closure of the divided ends as subsequently shown, is preferred.

K. A close-up and magnified view of the severed ends of the ductus to show the details of the suture closure as described by Potts.

L, M. The closure of the severed aortic end of the ductus is being completed (L), and the relation of the severed and occluded ends of the ductus to the surrounding structures is visible (M).

N. The mediastinal pleura is loosely sutured as demonstrated. The closure of the mediastinal pleura, originally stressed by Jones, is believed an important technical step in the prevention of postoperative complications, particularly aortobronchial fistulas.

DISCUSSION—DR. MAIER (cont.)

termine whether obliteration of the ductus is tolerated.

When the ductus is to be divided, it is essential that it be thoroughly dissected out so that advantage can be taken of its full length. The ductus appears longer after such dissection. The Potts multitoothed clamps are ideal for ductal division. The clamps should be tested from time to time to ascertain that misuse has not impaired the proper apposition of the fine teeth. The clamps must be placed sufficiently far apart to leave a good cuff of vessel projecting beyond each clamp after the ductus has been carefully transected midway between the two clamps. In order to obtain sufficient distance the clamps may have to "ride up" on the aorta or pulmonary artery. An extra set of Potts multitoothed clamps is a highly desirable safety measure in case the original clamps are found to be imperfectly placed after the ductus has been divided.

Failure to obliterate permanently a patent ductus arteriosus by operation is usually due to either infection or failure to occlude the ductus completely by encircling ligatures or tapes. When recanalization occurs because a ligature cuts through, infection often plays a role, except if transfixion sutures were placed through the ductus itself. We have never employed transfixion sutures, since their use seems unnecessarily hazardous to us.

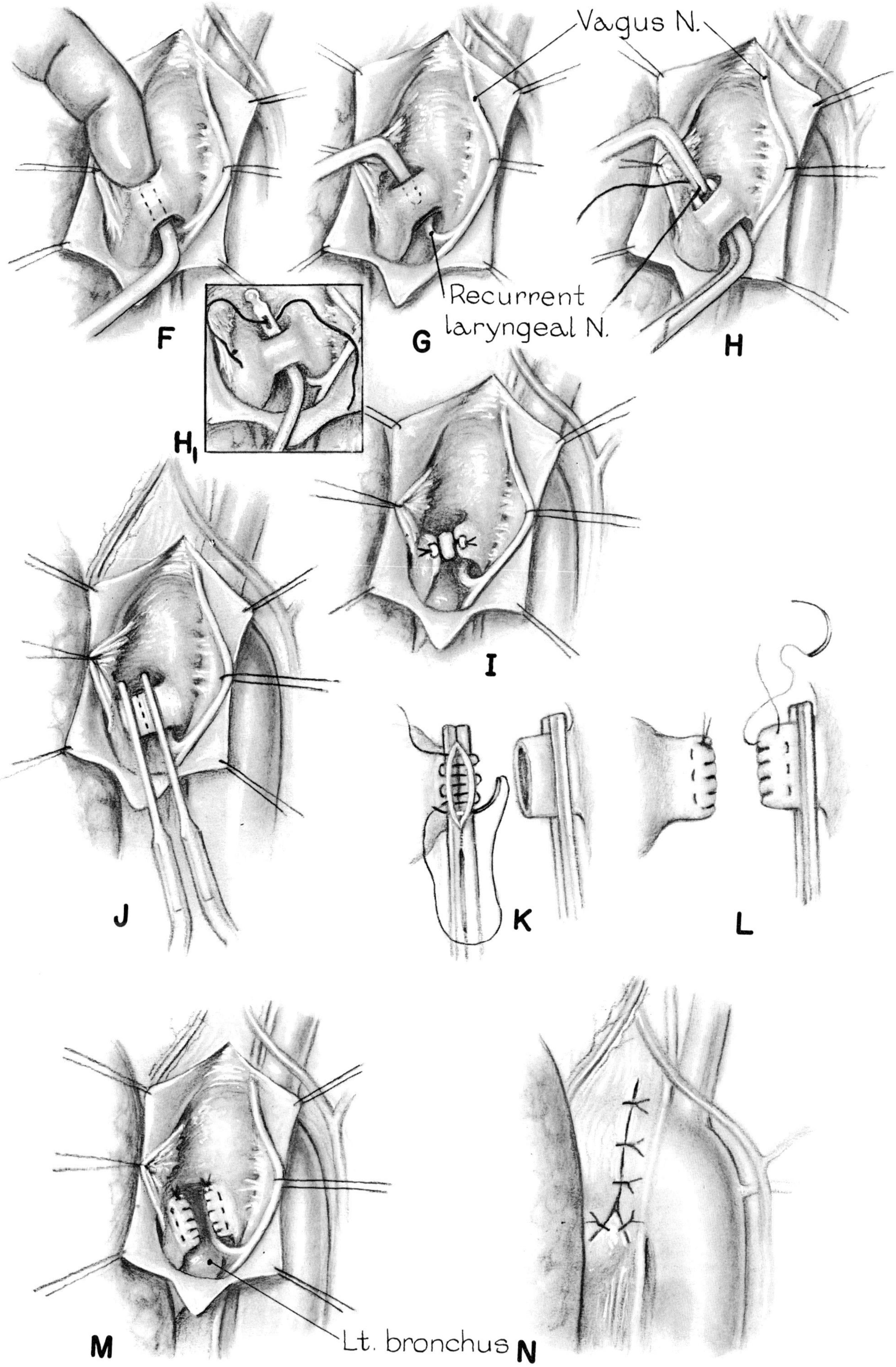
Vagus N.
Recurrent laryngeal N.
F
G
H
H1
I
J
K
L
M
Lt. bronchus
N

DISCUSSION—DR. ARTHUR S. W. TOUROFF. Two surgical approaches are commonly employed in cases of patent ductus arteriosus. The first is anteriorly and extends from the left lateral border of the sternum to the anterior portion of the axilla. The second approach is lateroposteriorly.

If an anterior incision is used, its site is best determined by the level of the under surface of the aortic arch as seen in an x-ray film of the chest. With the patient in the supine position, the incision usually is made along the third intercostal space. After the left hemithorax is entered, the third costal cartilage is divided close to the sternum. If additional exposure is required, the second costal cartilage may be divided. In adult females, the incision is made beneath the breast and the latter mobilized upward until the region of the third intercostal space is exposed. The postoperative cosmetic result is excellent.

If the lateroposterior approach is employed, the patient is placed in the right lateral recumbent position. A sweeping subscapular incision is made from the level of the third rib posteriorly and carried downward and around the angle of the scapula (Plate 95A). The pleural cavity is entered through the fourth intercostal space after dividing the fourth rib close to its posterior attachment.

Each incision has certain advantages and disadvantages with which the well-trained surgeon should be familiar. The anterior approach is shorter, more direct, divides relatively little muscle tissue and can be performed much more rapidly and with much less bleeding than the lateroposterior approach. Inasmuch as the patient does not lie on the incision following operation, there is apt to be considerably less pain than when the lateroposterior approach is employed. However, the surgical exposure of the ductus is not as good. The lateroposterior approach requires a long incision, and the scapula must be freely mobilized in order to expose the fourth intercostal space which lies beneath it. In order to accomplish this, a good deal of musculature must be divided. This requires considerably more time, and numerous bleeding vessels must be clamped and ligated. Similarly, the surgical closure is time-consuming. Since the patient frequently lies on his back, the incision is apt to be much more painful postoperatively than when an anterior incision is employed. However, the lateroposterior incision provides better exposure of the ductus, especially of its deep or posteromesial aspect. This area and the left branch of the pulmonary artery are the two structures which are most liable to be injured during the process of freeing the ductus from the surrounding structures.

The site of the ductus is best determined at operation by palpating the area in the concavity of the distal portion of the aortic arch. There, a thrill will be felt which is maximal directly over the ductus. Once discovered, firm pressure on the ductus with the index finger will cause the thrill to disappear and

DISCUSSION—DR. TOUROFF (cont.)

the heart to beat more slowly and forcefully. The vertical incision in the mediastinal pleura is made between the phrenic and vagus nerves (Plate 222B) and should be about 2 inches long. A few small mediastinal lymph nodes usually are encountered after the mediastinal pleura has been incised. The incision is best made with long, fine scissors. Scissors likewise are employed to incise the pericardial lappet (Plate 95C). Small "peanut" sponges on long artery clamps then are used to free the pericardial lappet from the ductus in a caudad direction. A search is made for the recurrent laryngeal branch of the vagus nerve, for this is the most important landmark available for determining the precise position of the ductus (Plate 95E).

From this point on, the surgeon's two most valuable instruments are a pair of fine (¼ inch wide) malleable retractors and a blunt, curved cystic duct clamp. The ductus is freed by repeatedly opening and closing the aforementioned clamp along the superior and inferior surface of the ductus. The clamp is thus worked slowly beneath the deep aspect of the ductus from above and below. As the ductus is freed progressively, the fine malleable retractors are introduced to hold the tissues above and below the ductus away from the latter structure. From time to time, counterpressure is made with the left index finger against the tip of the closed clamp as it is slowly advanced behind the ductus (Plate 95F). Sharp instruments such as a scalpel or ligature carrier never should be used in freeing the deep surface of the ductus from the underlying structures (left main bronchus, left branch of the pulmonary artery, and recurrent laryngeal nerve).

Once the ductus has been freed completely (Plate 96H), a ligature should be placed around it and the lumen of the ductus temporarily obliterated. This maneuver is valuable in determining whether or not the ductus is acting as a necessary bypass for some other congenital cardiac anomaly. If it is, the patient will become cyanotic, and, thus, permanent interruption of ductal flow will be contraindicated. Contrariwise, if the patient does not become cyanotic and the heart beat becomes slower and more forceful, ductal interruption may be performed.

The methods of ductal ligation and division illustrated in Plate 96 I, J, K, L, and M are those usually employed and are adequate.

I, personally, prefer the anterior approach with double ligation of the ductus using heavy braided silk and have found it to be adequate in the vast majority of cases. Should the ductus be unusually short and of large caliber, indicating ductal division as the method of choice, the anterior incision can be carried well posteriorly into the axilla to provide adequate exposure for safe ductal division.

TETRALOGY OF FALLOT

A. The patient is placed in the direct right lateral prone position and a pillow support is inserted between the extended arms. The lateroposterior thoracic incision employed is seen in dotted outline.

B. The latissimus dorsi muscle is first mobilized posteriorly and then compressed between the index fingers and thumbs of the surgeon and the first assistant respectively as it is transected (dotted lines). The digital compression is released intermittently for the identification of the severed vessels and the application of clamps for hemostasis. The clamps are subsequently replaced by suture ligatures of 000 silk. This particular technic for the transection of the muscles of the thoracic cage minimizes both blood loss and tissue trauma.

C. The severance of the latissimus dorsi and trapezius muscles is completed, and the underlying serratus anterior and rhomboideus major muscles are visible.

D. Prior to the transection (dotted line) of the serratus anterior (serratus magnus) muscle, the fingers of the right hand of the surgeon are inserted beneath the scapula, and the intercostal interspace to be entered (fifth) is identified. This is facilitated by counting downward from the highest rib palpable, the second rib.

E. The lower half of the periosteum of the fifth rib is removed, and by digital dissection the endothoracic fascia and the pleura are separated from the third, fourth, and fifth ribs and the intervening musculature. This particular technic, credited to Sir R. C. Brock of England, is used almost as a routine in the performance of a thoracotomy. It permits an adequate exposure of the intrapleural surgical field without the necessity of resecting a portion of a rib or severing the related intercostal muscle bundle. A portion of a gauze sponge located beneath the erector spinae muscle group is visible.

F. The fifth rib is retracted upward; the site of the incision in the subjacent endothoracic fascia and parietal pleura is indicated by the dotted line.

G. The left pleural cavity is entered, and the rib margins, covered by protective moist toweling, are separated by a self-retaining retractor (Tuffier) to expose the structures as depicted.

H. The deflated upper lobe of the left lung is covered by a moist gauze protective pad and retracted downward and posteriorly. The incision in the mediastinal pleura, which partially encircles the anterior and posterior aspects of the hilum (dotted line), and the related intrapleural structures are demonstrable.

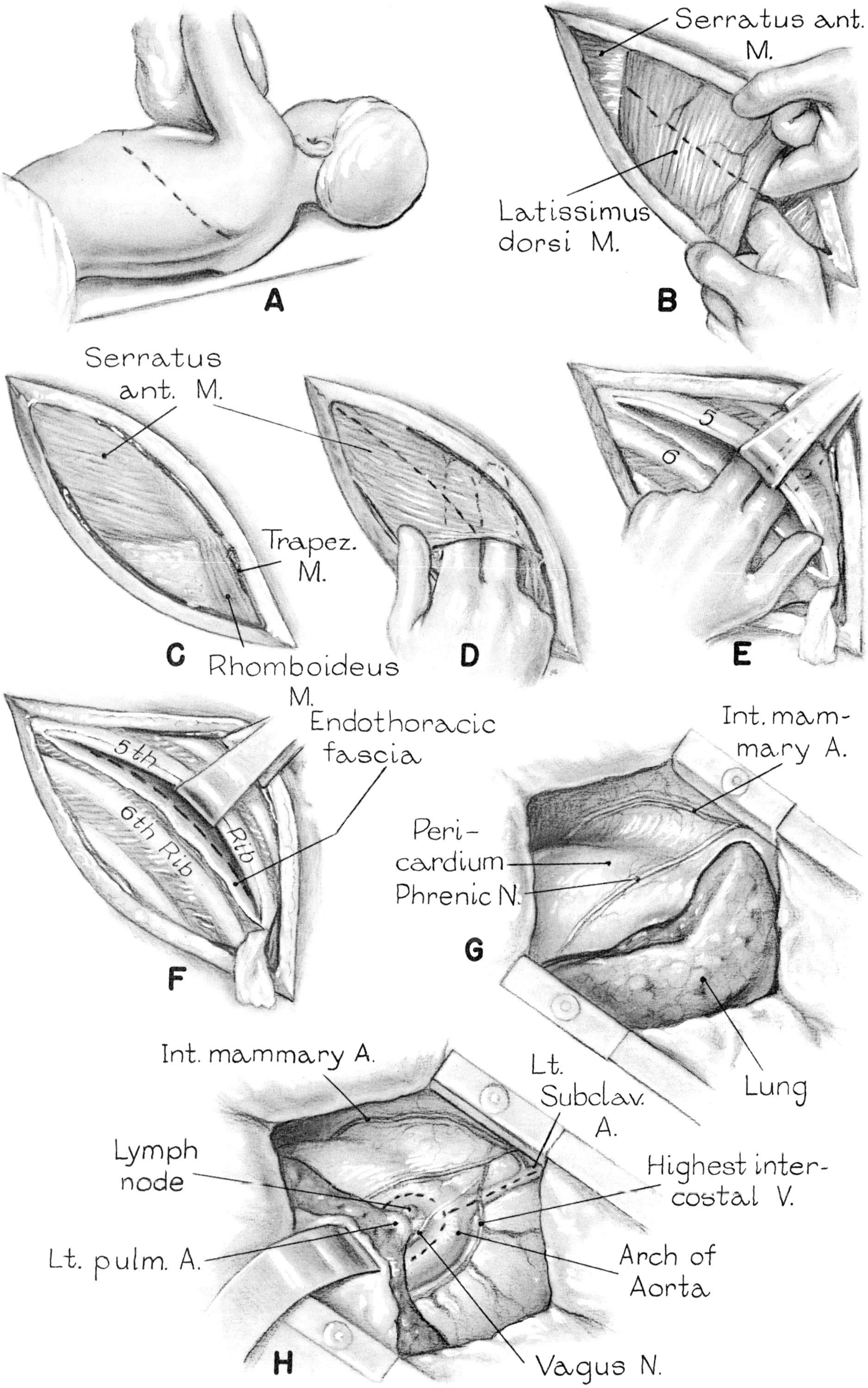
Serratus ant. M.
Latissimus dorsi M.
A
B
Serratus ant. M.
Trapez. M.
Rhomboideus M.
5
6
C
D
E
5th
6th Rib
Rib
Endothoracic fascia
Int. mammary A.
Peri-cardium
Phrenic N.
F
G
Lung
Int. mammary A.
Lt. Subclav. A.
Lymph node
Highest inter-costal V.
Lt. pulm. A.
Arch of Aorta
Vagus N.
H

I. In opening the mediastinal pleura, which is now completed, it is usually necessary to ligate doubly and sever the highest intercostal vein. The left pulmonary artery, mobilized completely about its circumference, is being encircled with a cotton (umbilical) tape. The relation of the artery to the surrounding structures is visible.

J. The pulmonary artery encircled by two cotton tapes is displaced medially to expose portions of both the left main stem bronchus and one of the bronchial arteries. The vagus nerve and its recurrent laryngeal branch, which arches upward beneath the lower border of the ligamentum arteriosum at its aortic end and then passes behind the arch of the aorta (dotted line) into the neck, are also visible.

K, L. One of the bronchial arteries, the upper three sets of intercostal arteries, and the branches of the subclavian artery within the thorax are doubly ligated and severed. The ligated ends of a small arterial branch from the base of the subclavian artery may be seen. In this patient, a four-and-one-half-year-old boy, an end-to-side anastomosis between the left subclavian artery and the pulmonary artery (Blalock) was originally planned. However, following exploration, the subclavian artery was believed too narrow in diameter to effect an adequate shunt, and, accordingly, a side-to-side aortopulmonic anastomosis (Potts) was the operation of choice.

K[1]. Inset showing the left pulmonary artery occluded proximally by a double encircling cotton tape ligature. A similar ligature, loosely encircling the artery distally, may be seen. This ligature will be subsequently tightened by traction to occlude completely the intervening segment of the left pulmonary artery.

M. The mobilized segment of the proximal portion of the descending aorta is partially occluded in a Potts–Smith clamp and approximated to the occluded segment of the left pulmonary artery. To maintain approximation, one strand of each of the occluding tape ligatures on the pulmonary artery is passed beneath the metal bar on either end of the jaw of the clamp, and, by traction on the tapes, both the arterial occlusion and the approximation of the vessels are adequately maintained. If preferred, the ligature strands may be tied to the jaws of the clamp. The sites of the incisions in the occluded segments of the aorta and the pulmonary artery are shown in dotted outline. The length of each of the incisions, measured by a caliper, is 6 mm. It is important not to make the anastomotic stoma too large, and yet it must be adequate in size to be effective.

N. The openings into the lumen of the aorta and the pulmonary artery are made, and the insertion of the posterior suture layer is completed. A continuous over and over suture of 00000 arterial silk, which starts from the "outside in" on the aorta and terminates from the "inside out" on the pulmonary artery, is used.

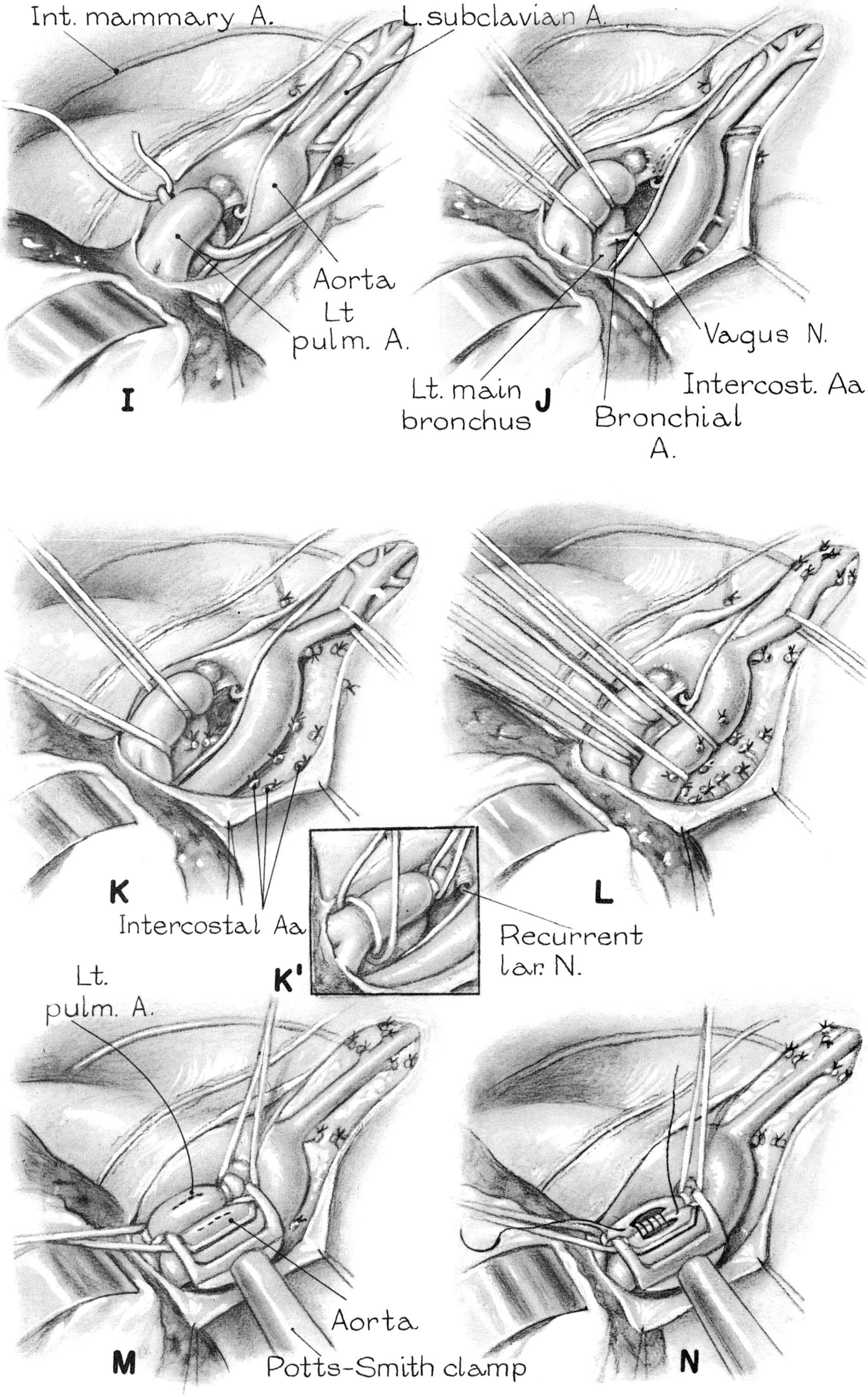
Int. mammary A.
L. subclavian A.
Aorta
Lt pulm. A.
I
Vagus N.
Lt. main bronchus
J
Intercost. Aa
Bronchial A.
K
Intercostal Aa
K'
Recurrent lar. N.
L
Lt. pulm. A.
Aorta
Potts-Smith clamp
M
N

O. Close-up view of the completed posterior layer of the anastomosis. The presence of the line of sutures within the lumen of the blood vessels, though theoretically objectionable, has not produced any untoward symptoms.

P, Q. Close-up views of the anterior layer of the anastomosis during (P) and following its completion (Q). A series of interrupted everting mattress sutures of silk (00000) is used for the closure of the anterior layer. If desired, either a continuous over and over or everting type of suture may be employed. At either end of the anastomosis one of the strands of the adjacent mattress suture is tied to the free end of the suture forming the posterior layer.

R^1, R^2, R^3, R^4. These close-up views illustrate an actual occurrence during the performance of an aortopulmonic anastomosis (Potts). Accordingly, it is believed that it may be of technical surgical interest. Following the completion of the posterior layer of the anastomosis, it was observed that the central portion of the anterior lip of the incised aorta had slipped beneath the upper blade of the Potts-Smith clamp (R^1). This technical difficulty was dealt with satisfactorily by first occluding the aorta completely, both proximally and distally, to the site of the anastomosis with angulated Potts ductus clamps (R^2). The Potts-Smith clamp was then quickly removed, and a series of simple interrupted sutures of silk (00000) were inserted (R^2) and drawn taut (R^3). The Potts–Smith clamp was then reapplied, and the angulated ductus clamps occluding the aorta were removed (R^3). Subsequently the anterior layer of interrupted sutures was tied to complete the anastomosis (R^4). In this patient the total time of complete aortic occlusion was six minutes. The convalescence of the patient was uneventful.

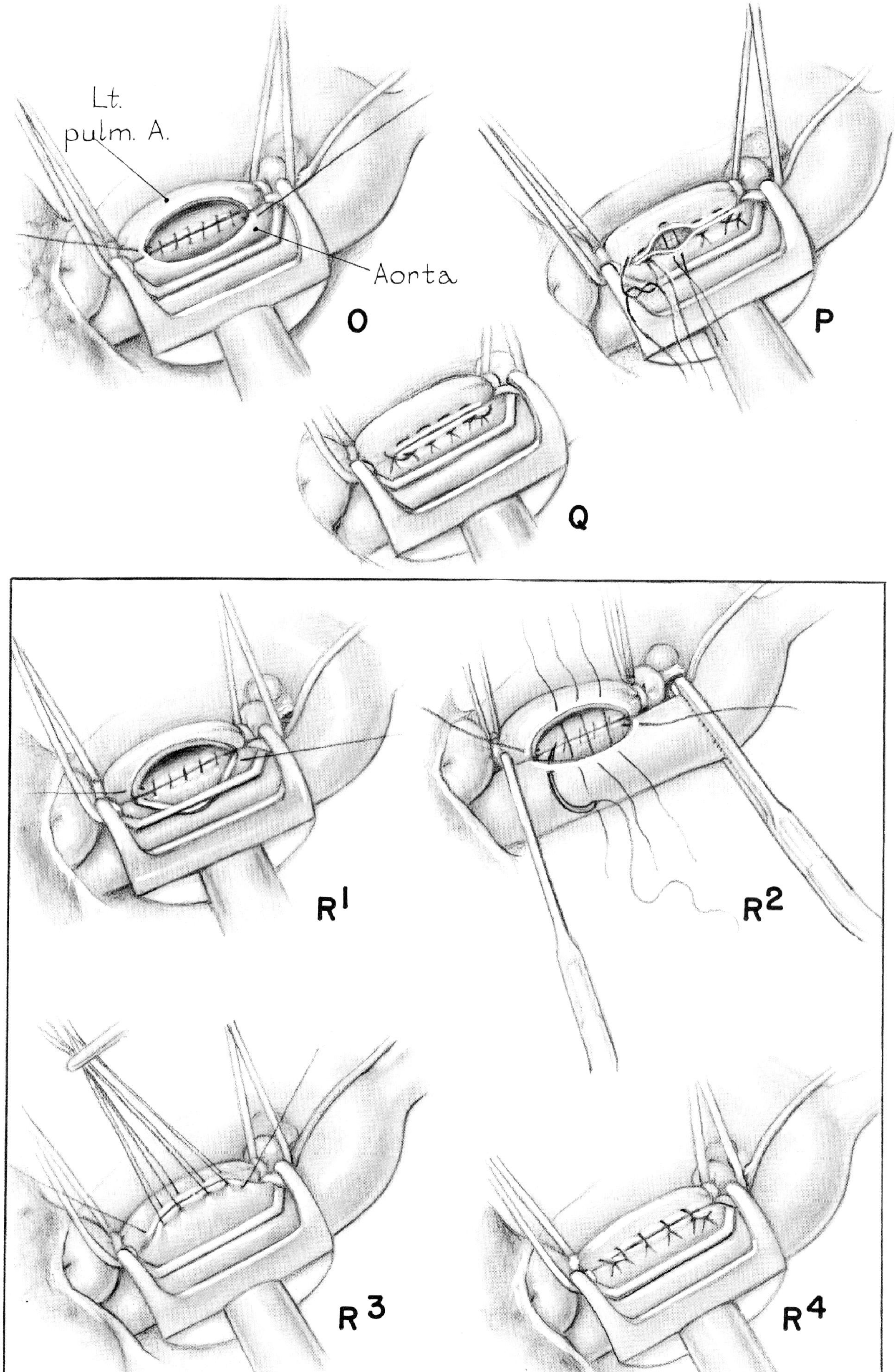
Lt.
pulm. A.
Aorta
O
P
Q
R1
R2
R3
R4

If both the diameter and the length of the subclavian artery are adequate in size, it may be used for an anastomosis to the pulmonary artery (Blalock technic). In fact, if given a choice, this method is preferred to the performance of a side-to-side anastomosis between the pulmonary artery and the aorta (Potts technic). Although the use of the right subclavian artery has been advocated by Blalock because of the unobstructed arch it forms with the innominate, the use of the left subclavian artery is preferred. Technically the left subclavian artery is easier to mobilize and the objection to the angulation that occurs at its origin from the aorta is believed more theoretic than real.

S. The proximal portion of the left pulmonary artery is occluded with a Blalock clamp, and a Potts angulated ductus clamp is applied across the base of the left subclavian artery, the branches of which have been previously ligated and severed. The subclavian artery is occluded distally by a ligature of silk (0) immediately proximal to which a transfixion suture ligature is being inserted. The site of transection of the subclavian artery is indicated by the dotted line.

T. The proximal transected end of the left subclavian artery is turned downward toward the pulmonary artery, which is doubly encircled distally by a cotton tape that will be used subsequently to occlude completely the lumen of the pulmonary artery. The site for the incision into the lumen of the pulmonary artery is shown by the dotted line.

U, U¹, The insertion of the continuous over and over suture (00000 silk) posteriorly is completed, but it is not drawn taut. This suture starts from the "outside in" at the proximal end of the opening in the pulmonary artery and terminates from the "inside out" at the lateral angle of the transected proximal end of the left subclavian artery. If preferred, a continuous everting mattress suture may be used (U¹). This suture starts from the "outside in" at the medial angle of the proximal transected end of the subclavian artery and finishes from the "outside in" at its lateral angle.

V. The posterior suture is drawn taut to complete the posterior layer of the anastomosis, and the insertion of the everting interrupted mattress sutures anteriorly is begun.

W. The insertion of the interrupted mattress sutures which form the anterior layer of the anastomosis is completed, and all but one are tied. At either angle of the anastomosis, one of the strands of the adjacent mattress suture anteriorly is tied to either free end of the continuous suture posteriorly (a, a¹ and b, b¹).

X. The completed end-to-side anastomosis of the left subclavian artery to the side of the left pulmonary artery is depicted. Although the angulation of the left subclavian artery at its site of origin from the aorta is theoretically objectionable, the clinical results obtained with its use have proved satisfactory.

DISCUSSION—DR. ALFRED BLALOCK. *Anesthesia.* The patient should not be deeply anesthetized. Control of respiration greatly facilitates the operation. The use of hypothermia is rarely indicated.

Incision. If a subclavian-pulmonary anastomosis is planned, an anterolateral incision is used. The pleural cavity is entered through the second or third interspace; the second is preferred. If an aortic-pulmonary anastomosis is planned, a posterolateral incision is used. The anterior incision has the advantage of interfering less with respiratory function.

Choice of systemic artery. In approximately 25 per cent of patients with the tetralogy of Fallot, there is a right aortic arch. In such patients the innominate is on the left instead of the right. Since we prefer when possible to use the subclavian that arises from the innominate, the incision generally is made on the right when there is a left arch and on the left when there is a right arch. At times we use the subclavian that arises directly from the aorta but much

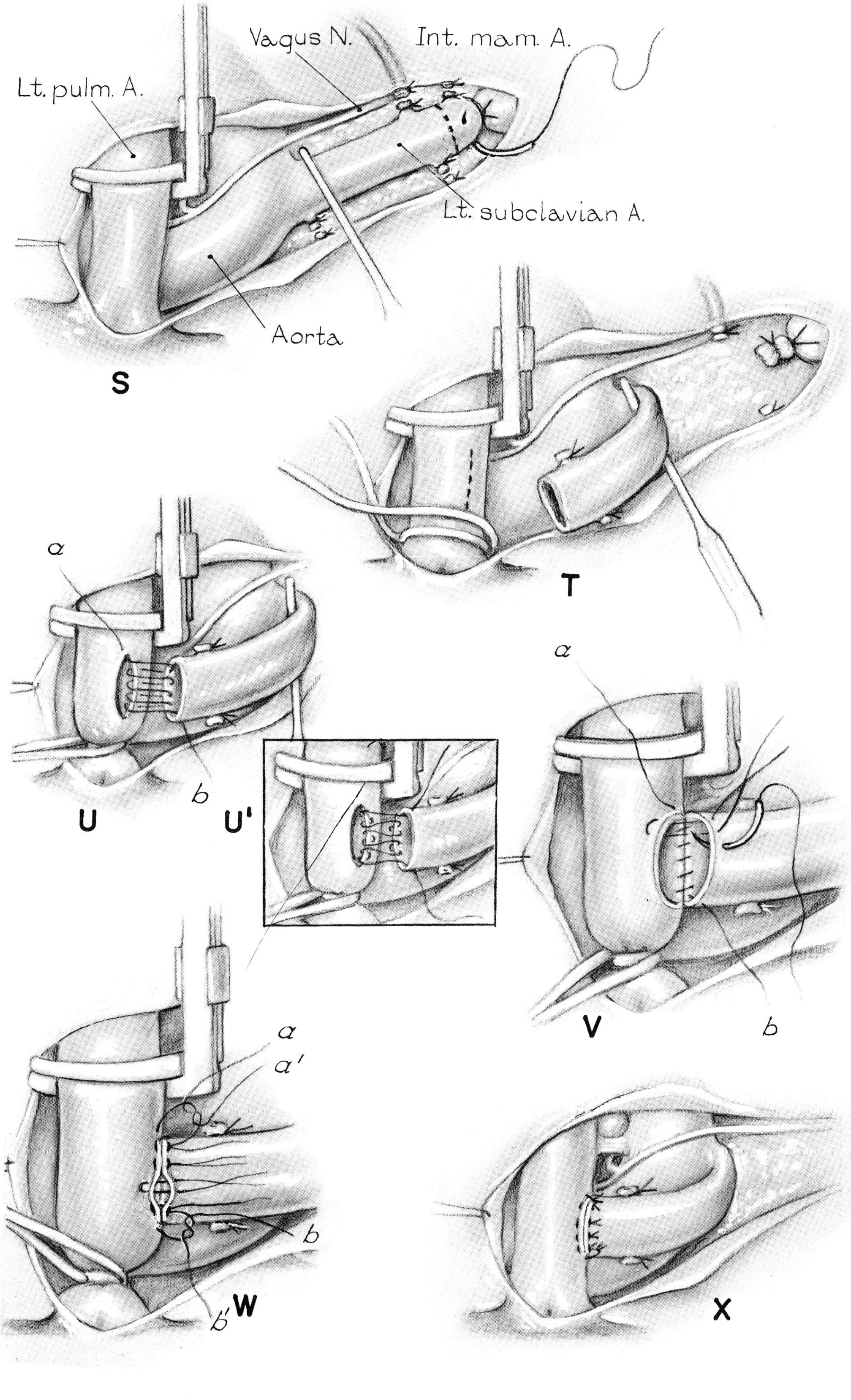
Vagus N.
Int. mam. A.
Lt. pulm. A.
Lt. subclavian A.
Aorta
S
T
a
b
U
U'
a
b
V
a
a'
b
b'
W
X

Y. The relation of the completed end-to-side anastomosis between the left subclavian artery and the left pulmonary artery (Blalock operation) to the surrounding structures in the operative field is visible.

Y^1. The same field as in Y after closure of the mediastinal pleura.

Z. The relation of the completed side-to-side anastomosis between the aorta and the left pulmonary artery (Potts operation) to the adjacent structures is shown. The previously isolated left subclavian artery, which at operation was considered too narrow in diameter to use, may be seen. It was this finding which indicated the performance of the Potts rather than the Blalock procedure.

DISCUSSION—DR. BLALOCK (cont.)

prefer that arising from the innominate. Sharp angulation is thereby avoided.

There are some exceptions to the following general statements. In children between the ages of 2 years and 12 years, an end-to-side anastomosis is performed between the subclavian branch of the innominate artery and the pulmonary artery. In infants the Potts aortic–pulmonary anastomosis is usually used because the subclavian is too small. In patients over the age of 12 years, the subclavian branch of the innominate may be too short, and we usually use the Potts type or the subclavian branch of the aorta.

Size of anastomosis. When using the subclavian artery, one need have little fear of causing heart failure. When using the aortic–pulmonary anastomosis one should not make the opening more than 5 or 6 mm. in diameter, or heart failure is apt to follow. We have the impression that a subclavian–pulmonary anastomosis of a given size is less apt to cause heart failure than an aortic–pulmonary union of the same size.

Bilateral operation. In approximately 110 of our 1500 patients with Fallot's tetralogy or some variation of it, a second operation on the opposite side has been performed. The indications have been closure of the first anastomosis or inadequacy of the shunt associated with growth of the patient. If the first operation consisted of a shunt between the right subclavian and pulmonary arteries, the second operation consists of an anastomosis between either the aorta or the left subclavian and the left pulmonary artery. If the patient has a right aortic arch and the first operation consisted of a shunt between the left subclavian and left pulmonary arteries, in performing a second operation on the right, one may have to use a graft in connecting the aorta with the right pulmonary artery.

Open heart surgery. When the operative mortality is reduced further and when the results of a longer follow-up period become known, it is likely that the direct open attack will largely replace the shunt procedures except in cases of tricuspid atresia, pulmonary atresia, and similar situations. The likelihood that this will occur is a point in favor of subclavian–pulmonary anastomosis rather than aortic–pulmonary anastomosis because the former can be closed more readily if it is advisable to do so in the future.

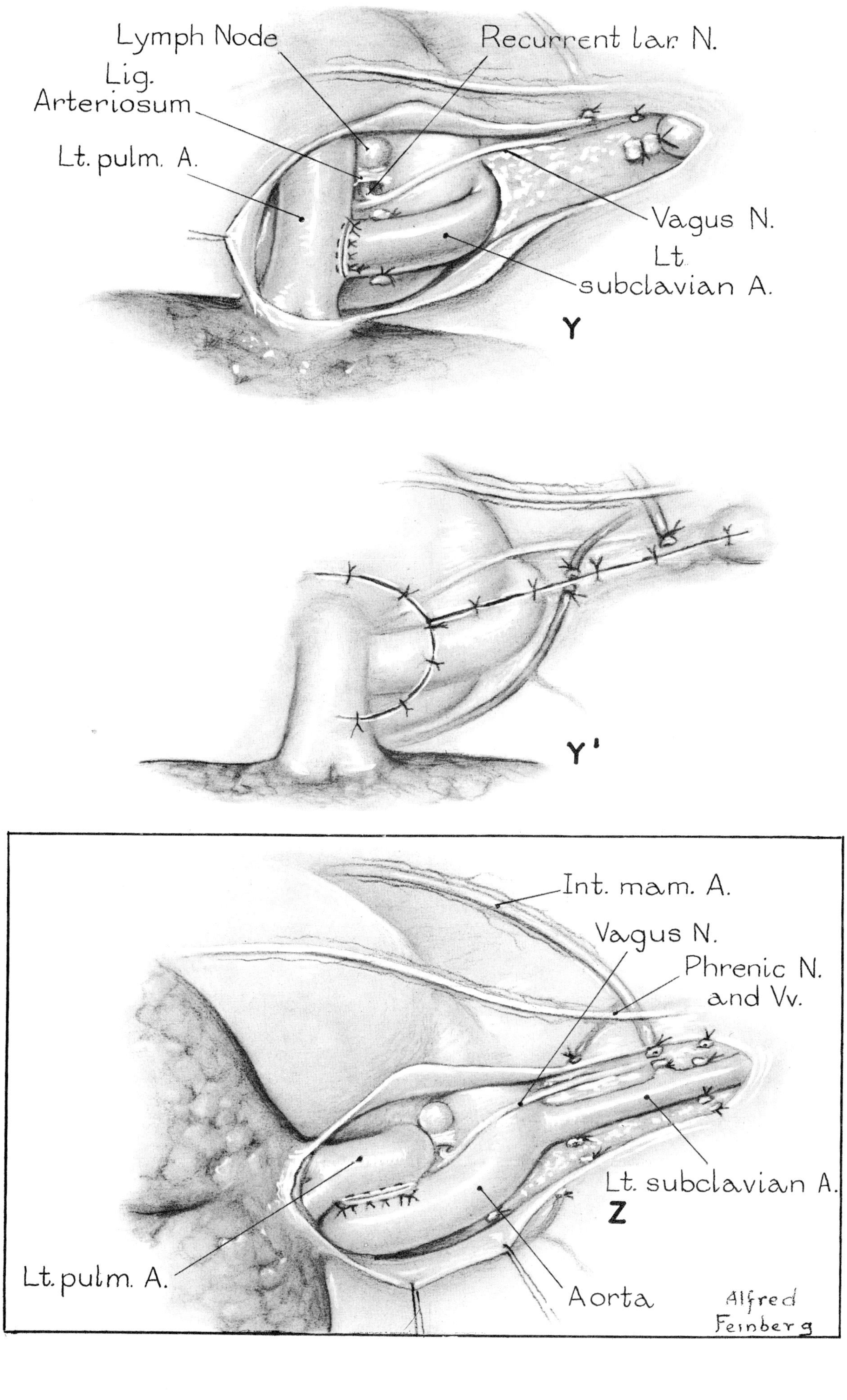
Lymph Node
Recurrent lar. N.
Lig. Arteriosum
Lt. pulm. A.
Vagus N.
Lt. subclavian A.
Y
Y'
Int. mam. A.
Vagus N.
Phrenic N. and Vv.
Lt. subclavian A.
Z
Lt. pulm. A.
Aorta
Alfred Feinberg

COARCTATION OF THE AORTA

A. The patient is placed in the direct right lateral prone position, and the site of the left thoracotomy incision is outlined and crosshatched to facilitate later closure.

B, C. The incision is deepened through the subcutaneous fat and fascia to expose the underlying musculature and the accompanying large collateral blood vessels.

D, E. The trapezius and latissimus dorsi muscles respectively are compressed between the thumbs and index fingers of the surgeon and first assistant, and the muscle fibers are severed with a scalpel. The muscles are incised for only short lengths at a time, and, as the digital compression is released, bleeding points are identified and clamped. Hemostasis is then secured with suture ligatures of silk (000). This method for severance of the muscles prevents excessive blood loss and its use is believed mandatory in all thoracotomies performed for coarctation of the aorta.

F. A subperiosteal resection of a long segment of the fifth rib and short segments of the fourth and sixth ribs is performed. The intervening intercostal bundles are clamped, severed, and ligated with suture ligatures of 00 silk. The incision in the bed of the resected fifth rib is depicted by the dotted line. In some instances resection of a long segment of the fourth rib and short posterior segments of the third and fifth ribs may prove more desirable.

Discussion—Dr. Ralph A. Deterling, Jr. In general, I have favored a curved incision for high thoracotomies. For repair of coarctation my incision begins horizontally, passing about 1 cm. below the tip of the scapula and curving cephalad between the scapula and the spinous processes of the thoracic vertebrae. Because of the very large subcutaneous collateral arteries, I develop the skin incision in lengths of about 10 cm., securing bleeding vessels before continuing. In this way blood loss may be minimal.

Regarding the division of the muscles of the chest wall in these patients, I, personally, prefer not to introduce instruments or fingers blindly beneath the muscles (Plate 102C, D, E). I have seen very troublesome bleeding occur because of injury to the dilated, thin-walled arteries entering the muscles from the chest wall. I prefer to cut the muscle with a gentle sawing action, deepening the incision slightly with each stroke. The arteries to the muscles may be readily observed before being cut and can be secured with clamps without blood loss. The slight extra expenditure of time is compensated for by the loss of only minimum quantities of blood.

I have generally resected only the fourth rib subperiosteally. In contrast to the method of standard thoracotomy, I do not separate the erector spinae muscle group from the posterior segment of the rib until the rib is completely freed from periosteum elsewhere. If the large perforating posterior branch of the intercostal artery is then opened inadvertently, the rib can be removed at once for better exposure and the control of hemorrhage. I have been satisfied with the use of ligatures of 0000 and 000 silk.

I have found two Tuffier retractors (Plate

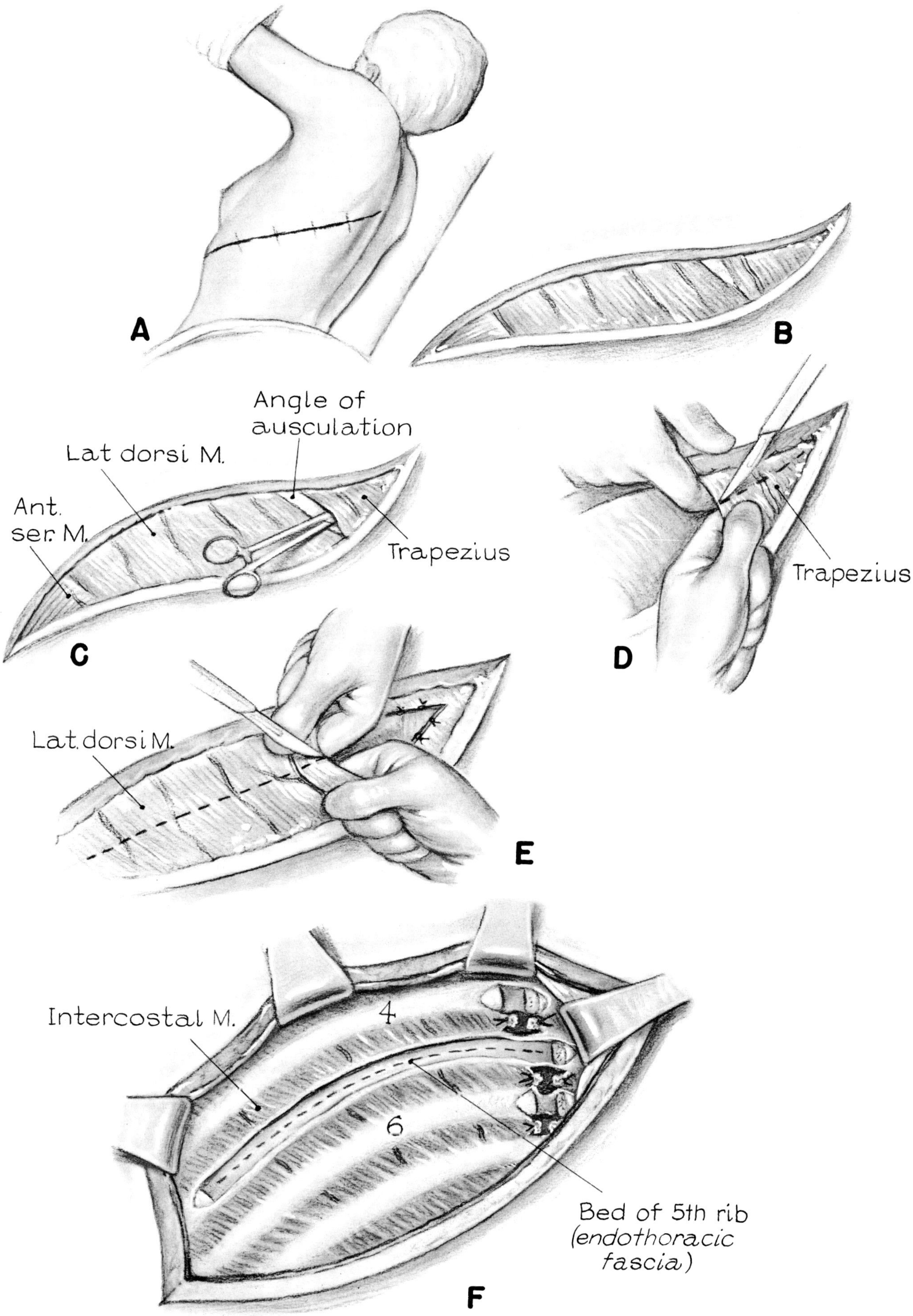
A
B
Angle of
ausculation
Lat dorsi M.
Ant.
ser. M.
Trapezius
C
Trapezius
D
Lat. dorsi M.
E
Intercostal M.
4
6
Bed of 5th rib
(endothoracic
fascia)
F

G. The wound margins and rib cage are separated with two self-retaining (Tuffier) retractors, and the operative field is exposed. An incision is made through the pleural covering of the aorta, and its cut margins are retracted by guy sutures of silk (0000) to show more clearly the underlying highest intercostal vein and the surrounding fibroareolar tissue layer.

H, I. The incision in the pleura is extended, and the highest intercostal vein is doubly ligated and severed. The dissection of the surrounding fibroareolar tissue is completed to demonstrate the coarcted segment of the aorta and its related structures. The poststenotic dilatation of the aorta and the enlarged intercostal arteries are visible. In this particular patient there were two branches from the segment of the aorta proximal to the site of the coarctation.

J. Inset showing the ligated stumps of two of the severed intercostal arteries and the insertion of a transfixion suture of silk (000) in the uppermost and largest of the three intercostal arteries. The site of severance of this artery is indicated by the dotted line. Clamps are not used because of the frequent friability of the vessels. Every precaution should be taken to secure adequate hemostasis and prevent the excessive bleeding that may accompany the slipping of a ligature. If hemorrhage should occur from a severed intercostal artery, the best method for hemostasis is for the surgeon to insert the index finger of the left hand behind the aorta, the circumference of which is always mobilized prior to ligation and severance of the intercostal vessels, and compress the aorta between the thumb and the index finger about the site of the hemorrhage. The operative field is then cleared of blood by irrigation with saline solution and suction siphonage. The bleeding site is visualized and hemostasis is obtained with suture ligatures of arterial silk (00000) swedged on a minimum trauma needle. Preservation of the collateral pathways through the enlarged intercostal arteries is frequently stressed, but the necessity for this is questioned if resection of the coarcted segment and restoration of aortic continuity, either by direct anastomosis or the insertion of a graft, is feasible.

K. The uppermost paired intercostal arteries and the bronchial arteries are ligated and divided, and the aorta, the coarcted segment, and the subclavian artery respectively are encircled with umbilical tapes. As mentioned previously, this is done prior to ligation and division of the intercostal arteries to facilitate the control of bleeding should hemorrhage occur. The relation of the recurrent laryngeal branch of the vagus nerve to the inferior surface of the ductus arteriosus (patent in this patient) is demonstrated. The operative field is now in readiness for division of the ductus arteriosus and resection of the coarcted segment of the aorta.

DISCUSSION—DR. DETERLING (cont.)

103G) difficult to keep in place, even with double thickness pads over the rib edges. Not infrequently one is opened wider than the other or else they angulate during the operative procedure. A single Burford retractor with a large blade above and small blade below has been simpler to keep in proper position in the midportion of the wound.

The author has done well to point out the variation observed in the minor aortic branches (Plate 230H, I). On occasion a branch passes posteriorly from the dilated subclavian artery at its origin and can be easily damaged during the mobilization of the subclavian artery.

I agree heartily with the author's admonition against the use of clamps on the intercostal arteries (Plate 103J, K). These friable arteries easily pull out of the wall of the aorta with merely the weight of a hemostat. Prior to the division of the first set of intercostal arteries and bronchial arteries (Plate 103J, K; Plate 104L), I have preferred to perform first the step subsequently described by the author (Plate 104M).

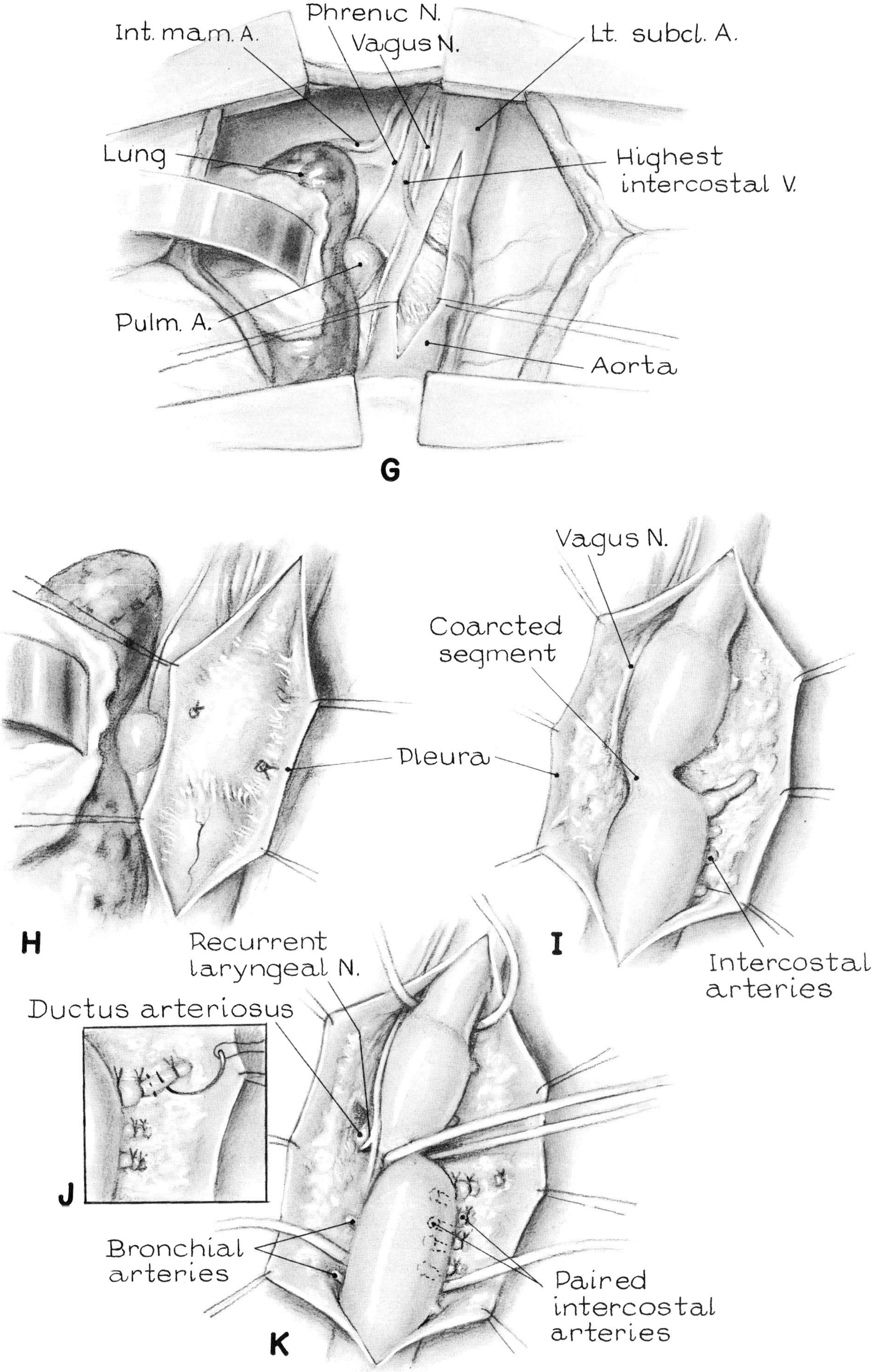
Int. mam. A.
Phrenic N.
Vagus N.
Lt. subcl. A.
Lung
Highest intercostal V.
Pulm. A.
Aorta
G
Vagus N.
Coarcted segment
Pleura
H
I
Recurrent laryngeal N.
Intercostal arteries
Ductus arteriosus
J
Bronchial arteries
Paired intercostal arteries
K

L. The thoracic aorta below the coarctation is rotated on its longitudinal axis, and the ligated stumps of the paired intercostal arteries are demonstrated.

M. The patent ductus arteriosus is isolated and doubly clamped prior to its division. The recurrent laryngeal nerve curves upward and passes inferior and posterior to the aortic end of the ductus. Its preliminary exposure provides an important landmark for the identification of the ductus. Furthermore, in the application of clamps and ligatures to the ductus one must be careful to avoid injury to this nerve.

N. The coarcted segment is completely mobilized, and Potts multitoothed straight clamps are applied across the aorta above and below the area of coarctation. The extent of the resection is indicated by the dotted lines. In the resection of the area of coarctation it is most important to remove a sufficiently long segment, both proximally and distally, to assure an adequate size of the aortic lumen upon completion of the anastomosis. However, if after the resection a direct anastomosis cannot be performed without undue tension on the suture line, a graft or prosthetic replacement should be employed. The use of a graft should always be considered in the older adults in whom extensive arteriosclerosis and concomitant friability of the aorta may be present.

O. The posterior suture layer of the anastomosis is inserted. This is a continuous eversion type of suture (silk, 00000) with intima to intima approximation. The suture is commenced from the "outside in" on the proximal segment of the aorta and terminates from the "inside out" also on the proximal segment of the aorta. Between its commencement and termination, the suture proceeds from the "inside out" to the "outside in" relative to the lumen of the aorta. Accordingly, the loops formed by the suture are always on the outside of the lumen.

P. The posterior suture, a–a, is drawn taut, and the intimal surfaces of the aortic segments are brought into close approximation. None of the silk suture is exposed within the lumen. The anterior layer of the anastomosis is commenced by the insertion of interrupted everting mattress sutures of silk (00000) at either angle of the anastomosis.

Q. The remaining interrupted everting mattress sutures are inserted anteriorly but not tied. The mattress sutures at either end are tied first, and one of the long ends of each of these sutures is in turn tied to either end, a–a, of the continuous everting suture of silk used for the posterior layer.

R. The intervening everting mattress sutures are tied to complete the anastomosis. Simple interrupted sutures are inserted between the mattress sutures to reinforce the closure.

S. The operative field following completion of the operation is depicted. The site of the aortic anastomosis may be seen in dotted outline beneath the line of closure of the incision in the pleura overlying the aorta.

Discussion—Dr. Deterling (cont.)

That is, after mobilizing the subclavian artery and securing it with a double loop of narrow braided cotton tape, I pass a similar loop about the arch of the aorta proximal to the ductus arteriosus for hemostatic control. I next develop the plane behind the aortic arch and region of the coarctation, and about the ligamentum arteriosum. The ductus arteriosus has been patent in only 15 per cent of my cases. I divide the ligamentum or ductus before mobilizing the dilated, friable aortic branches distal to this area because, if serious bleeding occurs while securing these branches, control can be effected simply by cross-clamping the mobilized aorta with two Potts coarctation clamps and dividing it. With the distal end elevated gently and rolled on itself slightly, the bleeding site can be easily and safely repaired with 00000 braided silk swedged on a taper point needle. The blind introduction of instruments or fingers beneath the aorta during its mobilization can lead to very serious and at times fatal hemorrhage. In dividing the ligamentum arteriosum (Plate 104L, M, N), I generally pass lengths of 00 silk about it, tying them at the aortic and pulmonary artery ends respectively before dividing it. If there is a patent ductus arteriosus, I place Potts ductus clamps on the aortic and pulmonary artery ends of the ductus, and after dividing it with a knife, oversew the ends with a continuous suture of 00000 braided silk.

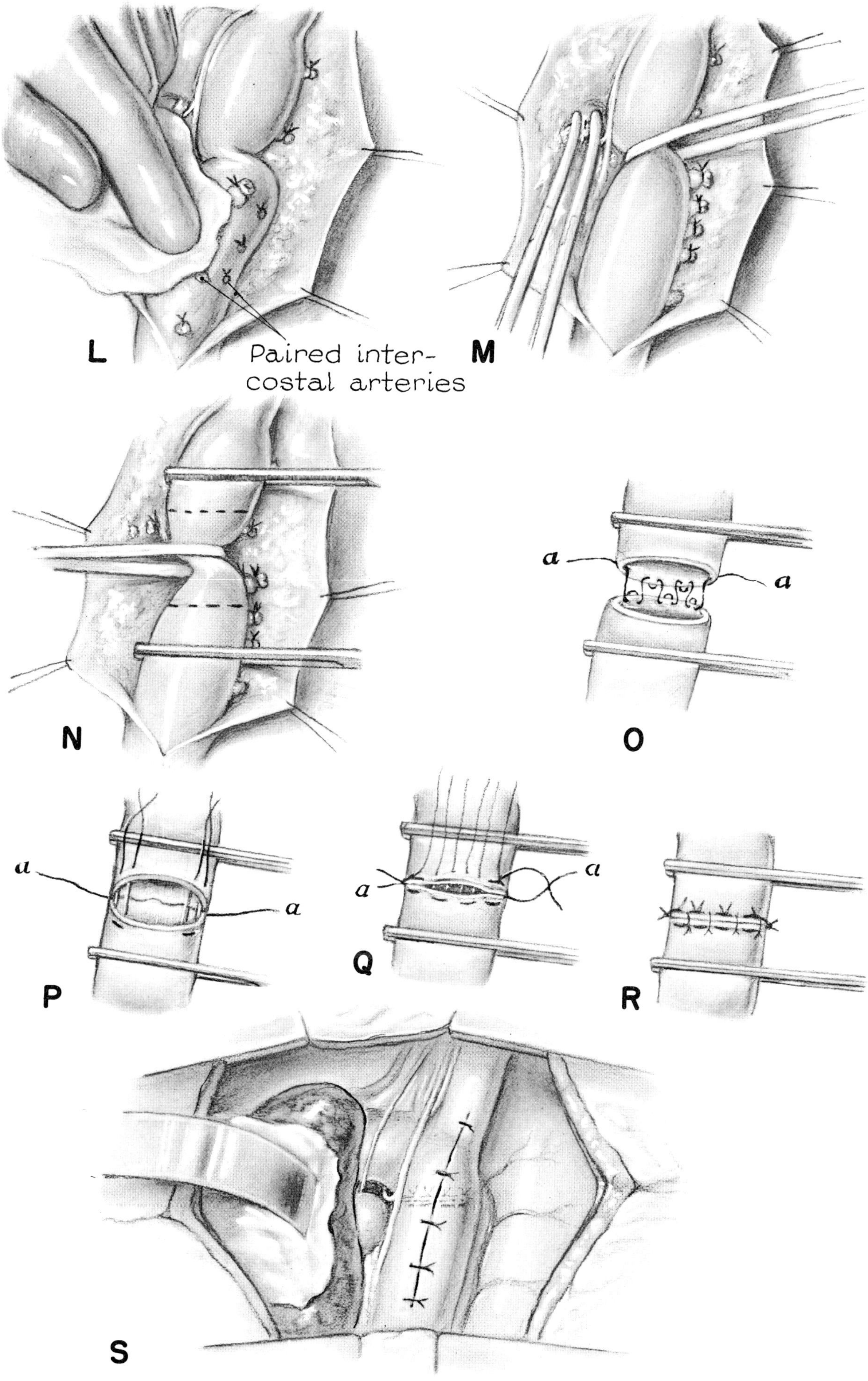
L
Paired inter-
costal arteries
M
a
a
N
O
a
a
a
a
P
Q
R
S

This plate depicts alternate methods for the resection of a coarcted segment of the aorta and the restoration of aortic continuity.

A, A^1, A^2, A^3, A^4. These illustrations demonstrate a high-lying coarctation in which mobilization of the aortic arch and cross-clamping of the arch and the left subclavian artery are required preliminary to resection and direct anastomosis.

B, B^1. In the presence of a long coarcted segment of the aorta, a resection and primary anastomosis is impossible. Accordingly, a graft is required to restore aortic continuity. This method is frequently employed in the older adults in whom the arteriosclerotic changes present may preclude a direct anastomosis. It is also preferred to the use of the proximal end of the severed left subclavian artery.

C, C^1, C^2, C^3. This series of drawings depicts the technic originally described by Gross and Hufnagel for direct aortic anastomosis following the resection of the coarcted segment. The cut ends of the aorta are rotated on their longitudinal axes, and a series of interrupted everting mattress sutures of silk (00000) are inserted posteriorly (C^1). The aorta is then derotated, and the anterior layer of interrupted everting mattress sutures of silk (00000) is inserted (C^2) to complete the anastomosis (C^3).

Discussion—Dr. Deterling (cont.)

When there is a moderate disproportion of the opposed aortic ends (because of hypoplasia of the proximal segment or poststenotic dilation of the distal segment), the use of everting mattress sutures reinforced with interrupted sutures is a very secure anastomosis (Plate 104O, P, Q, R). However, in most adult cases, I employ a simple continuous suture of 00000 braided silk. In infants I have used interrupted mattress sutures of 0000 chromic catgut with maximal growth as the goal. As an alternate method for infants, a simple continuous suture may be used for the posterior row with interrupted sutures anteriorly (Johnson and Kirby). If, even after dividing additional intercostal arteries, there is tension on the aorta while approximating the ends, I have placed the posterior continuous suture from within the aorta. This obviates the need for rotating the vessel and risking additional damage from the use of clamps.

Instead of two straight clamps (Plate 105A, A^1, A^2, A^3, A^4), a Potts-Beck clamp may be used as shown in Plate 106C. Circulation may thus be maintained from the aorta into the left subclavian artery and its collateral branches. In rare instances the coarctation may lie between the left common carotid artery and subclavian artery. In such instances the use of multiple straight clamps may be necessary.

I agree that a graft (Plate 105B, B^1) is indicated when a long stenotic segment is found. Since this cannot always be predicted, the surgeon should have available a graft for immediate use in all cases of coarctation in adults. In infants and children, an effort should be made to avoid the use of a graft which would not grow at a pace equal to that of the host vessel. By dividing additional intercostal arteries, enough length may be gained in most, if not in all, of the cases.

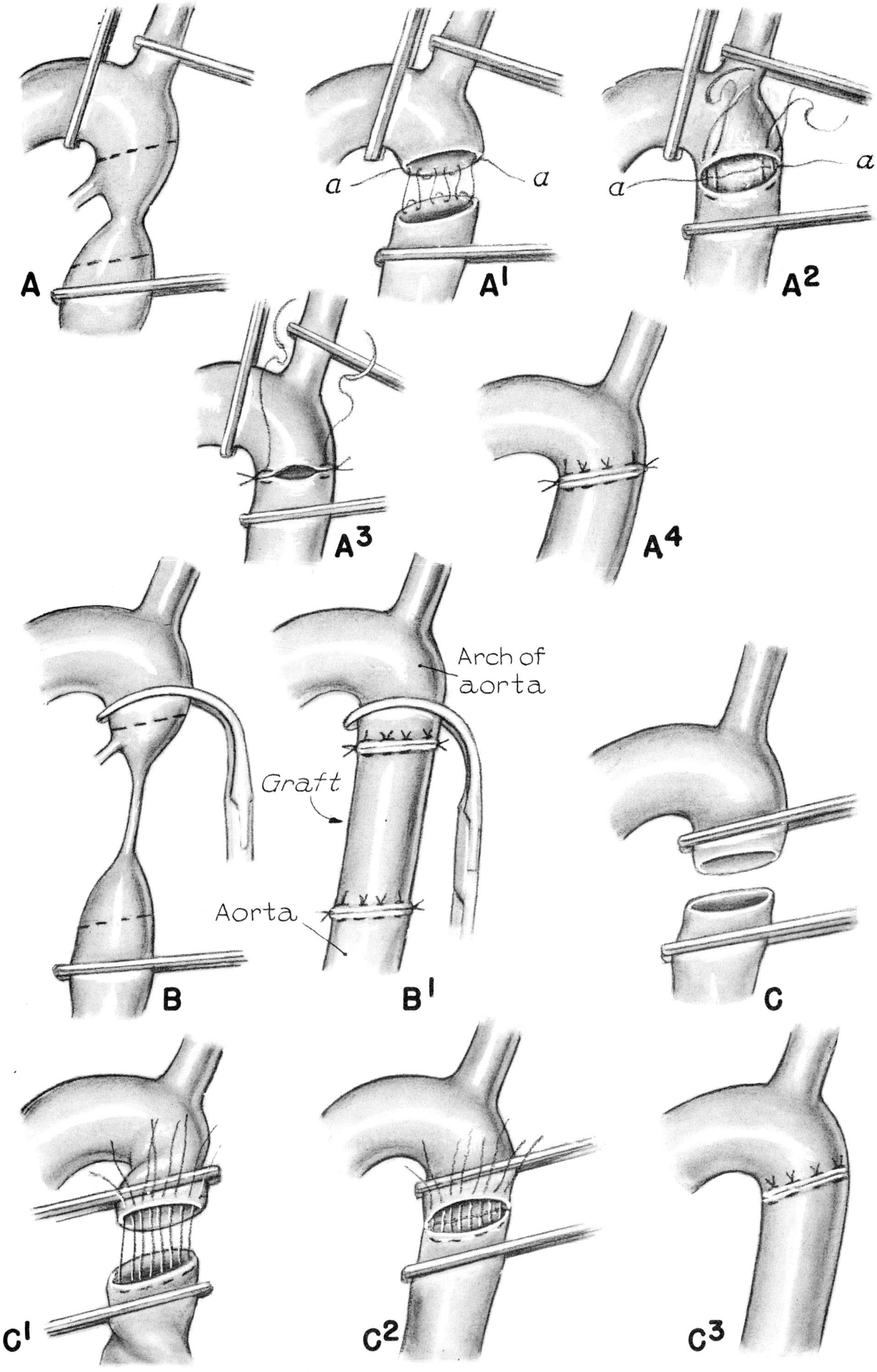
A
a
a
A1
a
a
A2
A3
A4
Arch of aorta
Graft
Aorta
B
B1
C
C1
C2
C3

A, B. In those instances in which the length of the coarcted segment precludes a direct anastomosis (A) and in lieu of a homologous aortic graft replacement or cloth prosthesis, the proximal end of the severed subclavian artery may be anastomosed to the distal severed end of the aorta (B) as originally suggested and practiced by Clagett.

C. In the presence of a high-lying coarctation of the aorta, the proximal or uppermost clamp, one of the Beck–Potts type, may be applied tangentially to occlude only partially the lumen of the aortic arch and the left subclavian artery.

Discussion—Dr. Deterling (cont.)

Although I assisted Clagett in his performance of the first subclavioaortic anastomosis in a patient with coarctation (August 6, 1946) and subsequently performed the same operation myself in patients with long stenotic segments at the time when grafts were not available, the final hemodynamic results have not generally been so good as those observed with end-to-end aortic anastomosis or with the use of an aortic homograft. However, I could conceive of this operation still serving a purpose in a young patient with a long stenotic segment (possibly as an interim procedure) or if graft material was unobtainable (Plate 106A, B). Usually the subclavian artery has a greater diameter than that depicted by the artist.

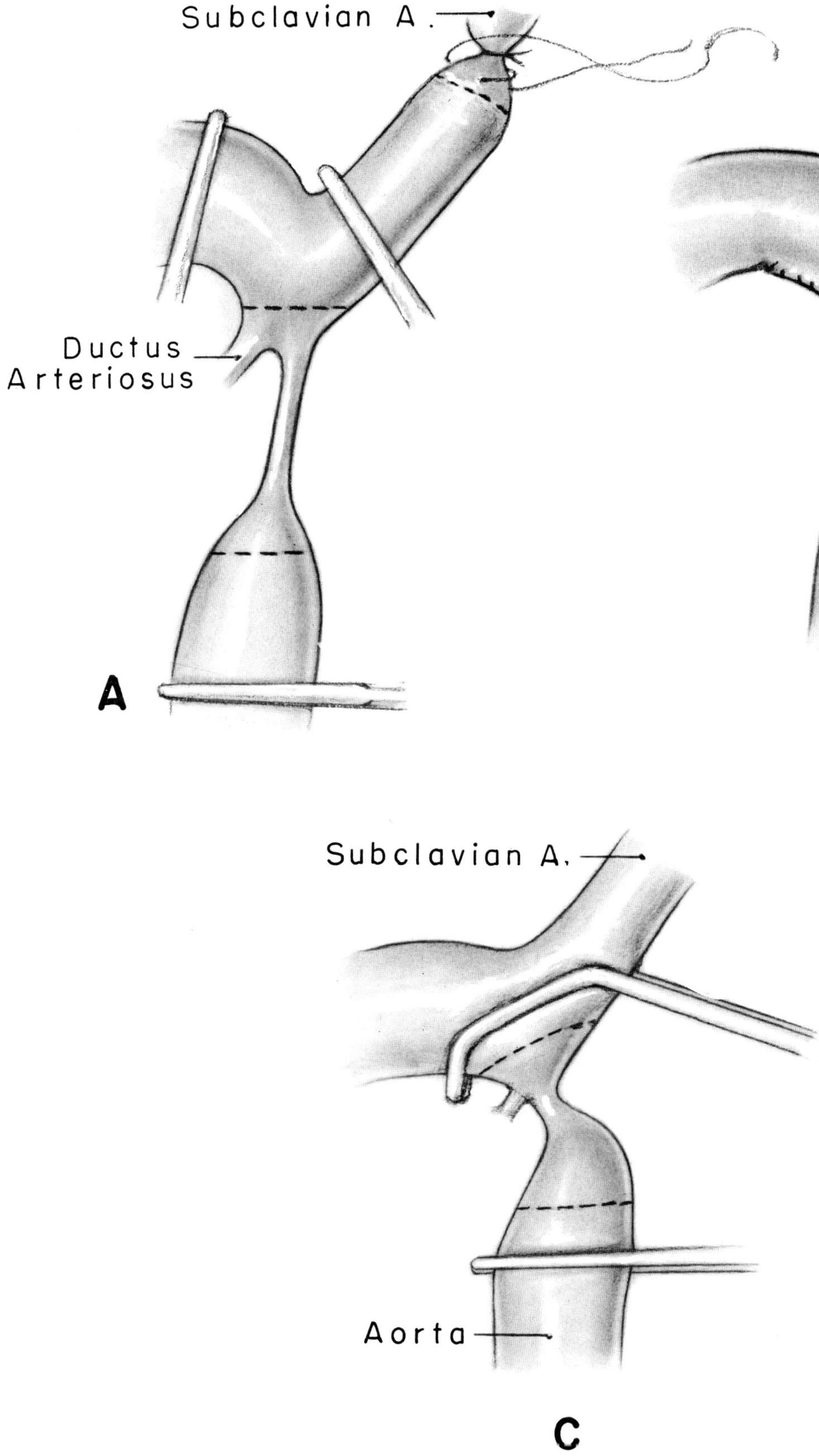
Subclavian A.
Ductus
Arteriosus
A
B
Subclavian A.
Aorta
C

DISCUSSION—DR. CHARLES DUBOST. In general, the technic I use is similar to the one illustrated. I use the same position but resect only the fifth rib without the additional resection of the fourth and sixth ribs. Similarly, the site of the coarctation is exposed as depicted. I make all efforts to preserve the maximum number of intercostal arteries. If necessary, the use of serrefine (bull-dog) clamps for temporary hemostasis is practiced. When ligation of the intercostal arteries is deemed necessary, usually there are no difficulties with the left intercostals. However, on the contrary, ligation of the right intercostals may prove difficult and annoying. Accordingly, for the ligation of the right intercostal arteries, I sever the aorta between two clamps placed at each side of the coarcted segment; the distal segment of the aorta is turned down and the ligation of the right intercostal vessels can be done easily and without danger.

In the performance of the anastomosis I use solely interrupted sutures, as I believe this technic is easier and safer.

In those patients with high lying coarctations I prefer to perform the operation under moderate surface hypothermia (31 to 32° C., 87.8 to 89.6° F.). This is done to avoid the risk pursuant to the clamping of the horizontal aorta and the subclavian artery.

When the coarctation is of a length that precludes resection and primary anastomosis, and in those patients with associated aneurysms, I prefer the use of a knitted dacron graft for restoration of aortic continuity.

My own series of patients in which a resection has been performed for coarctation of the aorta now numbers 450. Of this number the grafts represent approximately 8 per cent.

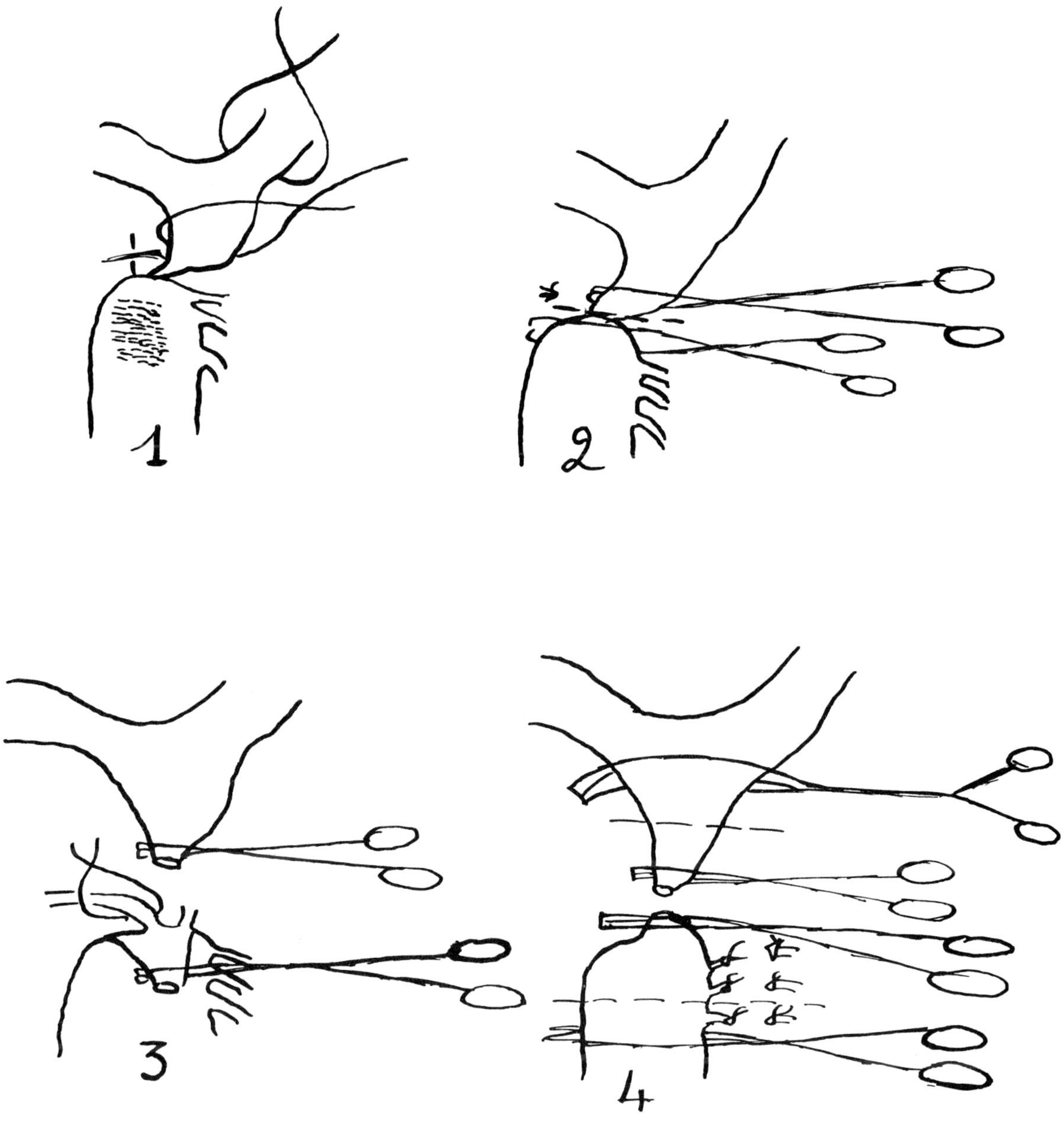

PULMONARY VALVOTOMY

A. The left side of the thorax is elevated slightly on a pillow, and a transverse curvilinear inframammary incision is depicted.

B. The mammary gland is elevated; the line of incision through the pectoralis major and serratus anterior muscles is shown in dotted outline.

C. The incised muscle layers are retracted, and the underlying fourth rib and adjacent intercostal muscles are visible.

D. The cephalad portion of the pectoralis major muscle is retracted upward to expose the pectoralis minor muscle, the angulated incision in the third costal cartilage, the partially resected fourth costal cartilage, and the line of incision in the fourth interspace.

E. The left pleural cavity is entered, and the intercostal neurovascular bundle subjacent to the fourth costal cartilage is doubly clamped, severed, and ligated. Portions of the pericardium and left lung may be seen.

F. The fourth and fifth ribs and the adjacent wound margins are retracted with a self-retaining retractor to expose more completely the underlying pericardium and adherent left lung.

Discussion—Dr. George H. Humphreys, II. A congenitally stenosed pulmonary valve may be opened either by the closed method devised by Brock and depicted in Plates 107 through 109, or by the open method advocated especially by Swan and demonstrated in Plate 110. Although each method is well illustrated, it should be noted that, even with the transverse double thoracotomy incision (Plate 110A), exposure of the heart and great vessels is not as complete as the illustration implies. When the valve is exposed in the open procedure, remnants of commissures may be seen and the surgeon may elect to restore a tricuspid valve rather than to make a simple transverse incision as illustrated (Plate 110). If the valve is irregularly distorted, care must be taken to avoid creation of incompetence. The valve annulus is frequently stenotic and will require dilatation in the open as well as in the closed procedure.

Consideration of the relative advantages and disadvantages of each method is important. The closed method of Brock is the older, and there is a tendency among many recently trained surgeons to consider it obsolete. However, it has the advantage of greater simplicity, and, when properly done in the appropriate cases, its results are equally good. Although published series do not show a greater mortality in the open procedure there is no question that the need for bilateral thoractomy and hypothermia or extracorporeal circulation add considerably to the risk of the operation and to the morbidity following it. Against this is the fact that the closed procedure is "blind." At best it cannot create a tricuspid valve, and the successive passage of knives and dilators may cause unnecessary damage to the delicate valve structure. It is also more difficult to be certain of an adequate relief of the stenosis, and the incidence of persistent or recurrent stenosis is presumably higher.

The open method has the advantage of direct vi-

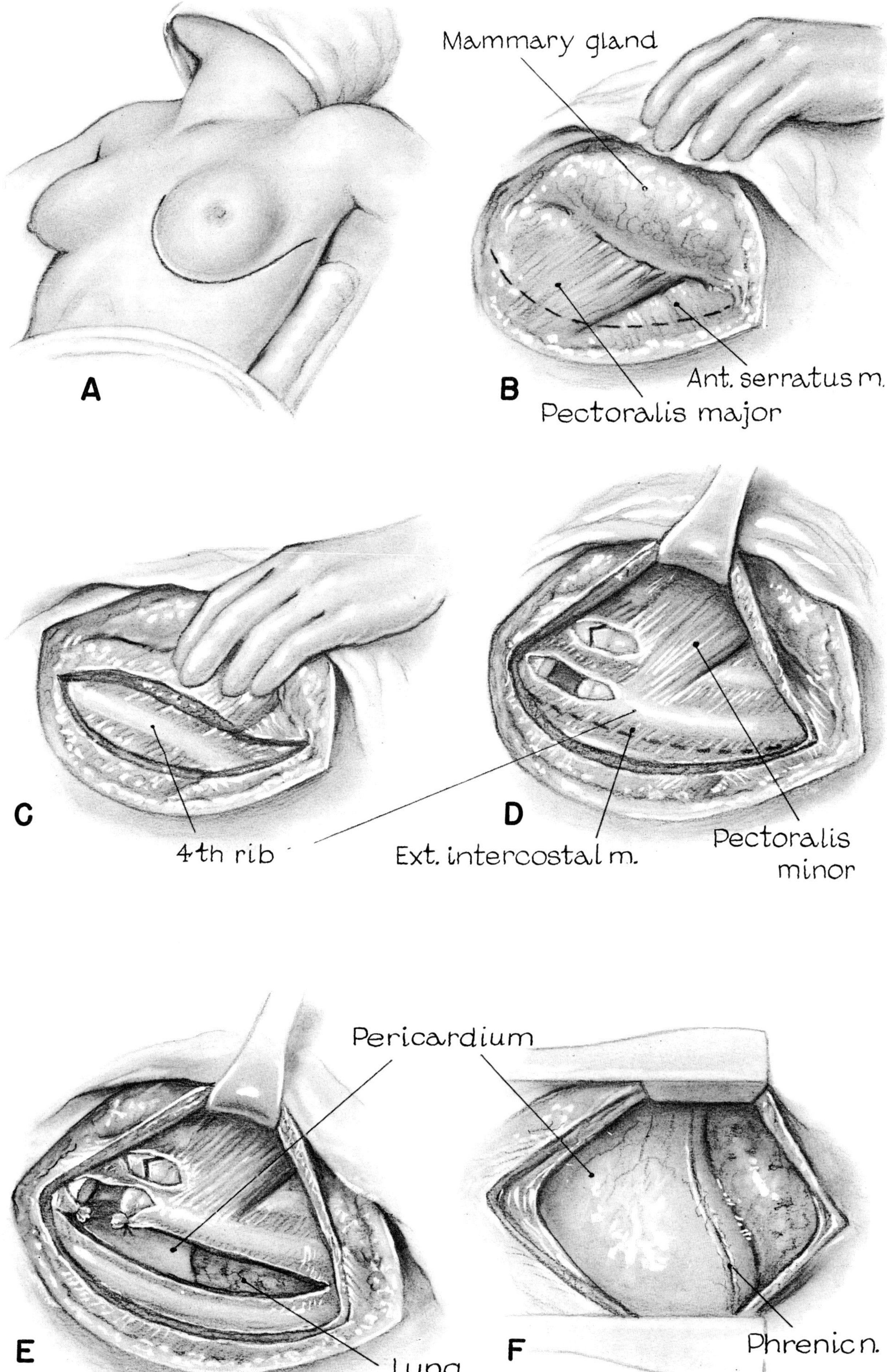
A
B
Mammary gland
Ant. serratus m.
Pectoralis major
C
D
4th rib
Ext. intercostal m.
Pectoralis minor
E
F
Pericardium
Lung
Phrenic n.

G. The left lung, having been dissected from the pericardium, is covered by a moist gauze pad and retracted laterally. The pericardial sac is entered between traction guy sutures of silk (000) medial to the phrenic nerve, and the opening in the pericardium is extended by scissor dissection to form a flap, the boundaries of which are indicated in dotted outline.

H. The formation of the pericardial flap is completed, and additional guy sutures of silk (000) have been inserted. Through the opening in the pericardium, portions of the anterior descending branch of the left coronary artery and the adjacent surfaces of the right and left ventricles are visible.

I. The flap and cut margins of the pericardium are retracted, and the anterior surface of the heart and its related structures are exposed. The anterior descending branch of the left coronary artery overlies the interventricular sulcus. An incision is being made through a portion of the wall of the right ventricle between guy sutures of silk (00) in close proximity to the pulmonary conus.

J. Close-up view to show a malleable probe with a ball-point protected tip being inserted by blunt force through the remaining portion of the incised wall of the right ventricle and through the stenotic orifice of the pulmonary valve into the lumen of the pulmonary artery. The characteristic and diagnostic jetlike stream of blood flowing through the stenotic orifice of the fused pulmonary valve and the tip of the probe as shown may be easily palpated by digital indentation of the anterior wall of the pulmonary artery.

Discussion—Dr. Humphreys (cont.)

sion, with the possibility of more nearly complete restoration to normal by division in the commissures and tailoring of the cusps. It avoids a ventricular incision and, in cases of poststenotic dilatation of the pulmonary artery, permits some correction of this abnormality by the "reefing" effect of the pulmonary artery closure. Aside from the inherent risks of hypothermia, the use of inflow occlusion without extracorporeal circulatory support introduces a time limitation which puts an undesirable premium on speed. For this reason, as well as those discussed below, there is an increasing tendency to use extracorporeal support rather than hypothermia in spite of the more elaborate technical problems and presumably greater risks of the method.

The correction of associated anomalies, especially infundibular stenosis or septal defects, is impossible with the closed method or with the open method using hypothermia and inflow occlusion. These methods are appropriate, therefore, only in cases of isolated valvular stenosis. Preoperative diagnostic tests to exclude other anomalies are essential, but, even then, an associated anomaly may be overlooked. Since secondary procedures to correct septal defects carry a higher risk than their correction at the first operation, it is highly desirable to correct all of the existing lesions at the first procedure. If, therefore, there is any suspicion that the problem includes more than a simple isolated valvular stenosis, complete cardiac exploration with extracorporeal support is indicated.

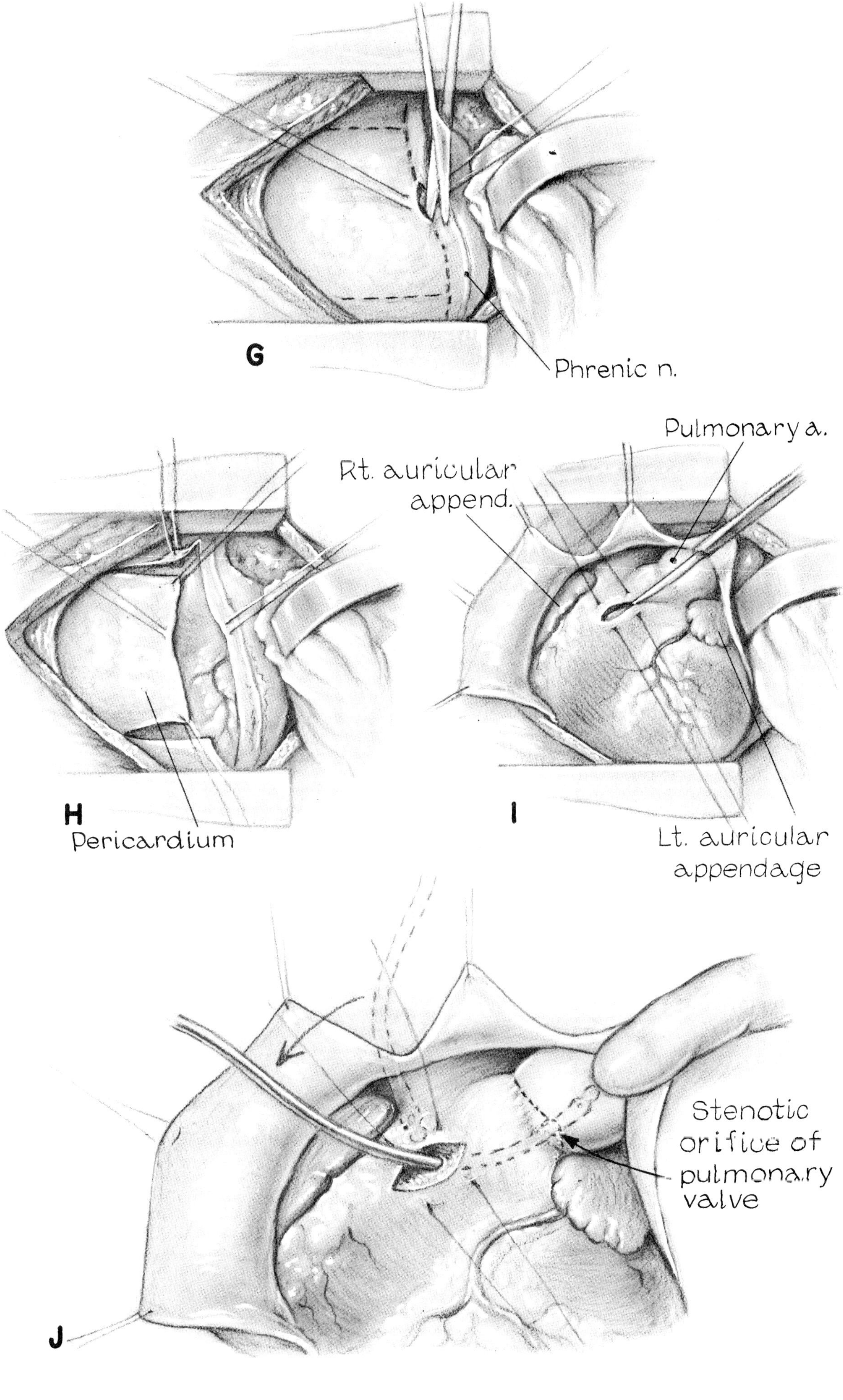
G
Phrenic n.
Pulmonary a.
Rt. auricular append.
H
Pericardium
I
Lt. auricular appendage
Stenotic orifice of pulmonary valve
J

K. The probe is withdrawn, and a small knife of the Brock type is inserted through the fused valves into the lumen of the pulmonary artery. Between the insertion and withdrawal of instruments, bleeding from the ventricle is controlled by a combination of cross-traction on the guy sutures and digital pressure over the incision.

L. The cut in the valve is further enlarged by the insertion of first a medium and then a large Brock knife as depicted in dotted outline. If preferred, a calibrated instrument as designed by Potts may be used.

M. A large urethral sound (29 F) is used to accomplish the final dilatation of the pulmonary valve orifice. This instrument is preferred to a clamp because it is associated with less blood loss.

N, O. For the control of hemorrhage after the removal of the sound, the guy sutures on either side of the incision in the myocardium are crossed, and finger compression over the incision is applied. Closure of the incision is obtained with sutures of silk (00) inserted through the myocardium immediately beneath the finger.

P, Q. The closure of the incision in the right ventricle is completed, and the pericardial flap is loosely approximated with interrupted sutures of silk (000). Small openings are present at either angle of the base of the flap to permit the escape of air and fluid collections into the pleural cavity.

R. The fourth and fifth ribs are approximated with one pericostal suture of heavy silk (No. 2) and a series of interrupted sutures of silk (000) in the intercostal muscle layer. These sutures are all first inserted and individually tied. If preferred, heavy chromic catgut may be used for the pericostal suture. The catheter (Foley No. 14 F), for water-seal drainage of the pleural cavity, has its exit through the intercostal incision.

S, T, U. The completion of the layer closure of the wound using interrupted sutures of silk throughout.

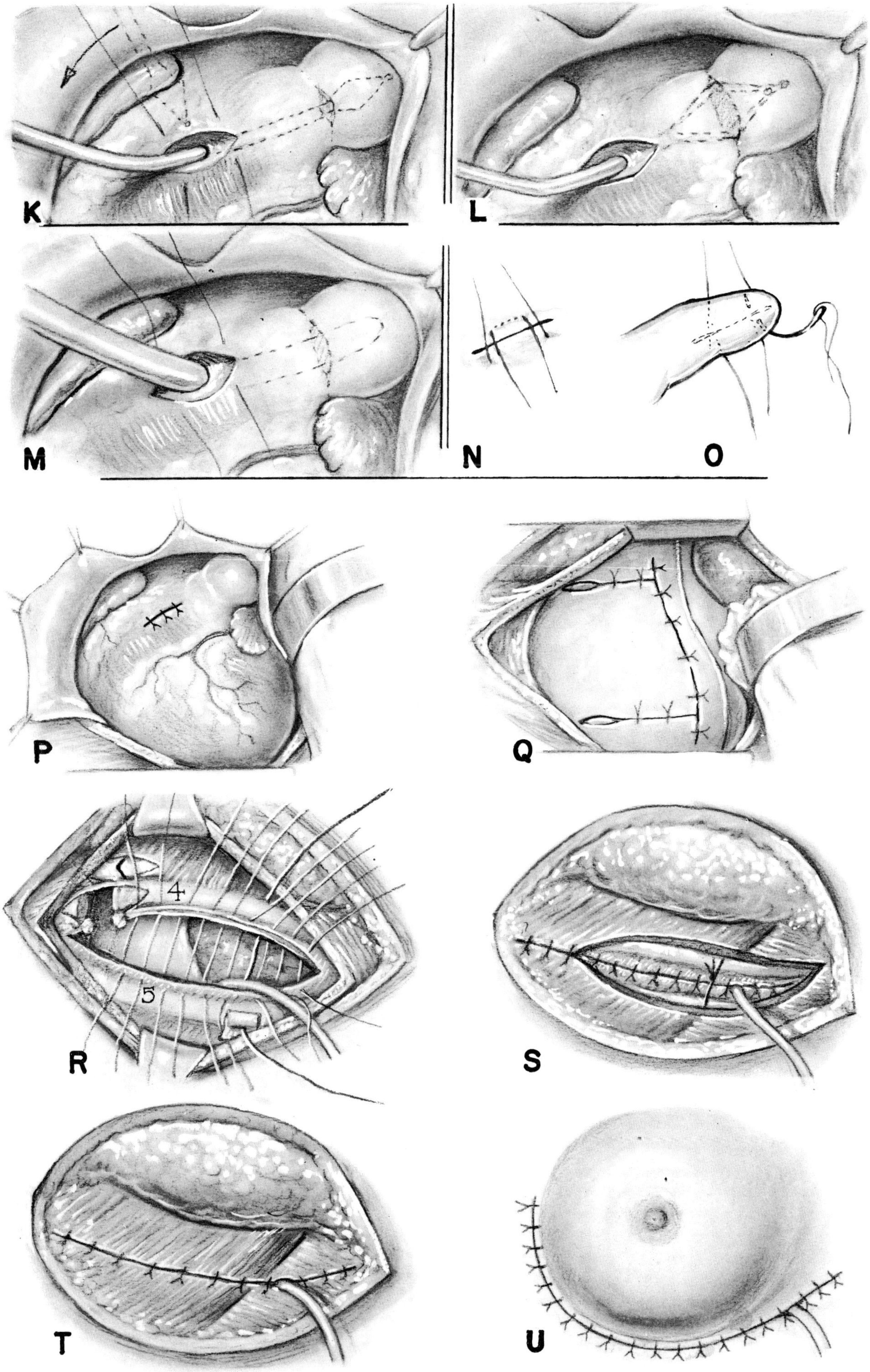
K
L
M
N
O
P
Q
4
5
R
S
T
U

The following illustrations depict an open or direct technic which may be employed in conjunction with either hypothermia as shown or with the use of a pump oxygenator and total bypass of the heart.

A. In the exposure of the heart, a Duval–Barasty longitudinal sternal-splitting incision (dotted line) or a trans-sternal cross-bow incision (solid line), entering the fourth interspace on the right and the third interspace on the left, may be employed.

B. Cardinal guy sutures of silk (0000) are inserted in the anterior wall of the pulmonary artery about the site of the incision (dotted line) to be made. Preliminary to making this incision, the superior and inferior vena cava are occluded with cotton tape ligatures, and the base of the aorta and the pulmonary artery just proximal to its bifurcation are cross-clamped (Potts). To conserve time relative to the occlusion of the inflow tracts, it is preferable to first apply a clamp (Beck–Potts), in a longitudinal direction, to a segment of the pulmonary artery which is tented by the traction sutures previously inserted. An incision is then made between the guy sutures into the lumen of the occluded segment of the pulmonary artery. Accordingly, when the clamp is subsequently released, immediate entrance into the lumen of the pulmonary artery and exposure of the valvular stenosis is obtained (C). Swan has advocated the application of a noncrushing clamp across the aorta about 2 cm. distal to its origin and the injection of 0.5 ml. of 1:4000 Prostigmin into the aorta between the valve and the clamp shortly following (30 seconds) occlusion of the inflow tracts. A duration of 15 to 20 seconds for this injection is advocated. The aortic clamp is then removed, and occluding clamps are applied to the base of the aorta and the pulmonary artery (B, C). The Prostigmin is used to prevent ventricular fibrillation in the hypothermic patient.

C. The incision in the pulmonary artery is retracted by the guy sutures, and the stenosis of the pulmonary valve is visible.

D, E. The pulmonary valvotomy is being completed by scissor dissection (D). Immediately following, the operative field is flooded with sterile saline solution, and the incised margins of the anterior wall of the pulmonary artery are approximated by the guy sutures preliminary to the application of the Beck–Potts clamp (E). The occluding tape ligature on the superior vena cava, the clamps on the aorta and the pulmonary artery, and finally the occluding tape ligature on the inferior vena cava are released in the order mentioned to restore the circulation in the heart and great vessels. The incision in the pulmonary artery is then sutured (00000), first down (E) and then back, to be tied at its starting point.

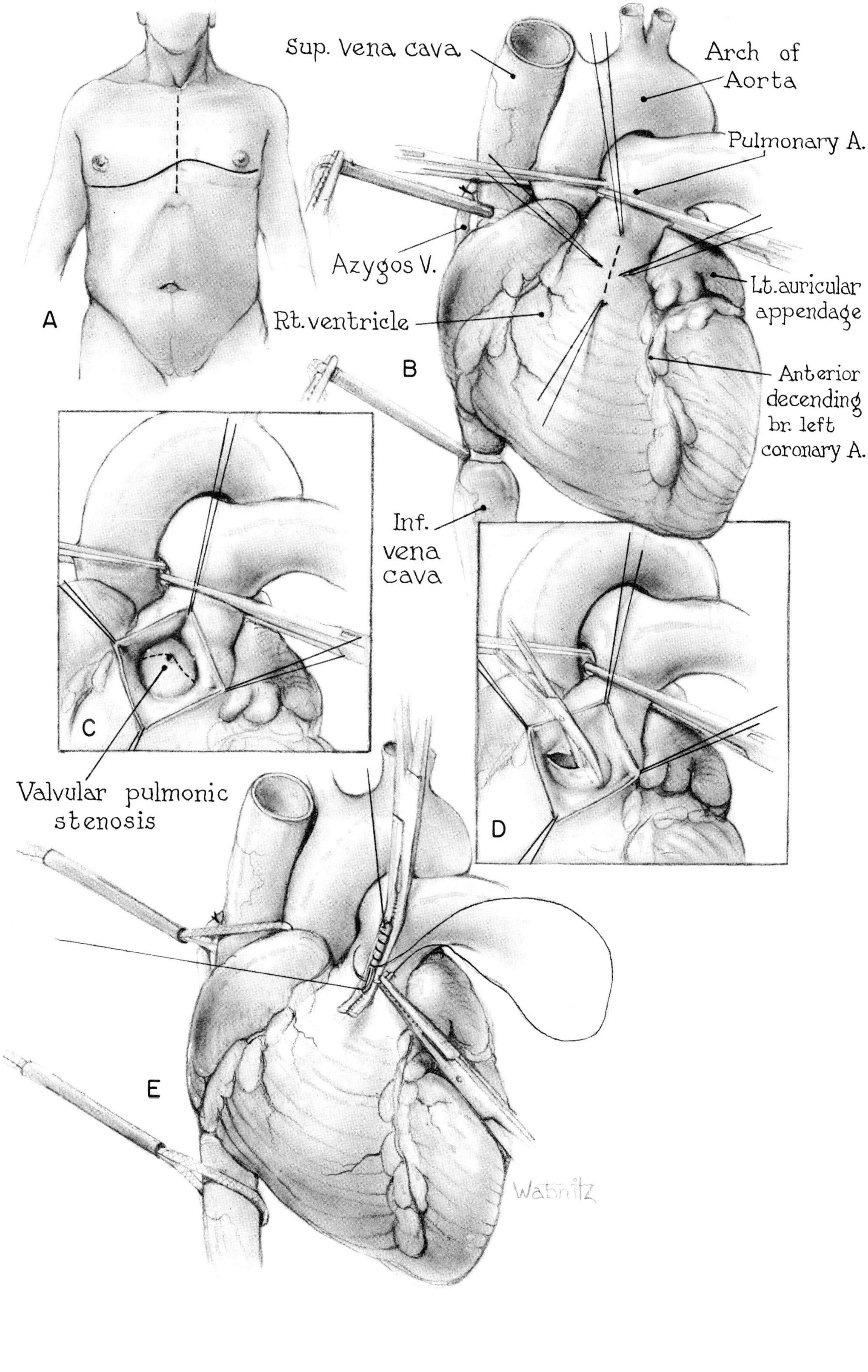

Sup. Vena cava
Arch of Aorta
Pulmonary A.
Azygos V.
Lt. auricular appendage
Rt. ventricle
Anterior decending br. left coronary A.
Inf. vena cava
Valvular pulmonic stenosis
A
B
C
D
E
Wabnitz

MITRAL COMMISSUROTOMY

A. The patient is placed in the direct right lateral prone position, and the thoracotomy incision immediately below the angle of the scapula is outlined.

B. The incision is deepened through the underlying musculature to expose the rib cage. A moist gauze sponge is inserted beneath the mobilized erector spinae group of muscles, and traction is maintained to demonstrate the angle of the fifth rib. The periosteum is removed from the lower half of the fifth rib anteriorly and the whole of the rib posteriorly after the manner of Brock. Posteriorly, the endothoracic fascia and pleura are separated from the fourth and fifth ribs throughout the extent of the incision to obtain mobility of the adjacent rib cage. The fifth rib is retracted upward, and the incision in its bed is shown in dotted outline. In this technic the intercostal muscle bundle is not incised, and accordingly there is minimal bleeding.

C. The left pleural cavity is entered, and the fifth and sixth ribs are separated by a self-retaining rib retractor. A portion of the pericardium either anterior or posterior (preferred) to the phrenic nerve is tented by traction sutures of silk (0000), and an incision is made into the pericardial cavity. The incision is extended upward, as indicated in dotted outline, and usually by scissor dissection to expose the anterior portion of the hilum of the lung and the dilated pulmonary artery.

D. Guy sutures of silk (000) are inserted through the cut margins of the pericardium, and, with traction on the sutures maintained, a portion of the left auricular appendage is visible within the pericardial cavity.

E. The tip of the left auricular appendage is mobilized with Babcock clamps, and a pursestring suture of silk (0) on a swedged-on minimum trauma needle is inserted. In the insertion of this suture, the full thickness of the wall of the appendage is included.

F. The insertion of the pursestring suture posteriorly is completed, and its relation to the subjacent circumflex branch of the left coronary artery is visible. This vessel is not seen at operation because of the overlying fatty tissue. The auricular appendage receives one, and occasionally two, arterial branches from the circumflex artery.

G. A Potts curved portacaval clamp is placed across the base of the auricular appendage immediately distal to the first pursestring suture, and the site of incision in the terminal portion of the appendage is indicated. Resection of the tip of the appendage is no longer practiced.

H. After the incision into the lumen of the appendage is completed, the cut margins on either side are grasped in Babcock clamps and a second pursestring suture of silk (0) is inserted. In utilizing this open technic for the insertion of the second pursestring suture, one is assured that the opposite wall is not included in the suture. This technical error may occur in the closed technic, and the suture may be inadvertently cut when the incision is made into the lumen of the appendage.

I. Inset to show an alternate technic that is preferred in patients in whom a history of recent thromboembolic episodes is obtained.

a. Guy sutures of silk are first inserted. A small incision is made between the sutures into the lumen of the appendage, and clots, if present, are allowed to extrude.

b. Active bleeding is controlled by crossing of the guy sutures and application of the curved Potts clamp proximally. The operation is then continued as previously described.

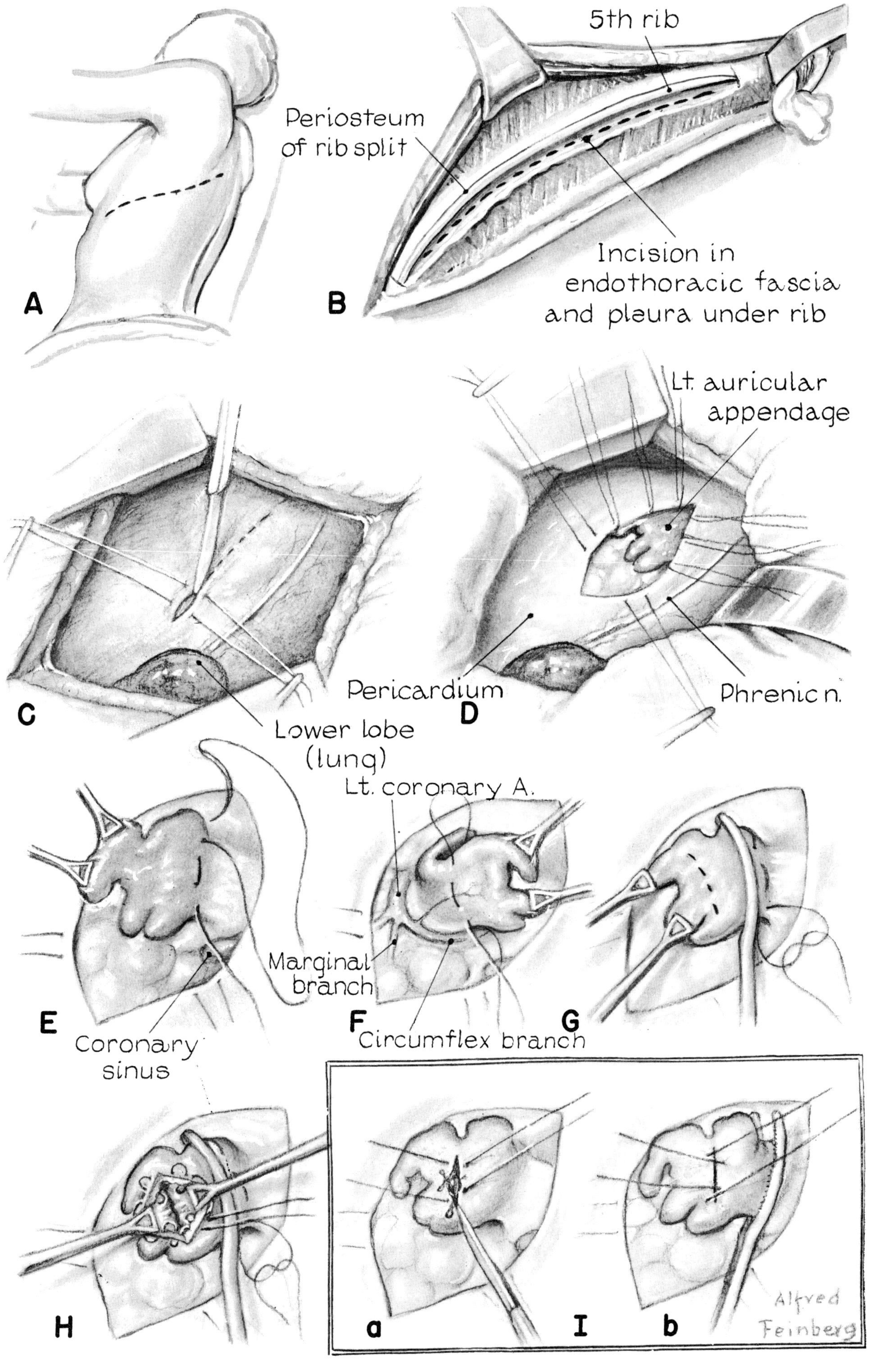
A
B
5th rib
Periosteum of rib split
Incision in endothoracic fascia and pleura under rib
C
D
Lt. auricular appendage
Pericardium
Phrenic n.
Lower lobe (lung)
E
F
G
Lt. coronary A.
Marginal branch
Coronary sinus
Circumflex branch
H
a
I
b
Alfred Feinberg

J. The right index finger is inserted through the incision in the left auricular appendage and into the lumen of the left atrium as the clamp on the appendage is released and subsequently removed. If necessary for the control of hemorrhage, though usually not, the pursestring suture may be drawn taut.

K, L. The tip of the index finger in dotted outline may be seen first engaging the stenotic orifice and then producing the "finger fracture" or avulsion tear through the anterolateral commissure. In some instances a preliminary subvalvular mobilization of the leaflets by avulsion of the chordae tendineae may be necessary before the commissurotomy may be performed. In other instances the use of a knife may be required. A unilateral, anterolateral commissurotomy may prove sufficient. However, in general, a posteromedial commissurotomy should also be done. In the performance of a mitral commissurotomy it is important that the split in the commissure extends out to the annulus of the mitral ring in order to obtain the maximum benefit of the operation. For clarity the pursestring suture has been deleted.

L′. The orifice of the mitral valve in the presence of pure stenosis. The dash and dotted outlines indicate the direction of the anterolateral and posteromedial separation respectively of the fused valve leaflets.

L″. The orifice of the mitral valve in the presence of a combination of stenosis and regurgitation. The typical "key hole" defect involving the aortic leaflet (baffle) is depicted. Through this defect, the typical regurgitant jet is readily palpable. In the presence of a combined lesion of the mitral valve a unilateral, anterolateral commissurotomy only is preferred (dotted outline) because of the danger of increasing the regurgitant jet if an extension in a posteromedial direction is performed.

M. The index finger is withdrawn from the lumen of the left atrium as the proximal pursestring suture, followed by the second pursestring suture, is tightened and tied by the first assistant. If desired, a Rumel tourniquet may be employed for tightening the first pursestring suture. If one pursestring suture only is used, the clamp may be reapplied to the auricular appendage just above the purse string as the finger is being withdrawn. In such instances, the use of the clamp is an extra safety factor in the prevention of hemorrhage.

N. The approximation of the left auricular appendage following the tying of the two pursestring sutures and the closure of the incision in the auricular appendage with interrupted sutures of silk (00) are shown.

O. The incision in the pericardium is partially closed with interrupted sutures of silk (000). The cut margins are loosely approximated, and small openings are present at either end of the incision to permit the escape of collections of both air and fluid into the pleural cavity.

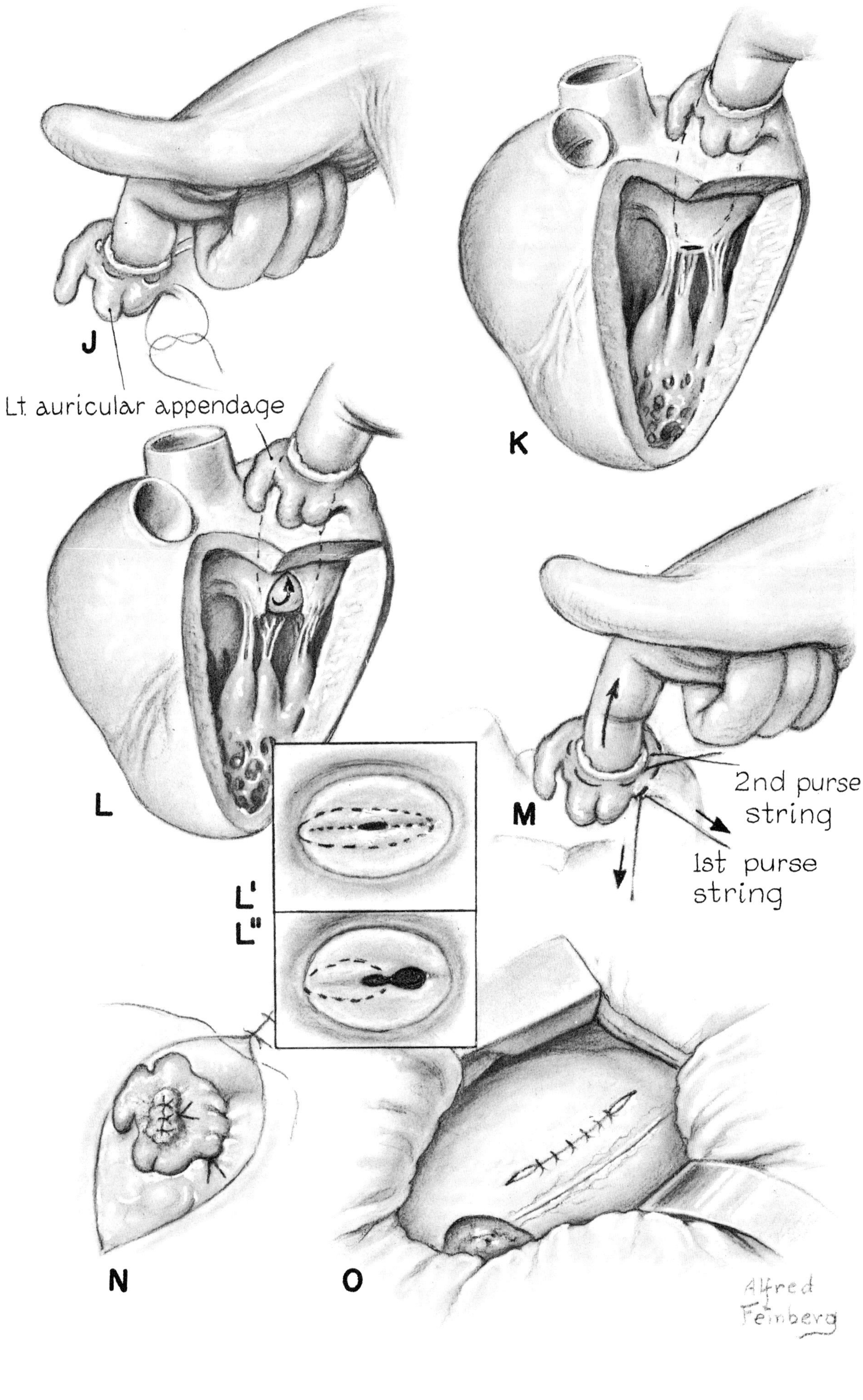
J
Lt. auricular appendage
K
L
L'
L''
M
2nd purse string
1st purse string
N
O
Alfred Feinberg

Discussion—Dr. Elliott S. Hurwitt. This is an admirable technic for opening the stenotic mitral valve. As performed at the Montefiore Hospital, the operation includes some variations that have proven to be extremely helpful. Many patients with advanced heart disease tolerate the lateral decubitus position poorly, and, occasionally, moderate elevation of the head and chest may be necessary to help prevent or control pulmonary edema. Consequently, the position of the patient is about 30 degrees posterior to the true lateral, and the incision is placed more anteriorly than depicted (Plate 111A), extending from beneath the breast to below the angle of the scapula. Adequate exposure may be obtained by entering the pleural cavity through the fourth intercostal space.

The vertical pericardial incision is made considerably closer to the phrenic nerve than shown (Plate 111C, D). Additional exposure may be obtained by mobilizing the phrenic nerve and making a short T-extension in the pericardial incision over the base of the auricular appendage. If the pursestring suture (Plate 111E, F) is begun and ended in the medial wall of the appendage, it may be controlled by the first assistant. Coordinated teamwork is of paramount importance in the subsequent maneuvers.

Of the wide variety of clamps available for application to the auricular appendage, the Satinsky clamp with the Glover grip has been highly satisfactory. Traction sutures in the lips of the auricular incision have been of considerable help in facilitating the exposure and in controlling the auricle. As the operator disengages the auricular clamp with his left hand and insinuates his right index finger into the heart, the pursestring and traction sutures are manipulated by the assistants. The effectiveness of the intracardiac finger may be augmented by pushing against the operator's left hand, placed over the upper portion of the anteromedial wall of the left ventricle. Pericardial drainage into the pleural space is promoted by a looser pericardial closure than illustrated (Plate 112O). Underwater drainage of the pleural cavity is accomplished by an intercostal tube.

Although time may not be of major importance in the performance of many operations, survival of the desperately ill patient with tight mitral stenosis and severe pulmonary hypertension may occasionally depend on the shortest possible lapse of time between induction of anesthesia and opening of the valve. Under such circumstances, it is wise to defer the ligation or electrocoagulation of the blood vessels in the thoracic wall until one is ready to close the chest.

ADDENDUM. Transventricular dilatation is frequently employed to augment a finger fracture commissurotomy that might otherwise be less than optimum. This is particularly applicable for valves with rubbery elastic margins that stretch rather than divide before the exploring finger, and for tough calcific valves. As illustrated in K, a dilator of the Tubbs or Gerbode type is inserted through a stab wound in the apex of the left ventricle. The surgeon, controlling the instrument with his left hand, manipulates the tip through the mitral orifice, where it is articulated against his right index finger within the left auricle. He then approximates the handles of the dilator to a preset gap, achieving a fracture resulting in an orifice with a diameter of approximately two fingerbreadths, which may then be increased as desired by the intra-auricular finger. The dilator is withdrawn from the ventricle, and hemostasis is effected by the assistant, either by tying previously placed pursestring or interlocking sutures, or by finger compression while myocardial sutures are inserted. The left auricular appendage is managed as described for the standard finger commissurotomy. Practiced coordination between the members of the operating team is essential.

Currently this type of "closed" cardiac surgery has been supplanted by "open" techniques, invoking cardiopulmonary bypass, when the problem involves the correction of mitral insufficiency or valve replacement. Since a wider commissurotomy for mitral stenosis could hardly be accomplished by an "open" method than that described above, there seems little indication at this time for cardiopulmonary bypass in the majority of cases of mitral stenosis. On the other hand, the equipment should always be available, on a standby basis at the very least, for all cases of mitral stenosis with substantial valvular calcification, where intra-auricular thrombosis is suspected, or where the mitral valve has previously been subjected to surgery.

CARDIOPERICARDIOPEXY

A. The relatively short (8 to 10 cm.) inframammary incision directly overlying the left fifth interspace is depicted by the solid line.

B. The skin incision is deepened through the underlying subcutaneous fatty tissue layer and the fibers of the pectoralis major muscle to expose the costal cartilage of the fifth rib.

C, D, E. The perichondrium of the fifth costal cartilage is incised (C), and perichondrial flaps are elevated (D, E). A long segment or the whole of the costal cartilage is then removed (E).

F, G, G^1. The bed or posterior perichondrium of the partially resected fifth costal cartilage is incised (F), and, after extension of the incision, the cut margins are secured by traction sutures of 0000 silk (G). Beneath the incision, portions of the pericardial fat and parietal pleura are visible. On occasions an opening may be accidentally made through the parietal pleura into the left pleural cavity. If this should occur, the opening is temporarily occluded with a moist gauze pad and the operation continued. At the completion of the poudrage, any pneumothorax present is removed by complete expansion of the lung while the chest wall incision is being closed. The inset (G^1) shows the internal mammary artery doubly clamped and being severed with a scalpel. This is done routinely as a technical expediency in the performance of a cardiopericardiopexy. If desired, the right internal mammary artery may be similarly clamped, severed, and ligated following the completion of the cardiopericardiopexy.

H, I, I^1. Guy sutures of silk (00) are inserted in the parietal pericardium (H, I), and, with traction maintained through the sutures, an incision is made into the pericardial cavity (I) and subsequently extended by scissor dissection (I^1).

Discussion—Dr. Samuel A. Thompson. Cardiopericardiopexy is a method of myocardial revascularization, and, as such, it is essentially a form of myocardial surface irritation. It stimulates the formation of extracardiac as well as intercoronary collateral circulation. It is a simple operation and attended with a low surgical mortality. The results over a period of 19 years have not been surpassed by any other method.

The operation is entirely extrapleural, and the approach is over the left fifth costal cartilage (Plate 113A). This cartilage is stripped of its perichondrium and then removed completely, from the sternal junction to the costochondral junction (Plate 113B, C, D, E). Opening the posterior perichondrium along the entire cartilage bed (Plate 113F, G) exposes the thin fibers of the transverse sterni muscle. The fibers are gently elevated and severed; this exposes the pericardium and parietal pleura. The parietal pleura is gently retracted laterally. Occasionally, in so doing, a small tear may occur in the pleura. No attempt should be made to repair this, but it should be temporarily covered with a moist gauze pad and the operation continued. Any pneumothorax which may be present is eliminated by complete expansion of the lung during closure of the chest wall structures. Ligation of the internal mammary artery (Plate 113G), which is done as a routine procedure in cardiopericardiopexy, appears to increase the vascularity of the pericardium. If the right internal mammary artery is to be ligated, it can be done through a separate small incision in the right second intercostal space at the conclusion of the cardiopericardiopexy.

The pericardium is elevated by two guy sutures (Plate 113H, I), and a small incision is made. If there is an abnormal amount of pericardial fluid present or if the fluid is under increased pressure, each myocardial beat will force a small jet of fluid from the incision. The pericardial incision is enlarged in a direction parallel to the skin incision or in a transverse direction (Plate 113 I^1), and thorough aspiration of all possible pericardial fluid is attempted by means of a soft rubber catheter. Frequent extra systoles may occur during this maneuver but are of no serious consequence. Thorough removal of the pericardial fluid is important since any quantity of residual fluid may wash the powdered talc to the dependent recesses of the pericardium, and the resulting myocardial surface irritation may be limited to the apical area instead of being generalized as is desired.

Magnesium silicate (U.S.P. talc) is the irritating material used to cover the epicardial surface of the heart. This is widely distributed over the anterior surface and borders of the heart by means of a special powder distributor (Plate 113J). Depending upon the size of the heart, from 2 to 6 gm. of talc are

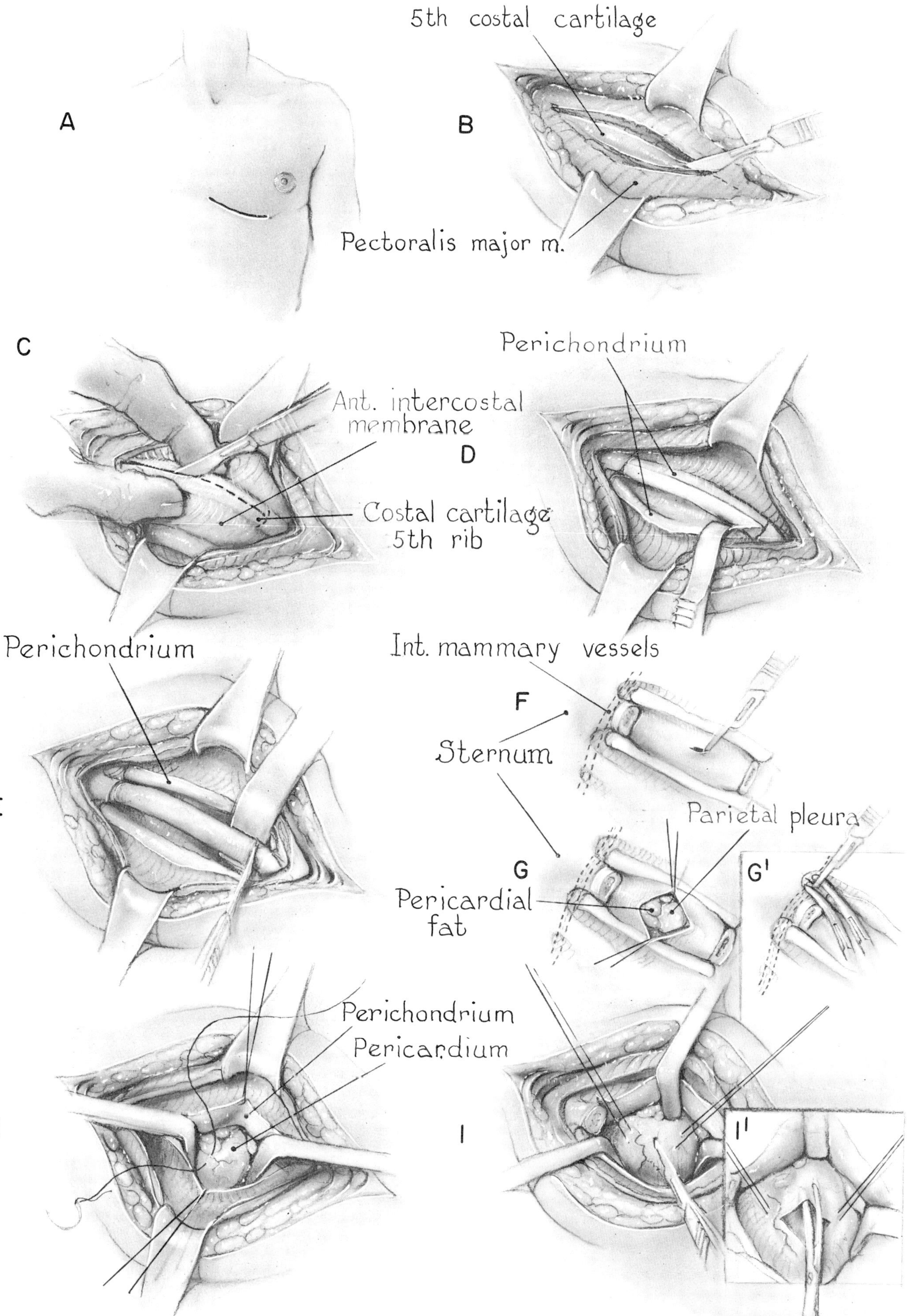
5th costal cartilage
A
B
Pectoralis major m.
C
Perichondrium
Ant. intercostal membrane
D
Costal cartilage 5th rib
Perichondrium
Int. mammary vessels
F
Sternum
E
Parietal pleura
G
G'
Pericardial fat
Perichondrium
Pericardium
H
I
I'

J. Three guy sutures of silk (000) are inserted at equidistant points in the incised margins of the parietal pericardium, and the adjacent surroundings are walled off with moist gauze pads. Upward traction is maintained on the three guy sutures as the dry, powdered talc is inserted into the pericardial sac and onto the epicardial surface of the heart covering the anterior surface and lateral margins. The various planes in which the talc is deposited are indicated by the varying positions of the Thompson powder distributor (dotted outlines). The moist gauze pads about the operative field serve to prevent the deposit of talc onto the adjacent tissues.

K. Upon completion of the insertion of the talc (2 to 6 gm.), the moist gauze pads are removed, and the interrupted silk (000) sutures used to close the incision in the anterior parietal pericardium are inserted but not tied.

L. The closure of the pericardial incision is completed, and the insertion of the silk (000) sutures in the incised bed of the fifth costal cartilage is begun. Portions of the pericardial fat and parietal pleura are also visible.

M, N. The closure of the incision in the costal bed is completed, and the beginning of the insertion of interrupted silk (000) sutures to approximate the cut margins of the pectoralis major muscle and the underlying flaps of anterior perichondrium as a unit layer is shown (M). The completed closure is depicted in N.

O. The closure of the skin incision with interrupted sutures of silk (000) completes the operation. No drains are used.

Discussion—Dr. Thompson (cont.)

used, and no attempt is made to cover the posterior surface, as the beating of the heart will carry a sufficient amount to this area.

Upon completion of the powder distribution, quite frequently there is a decided drop in the patient's blood pressure. The anesthetist should expect this, and, if it occurs, counteract it by the use of an intravenous pressor drug.

The pericardium is loosely closed with interrupted sutures, and the soft structures of the chest wall are closed in anatomic layers without drainage.

In a period of almost twenty years, there has been no evidence that cardiopericardiopexy produces any degree of constrictive pericarditis or becomes avascular.

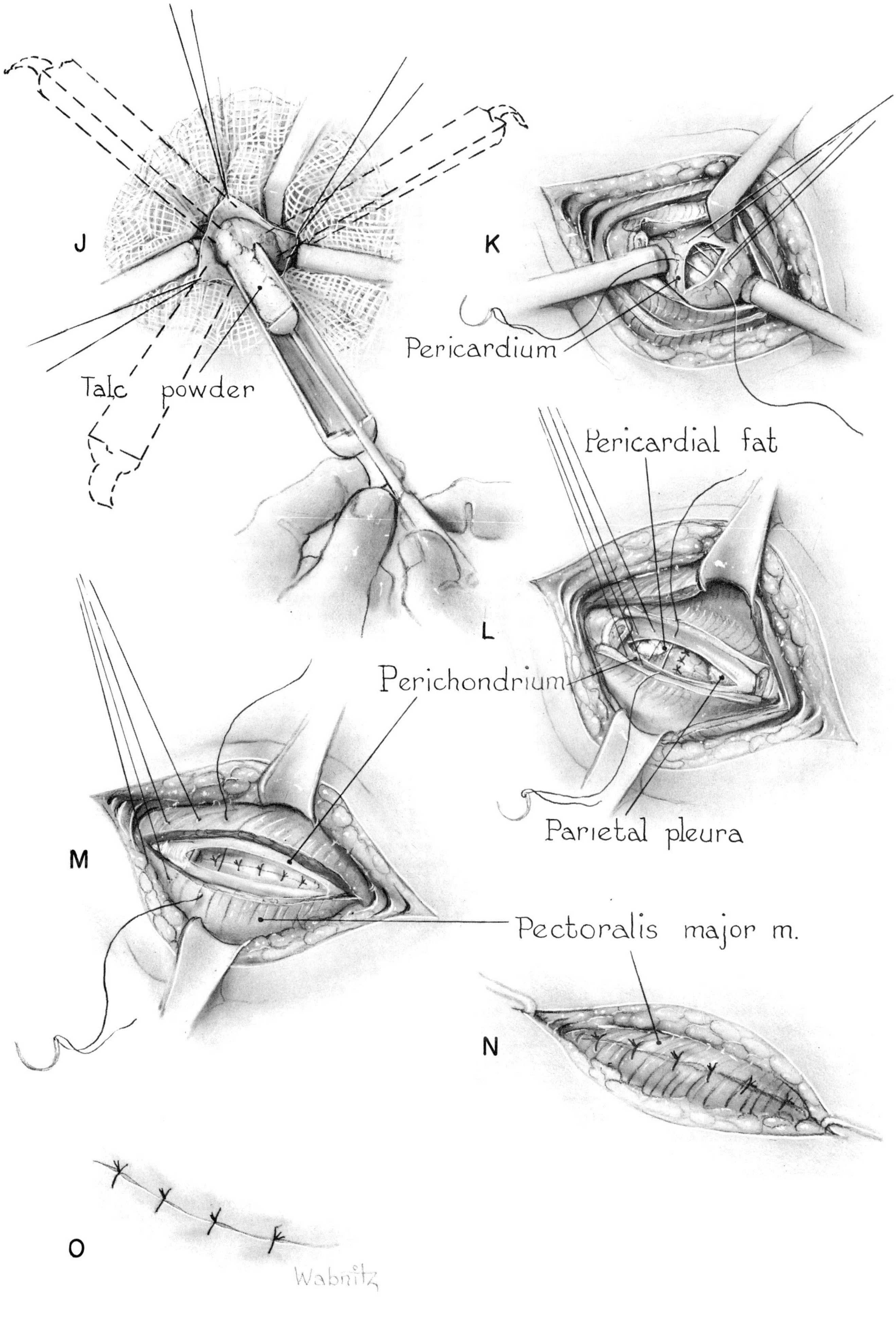
J
Talc powder
K
Pericardium
Pericardial fat
L
Perichondrium
Parietal pleura
M
Pectoralis major m.
N
O
Wabnitz

CORONARY THROMBOENDARTERECTOMY

A. The patient is placed in the supine position with the left side of the thorax slightly elevated. The anterolateral incision employed is indicated by the curvilinear dotted line.

B. The incised margins of the pericardium are retracted by guy sutures of silk (000) to expose the anterior descending branch of the left coronary artery. This artery, partially mobilized, is encircled by two silk (No. 1) sutures, between which the incision in the artery (dotted line) is subsequently made. The use of the encircling sutures in combination with finger compression for hemostasis is preferred to clamp (serrefine) occlusion.

B^1. This is a sketch of the instrument* of special design used for the dissection and mobilization of the thrombus.

C. The incision in the artery is completed, and the underlying thrombus which occludes its lumen is exposed. Four sutures of silk (00000) are inserted through either incised margin of the artery and will be used for later closure of the incision after completion of the coronary thromboendarterectomy.

D. The free ends of the four sutures previously inserted are separated into two groups, upper and lower, and grasped in clamps. The respective loops formed by the sutures are held in hook retractors and retracted cephalad and caudad respectively. A segment of the occluding thrombus is separated from the arterial wall and elevated on the dissecting instrument. The dotted lines indicate the segment of the thrombus to be resected.

E. A segment of the thrombus is resected, and the transected end caudad is grasped in a clamp for traction as dissection of this portion of the thrombus is being performed.

F. Following the removal of the caudad segment of the thrombus, free retrograde bleeding occurred. Similarly, the transected end cephalad is grasped in a clamp for traction as dissection of this segment of the thrombus is being performed. The thrombus was easily separated from the adjacent wall of the artery, the lining of which was characterized by a healthy glistening sheen. This finding, in conjunction with the ease with which the thromboendarterectomy was performed, is believed indicative of the technical feasibility of the operation.

F^1, G. Upon completion of the removal of the thrombus cephalad, a No. 6 ureteral catheter was inserted into the lumen of the coronary artery and through its orifice into the lumen of the aorta. As the catheter was slowly withdrawn, 10 ml. of a heparin–saline solution (100 mg. of heparin in 250 ml. of saline) was injected. When the withdrawal of the catheter was completed, a forceful ejection of blood through the coronary arteriotomy, which reached the level of the skin drapes, was observed. Hemostasis was obtained by digital compression overlying the arteriotomy preparatory to approximation of the incised margins of the artery by traction upon the sutures previously inserted (G). As traction is maintained, the sutures are tied individually (G) to complete the closure of the coronary arteriotomy. One additional suture was subsequently required. The use of this particular technic obviates the necessity for clamp occlusion of the coronary artery following the reestablishment of its blood flow. This is considered a desirable technical aid in the prevention of stasis thrombosis.

* Manufactured by Edward Weck & Co., Brooklyn, New York.

The patient, a 47-year-old man, was admitted to the hospital on February 10, 1957, because of severe angina on effort and resulting marked physical incapacitation. A previous history of a coronary occlusion in 1949 and again in 1952, as well as a bout of congestive failure in July of 1955, was obtained. Because of the severity of the symptoms and the limitation of physical activity, operation was advised and performed on February 21, 1957. Upon exposure of the heart, extensive atherosclerotic occlusive disease of both coronary arteries was present. Although initially a cardiopericardiopexy was contemplated, it was decided to attempt a coronary thromboendarterectomy, which was performed as illustrated. Shortly after entrance into the left pleural cavity, stoppage of the heart occurred which responded immediately to manual massage. Stoppage for the second time occurred before completion of the thromboendarterectomy and again responded to manual massage.

Postoperatively, the immediate progress of the patient was satisfactory with the exception of a persistent hypotension. Within three hours after the operation, he talked coherently and requested a cup of black coffee which was drunk and relished. However, seven hours postoperatively, irreversible peripheral vascular collapse occurred, and the patient died one-and-one-half hours later (eight-and-one-half hours postoperatively). At necropsy, 22 hours postoperatively, the appearance of the surgical field was completely satisfactory. To determine the patency of the coronary arterial system, a red-colored

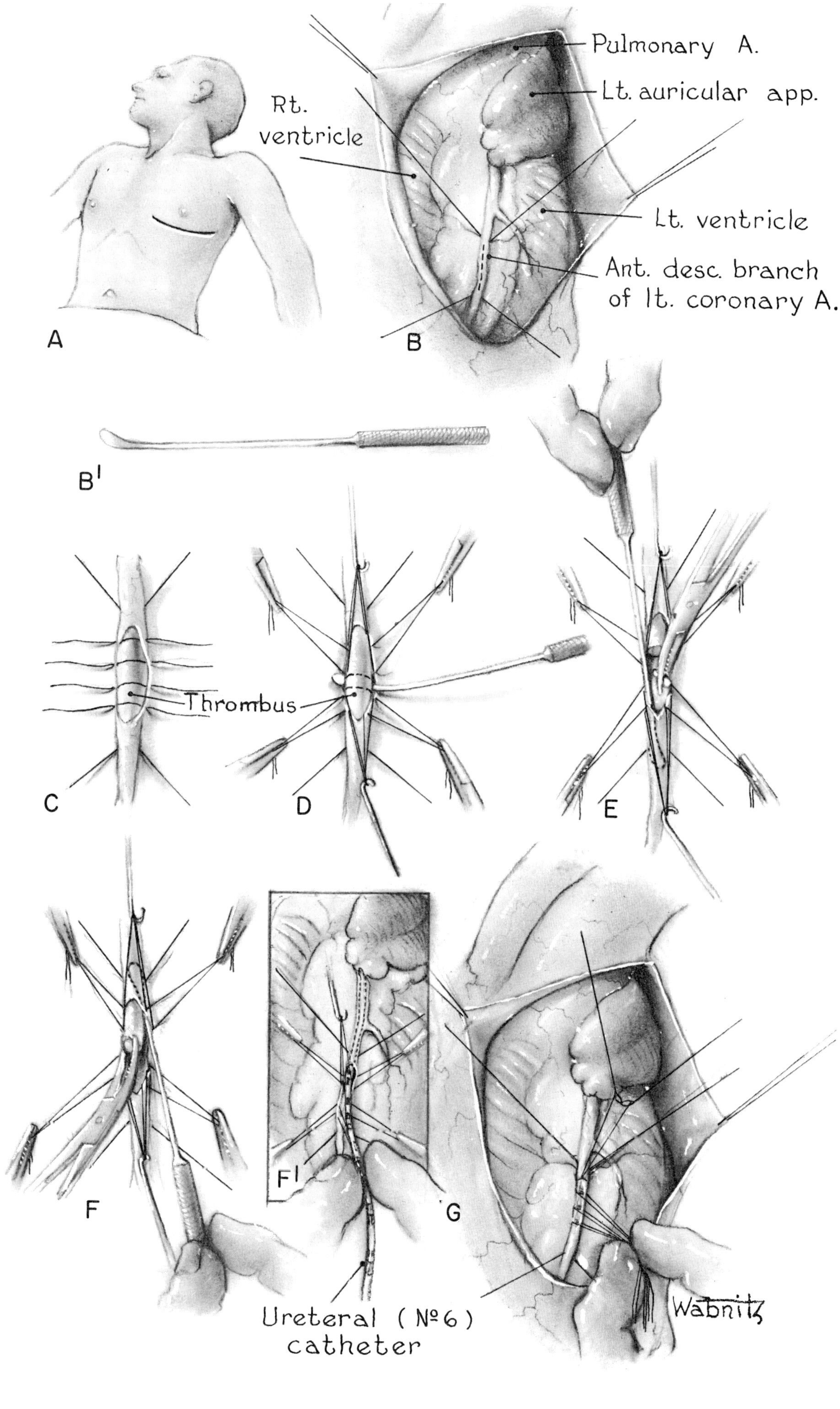
Pulmonary A.
Lt. auricular app.
Rt. ventricle
Lt. ventricle
Ant. desc. branch of lt. coronary A.
A
B
B'
Thrombus
C
D
E
F
F'
G
Ureteral (№6) catheter
Wabnitz

solution of neoprene latex type 571* was injected (with the heart in situ) in a retrograde manner into the ascending aorta which was cross-clamped immediately distal to the site of injection. The heart and the occluded segment of the ascending aorta were removed, and, 24 hours later, dissection of the coronary arteries was performed. It was of interest to observe that the left coronary artery and its anterior descending branch and related collateral vessels were filled with red-colored neoprene latex. Contrariwise, the circumflex branch of the left coronary artery and the right coronary artery, which were not operated upon, were occluded by atherosclerotic thrombi. Through the center of each of these thrombi, a faint red line of the latex dye indicative of the size of the lumen within the thrombus was discernible. The result of this study was considered positive evidence of the continued patency of the left coronary artery and its anterior descending branch for the duration of the short period (eight-and-one-half hours) of survival of the patient following the coronary thromboendarterectomy.

The objection that the coronary arteries are too small to maintain the patency of the lumen when reestablished may prove more of a theoretical than a practical objection. Certainly the central head of arterial pressure within the aorta in relation to the orifices of the coronary arteries is much greater than the head of pressure in relation to the orifices of peripheral arteries of similar diameter. Accordingly, it is believed a fallacy to negate the potential value of coronary thromboendarterectomy based on the poor results obtained in the performance of thromboendarterectomy in vessels of similar size in the peripheral arterial tree. Furthermore, despite the finding of extensive coronary atherosclerosis, as was present in this patient, the restoration of blood flow in one coronary vessel segment may prove beneficial. It is only by further cumulative experience that the practical value of coronary thromboendarterectomy will be either proved or disproved. Certainly the findings at operation in this particular patient proved that coronary thromboendarterectomy was technically a feasible operation. Following completion of the thromboendarterectomy, it was indeed most impressive to observe the force with which the blood was ejected and the volume of flow through the coronary arteriotomy with each systolic contraction of the ventricles.

* Supplied through the courtesy of E. I. du Pont de Nemours & Co., Elastomer Chemicals Department, New York City.

DISCUSSION—DR. CLAUDE S. BECK. The problem of coronary thromboendarterectomy is not so simple as it appears on the surface. It is scarcely comparable to cleaning out debris from other arteries. If you put a string on the descending ramus of the left coronary artery and keep it there for a half hour or so and then release the artery, the probability is that the heart will fibrillate as red blood enters this ischemic muscle. This was a worry to me for many years because I and my associates in the laboratory always considered arterial blood to be good for the heart and never bad. Here we had an indication that arterial blood could kill the heartbeat. Finally, the explanation became clear. If you anesthetize a dog and then clamp off the intratracheal tube for six to nine minutes, the dog becomes cyanotic and the heart becomes cyanotic. If you take a cotton electrode moistened with sodium chloride solution and sweep it across the ventricles, the electrogram is precisely the same as that obtained from a uniformly well-oxygenated heart. What does this mean? It means that the amount of oxygenated blood delivered to the heart has a relationship to the electrical condition, the electrical equilibrium, or electrical stability of the heart. A blue baby has a stable heart. If you put a string on a coronary artery, you create a blue or cyanosed area of muscle in a pink or well-oxygenated heart. If you canulate a coronary artery in a blue or asphyxiated heart and perfuse arterial blood into this artery, you create a pink area of muscle in a blue heart. Both of these hearts are electrically unstable and may fibrillate. The S–T segment of the electrogram is elevated over the blue area and depressed over the pink area. Pink or well-oxygenated muscle in juxtaposition with blue or cyanosed muscle creates an electrical condition that can fibrillate the heart. A baby with one coronary artery coming off the aorta and the other coming off the pulmonary artery has anginal pain and dies. This electrical situation is created because of differences in oxygen content or, as we have called them, oxygen differentials. It is not the amount of blood that kills; it is an uneven or checkerboard distribution of oxygen that kills. When the physiologist tied off a coronary artery and lifted electrical reactions from the heart, he called them "currents of injury." This concept is wrong. Creating pink and blue muscle in juxtaposition has nothing to do with "injury." This condition kills hundreds of thousands of men and women in this country every year. These are the people who die on the golf course, watching an exciting athletic contest, in the office, and so on. They are examples of self-electrocution of the heart. This often occurs in hearts that are too good anatomically to "die," and it often occurs without an infarct.

It is possible, therefore, to fibrillate the heart when one coronary artery is opened for a free flow of arterial blood and when the other two arteries are severely stenosed. Under certain conditions, red blood can kill the heartbeat.

This statement does not imply that there are no instances when the opening of an artery would not be beneficial to the heart. The writer has had numerous experiences in which the introduction of red blood would have been beneficial to the heart—cases in which the descending area of muscle would not contract because of inflow reduction. On many occasions, attempts were made to clean out the diseased artery without success. The disease was in the arterial wall, and to remove it would have required removal of the entire wall of the artery. The writer has operated upon 500 human beings for coronary artery disease. Almost always, the disease is in the primary, secondary, and tertiary branches of the coronary arteries—much too widespread for removal. Localized disease is rarely found.

The writer does not state that these attempts should not be made. This is the sort of approach that is easily understood. To take out something always has greater appeal than does a physiologic concept, especially if the concept is new and complicated. Surgeons have learned by experience that you cannot successfully clean out arteries so small as the coronary arteries elsewhere in the body, even in the presence of anticoagulants and hypertension with high-driving forward pressures. They clot again. Perhaps the experience with the coronaries may be different. This remains to be seen.

DISCUSSION—DR. WILLIAM P. LONGMIRE, JR. With the assistance of Dr. Albert Kattus of the Department of Medicine in the selection and preparation of patients, Dr. Jack A. Cannon and I have operated upon five patients for severe incapacitating angina pectoris without evidence of myocardial infarction by the technic of direct vision coronary thromboendarterectomy. Four of these patients survived the operative procedure. Over a short period of time, all seemed to have been improved. Improvement was noted, not only on the basis of subjective criteria, but also on the objective evidence of improved myocardial circulation; this evidence was obtained from electrocardiographic tracings taken during exercise both before and after operation. Operations designed to improve myocardial circulation and relieve symptoms of angina pectoris are notoriously difficult to appraise, and this procedure must await further evaluation before its true efficacy and future status can be estimated. The early results are encouraging.

The operative procedure, as described by Dr. Madden and also used by us in five patients, has proven that it is technically feasible to perform thromboendarterectomy of the major coronary vessels of the heart. Our limited experience has also demonstrated that it is possible to select patients for operation in whom the occlusive disease is limited to the major coronary vessels—i.e., vessels which may be attacked by direct surgical procedures. The crucial question to be answered by further observation pertains to the continued patency of these small vessels after thromboendarterectomy has been performed. The observation, as reported here by Dr. Madden, that patency of the thromboendarterectomized vessel could be demonstrated some eight-and-one-half hours after operation, supports the belief that the coronary arteries will remain patent following this procedure.

In the procedure we have used, the patient is placed in the supine position, the thorax is entered through a bilateral thoracotomy incision made at the fourth interspace, and the sternum is divided. The pericardium is opened widely, and all major coronary vessels are inspected and palpated. With this approach it is possible to open both the right main coronary artery and the left anterior descending artery. This incision is not suitable for an approach to the left circumflex artery. After the condition of the major vessels is evaluated, the smaller branches of the coronary arterial system are appraised by inspection and palpation. In only one case was there found to be slight "beading" of the smaller branches of the coronary arterial system. This was not felt to be sufficient reason, however, to occlude these smaller branches. The epicardial fat is dissected away from the major coronary vessels. In two cases, both the right main coronary artery and the left anterior descending artery were thromboendarterectomized; in two cases, only the right main coronary was so treated; and in one case, the left anterior descending artery alone was operated upon. As the epicardial fat is stripped away from the major vessels, the areas of disease inside the lumen of the vessel may be identified, owing to the marked adherence of the epicardial fat to the vessel at such a point.

In operations upon the right main coronary artery, the vessel is exposed from its origin at the base of the aorta for a distance of approximately 3.5 to 4 cm., at which point it breaks up into its terminal branches. The left anterior descending artery is exposed from its origin at the left circumflex artery peripherally until it also branches into several smaller vessels. After this artery is widely exposed, a ligature is passed about the vessel at its origin and again peripherally or about the major peripheral branches. A test period of complete occlusion of the vessel is then conducted by placing a "bulldog" clamp across the vessel for a period of six minutes. During this time, the color of the myocardium supplied by this branch is observed, as well as the rate and rhythm of the heart. The heart action is monitored by the electrocardiogram. We have not attempted to open any vessel if the heart did not tolerate complete occlusion of the vessel for a period of six minutes without showing any signs of regional cyanosis or arrhythmia.

A longitudinal incision is made in the vessel over the area which, by palpation, shows the most advanced disease, and the thickened intimal core is separated from the surrounding media and adventitia. It is not difficult to establish a good plane of cleavage between the structures and to isolate the obstructing core. Ligatures are then placed about the core at the proximal and distal ends of this incision. An elevator, similar to that described in Dr. Madden's article, but modified so as to permit the instrument to be adjusted to different angles, is used to elevate the core from the media and adventitia of the vessel. If necessary, additional longitudinal incisions are made in the vessel at the site of the major branches so that the branching core can be removed from these smaller vessels. When the limits of dissection with the elevator are reached, a circular stripper is inserted over the core and passed down the vessel between the core on one side and the media and adventitia on the other. The stripper is carried as far distally as possible; usually, when the thickened intima thins out and is freed from the surrounding layers of the vessel, it divides readily and is removed from the vessel intact. A similar procedure is then repeated in the proximal end of the vessel. In the case of the right coronary, the core is stripped up into the sinus of Valsalva at the mouth of the coronary artery. In the case of the left anterior descending coronary, the dissection is continued proximally into the lumen of the left circumflex artery. In all cases, a vigorous pulsatile flow has been established from the proximal end of the vessel, and abundant back bleeding from the distal end of the vessel has been obtained. A catheter has been inserted in the lumen of the coronary for the injection of heparin solution, as described by Dr. Madden, but in more recent cases a small amount of powdered heparin was placed directly into the lumen of the vessel following thromboendarterectomy.

The longitudinal incisions in the vessel are closed with continuous 000000 arterial silk sutures, the epicardial fat is resutured over the isolated artery, and the pericardium is closed loosely with interrupted sutures of silk. Two catheters are placed in both pleural spaces, and the thoracotomy incision is closed in layers in the usual fashion.

The one fatality in this series occurred in a 53-year-old, white, male patient, who was operated upon for severe incapacitating angina pectoris. In this case, an uneventful endarterectomy of the right main coronary artery was performed. During the subsequent removal of the thickened intima from the left anterior descending artery, sudden irreversible dilation and asystole of the heart occurred. Again, it should be stressed that this procedure is currently in the stage of evaluation, and its true place in the surgeon's armamentarium has not been clearly established.

CARDIAC RESUSCITATION

A. In this patient, acute cardiac arrest occurred during the course of an abdominal exploration. The abdominal wound was covered by a moist pad and towel. The left anterolateral thoracotomy incision overlying the fifth interspace is depicted by the dotted line.

B. The left pleural cavity is entered with a bold sweep of the scalpel, and the underlying intrapleural structures are demonstrable.

C, D. Immediate manual massage of the heart is performed and continued as a self-retaining rib retractor (Tuffier) is inserted. Concomitant with massage, artificial respiration is maintained, preferably through an intratracheal tube, either by rhythmic compression of the rebreathing bag using 93 per cent oxygen and 7 per cent carbon dioxide or by the use of a mechanical ventilator such as the Jefferson type. The placement of the patient in a 30-degree Trendelenberg position is a gravity aid in restoration of the circulation to the brain. Initially the pericardium is not opened (C) because this would entail an unnecessary waste of time in the establishment of an artificial circulation to supply the immediate tissue needs of the body. However, if desirable subsequently, the pericardium may be incised and intrapericardial massage continued (D). In the performance of manual massage, the heart is cupped in the hand with the apex directed toward the base of the palm. The fingers are inserted posterior and the thumb anterior to the heart, and rhythmic compression is performed. The rate of compression is 50 to 60 times per minute. Intermittently the epicardial surface of the heart is irrigated with warm saline solution as an aid to conduction. When a spontaneous rhythm is restored, manual massage is discontinued momentarily and the cardiac activity is observed. Frequently the heart rate will slow perceptibly and even come to a standstill unless manual massage is again performed. Under such circumstances, calcium chloride (5 ml. of 5 per cent solution) or epinephrine (1 ml. of 1:1000 solution) may be used. Following the use of such drugs, the restoration and maintenance of a forceful cardiac rhythm frequently occurs. In the event of ventricular fibrillation, cocaine (10 per cent) may be used topically in conjunction with the continuation of manual massage, or an electrical defibrillator may be employed.

E. A layer closure of the thoracotomy incision is performed about a Foley catheter (No. 16 F) which is used for water-seal drainage of the pleural cavity. If desired, the catheter may have its exit through a separate stab-wound drainage site below the incision.

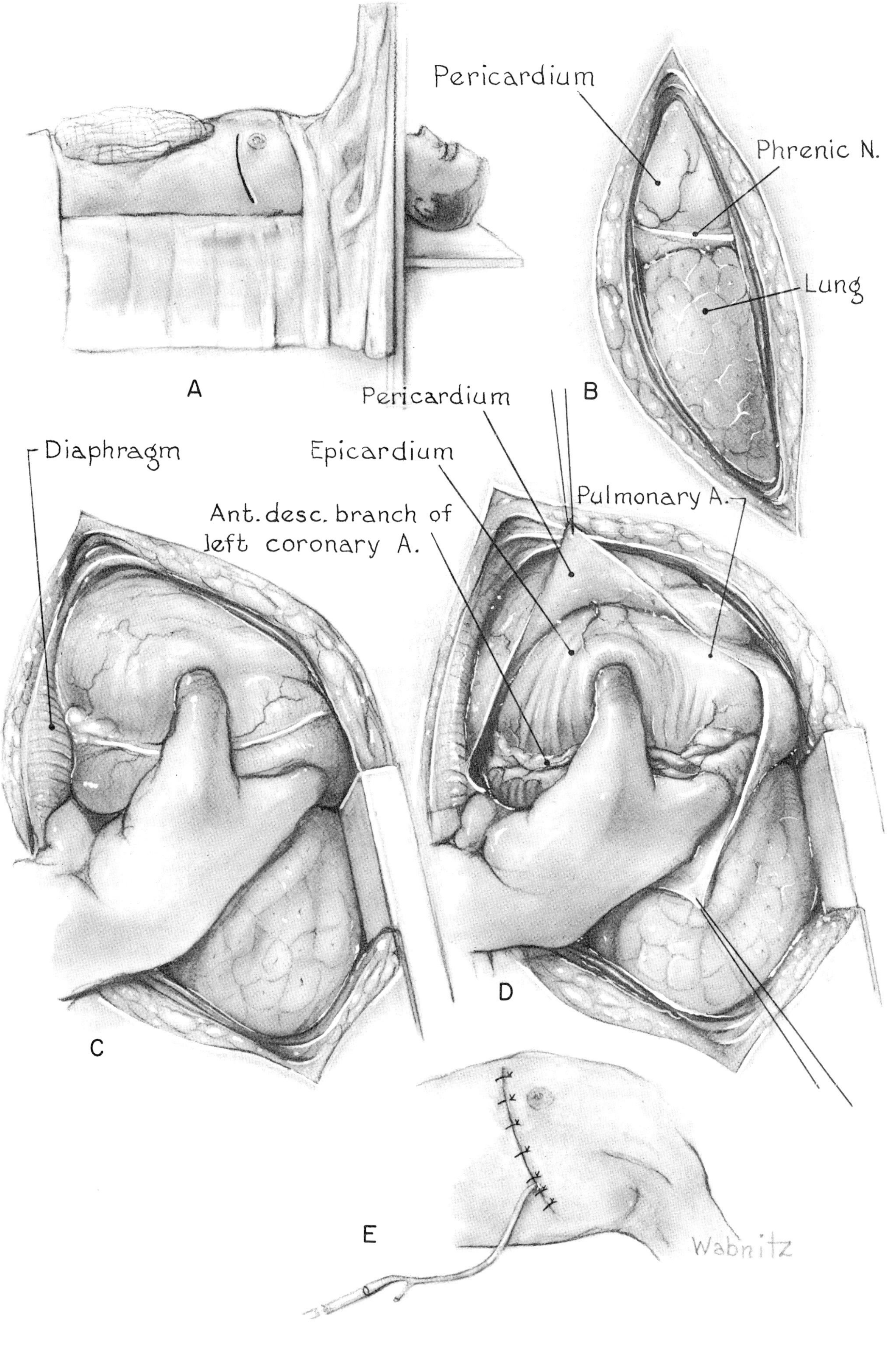
Pericardium
Phrenic N.
Lung
A
B
Pericardium
Diaphragm
Epicardium
Ant. desc. branch of
left coronary A.
Pulmonary A.
C
D
E
Wabnitz

PERICARDIECTOMY

The patient, a 45-year-old Negro man, was admitted to the hospital because of dyspnea on exertion and moderate pedal edema. Seven years previously a stab wound of the chest overlying the precordium was sustained. The immediate treatment was conservative, and the patient was discharged from the hospital six days later. Subsequent stays in the hospital were required after one and one-half years, three years, and five years, respectively, because of symptoms indicative of right-sided heart failure. Operation was advised on each occasion but was steadfastly refused.

The last admission to the hospital was in September, 1961. Dyspnea was severe on limited physical exertion but absent in full recumbency, a characteristic symptom in patients with constrictive pericarditis. Hydrothorax (right), hepatomegaly, ascites, and pedal edema were moderate. Interestingly, the heart sounds were neither muffled nor distant. The blood pressure was 110/90. Roentgenograms of the chest, in addition to the right-sided hydrothorax, showed a calcification of the pericardium that encircled completely the cardiac silhouette when viewed in the lateral projection.

The pressure in the left antecubital vein at the heart level was 245 mm. of water compared to the normal of 70-100 mm. The arm-to-lung (ether) and arm-to-tongue (decholin) circulation times were 25 seconds and 45 seconds, respectively, compared to the normal of 7-12 seconds and 9-16 seconds.

The operation as illustrated was done under general endotracheal anesthesia, and the patient actually improved as the decortication progressed. The postoperative course was satisfactory, and the patient was asymptomatic on discharge from the hospital three weeks after the operation. The venous pressure and circulation times (ether and decholin) were normal.

Tuberculosis and viral infections are the major causes for constrictive pericarditis. The occurrence of this complication following a traumatic hemopericardium is relatively rare but does occur as demonstrated in the patient presented. The rapidity of improvement and the complete relief of symptoms are believed related to the completeness of the decortication. Conversely, a protracted convalescence is frequently the result of an inadequate removal of the scar rather than myocardial weakness secondary to a muscle atrophy of disuse. Accordingly, the importance of completeness in the performance of decortication of the heart for chronic constrictive pericarditis cannot be overemphasized.

A. The patient is placed in the supine position, and the median sternotomy incision (Duval-Barasty) is depicted by the solid black line. Subsequently an extension of the incision to the left (broken line) was required to obtain optimum exposure.

B. The incision is deepened through the skin and subcutaneous tissue layers, and the periosteum overlying the sternum is incised.

C, C_1. The periosteum is separated from the sternum (C), the outer table of which is split longitudinally with a Stryker saw (C_1).

D, D_1. The median sternotomy is completed with a Lebsche knife (D), and the cut margins are separated (D_1).

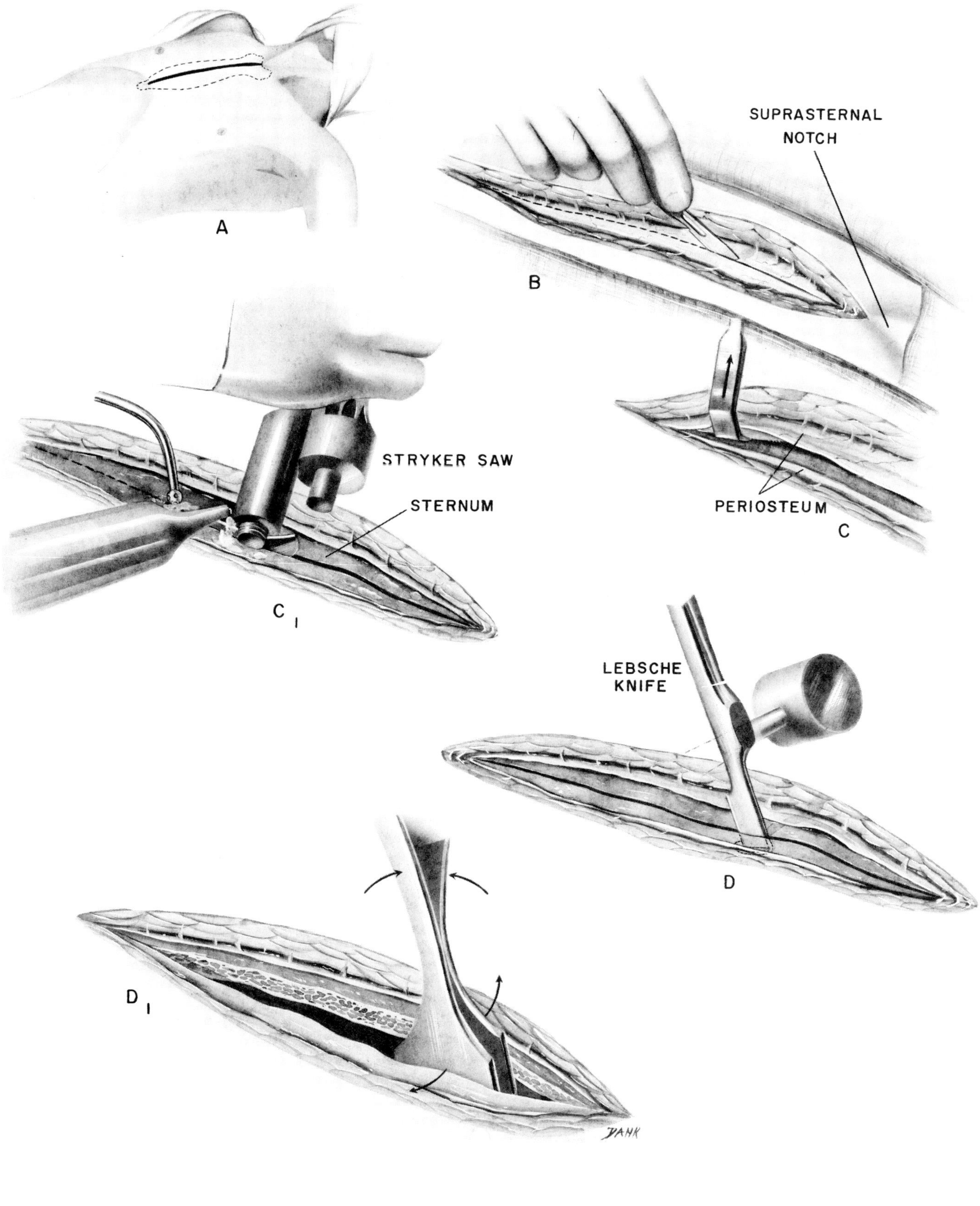
A
SUPRASTERNAL NOTCH
B
STRYKER SAW
STERNUM
C_1
PERIOSTEUM
C
LEBSCHE KNIFE
D
D_1

E. By blunt digital dissection the loose fibroareolar attachments between the pericardial scar and the posterior surface of the sternum are separated.

F. The wound margins are retracted, and the mediastinal pleura is separated from the surface of the pericardium by scissor dissection.

G. An opening was inadvertently made in the mediastinal pleura, which is elevated on the index finger to facilitate its further dissection from the pericardium.

H. The separation of the pleura from the pericardium is completed, and the opening previously made in the pleura is extended cephalad with scissors. A portion of the atelectatic lung is visible within the right pleural cavity, which contained 1500 cc. of serosanguinous fluid.

I. To obtain better exposure of the left border of the heart a transternal T extension of the incision into the fourth interspace is made.

Discussion—Dr. Emile Holman. The history of this patient's illness illustrates the not infrequent late development of cardiac constriction following the simple accumulation of blood in the undrained pericardial space, such as has been reported following an open heart operation, or a traumatic hemopericardium without laceration of the pericardium.

In effecting an adequate decortication the author has undertaken a so-called "radical" pericardiectomy, the successive steps of which are clearly shown: the freeing of the anterior and posterior aspects of the apex first; the liberation of the left border of the heart down to the left hilum [having displaced the phrenic nerve from the pericardium]; removal of scar beyond the inferior border of the heart, bringing into view the diaphragm and the inferior vena cava; extension of the decortication to free the base of the heart including the pulmonary artery, the superior vena cava, and finally freeing the right border of the heart down to the right hilar region. Adequate drainage must be provided both of the anterior mediastinum and usually the right pleural space to insure against the accumulation of blood clot over the surface of the denuded heart and recurrence of a contracting scar.

It should be recognized that the myocardial fibers and cardiac vessels are not always as clearly shown as illustrated (V) (W), particularly in a decortication performed in the presence of acute or chronic inflammation; but a complete and adequate removal of scarring over all possible critical areas is well stressed. Prompt reduction to normal venous pressure and circulation times provides convincing evidence of the adequacy of the decortication.

Discussion—Dr. Conrad R. Lam. The diagnosis in this case seemed to be well established by the history, roentgen finding of calcification of the pericardium and the markedly increased venous pressure. In some cases, confirmation by right heart catheterization will be indicated. Because of the lack of complete relaxation of the right ventricle, the diastolic pressure builds up quickly to equal the auricular pressure tracing.

The vertical sternum-splitting incision is definitely the incision of choice. I have found it satisfactory to split the sternum only to the third interspace, and to add a transverse incision to make a T-sternotomy. Since the great vessels do not need to be decorticated, this more conservative incision gives adequate exposure. Figures J through L show the use of traction sutures to hold up the thickened pericardium as it is separated from the underlying layer. I have preferred to grasp the edges firmly with clamps of the Allis type. It cannot be emphasized too strongly that a flap of at least one centimeter of pericardium should be left as dissection progresses so that it can be used to repair a tear in the ventricle if necessary. I believe that I have made an opening into the right ventricle in two-thirds of my cases, and in all the hemorrhage was easily controlled.

Figures M-O show that it was necessary to remove three layers of cortex before the myocardium of the right ventricle was completely exposed and freed. It has seemed to me that most of my cases have had two layers rather than three. At any rate, it is easy to see when he has done the proper amount of "peeling."

The extent of the decortication as shown in W seems adequate. Some previous writers on the subject of pericardiectomy for constrictive pericarditis have urged that the pulmonary veins be exposed. I am sure that manipulations this deep through the midline incision will result in injury to the phrenic nerves and perhaps auricular or venous bleeding which might be difficult to control. We have never failed to achieve what appeared to be a perfect clinical result when there was a complete decortication of the right ventricle and right auricle, and at least a partial decortication of the left ventricle.

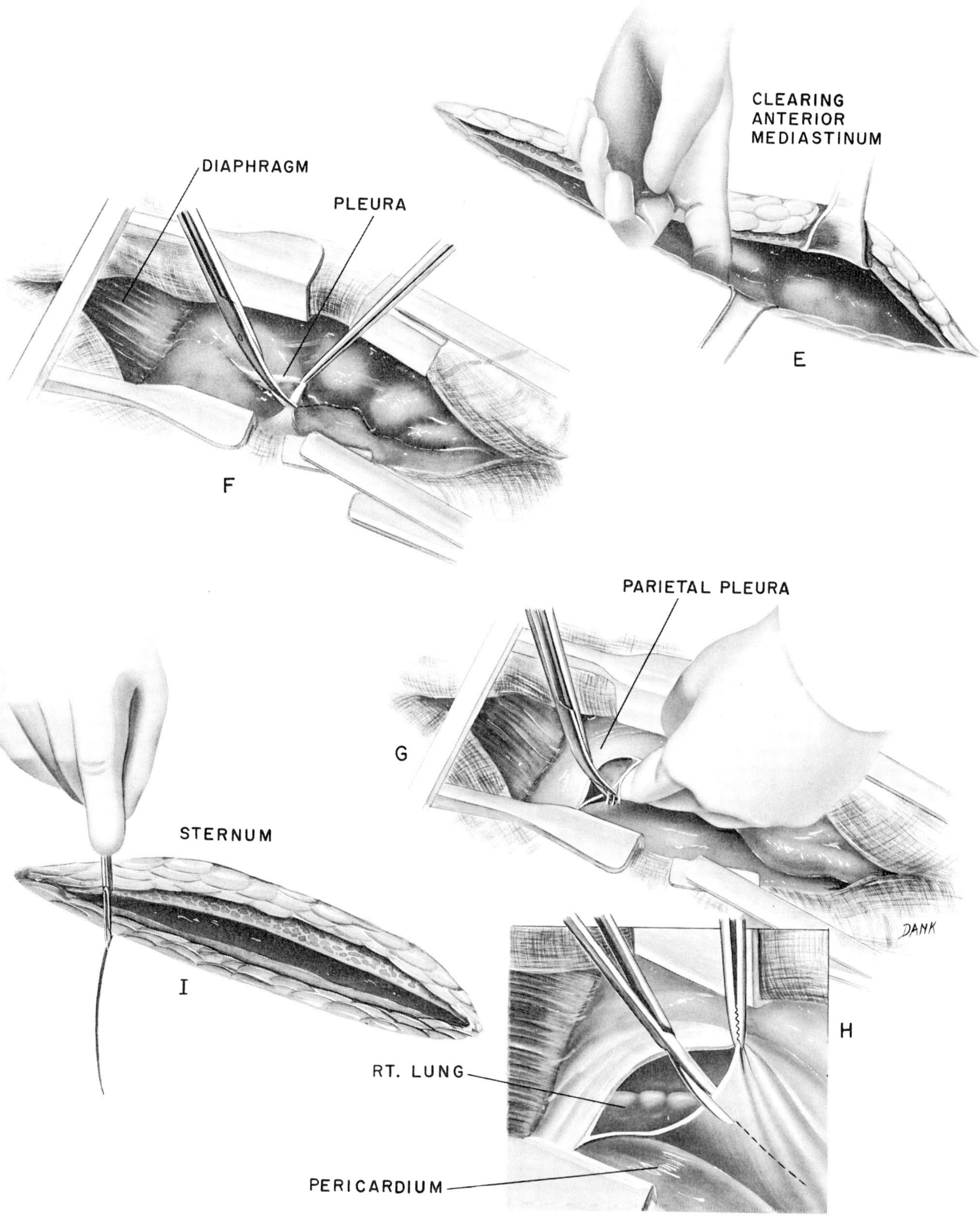
CLEARING
ANTERIOR
MEDIASTINUM
E
DIAPHRAGM
PLEURA
F
PARIETAL PLEURA
G
STERNUM
I
DANK
H
RT. LUNG
PERICARDIUM

J, J_1. Traction sutures of silk (000) are inserted through the thickened pericardium overlying the apical region of the left ventricle (J), and the pericardial scar is incised (J_1) between the sutures. Dissection is first begun over the left ventricle. This is based on the reasoning that the muscle fibers of the encased heart have undergone an atrophy of disuse. Accordingly, if the thinner-walled right ventricle were freed first, acute myocardial rupture might be more apt to occur with sudden distention of the ventricle with blood. Another objection to freeing the right ventricle first would be the potential hazard of producing acute pulmonary hypertension and resulting pulmonary edema. Blood would be permitted to enter the lungs, but its egress would be prevented by the compression scar about the left ventricle.

K, K_1. By blunt digital dissection a cleavage plane is entered beneath the first layer of the thickened pericardium (K), and the opening in this layer is enlarged by scissor dissection (K_1).

L. A second set of guy sutures (000 silk) is inserted in the second layer of the pericardial scar for traction. A portion of an adjacent circumscribed calcific plaque is visible.

Discussion—Drs. William H. Muller, Jr., and Gardner W. Smith. Despite the fact that pericardiectomy for chronic constrictive pericarditis is one of the oldest operations in cardiac surgery, the surgical technics remain controversial and are, to some extent, a matter of the personal judgment of the surgeon.

The case report presented in the text is typical in many respects, and the traumatic basis is certainly not unusual. Although constrictive pericarditis is commonly thought of as a sequel to tuberculous pericarditis, blunt and penetrating traumatic injury is being implicated with increasing frequency. The viral cause of benign pericarditis is still not thoroughly documented and the progression of this disease to the constrictive phase is difficult to prove. Rheumatic carditis seldom produces constrictive pericarditis. A great variety of other etiologic factors have occasionally been demonstrated, but the largest group of cases must still be classified as idiopathic.

A feature which bears emphasis is that these patients do not suffer from true congestive heart failure and digitalis therapy is of no benefit. Indeed, the preoperative use of this drug may be detrimental since it tends to slow the compensatory tachycardia, may decrease the stroke volume of the normal myocardium and often makes arrhythmias during operation more difficult to control. Thus, it is restricted to patients with auricular flutter or fibrillation whose ventricular response must be controlled. In contradistinction to these preoperative considerations, digitalis is essential during the postoperative period since a certain degree of myocardial atrophy is often present resulting in true congestive failure.

The incision represented in "A" is widely accepted. Greater exposure can be obtained if the skin and linea alba are divided inferiorly to a point one third of the way to the umbilicus. The Stryker saw facilitates accurate clean division of the sternum. Bleeding from the sternal periosteum may be diminished by dividing this structure with the cautery, and the problem of hemorrhage from the sternal marrow can be controlled with bone wax.

Many other approaches have been used but the most useful of these are the bilateral anterior thoracotomy and the left anterolateral thoracotomy. The former incision is most successful if made through the fifth intercostal space on the left and the fourth intercostal space on the right with an inverted V-shaped transverse division of the sternum. In recent years, the left anterolateral thoracotomy in the fifth intercostal space has been used frequently in this clinic. Excellent exposure of all but the superior vena cava and right atrium can be obtained and a thorough decortication performed. Most of the right atrium can be decorticated if the heart is slightly displaced. This incision is clearly less extensive and traumatic than either the median sternotomy or the bilateral anterior thoracotomy.

Certain features of the dissection in plate II should be emphasized. It is often impossible to avoid entering both pleural spaces and no effort should be expended to this end. The pleuropericardial separation is performed laterally to expose the phrenic nerve on either side, and on the left this structure should be elevated from the underlying pericardial scar and retracted from the field to avoid injury.

As regards the decortication itself, all layers of thickened pericardium must be removed for a successful operation. This usually includes distinct pericardial and epicardial surfaces which often have a tempting cleavage plane between them.

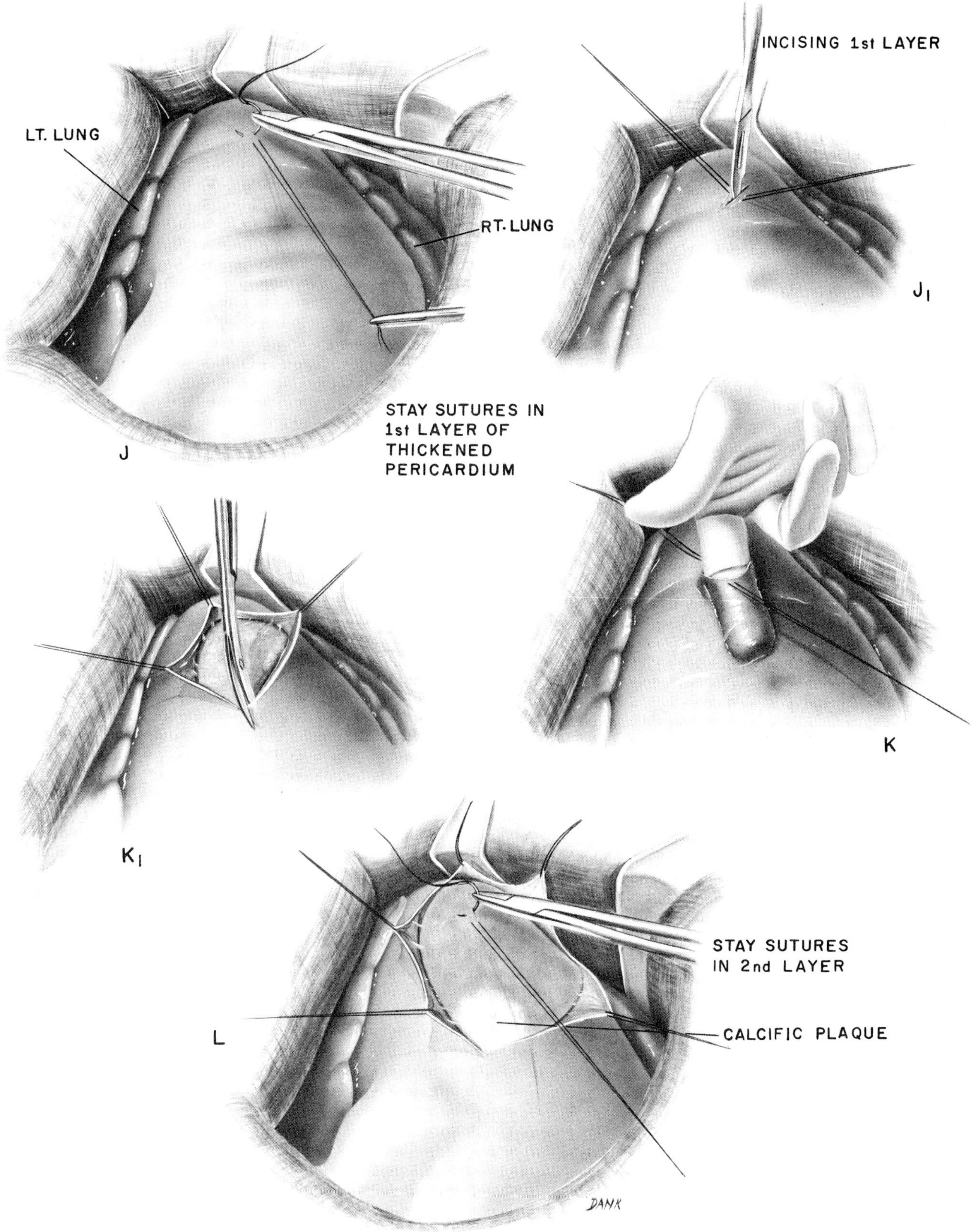
INCISING 1st LAYER
LT. LUNG
RT. LUNG
J
J_1
STAY SUTURES IN
1st LAYER OF
THICKENED
PERICARDIUM
K
K_1
STAY SUTURES
IN 2nd LAYER
L
CALCIFIC PLAQUE
DANK

M, M$_1$. The second layer is incised between the guy sutures (M), and the opening is extended by scissor dissection (broken lines) toward the apex of the heart (M$_1$). The circumscribed calcific plaque cephalad is again visible.

N. Through the opening in the second layer of the scar, the start of the incision (broken line) in the third layer is shown. On an anatomic pathologic basis one would expect to have only two layers within a pericardial scar—viz., visceral and parietal. However, in this patient there were three distinct cleavage planes between the surface of the heart and the overlying scar. It was not until the third layer was incised that a free expansile pulsation of the left ventricle was visible. The importance of removal of the whole thickness of the scar cannot be overly stressed.

O. The inset shows a circumscribed area of the freed apical portion of the left ventricle and the three layers of the pericardial scar.

P. A mobilized portion of the whole thickness of the pericardial scar is elevated on the left index finger and incised.

Q. By blunt digital dissection the whole of this apical region of the heart, including its diaphragmatic and posterior surfaces, is freed from the scar, which is then excised with scissors. The removal of the scar posteriorly is believed important to permit the maximum filling and emptying of the ventricle with each diastole and systole, respectively.

DISCUSSION—DRS. MULLER and SMITH (cont.)

Judgment as to the depth adequate for a complete decortication is determined by observing herniation of the myocardium through the defect created in the encasing scar.

The admonition to begin the dissection over the left ventricle, based largely on theoretical grounds, is commonly accepted and may be valid in some cases. It is prudent, however, to avoid the interventricular groove and its associated anterior descending coronary artery during the early phase of decortication before a well-defined plane is established at the myocardial level. The importance of maintaining all the pericardial flaps until the dissection is complete should be stressed since they are invaluable in repairing myocardial rents and in controlling bleeding.

The question of the extent of decortication is unsettled. Areas of deep myocardial infiltration by calcified plaques should be isolated and remain in place especially in the region of the coronary arteries. There is general agreement that the anterior surfaces of both ventricles should be decorticated completely, and as far laterally as the left phrenic nerve. The peel should be removed from the entire apex and from the diaphragmatic surface, even though proof is lacking that scarring in this area interferes mechanically with ventricular systole. The importance of caval and right atrial obstruction was overemphasized during the early history of pericardiectomy in this country. Significant caval obstruction has not been demonstrated by cardiac catheterization or by angiocardiography, nor has this phenomenon been found to occur experimentally. Isolated instances at operation have been described in which significant narrowing of the cavae was believed to be present. Furthermore, cases of impairment of function of the left atrium, the pulmonary veins, the great vessels at the base of the heart and the left atrioventricular groove have been recorded. The latter is further documented by catheterization evidence of functional mitral stenosis in some cases. Therefore, the question of decortication of the atria, the cavae, the great vessels and the pulmonary veins is still conjectural. There is little doubt that such an extensive pericardiectomy increases the operative risk, and the decision as to decortication in these areas must remain the judgment of the surgeon.

The control of arrhythmias during pericardiectomy, should be mentioned. As previously suggested, the avoidance of preoperative digitalis will reduce the risk of intractable arrhythmia. The pre-

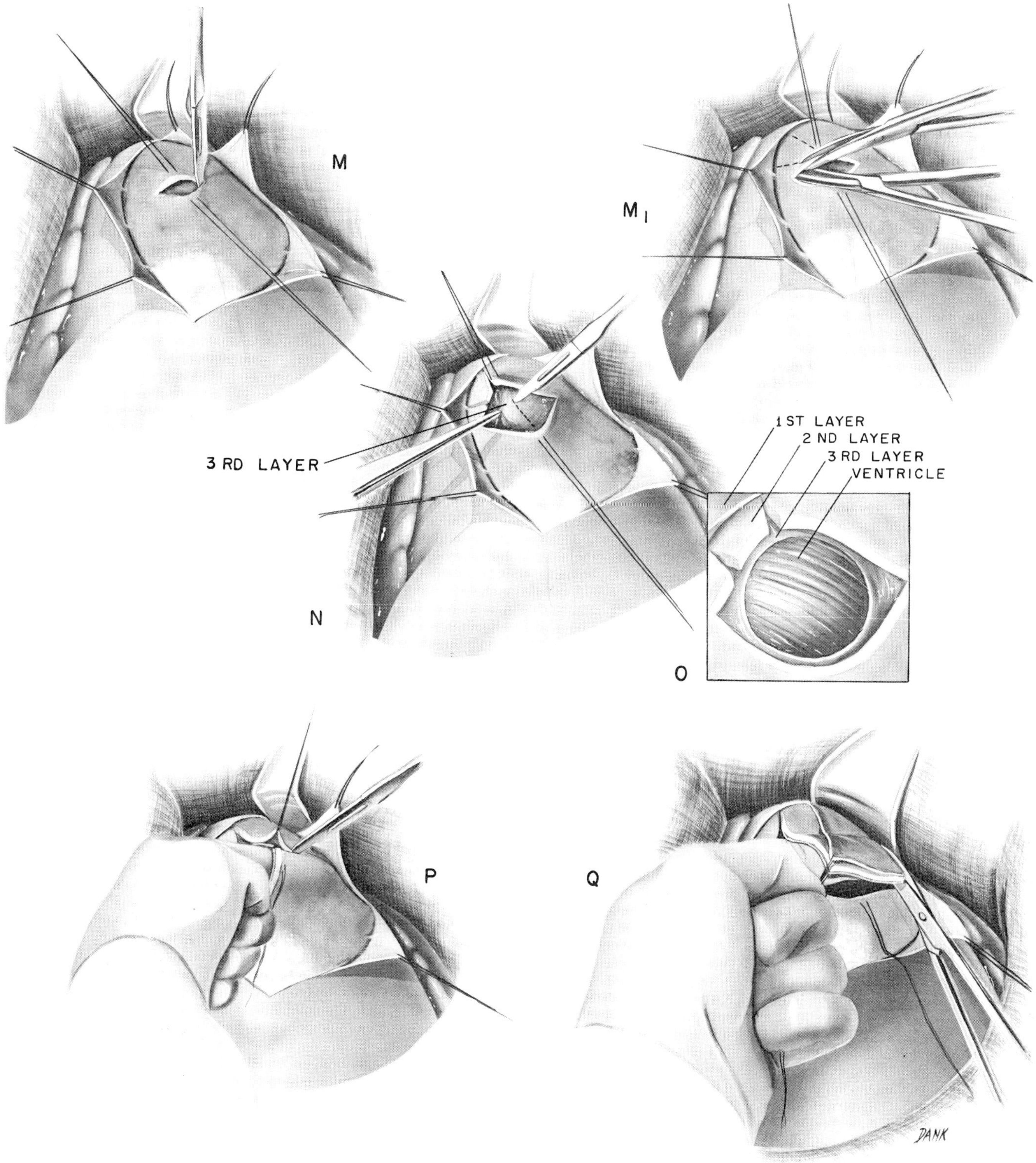
M
M_1
3 RD LAYER
1 ST LAYER
2 ND LAYER
3 RD LAYER
VENTRICLE
N
O
P
Q
DANK

R. The surgeon is now on the left side of the operation table. In this position the pericardial dissection cephalad is facilitated. A mobilized segment of the thickened pericardium, well beyond the area of the calcific plaque, is elevated on the index finger and severed with scissors in the direction indicated (broken line). When a calcific plaque is present, one should consider always the possibility that it has infiltrated the wall of the underlying myocardium. If this is proved, the surrounding pericardial scar should be tailored about the plaque, leaving it as a calcific island on the surface of the heart. An attempt to excise the plaque would risk the danger of severe or even fatal hemorrhage.

S. The cut margin of the mobilized portion of the pericardial scar is clamped and retracted upward to show the dissection beneath the plaque that did not infiltrate the myocardium. Dissection of the scar is aided by counterpressure on the surface with the use of moist cotton "paddies." The maintenance of a free flap of pericardium during the dissection is helpful for hemostasis in the event of accidental bleeding. Should it occur, the mobilized pericardium may be replaced immediately over the bleeding site and sutured in place.

T, T_1. By wide digital dissection beneath the scar the right border of the heart, including the area about the inferior vena cava, is freed (T), and the excision of the scar is continued toward the encased right auricular appendix (T_1).

U. A flap of thickened pericardium is maintained while the right auricular appendix, depressed by counterpressure over a moist cotton "paddie," is being freed by scissor dissection.

V. By combined blunt digital and scissor dissection the remaining attachments of the scar to the auricular appendix are severed to complete the decortication of the heart. It is frequently argued that the thin-walled auricular appendix should not be freed because of the danger of hemorrhage. In this patient the plane of cleavage was easily entered and the scar readily removed.

W. The operative field upon completion of the pericardiectomy is shown. The degree of clinical improvement postoperatively is believed directly proportional to the completeness of the operation. The decortication should include the anterior surfaces of both ventricles, the diaphragmatic and posterior aspects of the apex, the atria, the pulmonary hilar regions, the base of the pulmonary artery, and the areas about the entrance of the superior and inferior vena cava. The wound is closed and the pleural cavities drained as depicted in the illustrated technic for thymectomy.

DISCUSSION—DRS. MULLER and SMITH (cont.)

operative use of quinidine and the topical use of procaine or lidocaine have been widely tested and are found to be ineffective. The intravenous use of atropine sulfate will often control sinus bradycardia, and intravenous lidocaine helps to reduce mycocardial irritability manifested as ventricular ectopic beats or as ventricular tachycardia. However, the control of arrhythmias is best accomplished by rest periods during the dissection, allowing the irritability to subside.

As regards the results which can be expected from pericardiectomy for constrictive pericarditis there have been no recorded instances of recurrence of pericardial scarring. Thus, if re-exploration is required because of an unsatisfactory result, any residual scar tissue is evidence of a previously incomplete decortication. The over-all operative mortality is 12 to 15 per cent, but this increases to the vicinity of 30 per cent if a second procedure is required. Good results can be anticipated in 75 per cent of the patients, with 57 per cent cured and an additional 18 per cent improved. Late deaths account for 7 per cent of the remaining cases and 5 per cent of the cases will receive no benefit from surgery. Appropriate antibiotic preparation and early operation obviates myocardial atrophy and yields better results. It is apparent that a properly performed pericardiectomy can offer eminently satisfactory results.

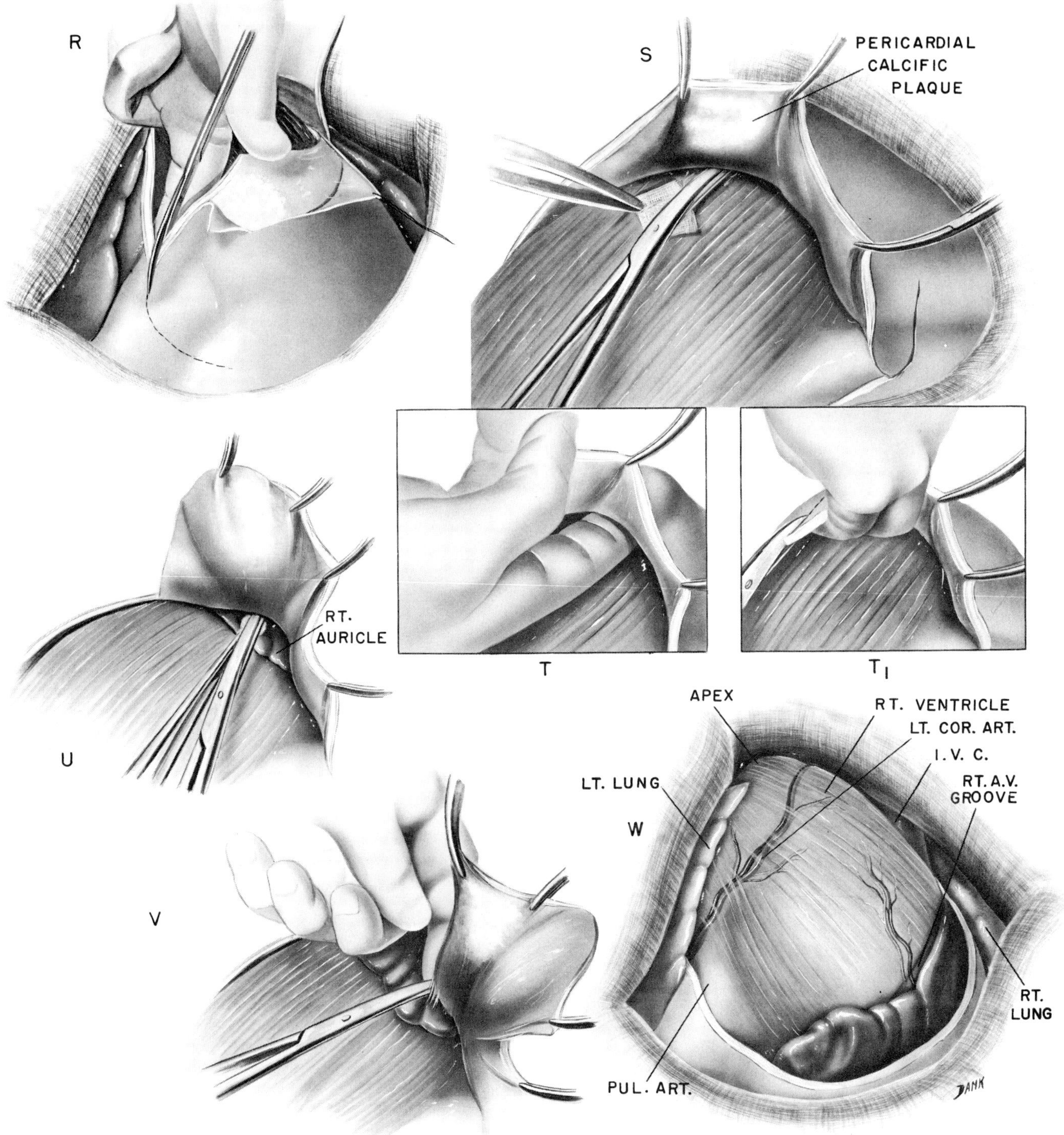
R
S
PERICARDIAL CALCIFIC PLAQUE
RT. AURICLE
T
T1
U
APEX
RT. VENTRICLE
LT. COR. ART.
I.V.C.
LT. LUNG
RT. A.V. GROOVE
W
V
RT. LUNG
PUL. ART.

AORTIC EMBOLECTOMY

A. A left paramedian incision as depicted is preferred. The incision extends approximately one third above and two thirds below the level of the umbilicus.

B. The peritoneal cavity is entered, the intestines are displaced upward, and the posterior parietal peritoneum is incised to expose the lower portion of the abdominal aorta and its bifurcation. The lumen of the aorta is occluded by digital compression,* and the anterior wall of the aorta overlying the contained thrombus is incised. The thrombus which extends distally into both common iliac arteries is herniated partially through the incision. This herniation of the thrombus causes an eversion of the incised margins of the intima and facilitates the subsequent insertion of the everting mattress sutures of fine (00000) silk. The spasm of the left iliac artery distal to the thrombus is visible.

* If for technical reasons the use of the index finger proves unsatisfactory, a 10-inch length anatomic tissue forceps may be conveniently substituted.

The surgical approach to the lower portion of the aorta and its bifurcation may be extraperitoneal, transperitoneal, or retrograde. The transperitoneal approach, spinal anesthesia being used, is preferred. Although objected to by many, the advantages are believed to exceed the proclaimed disadvantages.

The basic principles that are believed to underlie the successful surgical removal of an arterial embolus are: (1) an early operation, preferably within the first eight hours; (2) an adequate surgical exposure; (3) the production of a minimum of trauma, particularly in the intima; (4) the interruption of the circulation for a minimum period after the thrombus is removed.

In most of the surgical technics commonly employed for aortic embolectomy, mechanical devices or tape ligatures are used to occlude the aorta proximal to the blockage and the common iliac arteries distally. In the majority of patients with a saddle occlusion of the abdominal aorta, varying degrees of atherosclerosis are present. This is the reason why it is believed that most of the so-called saddle emboli in patients in the arteriosclerotic age group are in reality autocnthonous* thrombi. The degenerative changes occur predominantly in the posterior and lateral walls of the aorta. The occlusion of the lumen of the aorta by a mechanical device, a traction tape ligature, or an occluding tape ligature may produce a fracture of an atherosclerotic plaque with resultant injury to the intima. This predisposes to the formation of a local thrombus. In general, the use of such methods for hemostasis requires the complete mobilization of the distal portion of the abdominal aorta and its bifurcation. A notable exception is the technic described by Linton. This mobilization of the aorta prolongs the operation, risks the danger of dislodging a portion of the thrombus to form an embolus, and increases the likelihood of troublesome hemorrhage.

In the technic illustrated, mechanical devices or tape ligatures for hemostasis are not used. Instead, for this purpose, the left index finger of the assistant or an anatomic tissue forceps 10 inches in length is employed. Protective rubber shods predispose to slipping of the forceps off the walls of the aorta and are not used. The use of the index finger or tissue forceps produces a minimum of tissue trauma, does not require the mobilization of the aorta, and permits the immediate release or application of a compression force to the aorta, a desired technical aid. Furthermore, a delicate adjustment of the compression force applied may be obtained. The same principles of technic illustrated are employed for the removal of the more peripherally located arterial emboli.

* Thrombi which are formed where found.

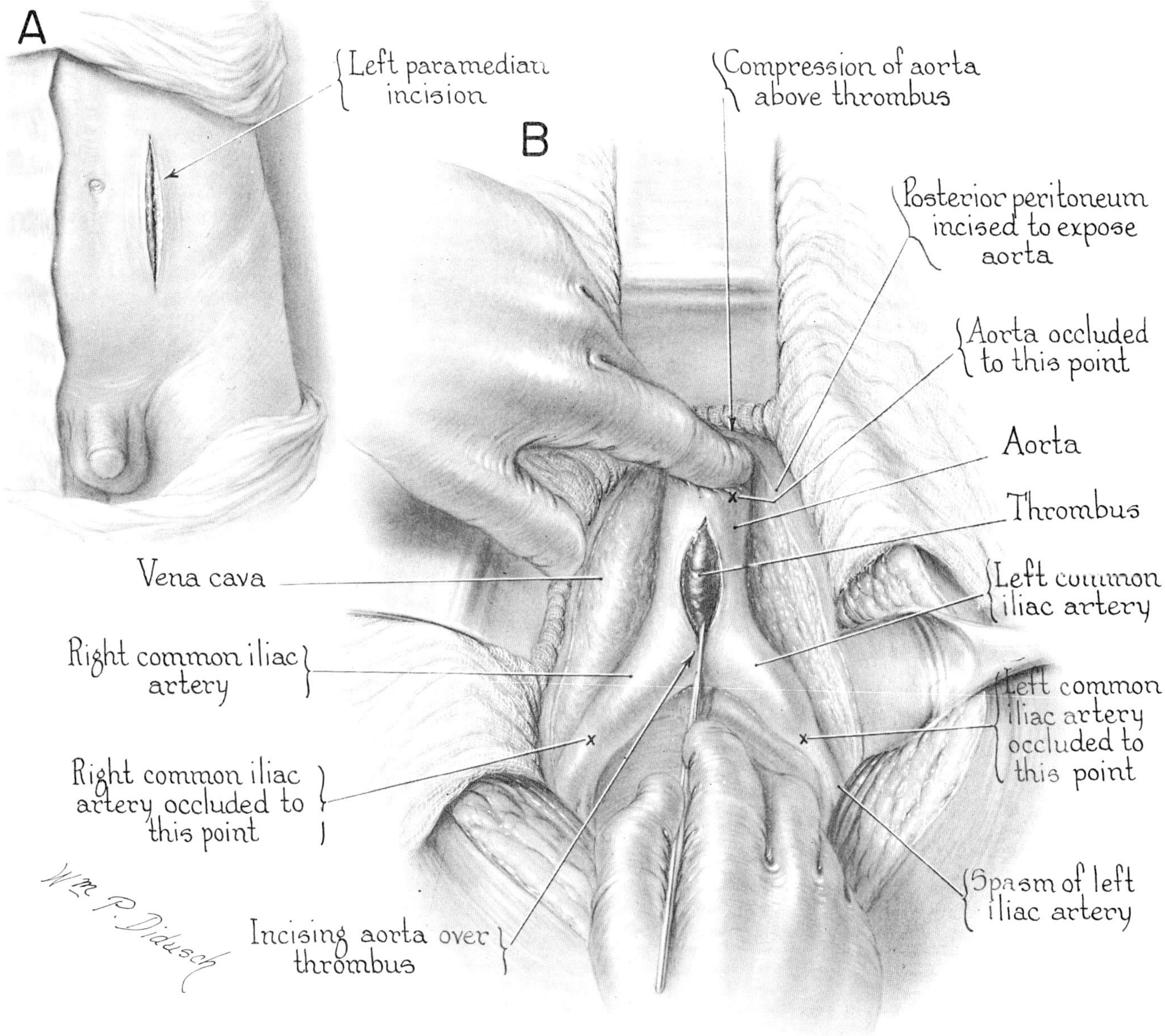
A
Left paramedian incision
B
Compression of aorta above thrombus
Posterior peritoneum incised to expose aorta
Aorta occluded to this point
Aorta
Thrombus
Vena cava
Left common iliac artery
Right common iliac artery
Left common iliac artery occluded to this point
Right common iliac artery occluded to this point
Spasm of left iliac artery
Incising aorta over thrombus
Wm. P. Didusch

C. Digital compression of the aorta is maintained proximal to the thrombus, and the untied strands of silk sutures are retracted on a nerve hook to allow the free escape of the blood clots. The thrombus, first in one then in the other common iliac artery, is "milked" upward and extruded through the opening in the aorta. The demonstration of free retrograde bleeding following this maneuver indicates the patency of the collateral vascular channels below the site of the aortic occlusion, which is a favorable prognostic sign.

D. The common iliac arteries are occluded by digital compression immediately distal to the bifurcation of the aorta, either by the right hand of the first assistant or the left hand of the surgeon, as the digital compression of the lumen of the aorta proximal to the thrombus is slowly released. Generally the pressure in the aorta is sufficient to expel forcibly through the aortic incision the remaining portion of the thrombus. If not, the thrombus may be evacuated by "milking" it downward from above by gentle digital compression. The discharge of the thrombus is followed by a forceful pulsatile flow of blood, the control of which is being initiated by traction on the untied strands of the silk mattress sutures. The digital occlusion of the common iliac arteries is done to prevent the dissemination of thromboemboli into the peripheral arterial bed.

Discussion—Dr. Ferdinand F. McAllister. I am in general accord with the principles outlined in this section, but have employed minor variations in technic. Lower abdominal midline incisions have been found very helpful in exposure of the aorta and both iliacs. The midline position allows equally good exposure for either iliac, can be rapidly extended upward if need be, and is more quickly closed. I have not observed any greater tendency to postoperative hernia through this incision than through a paramedian muscle-retracting incision.

I have felt that it is important to carefully encircle the iliac vessels with doubly looped umbilical tapes, distal to the area of obvious involvement with embolus before any manipulation of the involved area is attempted. With the use of these tapes it may be possible to prevent any fragmentation and passage of clot more distally. Whenever such occlusion is performed with the tapes, 2 to 3 ml. of heparin solution should be injected into the vessels distal to the area of occlusion. As far as proximal occlusion of the aorta goes, above the level of the embolus I have felt more secure with complete encirclement of the aorta with a tape and the employment of a Rumel type tourniquet. In some emboli which have been tackled after two to three days the clot is rather adherent and a good deal of manipulation may be required to loosen it. I have not felt that finger control is adequate for this, and I do not believe that the careful use of thick cotton tapes fragments the intima excessively. Again, whenever the aorta has been occluded proximally, 2 to 3 ml. of heparin solution should be injected proximal to the area of occlusion.

I have always felt that the best vascular closure was a simple over and over stitch of accurately placed 00000 arterial silk. I do not believe that the time factor here is as important as stressed by the author since the aorta has been occluded for some time anyway by the embolus. The entire lumen previously occupied by the embolus should be carefully and frequently and thoroughly flushed with heparin solution until the closure is complete. Once the closure is complete, the hemostatic tapes should be immediately released, and, unless drastic hemorrhage ensues through the wound, the vessel should never again be completely occluded, for this is sure to lead to clot formation. Care should be taken to control the proximal aorta digitally as the proximal tape is released in order to precipitate neither shock nor the reflexes which have been shown to lead ultimately to lower nephron nephrosis with renal shutdown.

Since additional distal emboli due to fragmentation of clot are not uncommon in such patients, two precautions should be taken before embarking on the performance of saddle embolectomies. First, the groins and thighs should be included in the prep and drape, so that if necessary the femoral arteries can be quickly exposed for the extraction of additional clots. Second, a selection of plastic and firmly polished catheters should be available to insert into the distal iliac vessels if back bleeding is poor following removal of the main thrombus. Frequently, a long complete slender thrombus can be extracted by the judicious use of such catheters and obviates the need for additional embolectomies at lower levels.

C

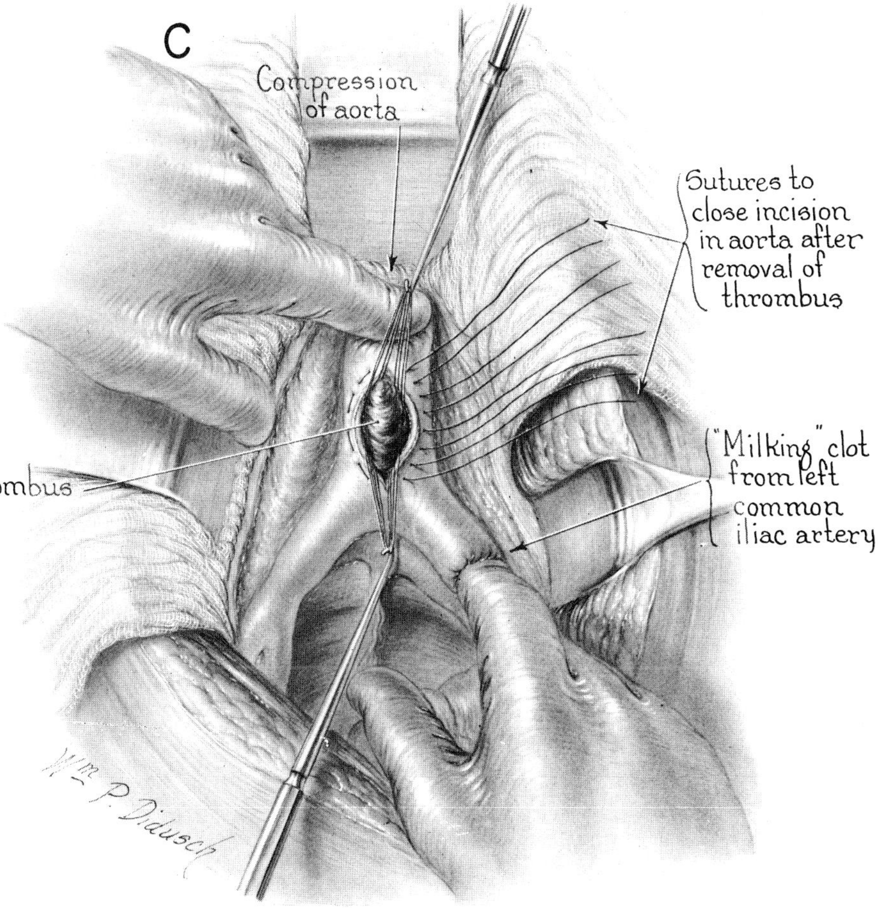
Compression
of aorta
Sutures to
close incision
in aorta after
removal of
thrombus
Thrombus
"Milking" clot
from left
common
iliac artery
Wm P. Didusch

D

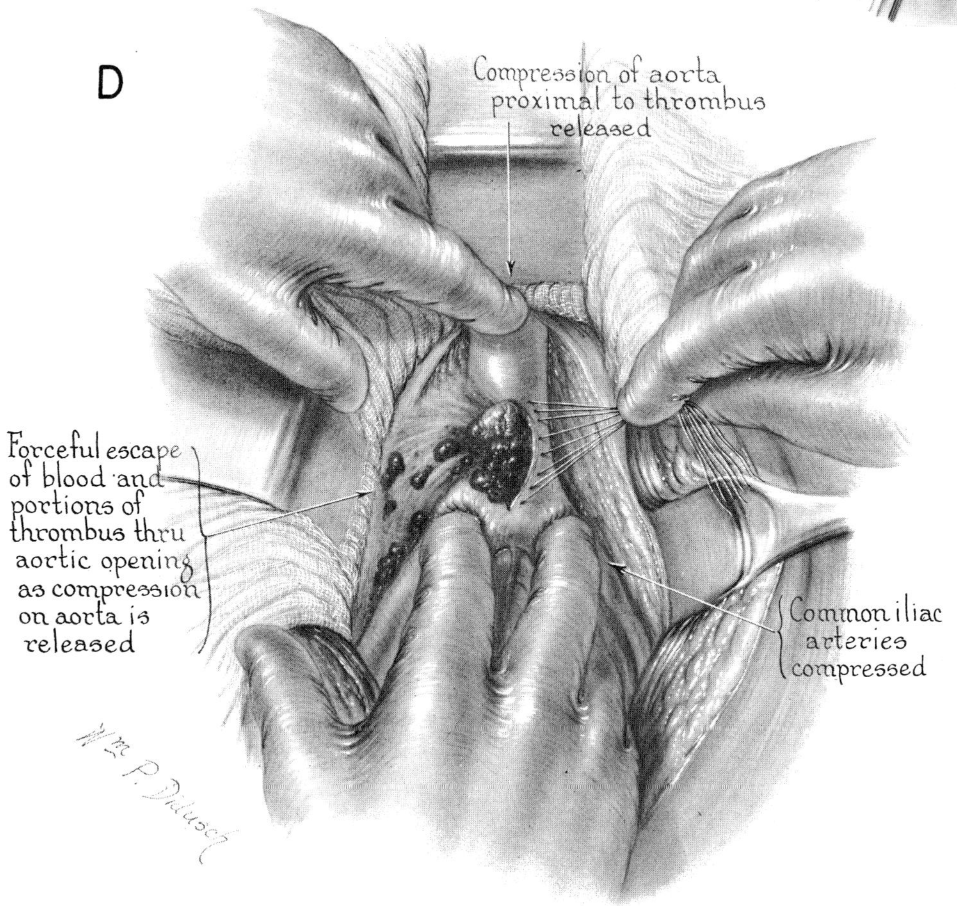
Compression of aorta
proximal to thrombus
released
Forceful escape
of blood and
portions of
thrombus thru
aortic opening
as compression
on aorta is
released
Common iliac
arteries
compressed
Wm P. Didusch

E. The thrombus is completely evacuated, and the lumen of the aorta is momentarily occluded proximal to the incision either by the index finger (first assistant), as depicted, or by an anatomic tissue forceps (10 inches) as the strands of silk mattress sutures are drawn taut to close the opening in the aorta. The operative field is toileted by irrigation with warm sterile normal saline solution which is removed by suction siphonage.

F. The compression of the aorta and the common iliac arteries is released, and the last of the everting mattress sutures of silk (00000) closing the aortic incision is being tied. If sites of bleeding in the incised aorta should persist, hemostasis is obtained either by gentle compression on the suture line for several minutes using a sterile dry gauze sponge or by the insertion of additional simple interrupted silk (00000) sutures, dependent upon the severity of the bleeding. The incised portion of the posterior parietal peritoneum is not sutured. A layer closure of the abdominal incision is performed using interrupted sutures of 00 silk for the peritoneum and fascia and 000 silk for the skin. Drainage of the wound is not employed. Because of the high incidence of complications due to hemorrhage, anticoagulant therapy postoperatively has been discontinued.

E

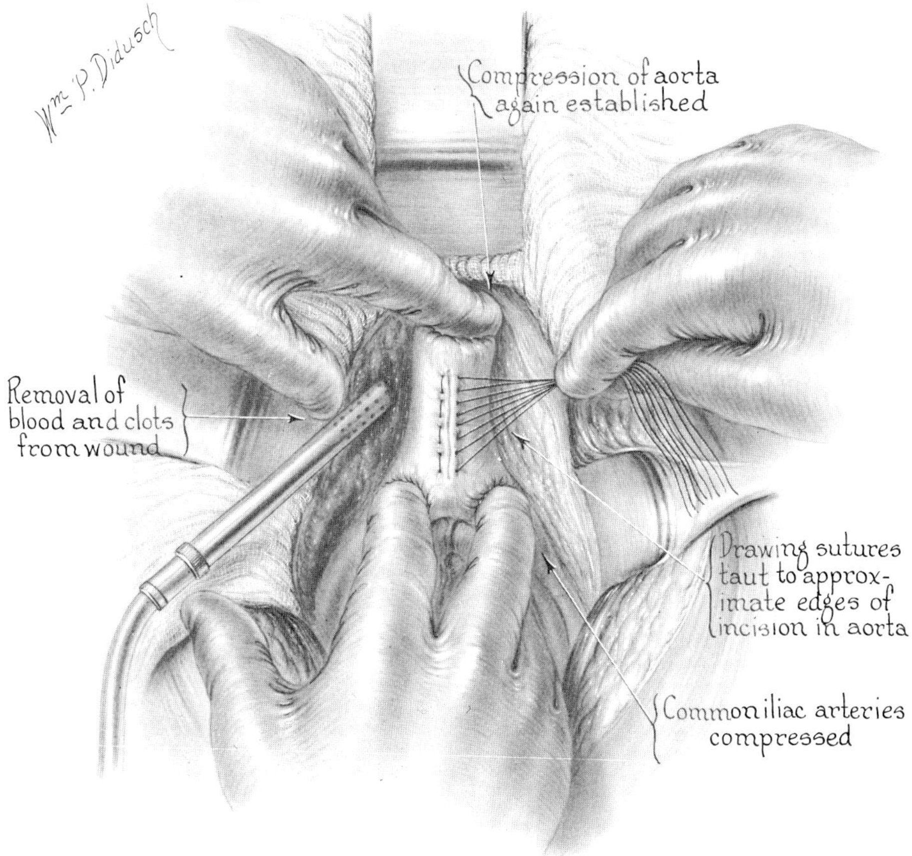
Wm P. Didusch
Compression of aorta again established
Removal of blood and clots from wound
Drawing sutures taut to approximate edges of incision in aorta
Common iliac arteries compressed

F

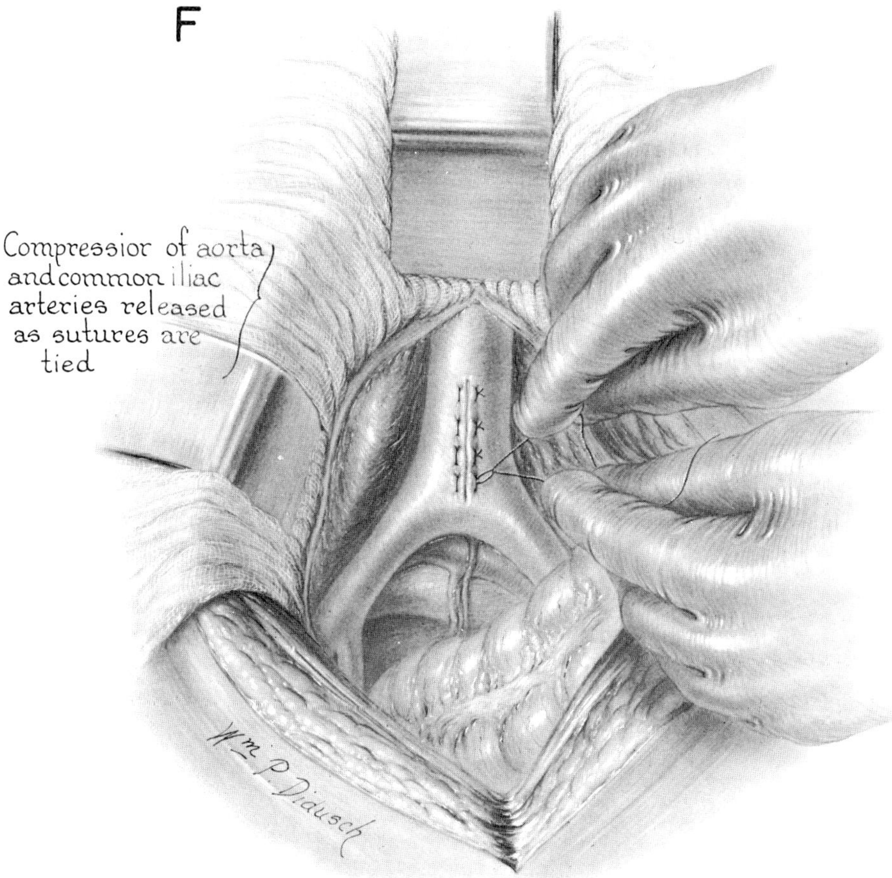
Compressior of aorta and common iliac arteries released as sutures are tied
Wm P. Didusch

EXCISION OF AN ANEURYSM OF THE THORACIC AORTA AND THE INSERTION OF A PRESERVED HOMOLOGOUS AORTIC GRAFT

A. The patient is placed in the direct right lateral prone position. The site of the left thoracotomy incision is depicted by the dotted line.

B, C. The skin incision is deepened through the underlying musculature of the lateral thoracic wall (B, C). The H-shaped incision to be made in the periosteum of the sixth rib (C) is shown in dotted outline.

D. A long segment of the sixth rib and a small segment of the posterior portion of the fifth rib arc resected subperiosteally. The severance of the intervening intercostal muscle layers and their neurovascular bundle is indicated by the dotted line.

E. The intercostal muscle layers and the related neurovascular bundle are severed and ligated with suture ligatures of silk (00). The wound margins are retracted, and a portion of the aneurysm which is partly covered by the overlying and adherent left lung is visible within the pleural cavity.

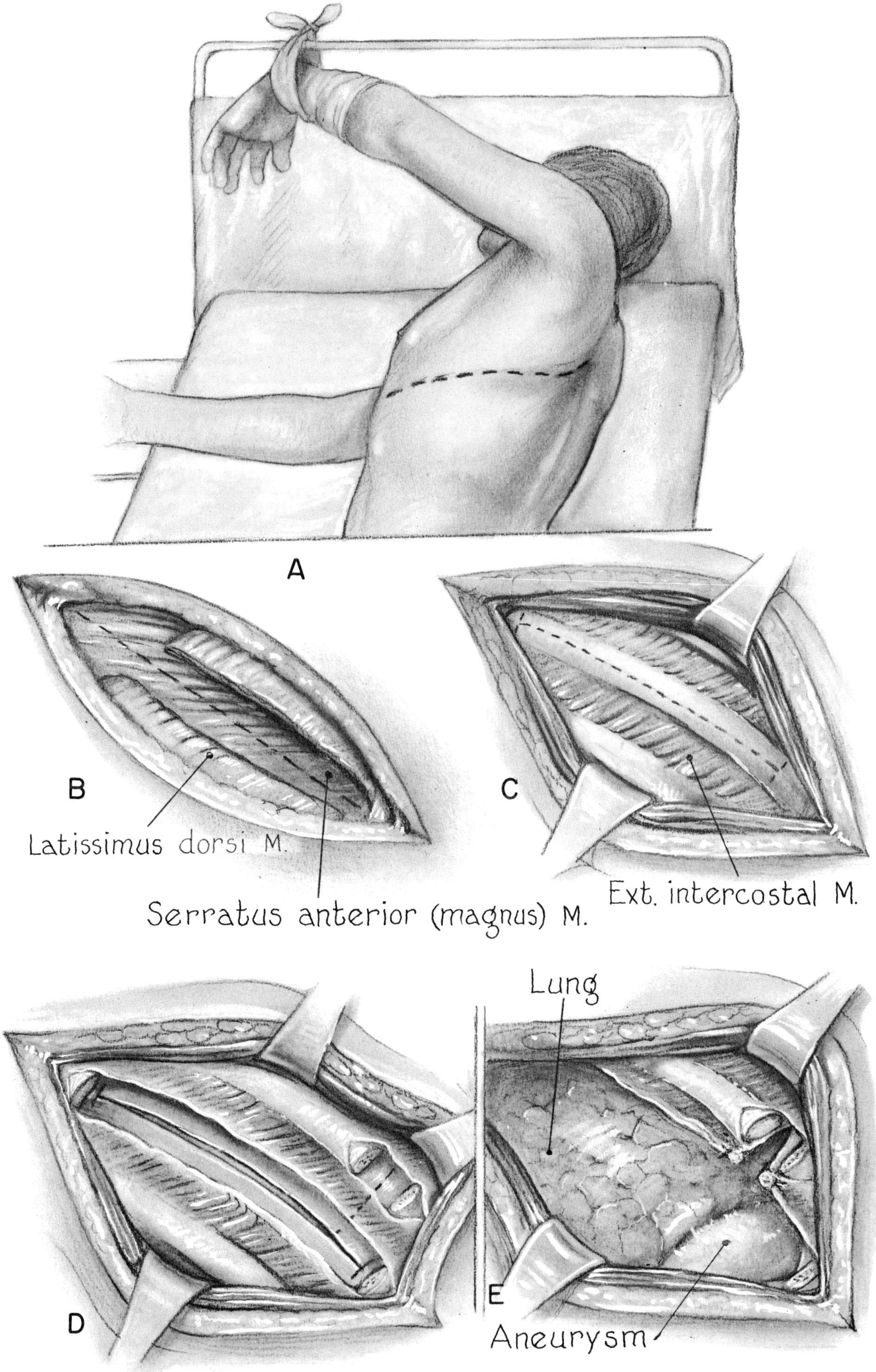
A
B
C
Latissimus dorsi M.
Serratus anterior (magnus) M.
Ext. intercostal M.
Lung
D
E
Aneurysm

F. The rib cage is widely separated with a self-retaining rib retractor (Finochietto) to expose more completely the underlying intrapleural structures. The adherence of the atelectatic lower lobe of the left lung to the wall of the aneurysm is visible. In this particular illustration, the cephalad extent of the aneurysm located in the middle segment of the descending aorta is somewhat higher than the actual level observed at the time of operation. This level is accurately shown in the subsequent illustrations.

G. The superior segment of the left lower lobe, partially dissected from the wall of the aneurysm, is clamped (Babcock) and retracted. The posterior parietal pleura, overlying the proximal portion of the descending aorta and the distal segment of the arch, is incised. The cut margins of the parietal pleura are retracted with guy sutures of silk (000), and the uppermost of the paired intercostal arteries are shown mobilized on a clamp and ligature carrier respectively.

H, I. Following the ligation and severance of the two intercostal vessels, a special ligature carrier* with a ball-point protected tip (H) is used to encircle the mobilized segment of the thoracic aorta proximally with a cotton tape (I).

* Manufactured by Edward Weck & Co., Brooklyn, N. Y.

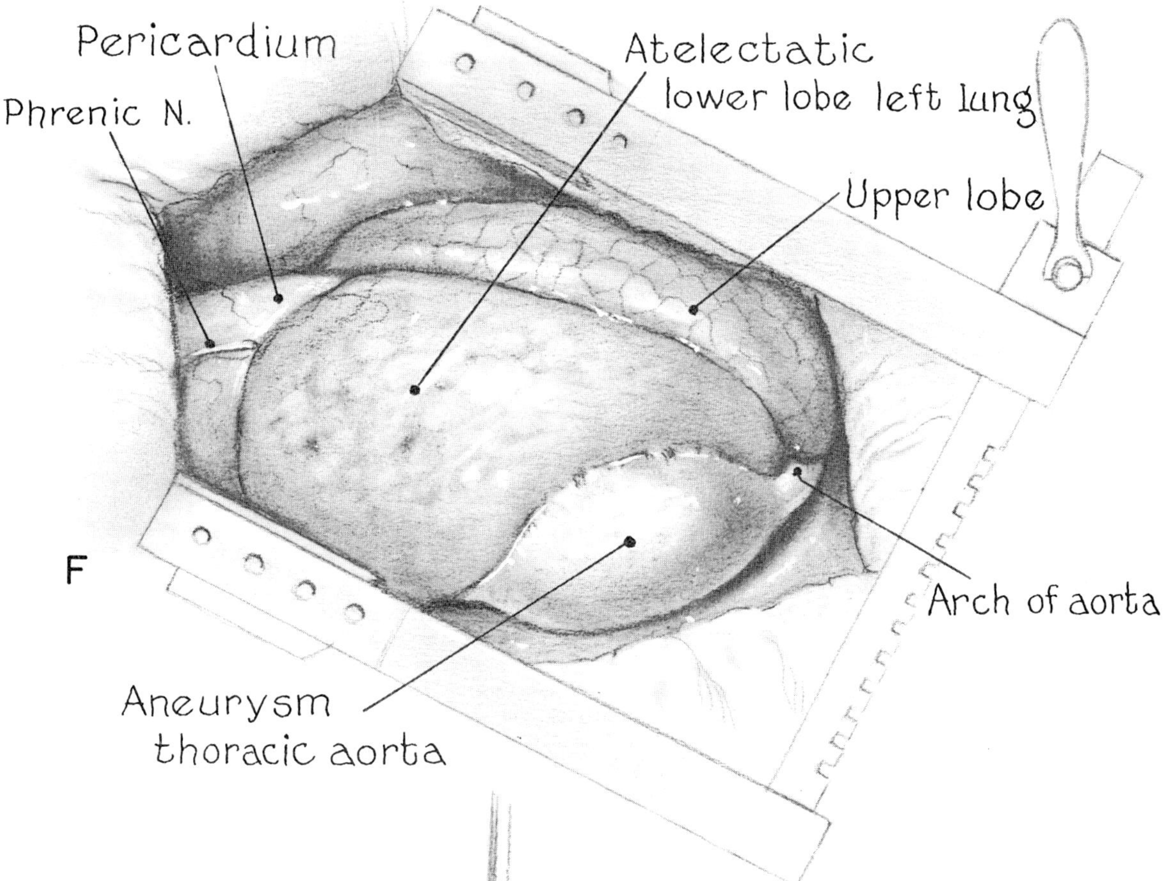
Pericardium
Phrenic N.
Atelectatic
lower lobe left lung
Upper lobe
Arch of aorta
Aneurysm
thoracic aorta

F

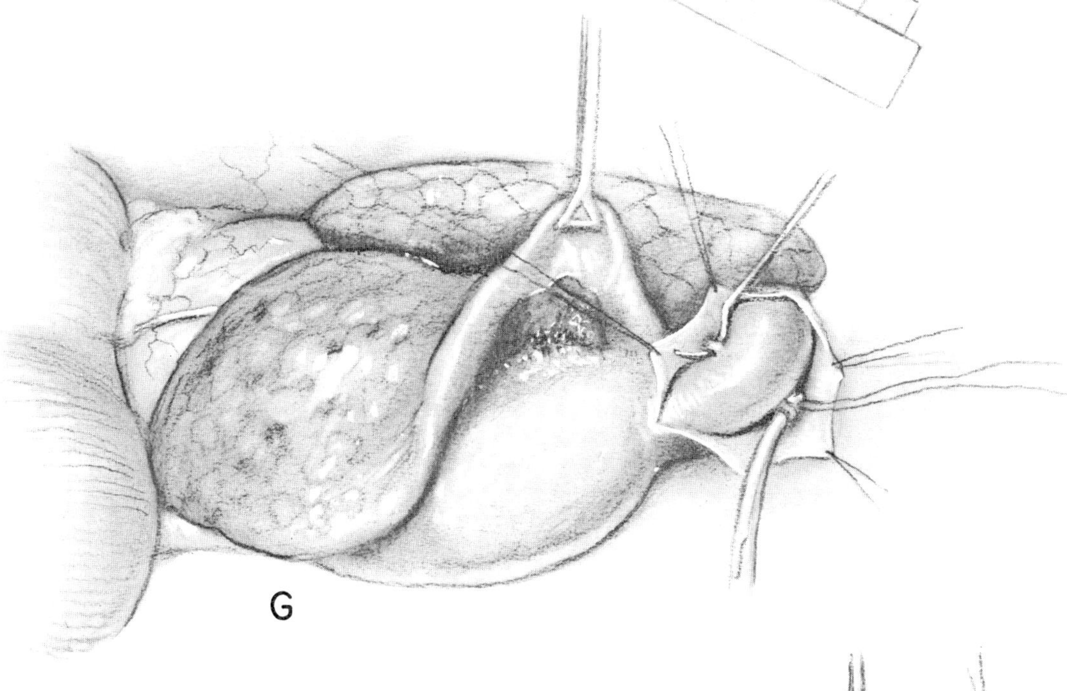

G

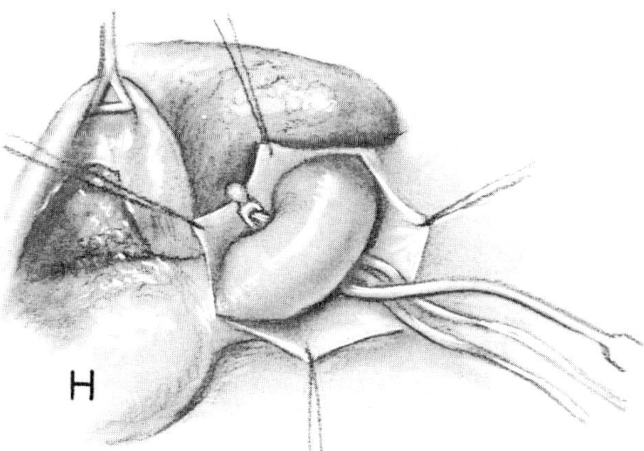

H

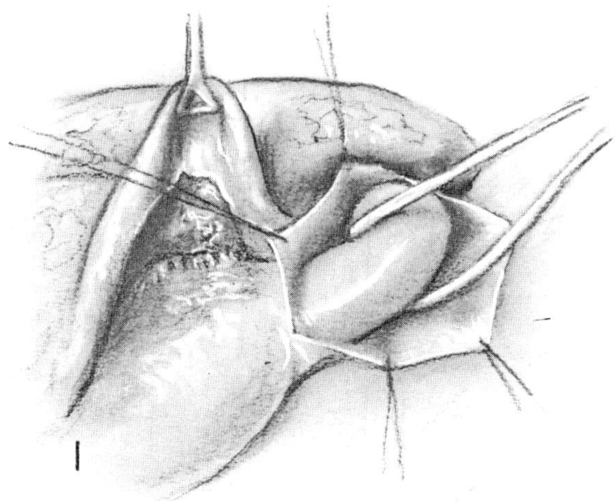

I

J. An incision is made in the posterior mediastinal and parietal pleura distal to the aneurysm, and the lower end of the esophagus is shown encircled by a cotton tape. A segment of the distal portion of the thoracic aorta is also visible.

K. The distal segment of the thoracic aorta is similarly encircled by a cotton tape, and the adherent lobe of the left lung is dissected completely from the surface of the aneurysm. The lines of closure of the openings in the small stem bronchi, made during the dissection, are visible. In retrospect, this was a technical error which could have been easily avoided by not performing the dissection as illustrated. Instead, at the time of the resection of the aneurysm, a portion of its wall that was intimately adherent to the lung could have been tailored to form a "patch" graft and the occurrence of bronchial air leaks obviated. The same reasoning applies to the separation of the wall of the aneurysm from the segment of the esophagus to which it was adherent. The use of a "patch" graft is ideally suited as a prophylaxis to injury of the esophagus.

L. Preparatory to mobilizing the aneurysm, the incision in the posterior parietal pleura is extended along the whole length of the posterior border of the aneurysm. By gentle manual manipulation the aneurysm is displaced anteriorly to show its mobilization by serially clamping, severing, and ligating the related intercostal arteries.

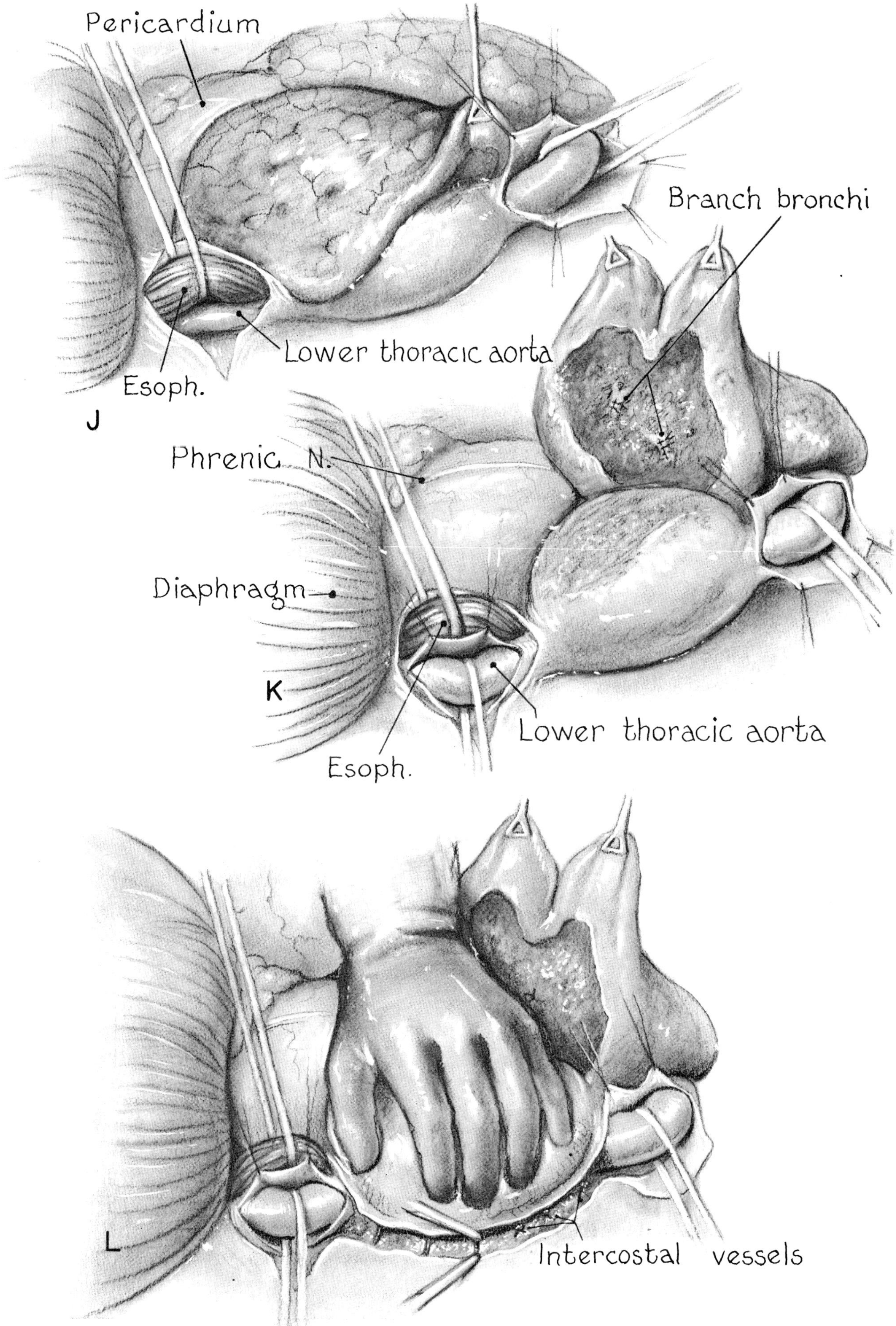
Pericardium
Branch bronchi
Lower thoracic aorta
Esoph.
J
Phrenic N.
Diaphragm
K
Lower thoracic aorta
Esoph.
L
Intercostal vessels

M. The thoracic aorta cephalad to the aneurysm is doubly clamped (Potts coarctation clamps), and the site for its transection is indicated by the dotted line.

N, N¹. The cephalad transection of the aorta is completed (N), and the site for its caudad transection between the occluding clamps is shown (dotted line). The denudation of the musculature of the segment of the proximal portion of the esophagus that was adherent to the wall of the aneurysm is visible. As previously stated, this could have been avoided by use of a "patch" graft of the wall of the aneurysm. The sites of the occlusion of the thoracic aorta are bypassed by the use of two large bore (12 gauge) needles which are connected through a Y-glass tube. The rubber tubing on the vertical stem of the Y-glass tube is used both as an air vent and for the instillation of heparin–saline solution (100 mg. of heparin in 250 ml. of saline solution) to prevent clotting within the tubing. These illustrations were made during the course of an operation performed early in 1952, and this particular bypass technic is no longer used. Although hypothermia may be employed successfully in resections of aneurysm of the thoracic aorta, the use of a temporary bypass shunt graft is preferred (N¹). In this regard preserved homologous and heterologous grafts or cloth prostheses may be employed.

O. The resection of the aneurysm is completed, and the insertion of a preserved homologous aortic graft is begun.

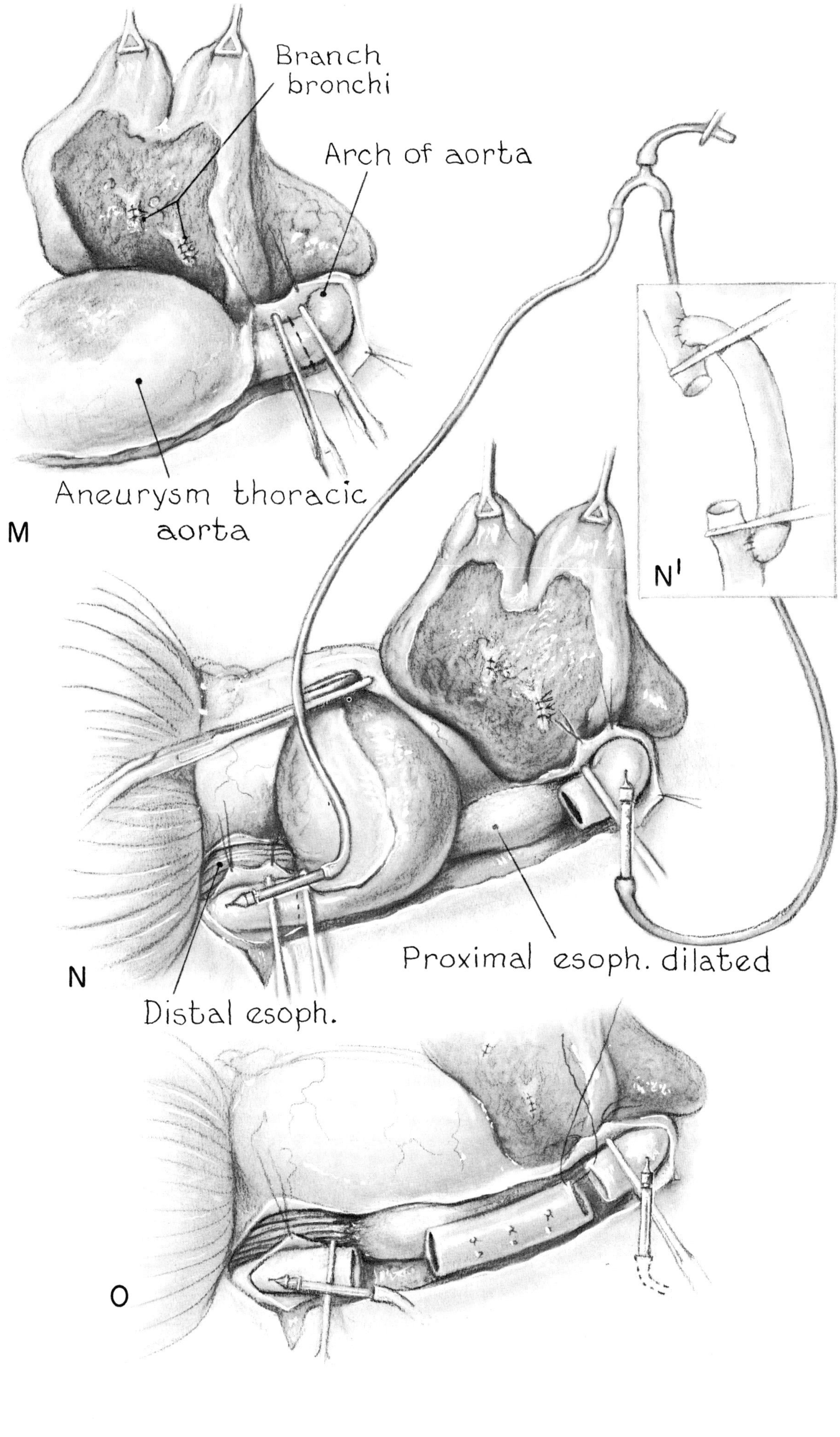
Branch bronchi
Arch of aorta
Aneurysm thoracic aorta
M
N'
N
Proximal esoph. dilated
Distal esoph.
O

O¹. Three cardinal guy sutures of 00000 arterial silk are inserted proximally, and the medial suture is tied.

O². The cardinal guy sutures are tied, and several of the intervening interrupted everting mattress sutures are inserted but not tied.

O³, O⁴. The everting mattress sutures are tied, and traction on the long strands of the medial and lateral cardinal guy sutures is used (O³) to facilitate the rotation of the aortic and graft segments for the insertion of the interrupted everting mattress and simple interrupted sutures posteriorly (O⁴).

P, P¹. In the event of a disparity in the size of the lumen of the segments to be anastomosed, a preliminary incision may be made in the anterior wall of the smaller vessel (P) to compensate for the discrepancy. When the anastomosis is completed and the sutures are tied, the flangelike effect on the end of the smaller vessel is evident (P¹).

Q. In this patient the original length of preserved homologous graft was too short. Accordingly, a second and smaller graft segment was required to restore continuity of the thoracic aorta. The needle openings in the cephalad and caudad portions of the host aorta are occluded with interrupted sutures of silk (00000).

R, S, T, U. A Foley retention (5 ml.) catheter is used for water-seal drainage of the pleural cavity (R), and a layer closure of the thoracic incision is performed using interrupted pericostal sutures of No. 2 silk (R, S) for the rib approximation and interrupted sutures of silk (00 and 000) for closure of the muscles and skin (T, U).

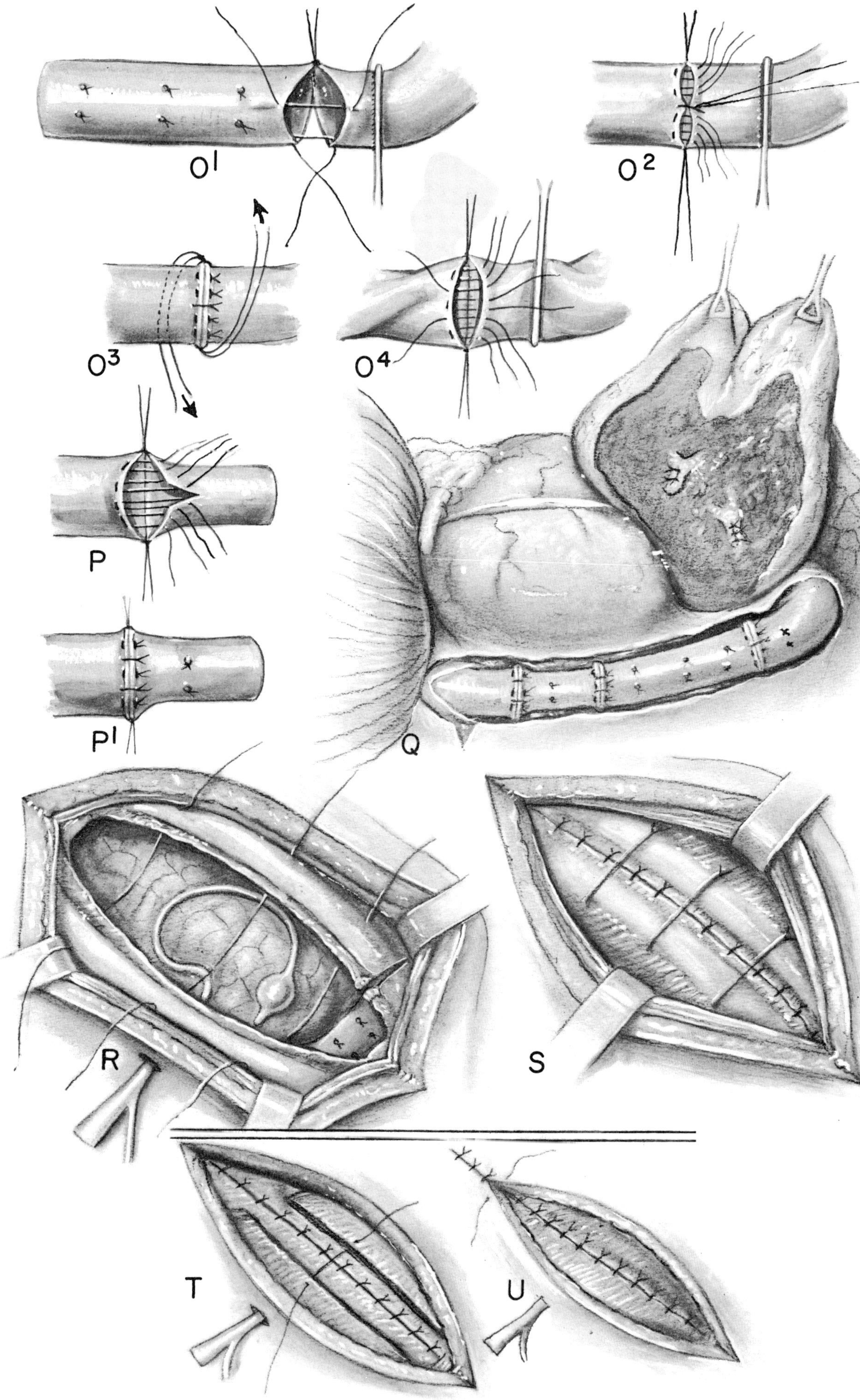

O1
O2
O3
O4
P
P1
Q
R
S
T
U

V. This is an enlarged diagrammatic illustration of the use of the partial by-pass employing an extracorporeal circuit as advocated and practiced by DeBakey. The left atrium is cannulated through the left auricular appendix and the arterial blood withdrawn is transferred by a pump mechanism into the left common femoral artery and the aorta distal to the site of its occlusion. The maintenance of flow is as described by Dr. DeBakey in his discussion of this operation. The monitoring of the venous and arterial pressures in the manner depicted is optional. The thoracic aorta is cross-clamped (DeBakey clamps) cephalad and caudad to the aneurysm. The aneurysm is then resected by transection of the aorta as indicated (broken lines).

W. The aneurysm is resected and aortic continuity is restored by the insertion of a woven teflon (or dacron) cloth prosthesis. This type of graft is used routinely in restoration of aortic continuity. The use of an homologous aortic graft as depicted in the illustrated technic (O-Q) is only of historic interest. These illustrations have been maintained because they show well the relation of the aneurysm to the surrounding structures, and in particular the extensive adherence to the lung and esophagus.

The technic that is shown (O-P′) for the anastomosis of the aortic graft, though acceptable, has been superseded by the use of a simple over and over suture, both anteriorly and posteriorly, with the knots of the sutures at each angle of the anastomosis (W). The anastomosis caudad is completed first and then the one cephalad. Just before the completion of the anastomosis cephalad, the distal aorta clamp is slowly released to permit retrograde filling of the graft and the escape of trapped air through the small opening remaining in the anastomosis. The closure of this anastomosis is then completed, and after removal of the distal clamp, the proximal clamp is slowly released concomitant with the occlusion of the left atrial cannula. The atrial cannula is withdrawn and the auricular appendix is ligated. Next the cannula is removed from the left common femoral artery and the opening in the artery occluded with interrupted sutures of 00000 silk. Finally, the heparin dosage (1 mg./1 kg. of body weight), administered prior to cannulation is counteracted by the administration of protamine sulfate (1.5 mg./1 kg. of body weight).

DISCUSSION DR. MICHAEL E. DEBAKEY. The major problem in the resection of aneurysms of the descending thoracic aorta at this level is concerned with the necessity of temporarily arresting aortic circulation and the consequent effect of the increased vascular resistance upon the heart and the potential ischemic effect upon the spinal cord. Several methods may be employed to overcome these difficulties —induced general body hypothermia to reduce metabolic requirements and the use of various types of temporary intraluminal and extraluminal shunts to provide circulation to the distal segment. We have employed all of these methods and have found them to be fairly effective. The fact remains, however, that all of them are associated with certain disadvantages, and, for this reason, our efforts were directed toward the development of a more satisfactory method of overcoming some of these technical problems.

This method, which we have employed in about 50 cases with highly gratifying results, consists of an extracorporeal circuit using a pump. In this method, oxygenated blood is removed from the left atrium through a plastic canula (3/16 inch inside diameter) and pumped into the distal aorta through a plastic canula inserted through the left common femoral artery. The rate of flow is adjusted to the blood pressure in the segment of aorta above the aortic clamp, attempting to maintain systolic pressure in this segment during the occlusion period at approximately 10 to 20 mm. Hg above normal pressure. Accordingly, from time to time during the period of occlusion, the rate of flow is adjusted to compensate for fluctuations in blood pressure varying in the range of 1000 to 2000 ml. per minute. Heparin 1 mg. per kg. body weight is administered intravenously before connecting the extracorporeal system, and a counteracting dose of protamine sulphate is administered after completing the procedure.

There are several other differences in technic which we consider preferable to that shown. First, in regard to the aortic occlusion clamps, we have found the Potts type of clamp to be unsatisfactory and prefer a clamp of our own design which is less likely to cause tearing or trauma to the aortic wall. Second, in regard to the graft, as indicated in the comment on resection of aneurysms of the abdominal aorta, we have completely abandoned the use of homografts and now prefer a flexible, crimped, knitted, dacron graft of our own design. Third, in regard to the anastomosis, we prefer to use a continuous through and through suture, as experience has demonstrated it to be functionally equally satisfactory to the so-called everting mattress suture, and technically it is easier and more rapidly performed.

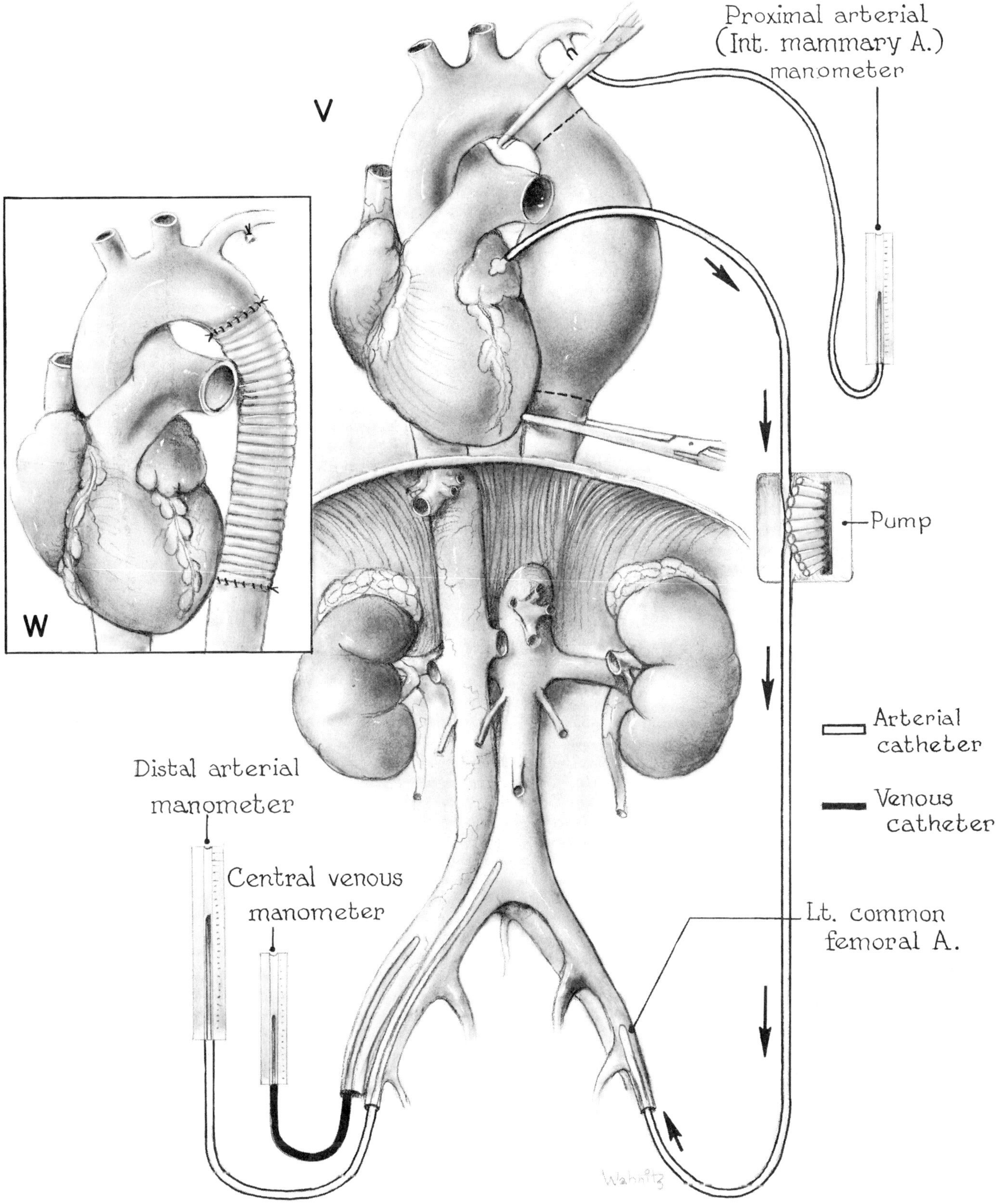
V
W
Proximal arterial
(Int. mammary A.)
manometer
Pump
Arterial
catheter
Venous
catheter
Distal arterial
manometer
Central venous
manometer
Lt. common
femoral A.
Wahnitz

EXCISION OF AN ANEURYSM OF THE ABDOMINAL AORTA AND THE INSERTION OF A PRESERVED HOMOLOGOUS AORTIC GRAFT

A. The long left paramedian muscle-retracting (lateral) incision, extending from the symphysis pubis to the left costochondral angle, and the short incision, overlying the left femoral artery, are shown in dotted outline. In this particular patient the femoral arterial pulsation was excellent on the right and absent on the left. Accordingly, it was deemed advisable to expose first the left femoral artery to determine the adequacy of the peripheral arterial "run off."

B, C. The thigh incision is deepened through the underlying fascial layer (B), and the sartorius muscle is retracted laterally to expose the common femoral artery and its deep (profunda) and superficial femoral branches (C). It may be observed that the common femoral artery is constricted and smaller in diameter than its superficial femoral branch. On palpation, the walls of the superficial femoral artery were pliable and the lumen patent although no pulsations were present. In contrast the deep (profunda) and common femoral arteries were calcific throughout and their lumens completely obstructed. It was evident at this time that the left external iliac branch of the bifurcation graft would of necessity be anastomosed to the left superficial femoral artery in the proximal portion of the thigh.

D. The cut margins of the short incision in the anterior parietal peritoneum are grasped in clamps, and the extension of the incision both cephalad and caudad is indicated by the dotted lines.

E. The entrance into the peritoneal cavity is completed, and the wound margins are retracted to expose the related subjacent intraperitoneal viscera.

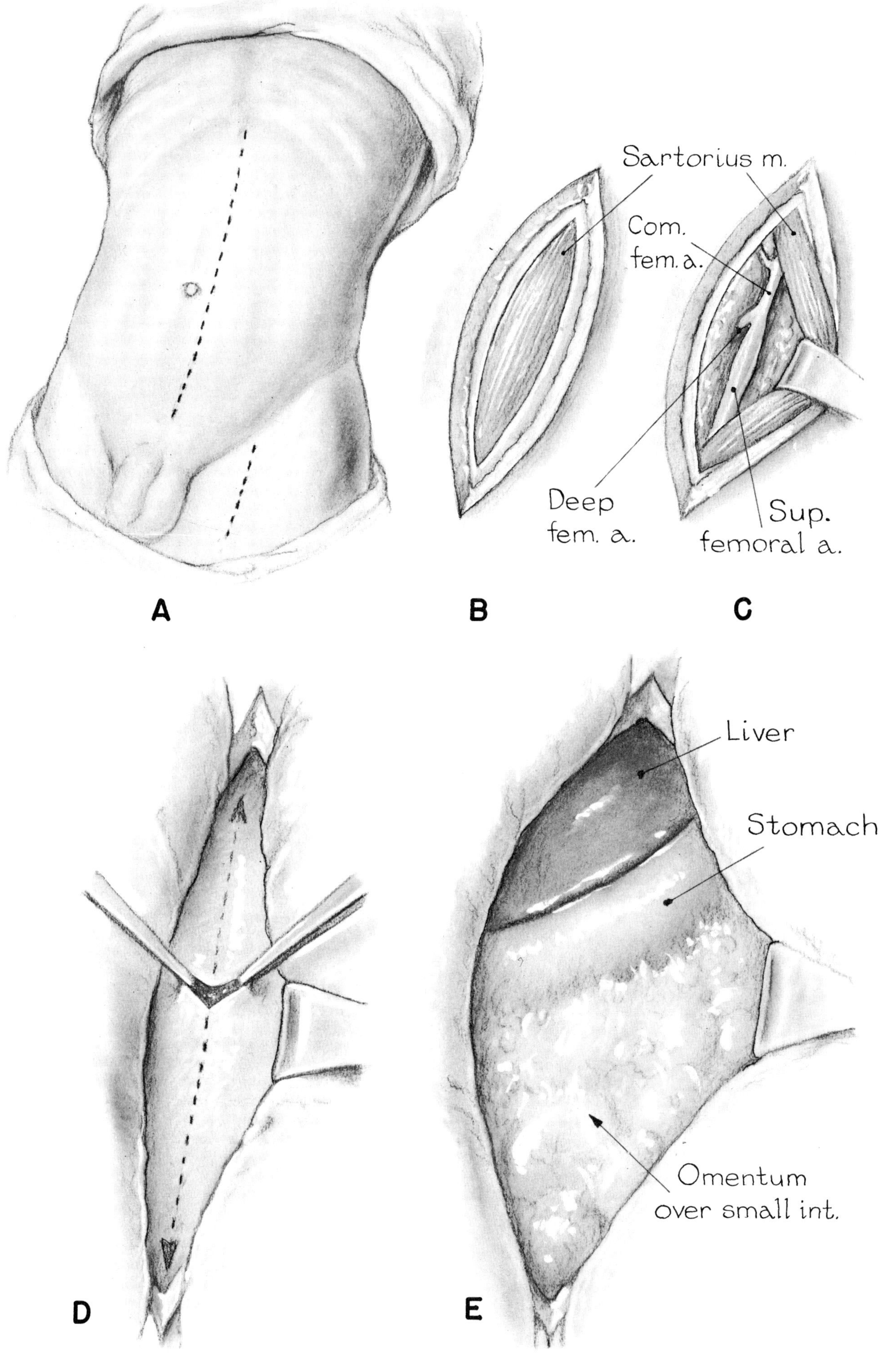
Sartorius m.
Com. fem. a.
Deep fem. a.
Sup. femoral a.
Liver
Stomach
Omentum over small int.
A
B
C
D
E

F. The omentum and transverse colon are elevated, and the completed incision in the posterior peritoneal attachment of the small bowel mesentery is visible. The extension of this incision around the cecum and upward along the peritoneal attachments of the ascending colon is shown in dotted outline. The peritoneal incision for mobilization of the duodenum and its horizontal extension (dotted line) along the inferior border of the fourth portion of the duodenum are also visible. The relation of the inferior mesenteric vein to the ligament of Treitz and the duodenojejunal junction is depicted.

G. The right side of the colon is mobilized, and the related structures posteriorly are shown. Although this mobilization of the colon is not an essential part of the operation, it has proved a technical aid in the exposure of aneurysms of the abdominal aorta.

H. The mobilized small bowel and colon are enclosed in a rubber bag (Lahey) and placed outside of the abdomen on the lower portion of the patient's chest. Before placing the bowel in the bag it is important to examine carefully the raw surfaces of the mesenteric attachments for bleeding sites. The failure to recognize and control bleeding may cause a loss of 800 to 1000 ml. of blood into the bag. In our own experience, this occurred on one occasion. The incision for severance of the remaining peritoneal attachment of the fourth portion of the duodenum is depicted (dotted line).

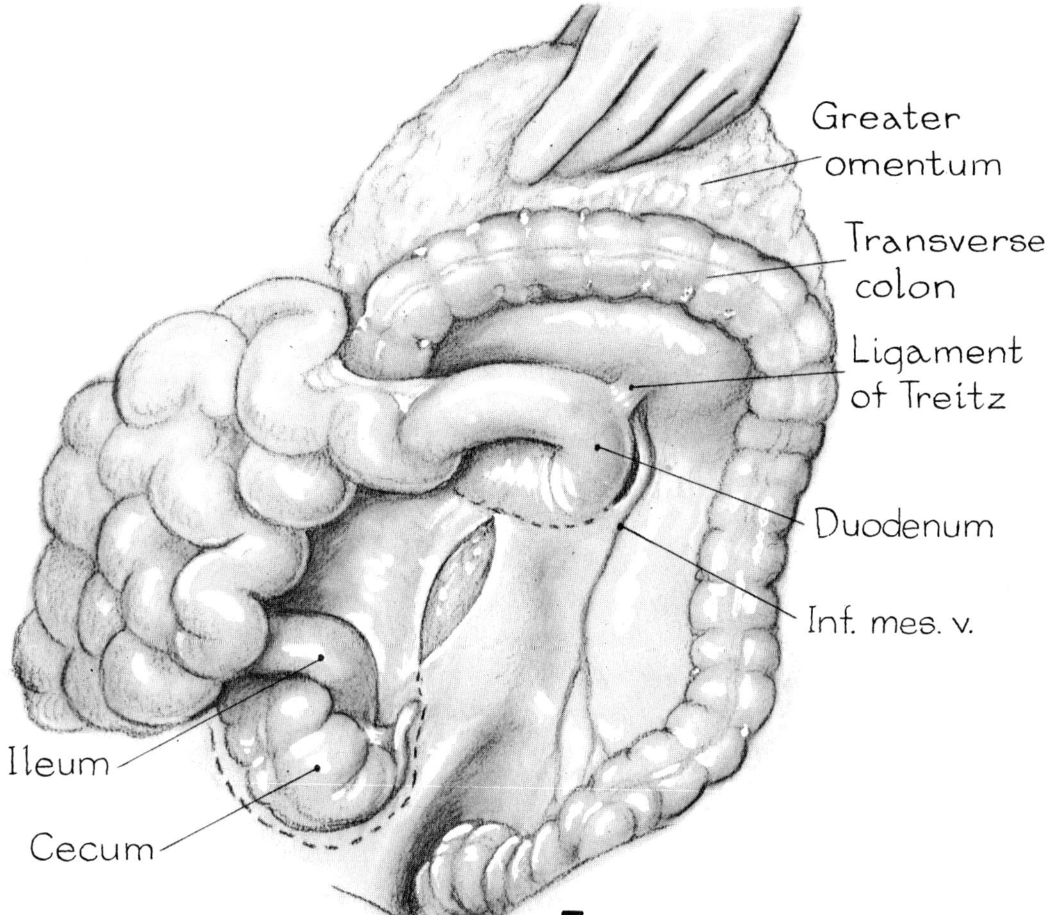
Greater
omentum
Transverse
colon
Ligament
of Treitz
Duodenum
Inf. mes. v.
Ileum
Cecum

F

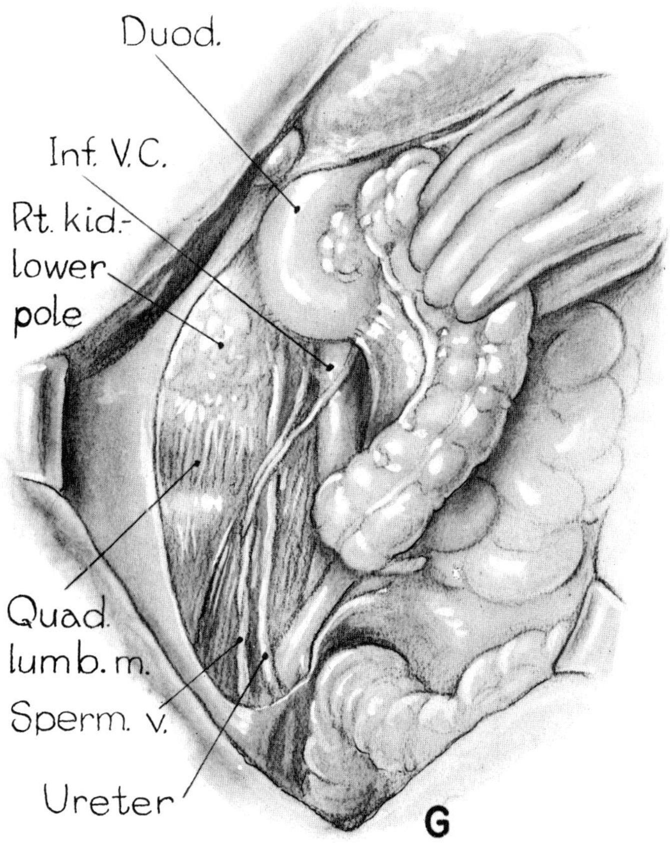
Duod.
Inf. V.C.
Rt. kid.-
lower
pole
Quad.
lumb. m.
Sperm. v.
Ureter

G

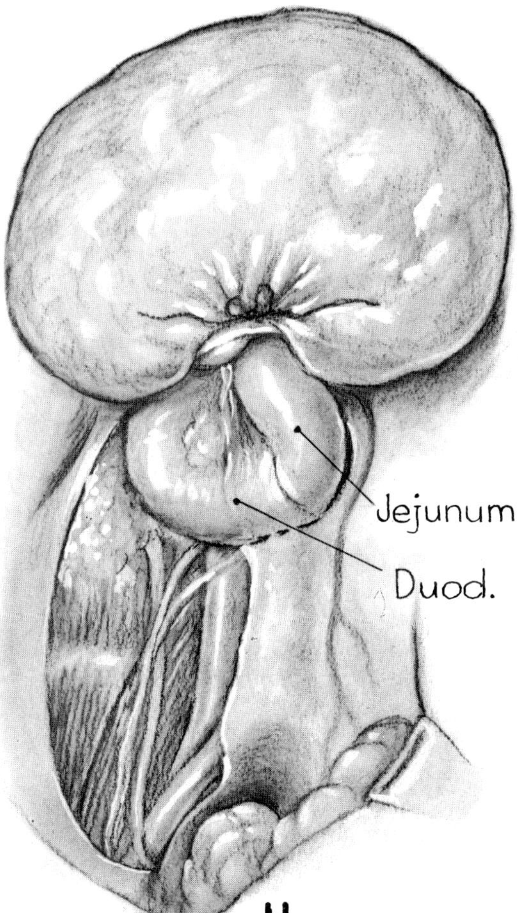
Jejunum
Duod.

H

I. The mobilized duodenum is retracted upward to expose the left renal vein which crosses over the abdominal aorta just proximal to the aneurysm and enters the inferior vena cava. The outline of the aneurysm beneath the posterior parietal peritoneum is visible.

J. The overlying posterior parietal peritoneum is elevated from the surface of the aneurysm, which is mobilized by scissor dissection from its attachment to the adjacent inferior vena cava. In some instances, the aneurysm is inextricably adherent to the inferior vena cava, and its separation without entrance into the aneurysm or the vena is impossible. Under such circumstances, further dissection in this area is discontinued until the aorta proximally and its common iliac branches distally are cross-clamped. The aneurysm is then incised and its contents evacuated. Bleeding from the orifices of the lumbar vessels entering the aneurysm posteriorly is controlled by suture ligatures of silk, and the wall of the aneurysm is tailored as it is excised by scissor dissection to leave a "patch graft" at its site of adherence to the inferior vena cava. This technic applies in particular to the treatment of the acutely ruptured aneurysm. To persist in the attempt to dissect an adherent aneurysm from the vena cava is not only time-consuming but may result in serious and even fatal hemorrhage. The site of the segmental occlusion of the left common iliac artery is visible. In this patient, four aneurysmal dilatations, the lowermost being the largest, were present in the segment of the aorta below the left renal vein. Furthermore, a dissection plane between the aorta and the inferior vena cava, which facilitated the separation of these structures, was easily obtained.

K. The dissection of the aneurysm from the inferior vena cava is completed. The aorta proximally and the common iliac arteries distally are encircled by cotton tapes. The inferior mesenteric artery is occluded proximally with a ligature of silk (00) and distally by two clamps between which the artery is subsequently severed. Each clamp is then replaced by a suture ligature of 000 silk.

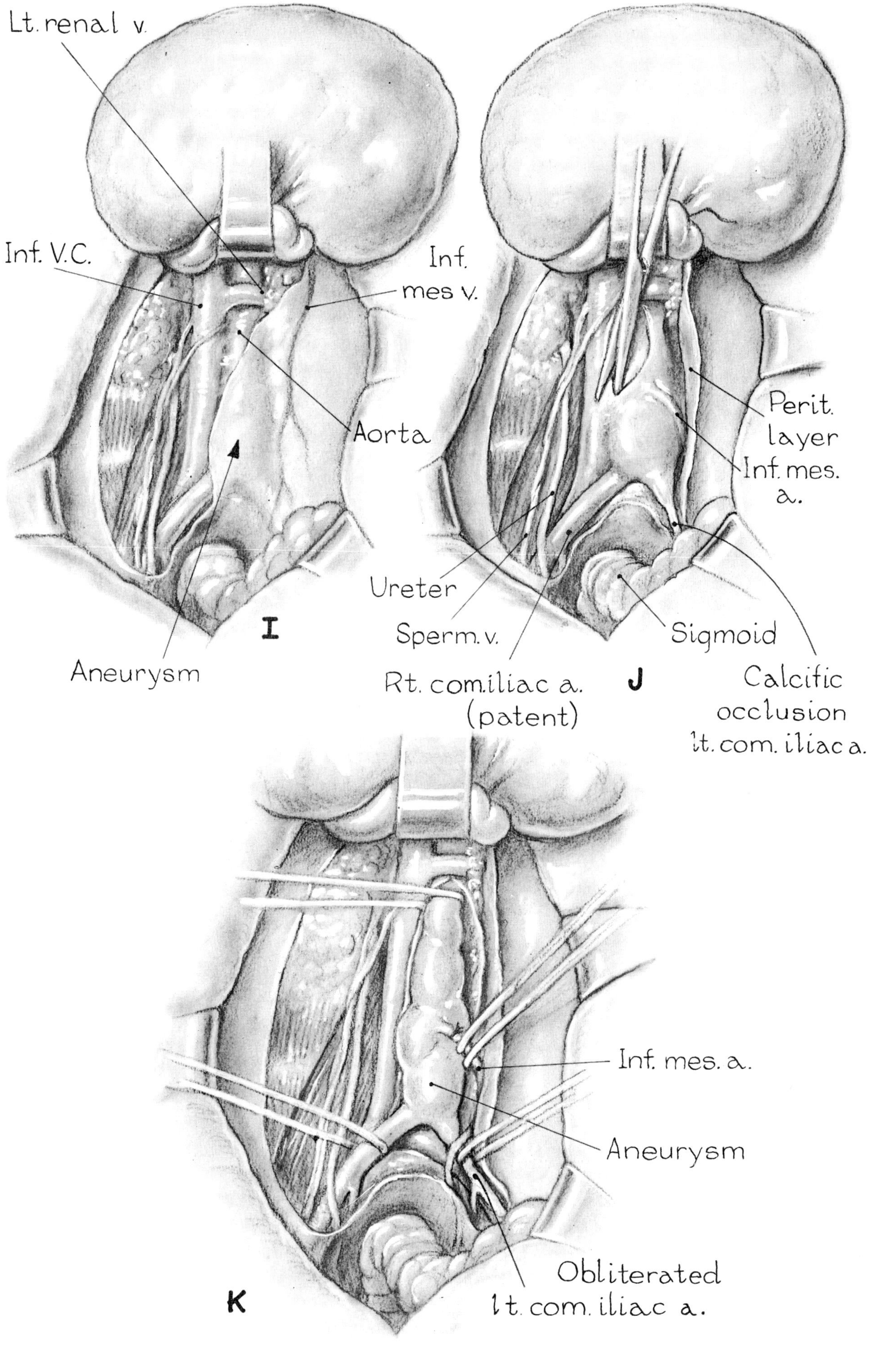
Lt. renal v.
Inf. V.C.
Inf. mes v.
Aorta
Aneurysm
I
Perit. layer
Inf. mes. a.
Ureter
Sperm. v.
Sigmoid
Rt. com. iliac a. (patent)
J
Calcific occlusion lt. com. iliac a.
Inf. mes. a.
Aneurysm
Obliterated lt. com. iliac a.
K

L. The ligation and severance of the inferior mesenteric artery is completed. The site of the segmental occlusion of the left common iliac artery is depicted. The left internal iliac artery was completely calcific throughout its whole length.

M. The sigmoid colon is partially mobilized by severance of its lateral parietal peritoneal attachment to expose a portion of the obliterated left external iliac artery.

N, N[1]. The aorta is manually displaced, first to the right (N) and then to the left (N[1]), for exposure, ligation, and severance of the paired lumbar vertebral arteries. Although this was readily accomplished as depicted, in some patients the size of the aneurysm precludes the use of this technic. Under such circumstances, the aorta is first transected, either cephalad to the proximal pole of the aneurysm or caudad to the aortic bifurcation, and the lumbar vessels are serially clamped and severed as the aneurysm is mobilized in either a cephalad or caudad direction.

N[2]. The mobilization of the aneurysm-containing segment of the abdominal aorta is completed, and the site of its transection cephalad is indicated by the dotted line.

Discussion—Dr. Michael E. De Bakey. Our experience with resection of aneurysms of the abdominal aorta now includes over 500 cases. In the first 100 cases in this series, the operative mortality was 17 per cent, whereas in the last 100 cases it was only 4 per cent. While there are undoubtedly a number of factors in the surgical management of this problem that have a bearing upon the risk of operation, we are convinced that certain technical considerations are particularly significant in this respect. Accordingly, we believe that improvements in technic derived from this experience have contributed to the progressive decrease in our operative mortality.

Although in principle, the method of resection and graft replacement shown here is similar to ours, there are certain differences in technic which, from our experience, we consider preferable. The first concerns exposure. We prefer a true midline incision rather than a paramedian. For one thing, it greatly facilitates both exposure and closure and thus minimizes operative time. For another, it has not been associated in our experience with significant early or late complications. After entering the peritoneal cavity, the small intestine and its mesentery are simply mobilized to the right and retracted with moist packs. We have abandoned the use of the Lahey bag and have found no advantage to mobilization of the right peritoneal attachment of the ascending colon. Indeed, this is considered an unnecessary maneuver.

Second, in regard to the graft, we have completely abandoned the use of homografts and during the past year have employed exclusively a flexible crimped knitted dacron graft of our own design. Our experience with this graft in approximately 400 cases of aortic and arterial replacements has convinced us of its advantages over homografts as well as other vascular replacements.

As regards occluding clamps, we have found the Potts type of clamp to be unsatisfactory, particularly for the aorta. The occluding clamps which we prefer are specially designed for this purpose and are made by the Pilling Company. Their main advantage lies in the fact that they provide secure occlusiôn with minimal trauma to the vessel wall.

It is highly desirable to minimize the period of arrest of aortic circulation, and this may be accomplished by the manner in which the procedure is performed. In this case, for example, after completing the anastomosis of the graft to the aortic opening, we would have performed anastomosis of the right iliac

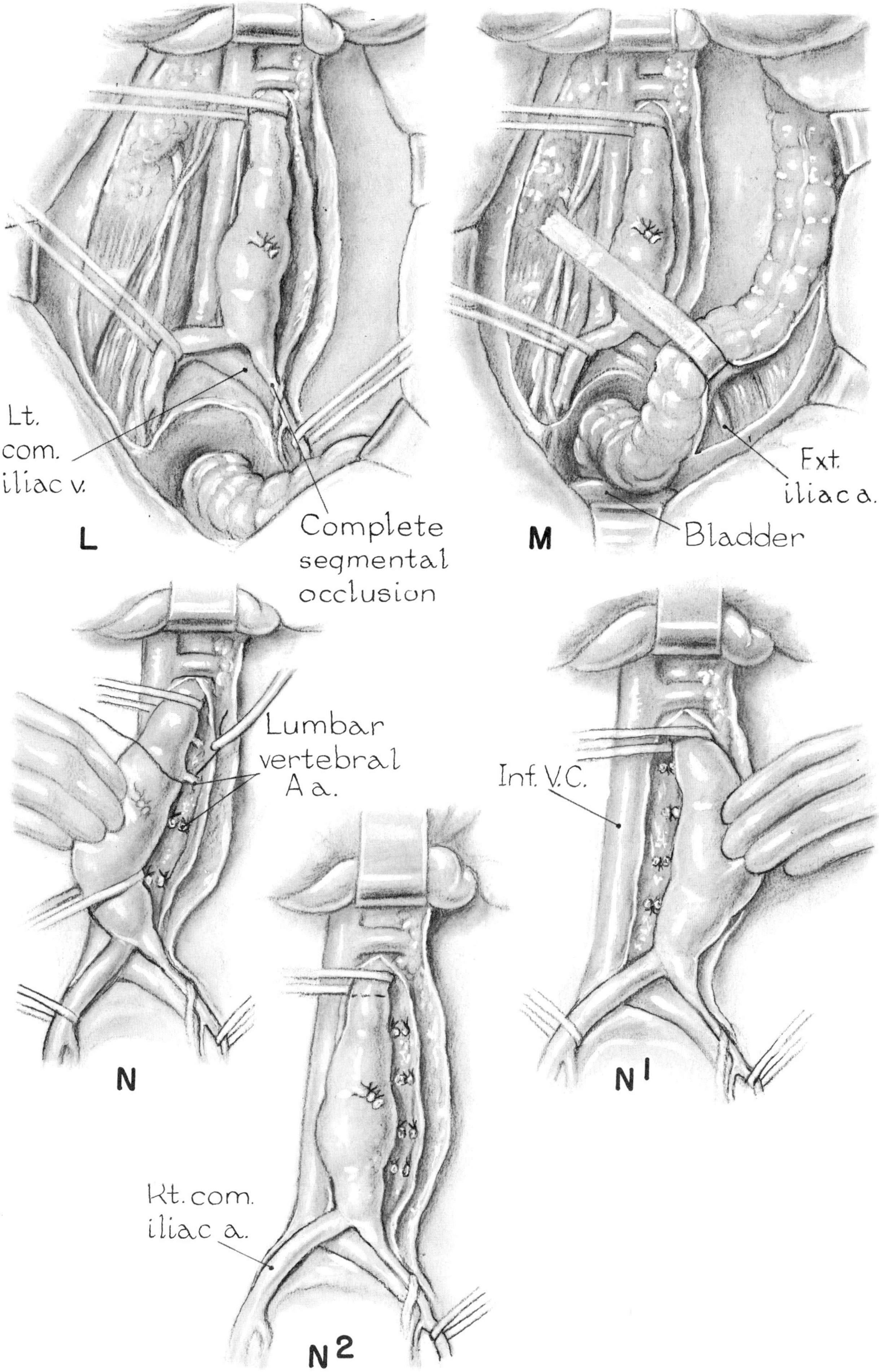
Lt.
com.
iliac v.
L
Complete
segmental
occlusion
M
Ext.
iliac a.
Bladder
Lumbar
vertebral
A a.
N
Inf. V.C.
N1
Rt.com.
iliac a.
N2

O. The left common iliac artery and the left external iliac artery are severed proximally and distally respectively to the internal iliac artery, and the distal transected end of the external iliac artery is partially withdrawn beneath the inguinal ligament into the thigh. The T-shaped appearance formed by the ligated stumps of the common and external iliac arteries in relation to the obliterated internal iliac artery is visible.

P. The withdrawal of the distal segment of the left external iliac artery beneath the inguinal ligament is completed, and the superficial femoral artery is cross-clamped with a straight Potts clamp.

Q. The obliterated left common iliac artery is severed just distal to the aortic bifurcation, and noncrushing clamps (Potts) are applied to the right common iliac artery and to the aorta proximal to the uppermost aneurysmal dilatation. The dotted lines indicate the respective sites for transection of the aorta proximally and the right common iliac artery distally.

R. The common iliac arterial branches of the preserved homologous bifurcation graft are clamped (Potts clamps) and elevated to show the initiation of the anastomosis between the aorta and the homologous graft by the insertion of two silk (00000) sutures in the midline posteriorly.

R¹, R², R³. The sutures posteriorly are tied, and one of the sutures proceeds to the patient's left (R¹) and the other to the patient's right (R²) to complete the insertion of the posterior layer of the anastomosis (R³). The insertion of each suture is begun on the graft side so that the needle, when inserted on the host aortic side, impinges the intima plaques which are usually present against the underlying coats of the aorta.

Discussion—Dr. De Bakey (cont.)

segment of the graft to the right iliac artery. After completing this latter anastomosis, the occluding clamp on the right iliac artery would be removed and an effort made to obtain retrograde flushing of the vessel to remove any debris or clots that may have accumulated distal to the clamp. After good retrograde blood flow was assured, an occluding clamp would be applied to the right iliac segment of the graft just distal to the bifurcation and the aortic clamp released for a few seconds to flush out the aorta through the graft and the remaining open end of the left iliac segment of the graft. This assures removal of any debris and clots that may have accumulated in the blind segment of the aorta proximal to the clamp. Following these maneuvers, the occluding clamp on the right iliac segment of the graft is removed and applied to the left iliac segment of the graft just distal to the bifurcation. The aortic clamp is then slowly released, permitting circulation to be restored through the graft and into the right lower extremity.

Attention may now be directed toward anastomosis of the left iliac segment of the graft. In this case, since the left common iliac artery was occluded, it is necessary to extend the left iliac segment of the graft beyond this level. Under these circumstances, our experience has led us to use the bypass principle. The occluded segment of the left iliac artery is allowed to remain undisturbed, and, instead of resecting the common femoral artery, we would probably have performed an endarterectomy in this region and attached the graft as an end-to-side anastomosis. This has the advantage of being a simpler and less time-consuming procedure and has proved effective in our experience. Significantly we have never encountered gangrene as a complication of this operation.

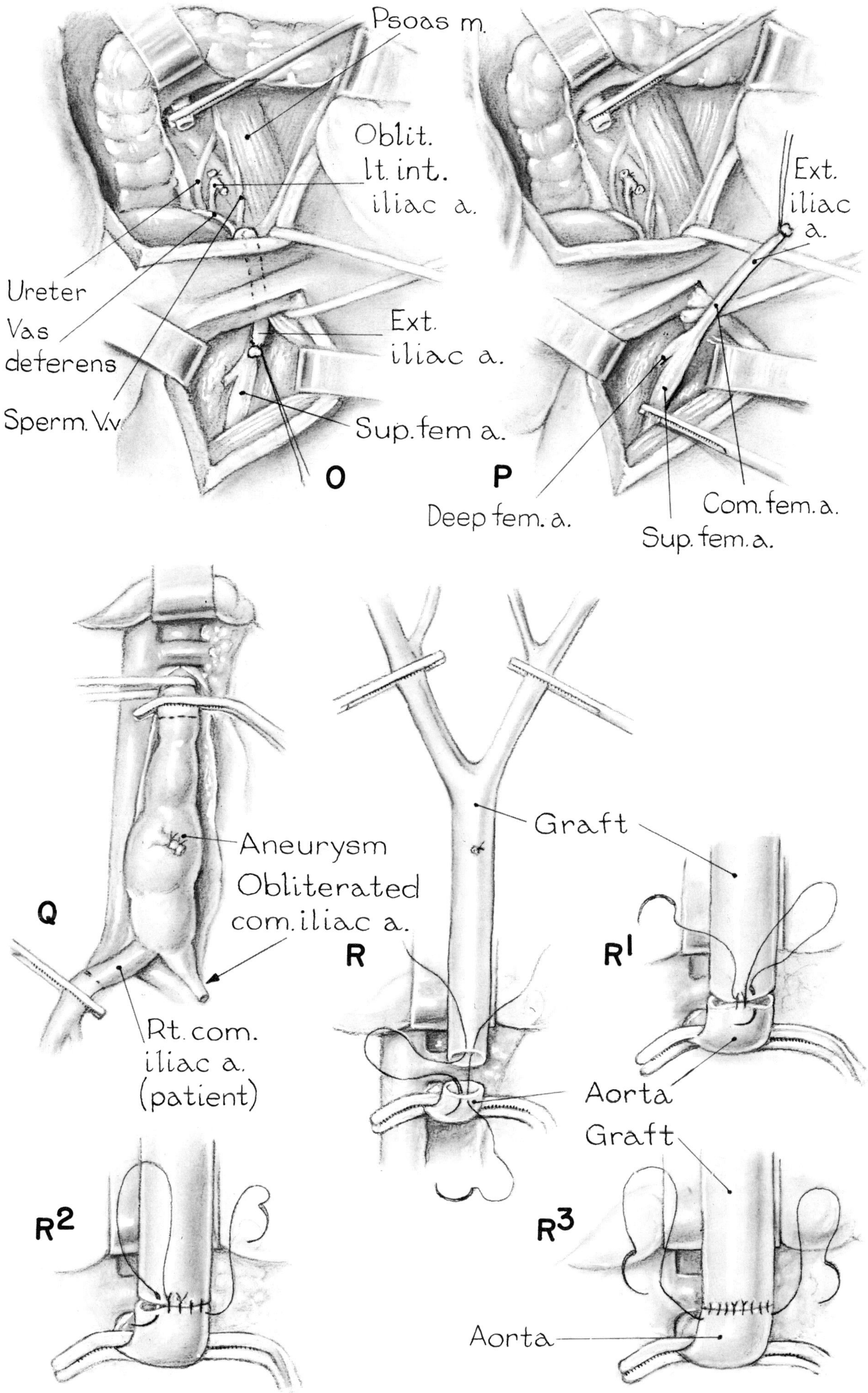
Psoas m.
Oblit.
lt. int.
iliac a.
Ureter
Vas
deterens
Sperm. V.v.
Ext.
iliac a.
Sup. fem a.
O
P
Ext.
iliac
a.
Deep fem. a.
Com. fem. a.
Sup. fem. a.
Aneurysm
Obliterated
com. iliac a.
Q
Rt. com.
iliac a.
(patient)
Graft
R
R[1]
Aorta
Graft
R[2]
R[3]
Aorta

R^4, R^5, S. The graft is displaced downward, and the insertion of the anterior layer of the anastomosis is continued from either side (R^4, R^5) to meet in the midline anteriorly where the sutures are tied together (S). As previously stated, the insertion of the needles on the host aortic side anteriorly is again in such a manner as to impinge the intima coat against the underlying coats of the aorta.

T. The external iliac segment of the aortic bifurcation graft was too short to reach to the level of the superficial femoral artery. Accordingly, the unused portion of the right common iliac artery of the graft and its bifurcation was used on the left side to gain the necessary length to complete the anastomosis with the superficial femoral artery. The substitute graft segment was inserted in a reversed direction, and its terminal external iliac segment was anastomosed to the terminal portion of the left external iliac artery. The terminal segment of the common iliac artery (right) of the substitute graft segment is in readiness to be anastomosed to the superficial femoral artery.

U, V. The three cardinal guy sutures of silk between the common iliac artery segment and the superficial femoral artery are inserted (U), and the end-to-end anastomosis in the proximal portion of the left side is completed (V). In this particular patient, anastomosis of the graft with the internal iliac arteries was not required. However, in the excision of aneurysms of the abdominal aorta in which transection distal to the common iliac arteries is done, anastomosis of the internal iliac arteries, if patent, to the graft is practiced. In one patient in whom ligation rather than anastomosis of the internal iliac arteries was done, two large areas of tissue necrosis of the tissues deep within the buttocks with secondary skin necrosis occurred. Furthermore, in some patients, compromise of the blood supply to a segment of the colon may result from failure to anastomose the graft with the internal iliac arteries.

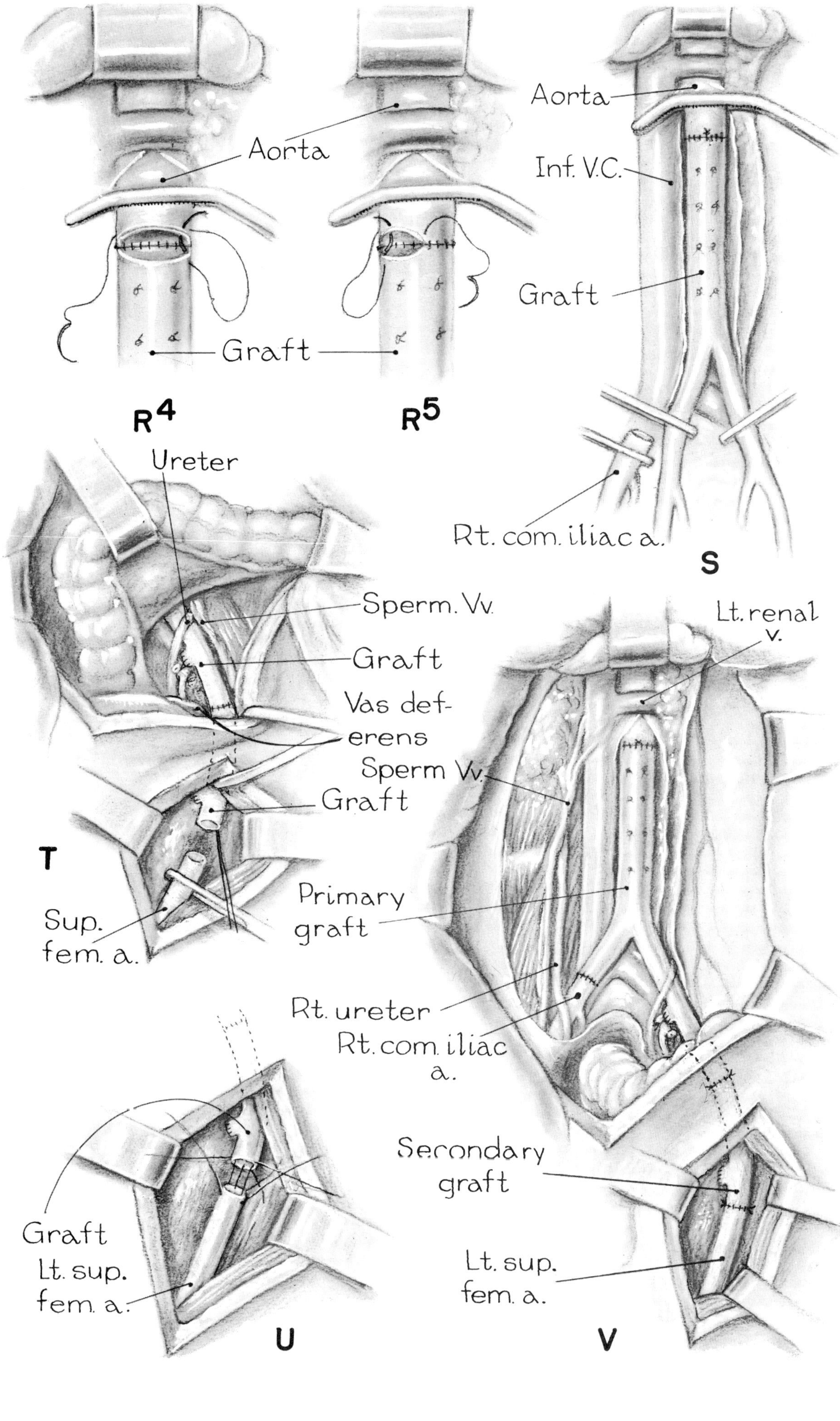
Aorta
Graft
R4
R5
Aorta
Inf. V.C.
Graft
Rt. com. iliac a.
S
Ureter
Sperm. Vv.
Graft
Vas deferens
Sperm Vv.
Graft
T
Sup. fem. a.
Lt. renal v.
Primary graft
Rt. ureter
Rt. com. iliac a.
Graft
Lt. sup. fem. a.
U
Secondary graft
Lt. sup. fem. a.
V

W, X. The insertion of the preserved homologous bifurcation graft and the substitute extension graft is completed. The anastomosis on the right side is to the common iliac artery and on the left to the superficial femoral artery in the thigh (W). The closure of the incision in the proximal portion of the left thigh is completed, and the abdominal wound is being closed, using both interrupted mattress sutures and simple interrupted sutures of 00 silk for the peritoneum and interrupted sutures of 00 silk for the anterior rectus sheath (X). The skin incision is subsequently closed with interrupted sutures of 00 silk.

Y. The restoration of continuity of the abdominal aorta by the insertion of a woven dacron cloth prosthesis is depicted. Woven dacron (or teflon) grafts are now used routinely. The use of homologous aortic grafts as illustrated (R-V) is no longer practiced and is considered only of historic interest. However, the suture technic employed, simple over and over sutures, remains the one of choice.

The patient, a 55-year-old white man, was admitted to the hospital with the history that, during the preceding year, pain in the left leg on walking, relieved by rest, was noted. The symptoms persisted, and, during the two months prior to admission to the hospital, pain in the left hip and the low back was observed. Examination at this time demonstrated a palpable pulsatile mass in the lower abdomen and the absence of pulsations in the left femoral artery. The pulsations in the right femoral artery were normal. A diagnosis of an aneurysm of the abdominal aorta with segmental occlusion of either or both the left common and external iliac artery was made. At operation, multiple (four) relatively small aneurysms of the abdominal aorta were present in conjunction with atherosclerotic obliteration of the left common iliac, the internal iliac, the external iliac, and the common and profunda femoral arteries. The local pathologic findings in the aorta and its peripheral arterial branches on the left side were consistent with the diagnosis of juvenile arteriosclerosis (Leriche). The pathologic findings present accounted for the relative ease with which the involved segment of the abdominal aorta was freed from the adjacent inferior vena cava. Following the insertion of the preserved homologous aortic graft as depicted in the illustrations, an excellent arterial pulsation was restored in the left superficial femoral artery. The subsequent postoperative course was without incident, and the patient was discharged from the hospital in satisfactory condition on the 16th day after operation.

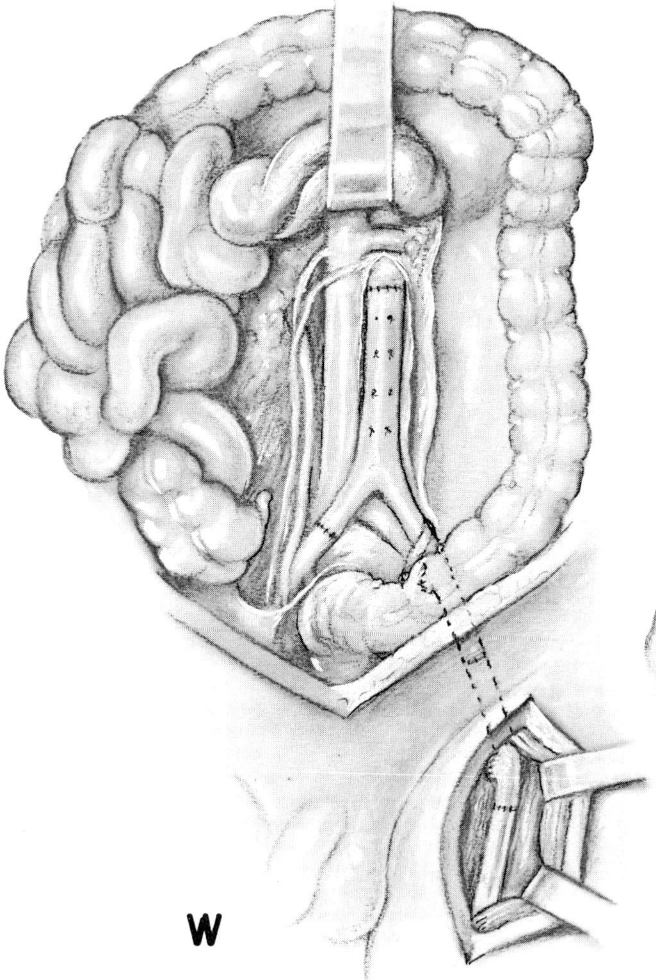

W

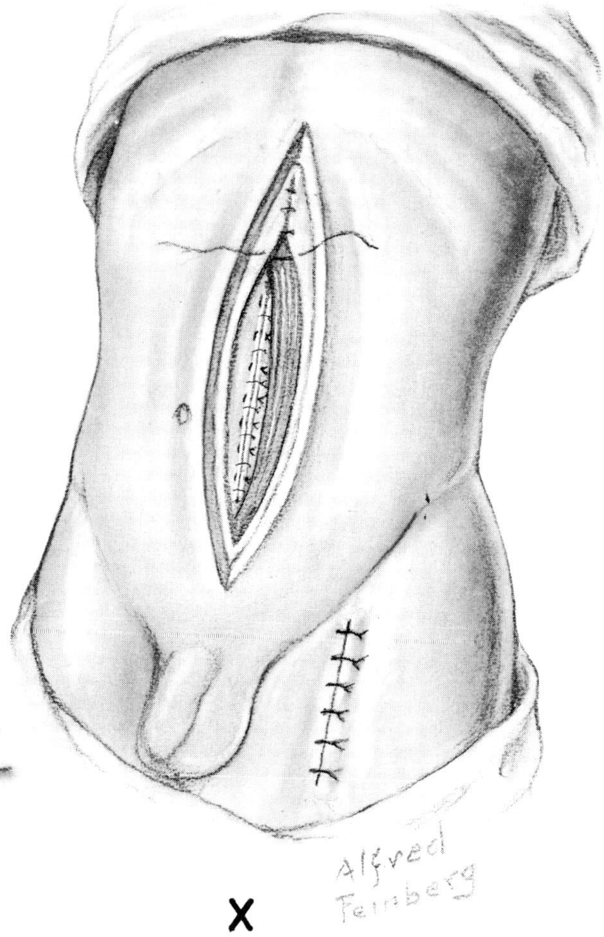

X

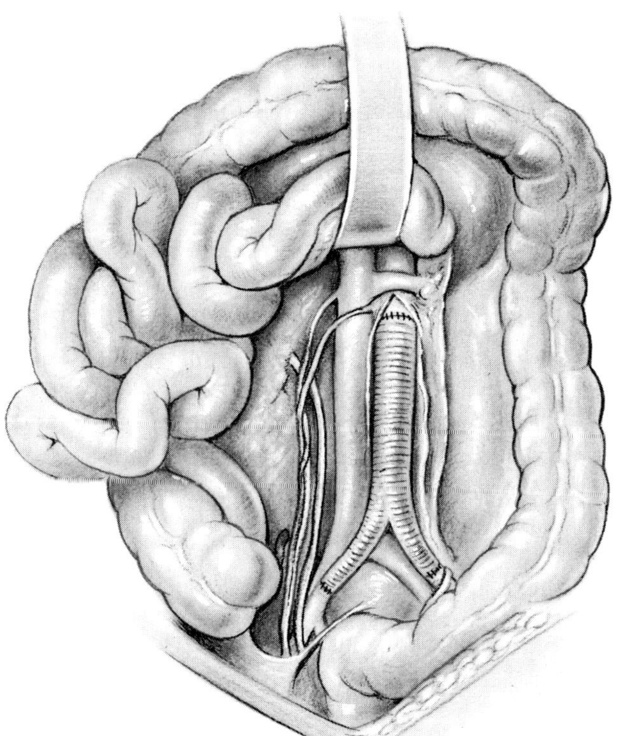

Y

EXCISION OF AN ANEURYSM OF THE POPLITEAL ARTERY AND THE INSERTION OF AN ALCOHOL (70 PER CENT) PRESERVED HOMOLOGOUS AORTIC (THORACIC) GRAFT

A. The incision employed, depicted in dotted outline, is preferred to one of the midline longitudinal type.

B. The mobilized flaps of skin and subcutaneous fatty tissue are retracted to expose the posterior crural fascia and the underlying muscles. The perforation of the crural fascia by the short saphenous vein (saphena parva) is visible.

C, D, E. The incised margins of the linear incision in the posterior crural fascia are retracted in clamps (C), and, by scissor dissection in the underlying tissue, the popliteal vein and the entrance of its tributary, the short saphenous vein, are demonstrable. A portion of the tibial nerve and its branches, as well as portions of the surrounding musculature, are also delineated (D, E).

F. The dissection is continued within the deeper tissue, and the superior pole of the popliteal artery and the outline of its "dumbbell" aneurysm immediately distal are visible. A greater length of the tibial nerve is now exposed, and its branch to the medial head of the gastrocnemius muscle may be seen arched across the lower portion of the popliteal vein.

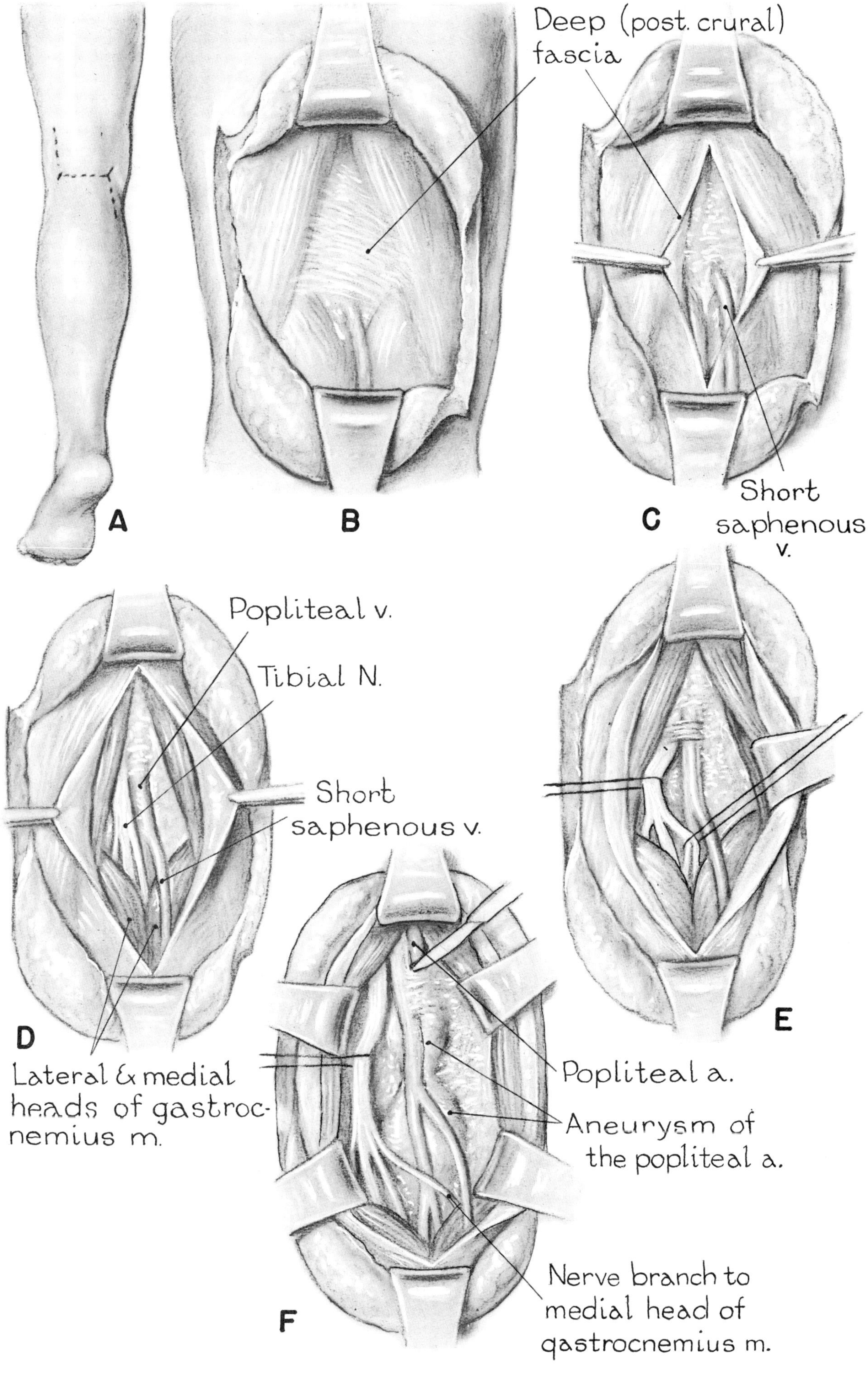
Deep (post. crural) fascia
A
B
C
Short saphenous v.
Popliteal v.
Tibial N.
Short saphenous v.
D
Lateral & medial heads of gastrocnemius m.
E
Popliteal a.
Aneurysm of the popliteal a.
Nerve branch to medial head of gastrocnemius m.
F

G, H. The operative field is more widely exposed, and the bifurcation of the branch of the tibial nerve to the medial head of the gastrocnemius muscle may be seen. The popliteal vein, inextricably adherent to the posterior wall of the aneurysm, was removed with the specimen. Accordingly, its lowermost tributaries and the short saphenous tributary were doubly clamped, severed, and ligated (H). In doing this, care was observed to avoid injury to the overlying nerve branch to the gastrocnemius muscle.

I. Scissor dissection is continued to mobilize completely the "dumbbell" aneurysm from its surrounding structures.

J, J¹, J². In mobilizing the aneurysm, it is deflected first to one side (J) and then the other (J¹) to expose the arterial branches which are doubly clamped, severed, and ligated (00 silk). The majority of the arterial branches were in the lower aneurysmal dilatation of the popliteal artery (J²).

K. The aneurysm is completely mobilized, and its superior pole is encircled with a ligature of silk (0). The cephalad portion of the popliteal vein is doubly clamped prior to its severance and ligation (00 silk).

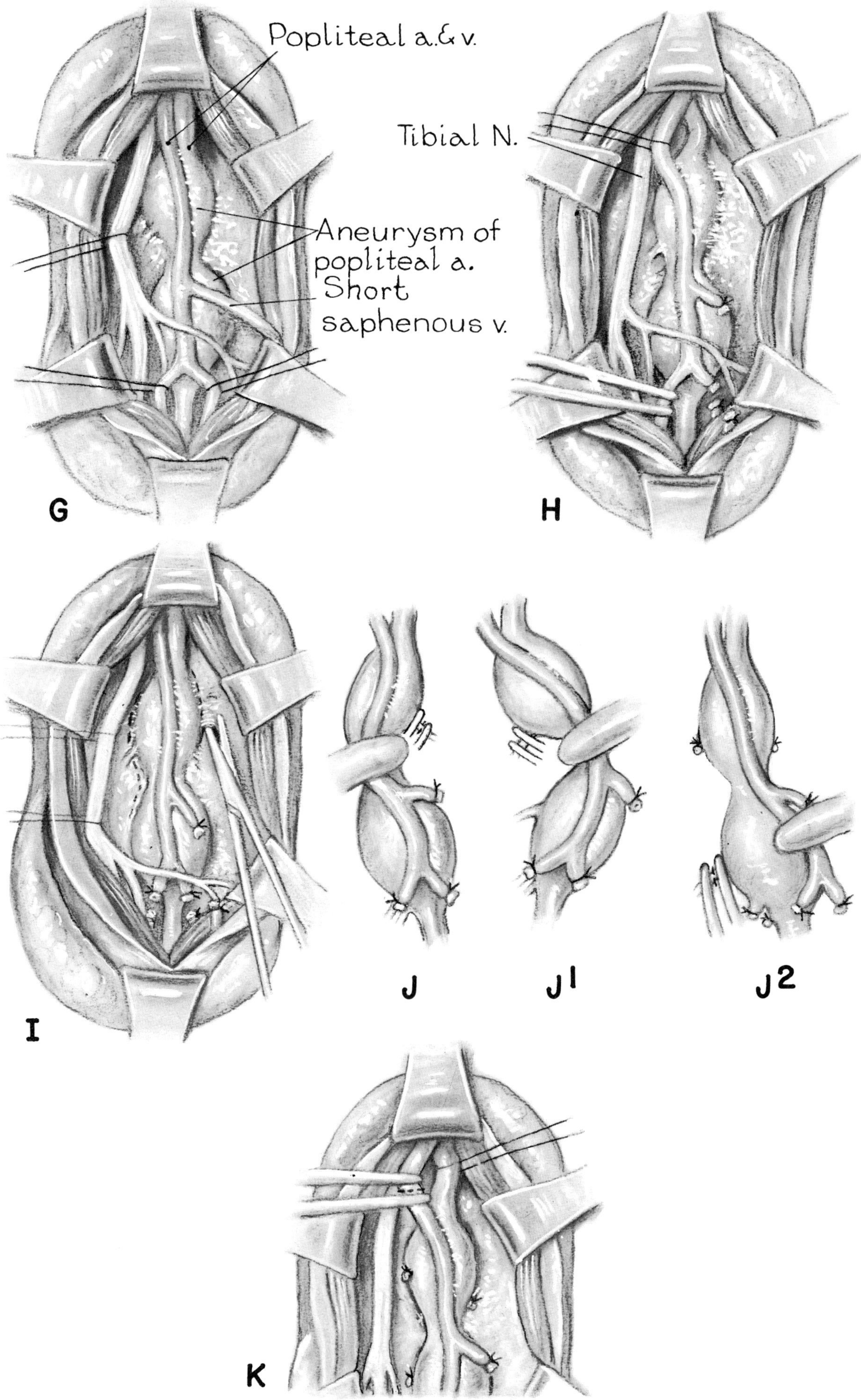
Popliteal a.& v.
Tibial N.
Aneurysm of popliteal a.
Short saphenous v.
G
H
I
J
J1
J2
K

L. The superior and inferior poles of the "dumbbell" aneurysm are clamped (Potts clamps) prior to transection (dotted lines) and removal of the aneurysm with the attached popliteal vein.

M. In this patient, the diameters of the lower portion of the femoral artery and the distal segment of the popliteal artery were extremely large and required the use of the thoracic segment of an alcohol (70 per cent) preserved homologous aortic graft to obtain a proper fit. The three cardinal guy sutures (00000 arterial silk) are inserted, one posteriorly and one at either lateral angle, but not tied.

N, N^1, N^2, N^3, N^4, N^5. The guy sutures are tied, and the suture strands are left long (N). The lower end of the graft is elevated to show the start of the posterior layer of the anastomosis (N^1). One of the lateral angle sutures is inserted as a continuous over and over suture to the midline posteriorly where it is tied to the free end of the posterior cardinal guy suture (N^2). The needle attached strand of the posterior cardinal guy suture is similarly continued as an over and over suture (N^3) and tied to the free end of the remaining lateral angle cardinal guy suture (N^4, N^5).

O, O^1. The aortic (thoracic) graft segment is turned downward to show the insertion of the sutures forming the anterior layer of the anastomosis. The needle attached strand of one of the lateral angle cardinal guy sutures (N^5) is continued anteriorly as a continuous over and over suture (O) and tied to the free end of the opposing lateral angle guy suture (O^1). The needle is inserted from the "inside out" on the host popliteal artery to impinge the calcific plaques which are frequently present in the intima against the underlying coats of the vessel.

O^2. The proximal anastomosis is completed, and the three cardinal guy sutures are similarly inserted distally but not tied.

O^3. The use of the free ends of the lateral angle cardinal guy sutures to rotate the graft and arterial segments for the insertion of the posterior layer of sutures, as previously depicted, is shown.

P. The insertion of the thoracic segment of the alcohol (70 per cent) preserved homologous graft to restore continuity of the popliteal artery is completed, and its relation to the surrounding structures is visible.

Q. A rubber tissue drain is inserted into the popliteal fossa, and the incision in the posterior crural fascia is closed with interrupted sutures of 000 silk. The closure of the skin incision and the application of a sterile gauze compression dressing complete the operation.

Discussion—Dr. Ormand C. Julian. The very marked tendency for thrombosis to occur in a popliteal aneurysm provides the absolute indication for their removal as soon as the diagnosis is made. In spite of their location, which subjects them to a peculiarly constant movement as the knee flexes and extends, they rarely rupture. Obstruction to arterial flow into the leg associated with aneurysm also results from occlusion of the popliteal artery just beyond the aneurysm, usually very close to the popliteal artery bifurcation. In this instance, the arterial pulses are absent at the ankle while at the same time the aneurysm continues to exhibit expansile pulsation. Whether this occlusion is entirely the result of an arteriosclerotic change in the popliteal artery beyond the aneurysm, or due primarily to kinking of the vessel in this area associated with elongation of the aneurysmal segment of the popliteal artery, is not clear. However, the blood supply to the leg may remain adequate for survival by way of collaterals which probably arise proximal to the aneurysm rather than from it. Actually, a complete thrombosis of a popliteal aneurysm is not always associated with a severe degree of acute ischemia of the leg.

The additional fact that popliteal aneurysms may be resected without loss of the extremity, even if continuity is not restored by a graft, if (1) a lumbar sympathectomy is done in preparation and (2) maximum care is taken to avoid damage to collaterals in the knee area, has led us to vary the technic of popliteal artery aneurysm resection. This variation, which will be mentioned in the discussion of specific elements of the illustrated oper-

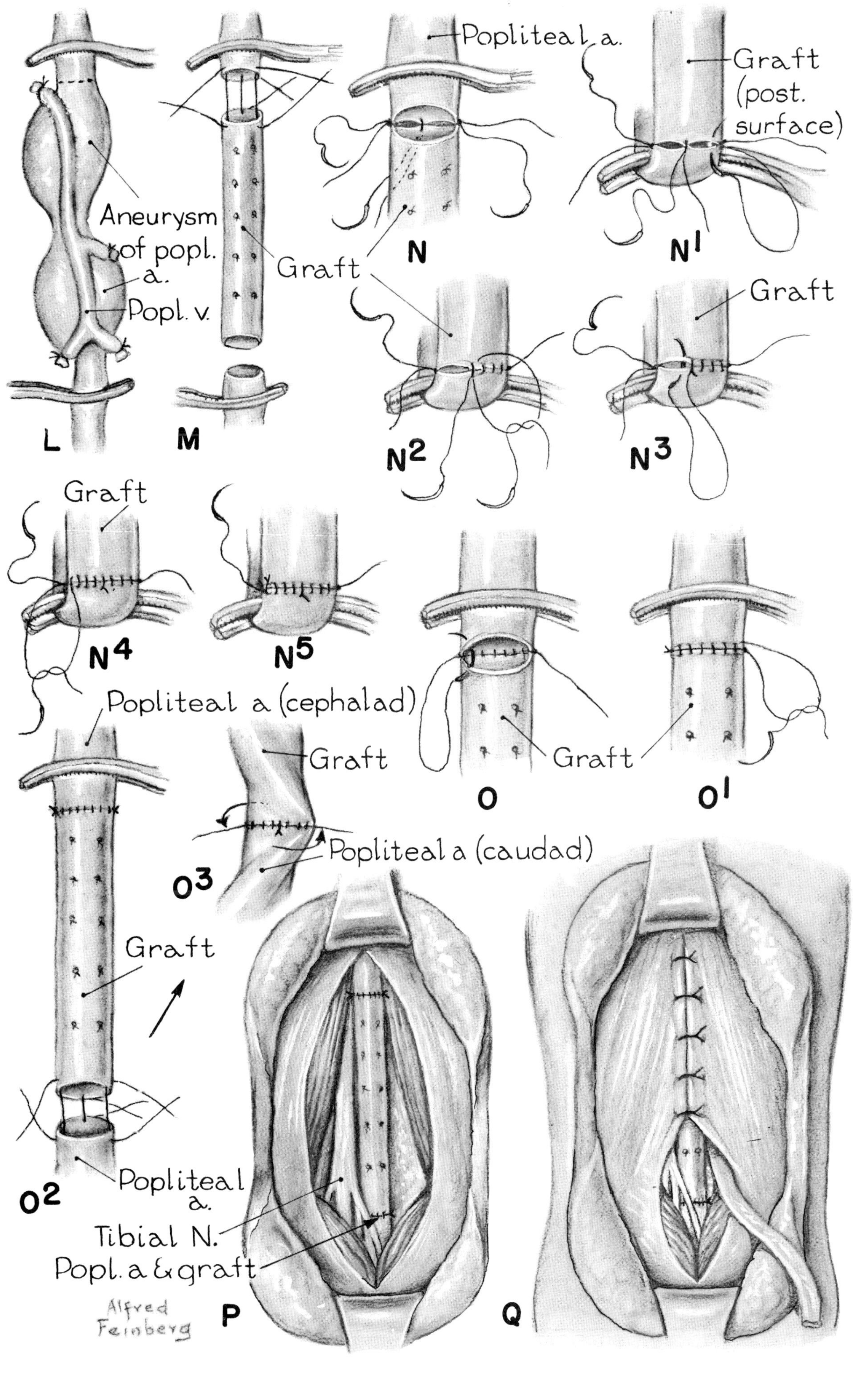
Aneurysm of popl. a.
Popl. v.
L
M
Popliteal a.
Graft
N
Graft (post. surface)
N1
Graft
N2
N3
Graft
N4
N5
O
Graft
O1
Popliteal a (cephalad)
Graft
Popliteal a (caudad)
O3
Graft
Popliteal a.
O2
Tibial N.
Popl. a & graft
Alfred Feinberg
P
Q

DISCUSSION—DR. JULIAN (cont.)

ation, consists of opening and thromboendarterectomizing the aneurysmal sac after obtaining close proximal and distal control of the afferent and efferent popliteal segments. Branches of the vessel which arise in the aneurysmal portion may then be tied or sutured from within the sac, thereby avoiding in the greatest degree possible damage to collateral vessels. Then, if re-establishment of vascular continuity proves impossible or insecure, as is sometimes the case if occlusion has already developed, ischemic necrosis of the extremity is avoided. In patients having prior occlusion either by thrombosis of the aneurysm or arteriosclerotic obstruction of the vessel distal to the aneurysm, a lumbar sympathectomy is done at some time in relation to the operation for aneurysm.

The selection of a segment of the patient's saphenous vein or one of woven dacron tubing for restoring circulation is optimum. The defect resulting from removal of the popliteal aneurysm is usually not very long and the graft used to fill it does not really cross the active flexion area of the knee. Since the lesser saphenous vein is not to be depended upon for size and muscularity, and the long saphenous vein may be difficult to obtain in the semi-prone position most often used, a Dacron prosthesis is frequently our choice.

A Z-shaped incision, such as that illustrated in Figure A, is most often used, except that the proximal limb would seem better placed on the medial side of the thigh where an extension even further proximally will allow for higher control of the popliteal artery if the aneurysm is an extensive one. Indeed, proximal control in the thigh at the level of the adductor hiatus is sometimes convenient in very large aneurysms. Another variation which we have found valuable has been to carry the distal limb of the incision downward in the midline of the calf which obviates the need for any elevation of a distal flap as shown in Figure B.

The odd dumbbell shape of the popliteal aneurysm illustrated has been present in several cases in our series. It seems to be produced by an especially firm area of the fascia of the popliteal fossa which crosses the waist of the lesion. A careful definition and dissection of the nerve and its branches is essential. However, it is often difficult to free the displaced and compressed popliteal vein from the aneurysm and this is not essential at this stage if the aneurysm is to be opened and cleared out after clamping the popliteal artery above and below it. It is believed that preservation of the popliteal vein is worthwhile in preventing the postoperative edema of the leg which occasionally otherwise occurs.

In small aneurysms, the dissection and removal can easily follow the steps illustrated in Figures G through J_2. The mobility of a small lesion is such that arterial branches originating from it can be controlled close to the wall but at the same time the compression of the popliteal vein is usually not so great but what it can be freed and preserved. In large aneurysms much time may be spent without real advantage in freeing the wall of the aneurysm from outside, and if the sac is instead opened and evacuated, much of the wall may be then removed far more easily, arterial branches controlled more quickly, and the vein which can assume its normal size with the compressing force relieved be dissected without damage from the loose aneurysm wall.

Whether the aneurysm is removed intact or after incision and thromboendarterectomy, the artery proximally and distally is transected and the stage indicated in Figure M reached. The technic used in doing each of the two anastomoses is subject to great variation. They are almost always carried out using continuous sutures, interrupted as shown at two points in the circumference. The first anastomosis is more easily accomplished because the other end of the graft is free and, therefore, it may be advantageous to do the distal one before the proximal. This is because the transection is often quite close to the popliteal artery bifurcation, or because thromboendarterectomy may have been required at this point to fashion a proper lumen through which good backflow occurs in patients with distal occlusive disease.

Arteriosclerotic changes in the patient's vessel may make it unwise to rotate it in constructing the posterior row of the second anastomosis, as shown in Figure O_3, whether this be at the proximal or the distal end. An alternative to rotation is to place the holding sutures at dorsal and ventral points rather than at lateral points.

Two additional points deserve mention as maneuvers designed to prevent thrombotic or embolic occlusion of the distal arteries during the operation. One concerns early clamping of the efferent popliteal artery, avoiding firm retraction of the aneurysm before this is done. The obvious purpose is to prevent downward displacement of some broken off piece of the mural thrombus that these aneurysms almost always contain. The second point concerns the use of heparin during surgery. This is administered at the time that circulation through the aneurysm into the leg is interrupted by clamping. It may be given as a single systemic dose of 0.25 to 0.5 mg. per kilogram, or injected in dilute solution into the distal popliteal arterial lumen which is opened early for this purpose.

Even with careful hemostasis, the use of a soft drain led from beneath the deep fascia through the skin wound is certainly desirable. It should, however, be removed in four to six hours to minimize the slight possibility that it might permit contamination of the graft.

DISCUSSION—DR. ROBERT R. LINTON. Popliteal aneurysms, whether of luetic, arteriosclerotic, or traumatic origin, should be excised as described and illustrated in the text because they are a risk to both limb and life if not treated. Secondary thrombosis eventually occurs if they are left in place, with resulting gangrene of the leg necessitating amputation in the majority of cases. This can be prevented in all cases by resection of the aneurysm with the insertion of some type of graft to restore arterial continuity. It has been found possible to excise these aneurysms safely, prior to grafting procedures, by first protecting the limb by a preliminary lumbar sympathetic ganglionectomy.

In more recent years, it has been possible, with the advance in the technic of arterial grafting procedures, to restore arterial continuity in these cases by the implantation of some type of graft. By this newer method, it has not been necessary to perform the lumbar sympathectomy in the majority of cases. In addition, the intermittent claudication which inevitably followed the resection of the aneurysm has been prevented by the restoration of arterial continuity, so that, in general, the method as described and illustrated is to be highly recommended.

It is believed that some of the details of the technic, as shown in the illustrations, can be improved upon in the performance of this procedure. In addition, the type of homograft that is recommended is open to some question. The type of incision used to expose a popliteal aneurysm has never been completely agreed upon. The S-type that is shown in Plate 137A is recommended by some, but it is the opinion of many vascular surgeons that the best incision for operations on major blood vessels is an incision which parallels the course of the blood vessel. Therefore, if the S-type of incision is to be used, it would seem better if the upper extension of it were on the inner side of the thigh rather than on the outer, as is shown, since that is the direction and course of the popliteal and femoral arteries. My preference, on the other hand, is a longitudinal incision without the S-type of configuration. This has been used in several hundreds of cases and has not been the cause of any contracture difficulty, providing the incision is resutured properly and the limb is placed in a posterior splint for a week after the operative procedure.

Retraction of the posterior tibial and peroneal nerves, as shown in Plate 137E, can be less traumatic if a thin piece of Penrose drain is used instead of the ligatures as shown. It is frequently necessary, especially with large aneurysms, to divide the nerve supply to either head of the gastrocnemius muscle. If such is the case there should be no hesitancy in doing this because it results in little, if any, incapacity. Rarely is it necessary to sacrifice the nerve supply to both heads of this muscle.

The popliteal vein is beautifully shown in the Plate 138G, H, and I, and, if possible, preservation and utilization of this vein as an autogenous venous graft to replace the portion of popliteal artery that has to be resected is recommended. In some instances, this is not possible because the vein is so firmly adherent to the aneurysm it cannot be dissected free without injuring it. When this can be accomplished, however, the popliteal vein is believed to make the most satisfactory reconstruction graft that can be found. In other instances, it is recommended that the saphenous vein be utilized if it is found to be of large enough caliber. Autogenous blood vessels are found to serve much more satisfactorily than any other type of arterial replacement, whether it be homologous venous or arterial grafts, or artificial prostheses.

In reviewing the illustrations, there is one very important step in the procedure which is not shown until Plate 139L. This is the application of an occlusive clamp to the popliteal artery distal to the aneurysm. It is recommended that one should be applied before any dissection of the aneurysm is commenced because, if it is not, there is great danger of breaking off portions of an intraaneurysmal clot and causing embolic occlusions of the arteries distal to the aneurysm with resultant serious impairment of the circulation to the lower leg. In my opinion the best type of clamp is a small "bulldog" one; it should be applied to the popliteal artery just distal to the aneurysm before carrying out any extensive dissection elsewhere.

There are various technics of implanting a venous autograft, an arterial homograft, or an artificial synthetic prosthesis. The method illustrated in the plates is one that has been discarded because, with the use of a running suture as demonstrated, stenosis inevitably results at the site of the anastomosis. Instead of the method as depicted, it is recommended that longitudinal slits be made in the host artery and the graft, which permit a much more easily accomplished end-to-end anastomosis without stenosis, even with a running over and over suture. This method of anastomosis also permits one to utilize a blood vessel of smaller caliber than one can use by the end-to-end technic as shown in the illustrations.

The utilization of aortic grafts preserved in alcohol is open to some question. The chief advantage is the availability of them. In the majority of cases, it is believed that a thoracic aorta is much too large in caliber to utilize satisfactorily for the replacement of a peripheral artery such as the popliteal. This may be possible as the result of the sclerosing and shrinking action of the alcohol on the aortic graft.

Drainage of the operative field is of doubtful value, and especially so if one is utilizing a homograft, because of the danger of infection. It is recommended that extreme care should be exercised to obtain complete hemostasis so that drainage will not be necessary. After closure of the incision and the application of a sterile gauze dressing, a posterior splint of either wood or plaster should be applied to keep the knee in extension and so prevent a contracture in the scar. It is recommended that it should not be removed until the fifth postoperative day.

EXCISION OF AN ANEURYSM OF THE COMMON CAROTID ARTERY AND THE INSERTION OF AN AUTOGENOUS VEIN GRAFT

A. The oblique cervical incision paralleling the anterior border of the left sternomastoid muscle is indicated by the solid line.

B. The incision is deepened through the subcutaneous fatty tissue, the platysma muscle, and the anterior layer of the deep cervical fascia to expose portions of the sternothyroid and sternomastoid muscles.

C. The muscles are retracted, and the summit of the traumatic aneurysm of the left common carotid artery is visible beneath the retracted margin of the sternomastoid muscle.

D. The aneurysm and its collateral arterial branches are mobilized from the surrounding tissues by a combination of sharp and blunt dissection. The common carotid artery, both cephalad and caudad to the aneurysm, is encircled by cotton tapes for traction and, if necessary, for temporary mechanical occlusion of the arterial lumen. Guy sutures of silk (000) for traction are also inserted in the wall of the aneurysm.

E, F. The collateral arterial branches are ligated and severed, and mobilization of the aneurysm is continued by scalpel dissection. The adherence of the aneurysm to the internal jugular vein is visible.

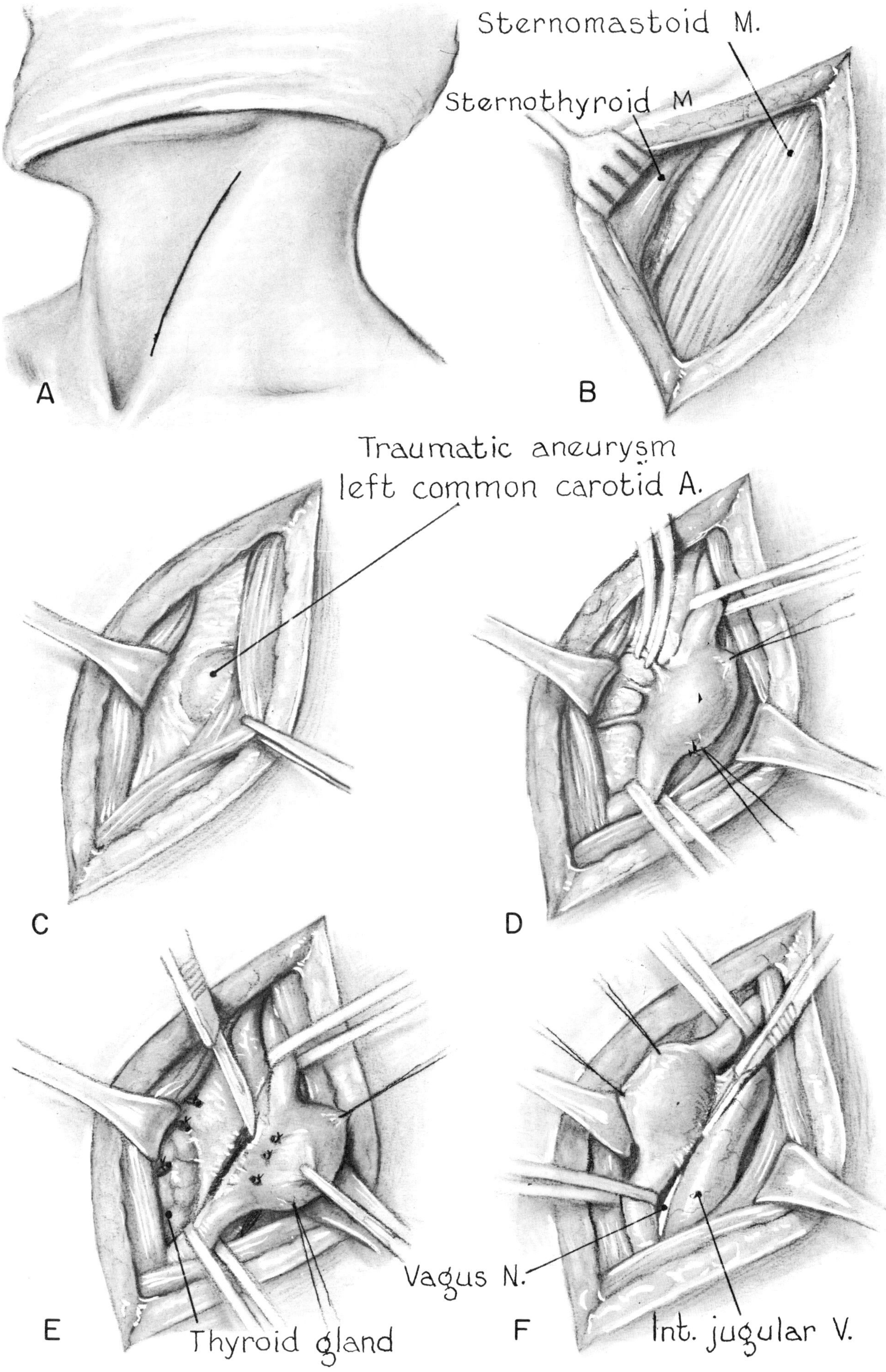
Sternomastoid M.
Sternothyroid M
A
B
Traumatic aneurysm
left common carotid A.
C
D
E
F
Vagus N.
Thyroid gland
Int. jugular V.

G. The mobilization of the aneurysm and portions of the common carotid artery, both cephalad and caudad, is completed. The common carotid artery is occluded by Potts serrafine or "bull dog" clamps on either side of the aneurysm preparatory to its excision. A cuff of the adventitia layer of the artery is removed at each site of election for its transection. This maneuver is more readily accomplished with the artery in continuity as depicted. The carotid artery caudad is being transected with a scalpel over an underlying sterile tongue depressor. The site of arterial transection cephalad is indicated by the dotted line.

G¹, G², G³. The excision of the aneurysm is completed, and the free graft of saphenous vein, which is reversed (cephalad portion is caudad), is aligned between the transected ends of the common carotid artery by three equidistantly placed cardinal guy sutures (00000 silk), which are inserted but not tied (G¹). The guy sutures are tied (G²), and the long strands are used for traction to facilitate the rotation of both the graft and the transected ends of the carotid artery for the insertion of the silk (00000) sutures posteriorly (G³).

H. The excision of the traumatic aneurysm of the left common carotid artery and the insertion of the reversed free graft of the great saphenous vein are completed. The relation of the graft to the surrounding structures is visible.

I. The anterior layer of the deep cervical fascia and then the skin are closed with interrupted sutures of 000 silk.

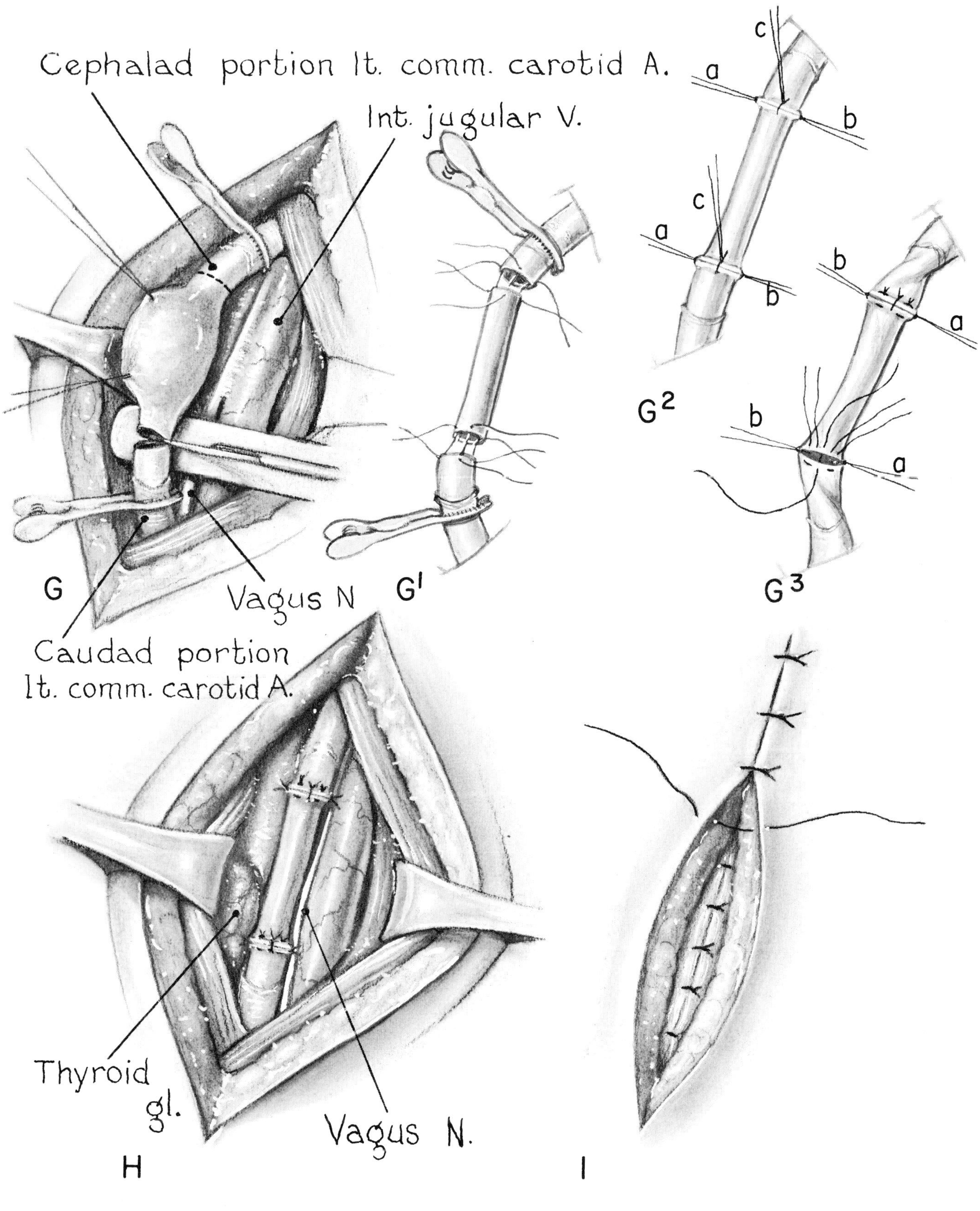
Cephalad portion lt. comm. carotid A.
Int. jugular V.
G
Vagus N
Caudad portion
lt. comm. carotid A.
G'
a
b
c
G2
G3
Thyroid
gl.
Vagus N.
H
I

A. The incision for the removal of a free graft of the great saphenous vein is shown by the solid line. The center of the incision is located at a position 1 inch below the inguinal ligament and 1 inch medial to the femoral arterial pulsation. This has proved an excellent site for the exposure of the cephalic portion of the saphenous vein.

B. The skin incision is deepened to expose the deep layer of the subcutaneous fascia beneath which the saphenous vein is located.

C. The deep layer of the subcutaneous fascia is incised, and the saphenous vein is isolated from the surrounding fatty areolar tissue. A guy suture of silk (00000) is inserted in the adventitia coat of the saphenous vein as a landmark for its proximal level of transection. The vein is doubly clamped. The site for transection of the intervening segment is indicated by dotted lines.

D. The resection of the segment of vein to be used as a free autogenous graft is being completed.

E, F, G. The transected ends of the saphenous vein are occluded proximally and distally with ligatures of 000 silk (E), and a layer closure of the wound is performed, using interrupted sutures of 000 silk (F, G).

H. The length of free graft of saphenous vein obtained is shown. Prior to its insertion, the vein graft is washed thoroughly in a heparin–saline solution (100 mg. of heparin and 250 ml. of normal saline solution).

It should be emphasized that the cephalic portion of the great saphenous vein, because of the comparable diameter of its lumen, is an ideal donor for restoration of continuity of the common carotid artery.

DISCUSSION—DR. HENRY T. BAHNSON. Aneurysms of the carotid artery are not common but in some instances will require treatment because of the danger of thrombosis or embolism from the lesion and a rare danger of rupture.

I would not consider the branches shown arising from the aneurysm as "collateral" branches, as there is no reason for collateral circulation in a simple arterial aneurysm. Indeed, one wonders whether these actually arose from the aneurysm itself as, there are normally no branches from the common carotid. Sometimes vessels in the adjacent tissue become adherent to such an aneurysm but can be dissected off without actually entering the lumen.

Inasmuch as both the common carotid below and the internal carotid above have no branches for some distance, heparin probably should be instilled both proximally and distally to avoid clotting in the blind segment when the vessel is occluded.

The type of suture one uses is largely a matter of personal preference. My own is for an everting mattress suture, usually continuous, or an over-and-over continuous suture. The latter is particularly useful when duration of occlusion is important and one must expedite the anastomosis. In any instance small size suture material should be used, and this is perhaps more important than the exact way of placing it.

In many instances sufficient mobilization of the carotid arteries can be obtained so that anastomosis might be done without a graft. If a graft is required, the saphenous vein is believed preferable. The graft should be treated as a fragile bit of living tissue and, hence, handled gently, grasping only adventitia with forceps if it must be grasped. I would question the artist's illustration of the saphenous vein as I think it runs in a more vertical direction than shown.*

With a satisfactory anastomosis and lumen, one normally would not need heparin or other anticoagulants in the postoperative period.

---

* Lower down, yes; but at this level the obliquity of the saphenous vein as depicted is believed characteristic [J. L. M.].

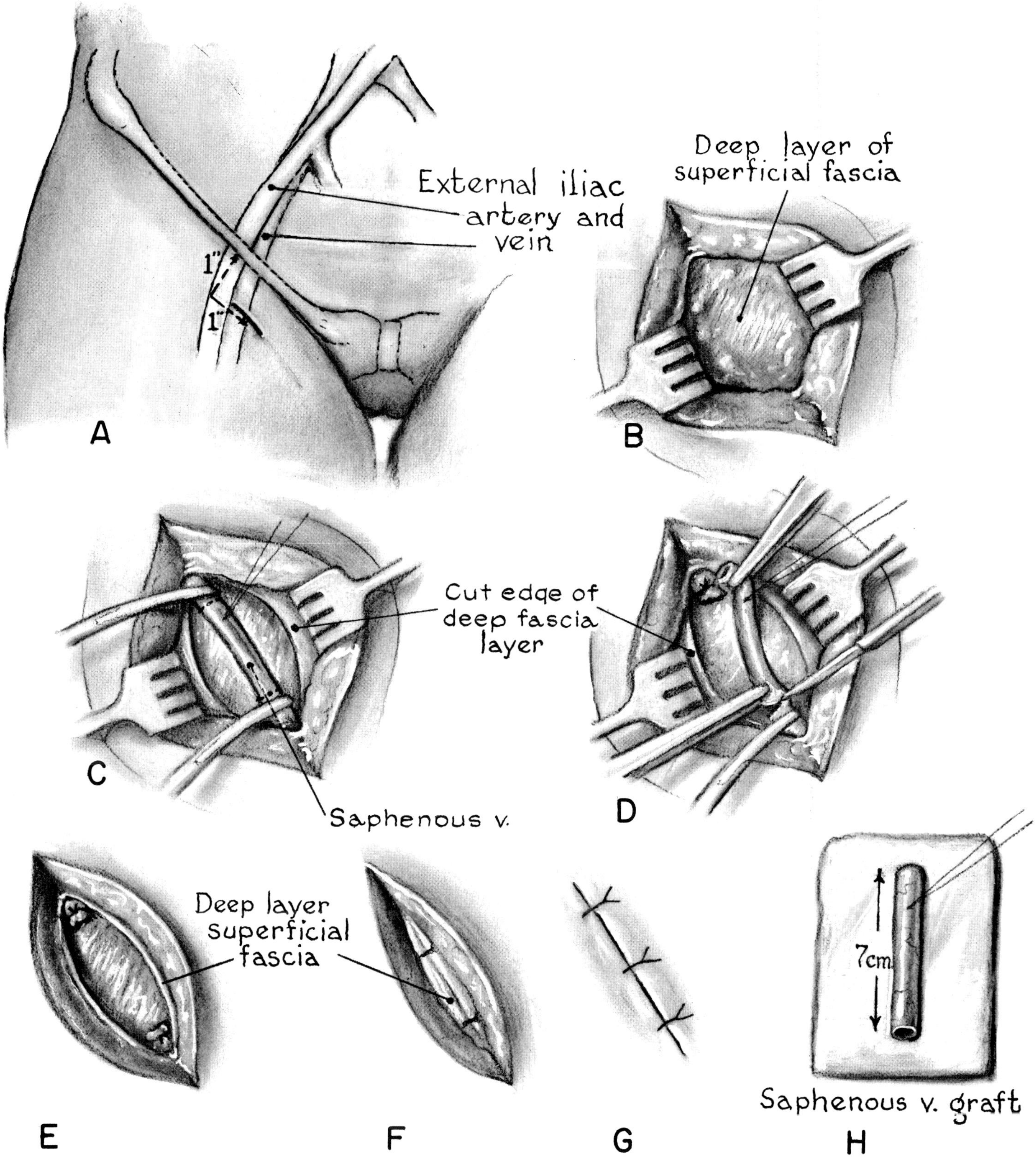
External iliac
artery and
vein
1"
1"
A
Deep layer of
superficial fascia
B
Cut edge of
deep fascia
layer
C
Saphenous v.
D
Deep layer
superficial
fascia
7cm.
Saphenous v. graft
E
F
G
H

CAROTID THROMBOENDARTERECTOMY

A. The patient is placed in the supine position, and the head is rotated to the right. The oblique cervical incision, paralleling the anterior border of the sternomastoid muscle, is indicated by the broken line.

Although local anesthesia is recommended by many for this operation, general anesthesia is preferred. Since these patients are frequently restless and uncooperative, the admitted advantage of having the patient awake to detect the signs of cerebral ischemia on occlusion of the common carotid artery, is not infrequently offset by his restlessness.

B. The platysma muscle layer is incised, and a portion of the underlying anterior or investing layer of the deep cervical fascia is visible. An unusually wide exposure of the platysma muscle, the fibers of which are accentuated, is shown.

C. The anterior layer of the deep cervical fascia is incised, and the sternomastoid muscle is retracted posteriorly to expose the dissection of the fascia and fibroareolar tissue layers that overlie the carotid sheath. In the lower part of the wound, the inferior belly of the omohyoid muscle may be seen lying on its "fascial carpet," the middle layer (pre-thyroid) of the deep cervical fascia.

D. The carotid sheath is opened, and a tributary of the internal jugular vein is being severed between clamps.

E. The mobilized segment of the internal jugular vein is retracted posteriorly, and the adventitia of the common carotid artery is removed by scalpel dissection. The vagus nerve is visible between and deep to the vein and artery. The superior thyroid artery, which usually is the first branch of the external carotid artery, is also visible. In this patient it arose from the common carotid artery just proximal to its bifurcation.

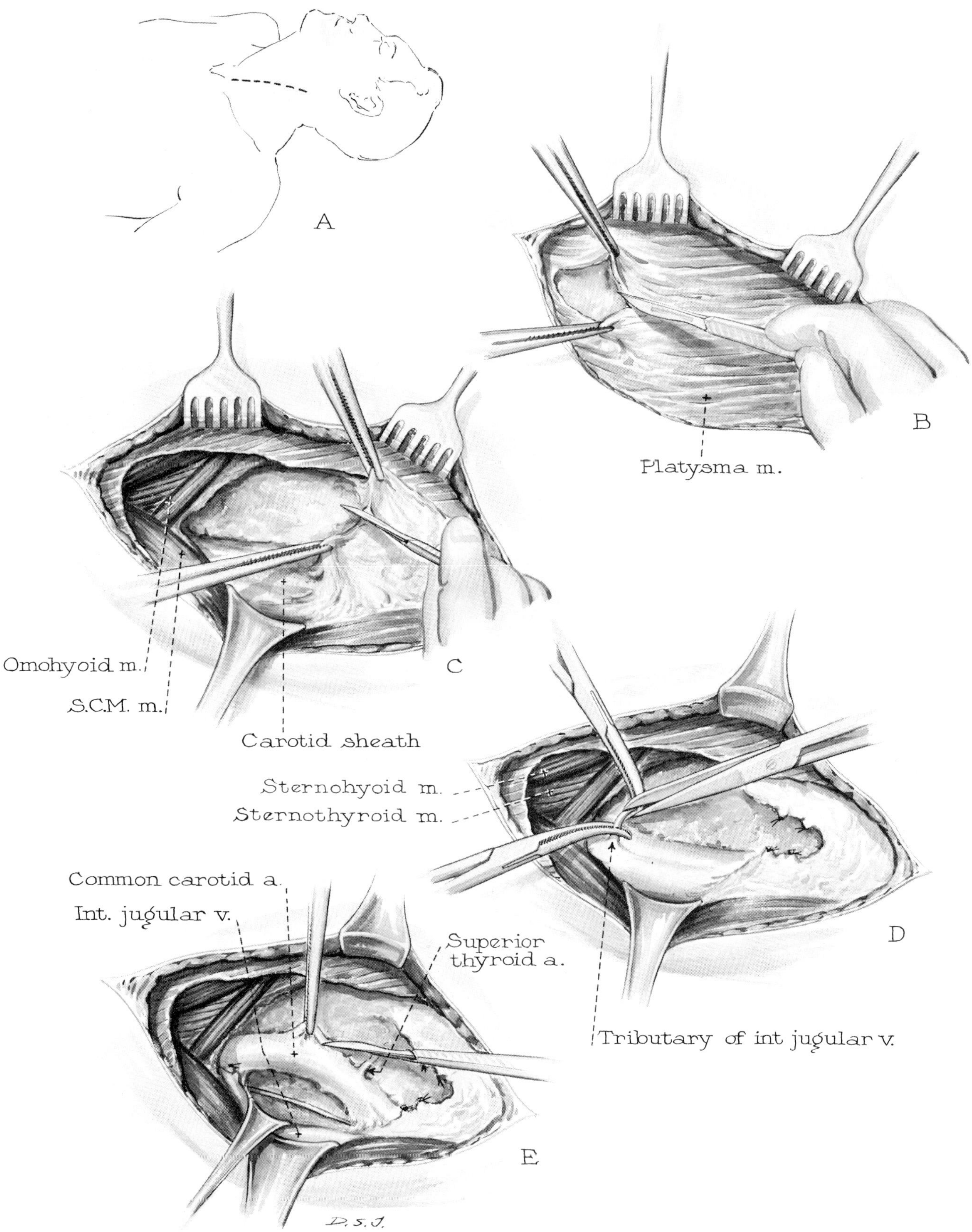

A
B
Platysma m.
C
Omohyoid m.
S.C.M. m.
Carotid sheath
Sternohyoid m.
Sternothyroid m.
D
Tributary of int jugular v.
Common carotid a.
Int. jugular v.
Superior thyroid a.
E
D.S.J.

F. The common carotid artery is retracted medialward, and the vagus nerve is elevated on a clamp that overlies the internal jugular vein.

G. The superior thyroid artery is doubly clamped and is being severed between the clamps.

H. The external and internal carotid arteries are mobilized by blunt dissection, and a cotton tape is shown being withdrawn beneath the proximal portion of the external carotid artery.

I. The common carotid artery and its branches are encircled by cotton tapes, and the relative size and shape of the occluding thrombus is depicted. A pulsatile blood flow was present in the external but not in the internal carotid artery. Potts' serrefine clamps are open and held in readiness to occlude the common and external carotid arteries after exposure and partial freeing of the thrombus. The duration of occlusion of the carotid arterial flow should be kept to a minimum.

J, K. An incision (broken line) is being made over the site of the thrombus and extends caudad from the origin of the internal carotid artery onto the common carotid artery for a distance of approximately 5 cm. (J). The incision is deepened to the level of the thrombus and a guy suture of silk (00000) is inserted through the center of each cut margin. The common and external carotid arteries are still unoccluded.

DISCUSSION—DRS. B. EISEMAN AND FRANK SPENCER. In positioning the patient extensive rotation of the head must be avoided, particularly with the neck extended, since this has been shown to decrease markedly blood flow through the carotid-vertebral axis. Though of little importance with a normal circulation, it may be a critical factor in patients with carotid or vertebral artery insufficiency. A preoperative and preanesthetic trial of such an exaggerated position may be warranted.

The use of local anesthesia is preferred, utilizing a posterior cervical block. Its advantages are (1) the constant ability to monitor the neurologic status of the patient to ascertain that there is no cerebral hypoxia requiring alteration or cessation of the operative procedure, (2) the (hypothetical) advantage of stellate and sympathetic block in increasing cerebral blood flow, and (3) its simplicity.

General anesthesia has the advantage of keeping the patient quiet, but restlessness may be and usually is a sign of cerebral hypoxia—a danger warning. There is no good evidence, either clinical or experimental, that anesthesia, or even deep anesthesia, decreases the metabolic demands of cerebral tissue. Indeed, all experimental evidence is to the contrary, so that its use must be justified on technical, not metabolic, grounds. If general anesthesia is used, an internal shunt should be employed, because some patients with bilateral arterial disease may develop serious neurologic injury from a very short period of occlusion.

In order to attain maximum cerebral blood flow through all existing collateral vessels during occlusion, it is advised to maintain a systolic arterial hypertension of approximately 180 to 200 mm. Hg during the period of carotid occlusion. Obtainable by the anesthesiologist in a number of ways, we advise an intravenous drip of neosynephrine.

Atherosclerotic plaques may contain friable granulations that can be dislodged by manipulation of the unopened vessel and cause cerebral emboli. It is, therefore, advised that encircling tapes and occluding clamps be placed at a distance from the plaque and that the bulb be left undisturbed without circumferential mobilization. Thus properly isolated, the incision can be made on its anterior surface.

As with any endarterectomy, the distal end of

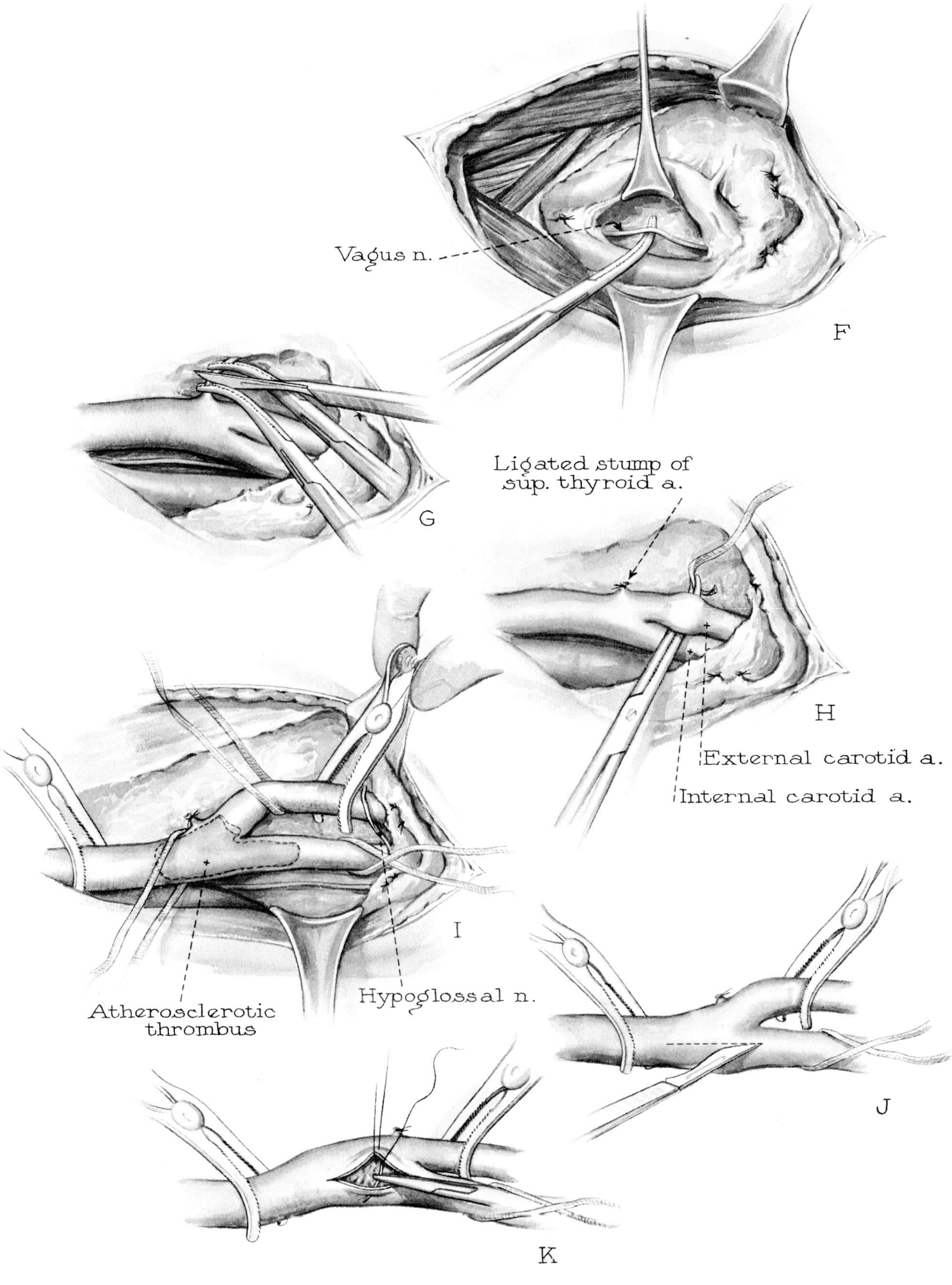
Vagus n.
F
G
Ligated stump of
sup. thyroid a.
H
External carotid a.
Internal carotid a.
I
Atherosclerotic
thrombus
Hypoglossal n.
J
K

L, M, N. The thrombus is mobilized from within the lumen of the artery by an instrument * of special design. When completely mobilized about its whole circumference, the thrombus is elevated on the dissector (M). Gentle traction is made on the liberated caudad portion of the thrombus as its extension cephalad into the internal carotid artery is being dissected free (N).

The absence of a retrograde flow in the internal carotid artery after the removal of a thrombus is not of the same grave prognostic import as when it occurs in the lower extremity. Repeatedly, patients have shown marked clinical improvement upon restoration of the blood flow in the internal carotid artery even though a retrograde flow was absent.

Upon removal of the segment of thrombus within the lumen of the external carotid artery, active retrograde bleeding occurs. Accordingly, the immediate occulusion of the artery with a serrefine clamp is required to prevent both the unnecessary loss of blood and imbalance of the cerebral circulation. Although extension of the thrombus into the external carotid artery frequently occurs, occlusion of its lumen is rarely present.

O. Inset shows the thrombus after its removal.

P, Q. The lumens of the common carotid artery and its branches are first flushed with a heparin-saline solution (100 mg. of heparin in 250 cc. of saline), and a series of interrupted sutures of silk (00000) are inserted but not tied (Q).

R. Upward traction is maintained on the sutures for hemostasis as the serrefine clamps are removed.

* Manufactured by Edward Weck & Co., Long Island City, N.Y.

DISCUSSION—DRS. EISEMAN and SPENCER (cont.)

the intimal dissection should be beveled and made as smooth as feasible, utilizing one or two anchoring mattress sutures if necessary, with the knots on the outside of the vessel. In closure of the arteriotomy a continuous suture is both simple and satisfactory.

Long bilateral cervical incisions made at the same operation may cause sufficient laryngeal edema to require tracheostomy. If the first operative procedure requires an extensive dissection, the operation on the opposite carotid artery should be postponed a few days.

In the rare patient who will not tolerate the short period of carotid occlusion that is necessary, an internal rather than an external shunt is advised. Anastomosis of an external shunt to the internal carotid for temporary use is awkward and occasionally requires periods of occlusion approximately equal in length to that required for removal of the plaque itself. Also, closure of the distal temporary shunt site may stenose the internal carotid artery.

An internal shunt of siliconized thin-walled plastic of a proper diameter can easily be slipped beyond the occlusive area and permits adequate blood flow for a major portion of the operation. This is a technic that seldom is required.

The operation depicted is that of a complete occlusion of the carotid artery of recent duration. Unfortunately, the majority of complete carotid occlusions are inoperable because of the cephalad extension of the thrombus in the internal carotid into the skull. Most of the carotid artery lesions that are operable are those that have stenosed but not completely occluded the lumen of the artery.

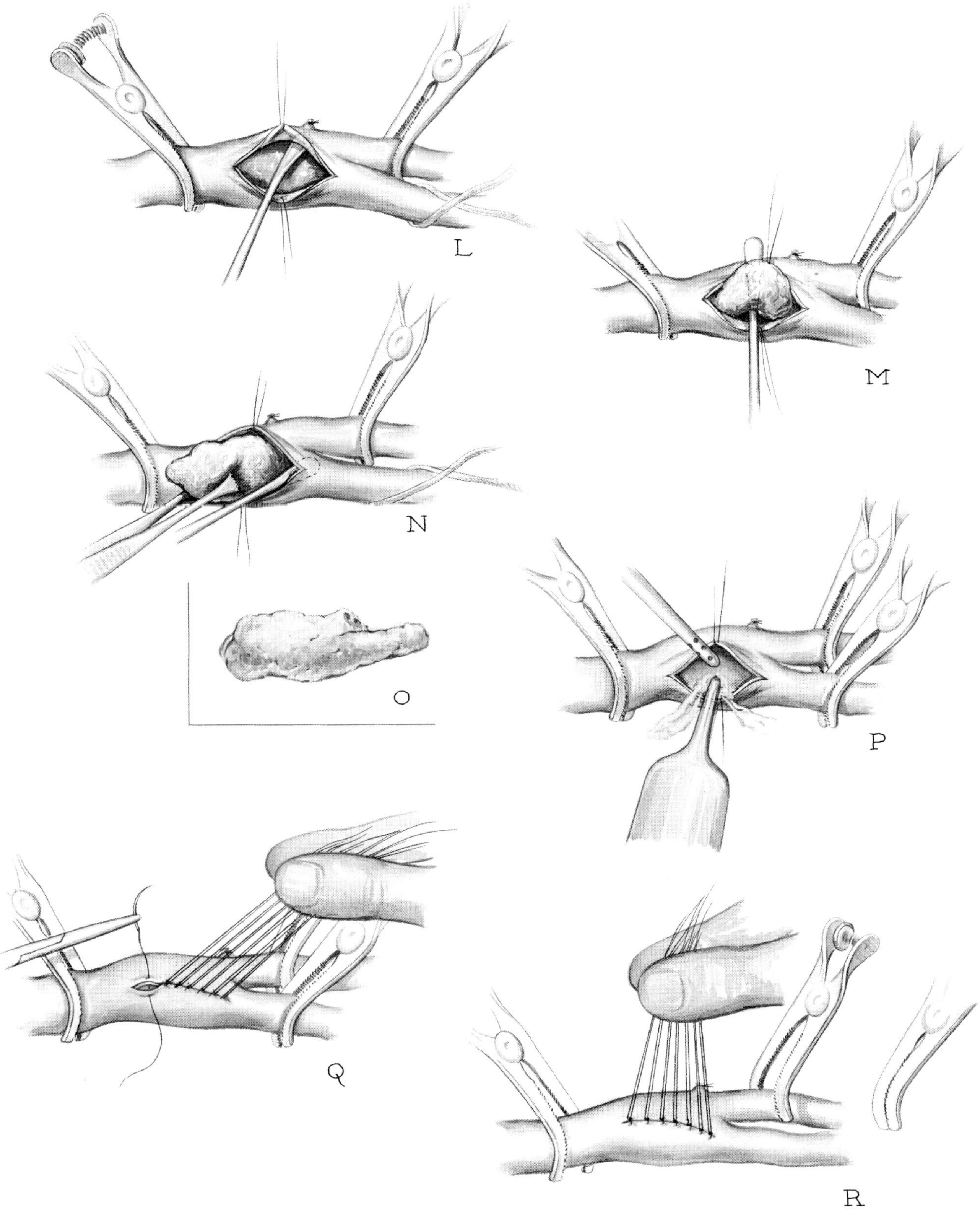
L
M
N
O
P
Q
R

S, T. The arterial circulation is restored and the series of interrupted sutures are tied (S) and cut (T).

U. The platysma muscle layer is approximated with interrupted sutures of silk (000).

V. The skin margins are coapted with a series of fine straight needles (cambric), which are withdrawn individually, and the accompanying suture is tied.

W. The appearance of the incision on completion of the operation is depicted.

DISCUSSION—DR. CHARLES ROB. The incision shown follows the line of the anterior border of the sternomastoid muscle, thus providing excellent exposure of the distal common carotid artery and the cervical portions of the internal and external carotid arteries. When a more limited exposure gives adequate access, as in localized plaques at the carotid bifurcation, a transverse incision centered upon the artery and following the line of the skin folds of the neck gives sufficient exposure and a better scar.

The platysma muscle is divided throughout the whole length of the incision; bleeding points in this layer and in the superficial fascia are secured in the usual manner. The carotid sheath is opened longitudinally to expose the internal jugular vein and carotid arteries. Any tributaries of the jugular vein that cross the anterior surface of the carotid arteries must be divided. These include the common facial vein, which usually enters the jugular vein at approximately the level of the bifurcation of the common carotid artery.

The common carotid artery together with its bifurcation into the internal and external carotid arteries are mobilized, and a tape is passed around the common carotid artery. The internal and external carotid arteries are now separated and mobilized completely. This is made possible by division of the carotid sinus nerves and of all fibrous bands surrounding these vessels. The vagus nerve lies behind the carotid bifurcation and should be carefully identified and preserved. The same applies to the hypoglossal nerve, which crosses in front of both the internal and external carotid arteries close to the digastric muscle.

Greater mobility of the carotid arteries is achieved by division of the superior thyroid artery. In many patients this is unnecessary, sufficient exposure being possible without sacrificing this vessel. Tapes are now passed around the internal and external carotid arteries. By palpation and inspection the extent of the plaque of atheroma can now be determined. This usually involves the distal 1 cm. of the common carotid artery and the proximal 2 cm. of the internal carotid artery.

Clamps are applied first to the external then to the common and internal carotid arteries. Just before the internal carotid artery is clamped 50 mg of heparin may be injected directly into the lumen of this vessel. In addition, any other branches such as the superior thyroid artery should be clamped if they have not previously been ligatured. An incision is now made through the wall of the artery overlying the area of disease. This incision lies in the long axis of the internal carotid artery. A plane of cleavage is now established in the layers of the media. A thromboendarterectomy is performed so that the atheroma, the intima, the internal elastic lamina, the inner layers of the media, and any blood clot are removed. The adventitia, external elastic lamina, and outer layers of the media are left in position.

The plane of cleavage in the media is developed by blunt dissection, and a thromboendarterectomy of the distal common carotid and proximal internal carotid arteries is performed. After completing the thromboendarterectomy, it is important to remove all loose fragments and debris, thereby reducing the risk to subsequent embolization. This is best accomplished by thorough flushing with saline.

Before closing the arteriotomy incision, the clamp on the internal carotid should be opened for a few moments to flush out this vessel. The incision is then closed with 0000 silk, either continuous or interrupted sutures being satisfactory. The former have the advantage that the force of the blood flow will tighten further the suture line. If it appears that the suture line will narrow the lumen, then a patch graft, preferably a segment of autogenous vein, may be used. The clamp on the internal carotid artery is removed followed by those on the common and external carotid arteries. At this point there is frequently some bleeding from the suture line, but firm pressure with a gauze square for five minutes usually stops this. If it is not sufficient extra sutures may be required.

The wound closure is in two layers, using interrupted sutures of fine silk for the platysma muscle and interrupted sutures for the skin. In many patients a drain inserted for 24 hours reduces the risk of hematoma formation.

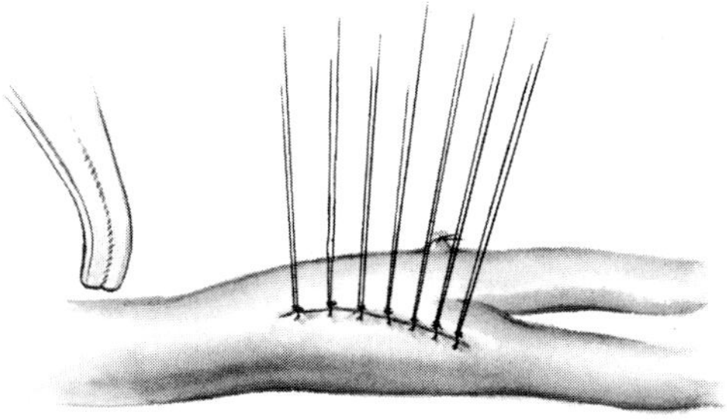

S

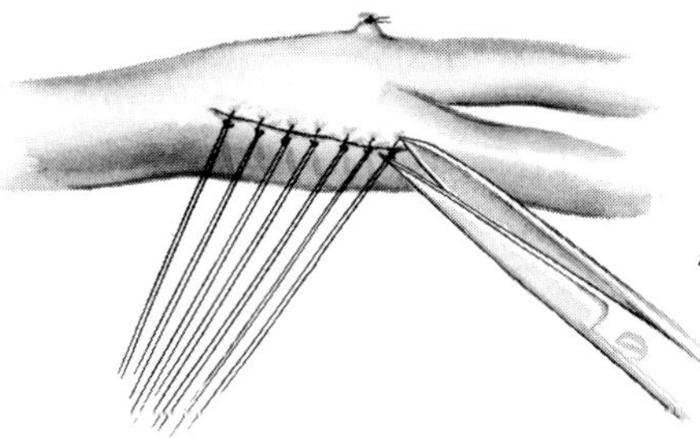

T

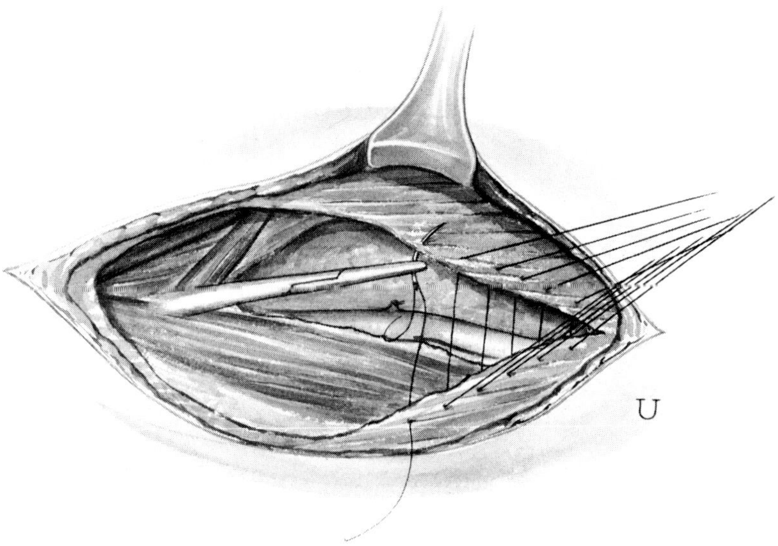

U

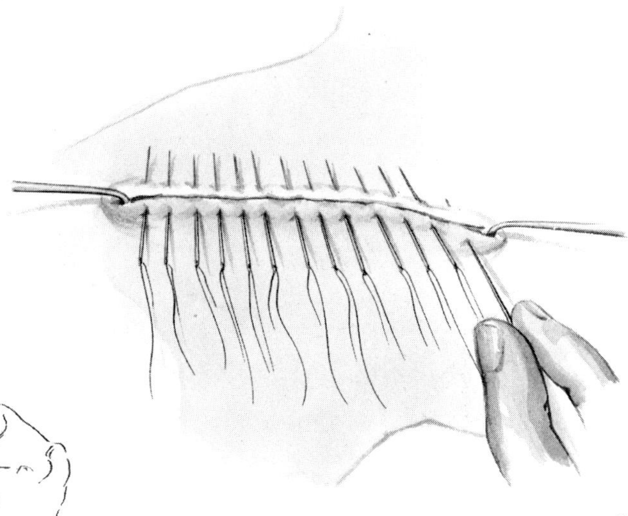

V

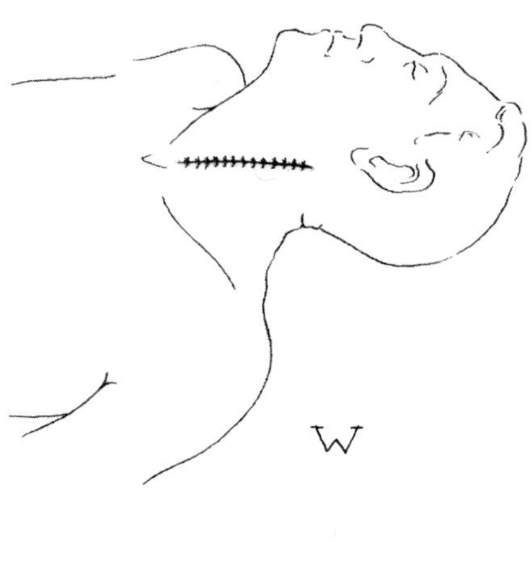

W

CAROTID ARTERIAL BYPASS GRAFT (DACRON)

A. This patient, a 58-year-old man, had recurrent episodes of momentary "blackouts" over a period of 18 months. Right carotid and right radial arterial pulsations were diminished to absent. The diagnosis of an aortic arch syndrome (Martorell) being a likely possibility, a supraclavicular incision (1) was first made after marking out (broken line) the anterolateral chest incision. Excellent carotid arterial pulsations were present proximally, and a second, more cephalad, transverse cervical incision (2) was made. Because of the inadequate exposure, a vertical connecting incision (3) was required. The primary supraclavicular incision (1) is completed and the cervical incisions subsequently made are indicated (2, 3). The chest incision (broken line) was not required.

B. The incision is deepened through the subcutaneous fatty tissue and platysma muscle layers, and the underlying related structures are exposed. The severance of the tendon of the omohyoid muscle is indicated (broken line).

C. The muscle structures are retracted, and the line of incision in the middle layer of the deep cervical fascia (omohyoid fascial carpet) is shown (broken line). The transverse cervical vessels in the upper portion of the wound are visible.

D, E. Upon incising the omohyoid fascial "carpet," the subjacent fat herniates into the incision. This is displaced to expose the underlying anatomic structures.

F. The previously isolated internal jugular vein and common carotid artery are retracted, and their relation to the vagus nerve posteriorly is seen.

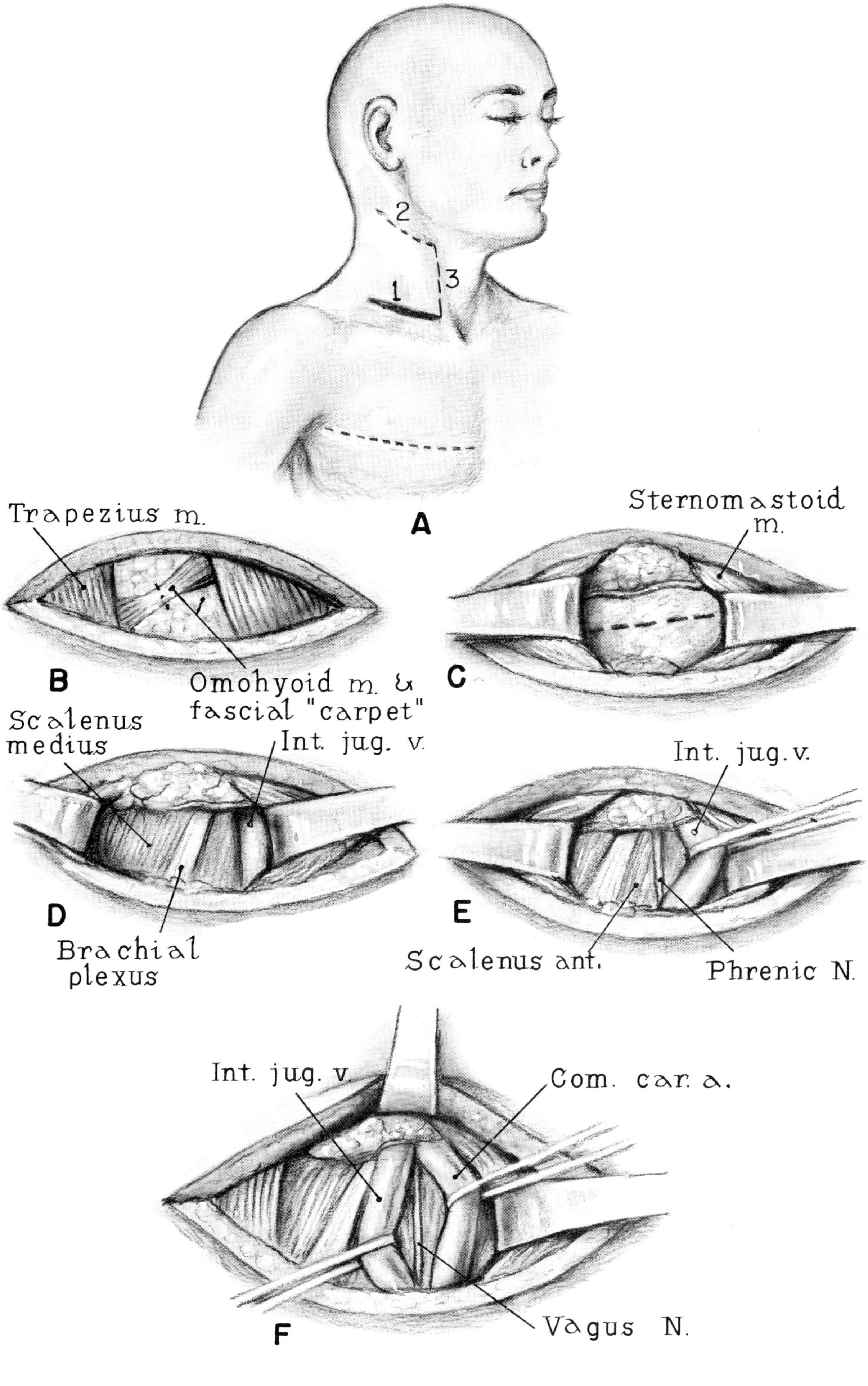
2
3
1
A
Trapezius m.
B
Omohyoid m. & fascial "carpet"
Sternomastoid m.
C
Scalenus medius
Int. jug. v.
D
Brachial plexus
Int. jug. v.
E
Scalenus ant.
Phrenic N.
Int. jug. v.
Com. car. a.
F
Vagus N.

G. Because of the excellent pulsation in the common carotid artery at the level of the supraclavicular incision, a second transverse cervical incision was made more cephalad and overlying the bifurcation of the common carotid artery. To obtain better exposure, the two cervical incisions were later connected by a longitudinal incision as indicated by the broken line.

H, I. The incision is deepened through the platysma muscle (H) to expose the underlying structures (I).

J. The external jugular vein is doubly ligated in continuity and severed. The sternomastoid muscle is retracted to show the mobilized carotid "bulb" and the atherosclerotic thrombotic occlusion (complete) of the proximal portion of the internal carotid artery. The ligated stump of the superior thyroid artery in relation to the carotid bifurcation is visible.

K, L. For better exposure of the operative field, a longitudinal incision is made anteriorly to connect the transverse cervical incisions (K), and the resulting skin and subcutaneous tissue flap is retracted posteriorly (L) to obtain an excellent exposure of the operative field.

Discussion—Drs. B. Eiseman and Frank Spencer. An endarterectomy, with or without a patch graft reconstruction, is always preferred to a bypass graft for a localized obstruction of the carotid artery. About the only situation where such a graft might be required is in a patient where attempted endarterectomy (or excision of the carotid body tumor) so injured the artery that it could not be sutured or patched. Under such unusual conditions systemic or regional heparinization should be employed while the graft is being inserted; this avoids thrombus formation in the occluded arterial segment, which subsequently could embolize to the brain when the occluding clamps were released.

Where, for some reason, an end-to-side jump graft to the carotid artery is necessary, every precaution possible should be taken to avoid the necessity for complete cross-clamping of the internal carotid during the anastomosis.

Bypass grafts of this type are occasionally indicated in extensive lesions of the aortic arch and its major branches to "jump" a series of obstructive segments. When thus employed, accurate preoperative roentgenographic visualization of the block should obviate the need for "searching incisions." Indeed, external inspection and palpation of these large vessels at operation may not give an accurate evaluation of the degree of obstruction. Open arteriotomy may be required to appreciate the extent of localized blocks of the "take-off" of the innominate or the common carotid arteries.

Incision for exposure of the aortic arch and its major vessels to the head and upper extremities is best obtained by a supraclavicular and a second interspace incision as illustrated, but connected by a median sternotomy. The sternoclavicular joint is thus not defiled. The incision is kept open by small chest retractors.

Occasionally in a high-lying aortic arch sufficient length of the distal innominate artery can be exposed solely from the supraclavicular approach after its thorough mobilization. This is not, however, an area where loss of proximal arterial control is either desirable or conducive to careful technic.

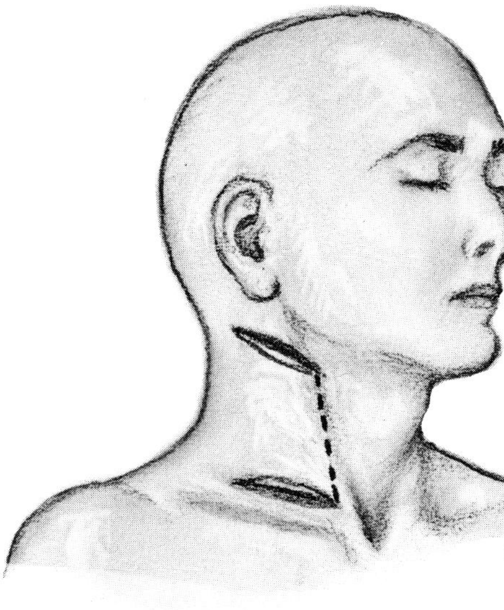

G

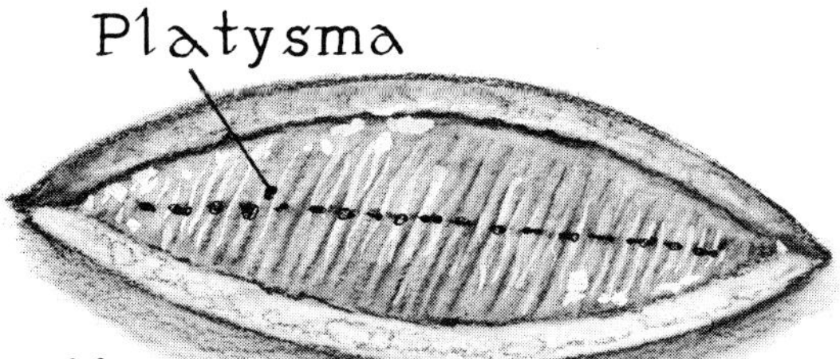
Platysma

H

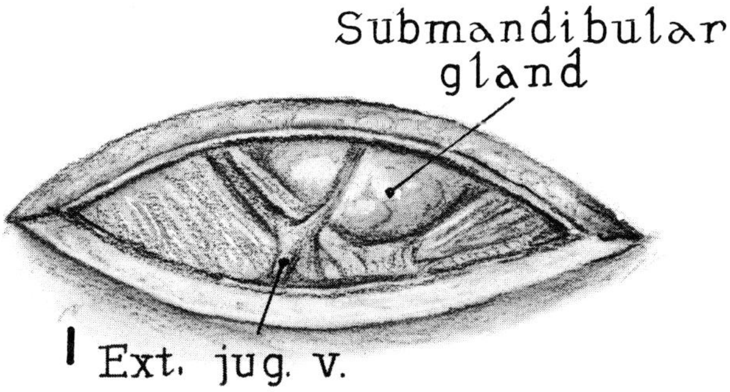
Submandibular gland
Ext. jug. v.

I

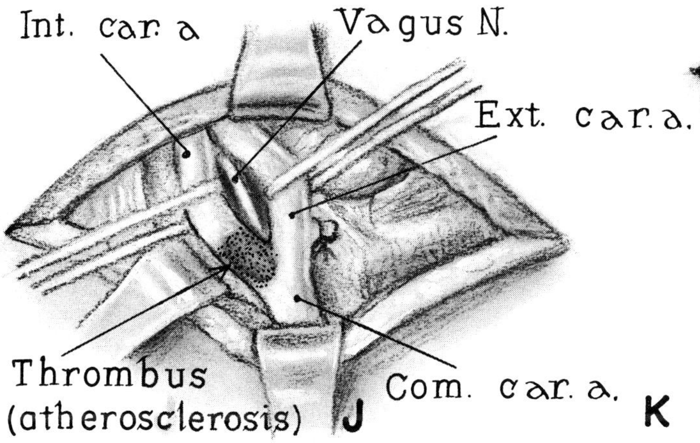
Int. car. a
Vagus N.
Ext. car. a.
Thrombus (atherosclerosis)
Com. car. a.

J

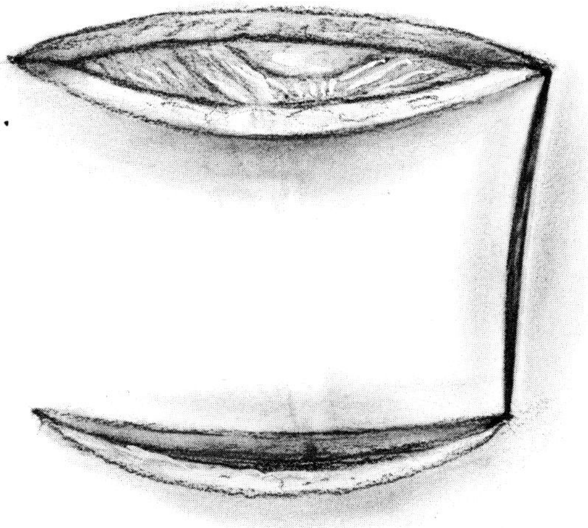

K

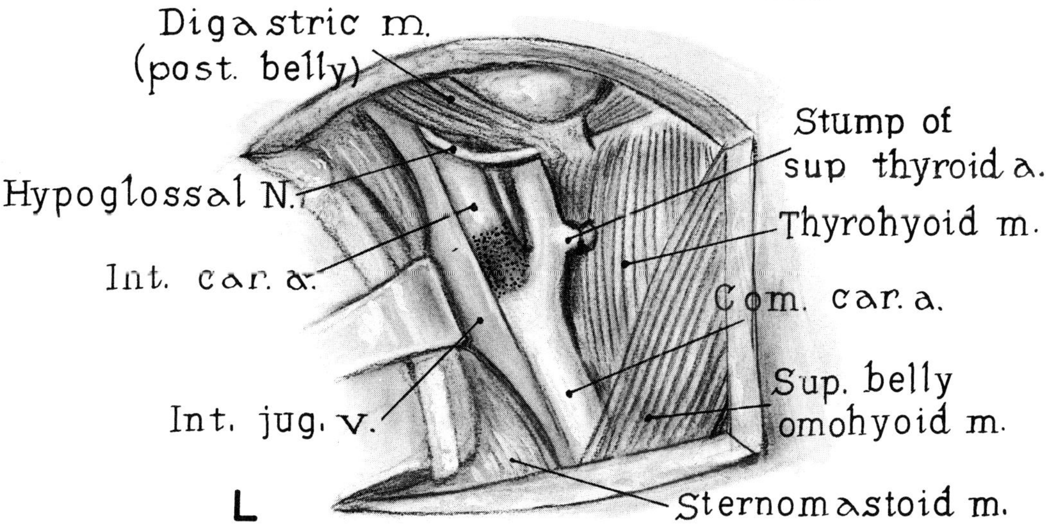
Digastric m. (post. belly)
Stump of sup thyroid a.
Hypoglossal N.
Thyrohyoid m.
Int. car. a.
Com. car. a.
Sup. belly omohyoid m.
Int. jug. v.
Sternomastoid m.

L

M. The lumen of the common carotid artery is partially occluded with a Beck-Potts clamp and the incision to be made into the lumen of the occluded segment is indicated by the broken line.

N, O, P. The ends of the graft are severed obliquely at an angle of 45° (N, O) and the "angle" sutures for the anastomosis caudad are inserted (P).

Q, R. The lower "angle" suture is tied, and its needle strand (a) is continued cephalad as an over-and-over suture (Q) and tied to the needle free strand (b) of the upper "angle" suture (R).

S, T. Similarly, the needle strand (b) of the upper "angle" suture is continued caudad as an over-and-over suture and will be tied to the needle free strand (a′) of the lower "angle" suture.

U. The anastomosis caudad is completed, and after the application of clamps to the graft and to the internal carotid artery distally, the clamp on the common carotid artery is removed. The "angle" sutures for the anastomosis cephalad are inserted, and the anastomosis is completed as previously demonstrated.

V. The operative field on completion of the insertion of the by-pass graft (teflon) is shown. An arteriogram 14 months postoperatively showed complete patency of the graft.* The patient has been asymptomatic since the operation.

* Eighteen months postoperatively, complete thrombosis within the lumen of the graft occurred and was associated with the recurrence of cerebral symptoms. The graft was replaced with an autogenous vein (saphenous) graft, and concomitant clinical improvement was observed. Because of the delayed and imperfect maturation of the pseudointima in the teflon grafts, their use in the small peripheral arteries (e.g., carotid, femoral) is not advocated.

Discussion—Dr. Charles Rob. A bypass graft for occlusion of the carotid arteries is most frequently used where there is an extensive disease of the distal common carotid as well as the proximal internal carotid artery. Two incisions are required over the common carotid artery at the base of the neck and the other over the carotid bifurcation.

In the exposure of the common carotid artery, the incision is placed about 1 in. above the clavicle and over the sternomastoid muscle. After division of the platysma muscle, the sternomastoid muscle is identified, behind which the carotid sheath lies. The common carotid artery may be exposed, as illustrated, by retraction medially of the lateral border of the sternomastoid muscle. An alternative and perhaps a better way is to retract the medial border of the sternomastoid muscle laterally. Once identified the common carotid artery is mobilized for a distance of about three inches.

In the exposure of the carotid bifurcation, the incision follows the lines of the skin folds of the neck and is centered upon the carotid bifurcation. The platysma muscle is divided, as is the external jugular vein. The sternomastoid muscle is retracted posteriorly and the carotid sheath identified. At this point it is often necessary to divide the common facial vein. The distal common carotid artery together with the proximal internal and external carotid arteries are then mobilized, great care being taken to preserve the vagus and hypoglossal nerves. Sufficient of the internal carotid artery must be mobilized to permit of an end-to-side anastomosis distal to the area of arterial disease.

A tunnel for the graft is then made between the two incisions. The bypass graft is anastomosed end-to-side to the common carotid artery proximally and to the internal carotid distally. A variety of materials have been used to bypass the carotid artery; these include prostheses of teflon and dacron and segments of autogenous vein. A teflon prosthesis, as illustrated here, gives good early results, but long-term follow-up studies show that the use of an autogenous vein is better. A suitable length of the long saphenous vein is removed and reversed so that the proximal end is anastomosed to the side of the internal carotid artery and the distal end to the side of the common carotid artery.

The anastomosis is performed with a continuous over-and-over suture of 0000 silk if a vein graft is used or merselene if a plastic prosthesis is inserted. After completion of both anastomoses, the distal clamp is removed first, followed by the proximal clamp. If bleeding occurs firm pressure is applied with a gauze square for five minutes. Later, if haemostasis is not complete, further sutures may be needed but these are rarely necessary.

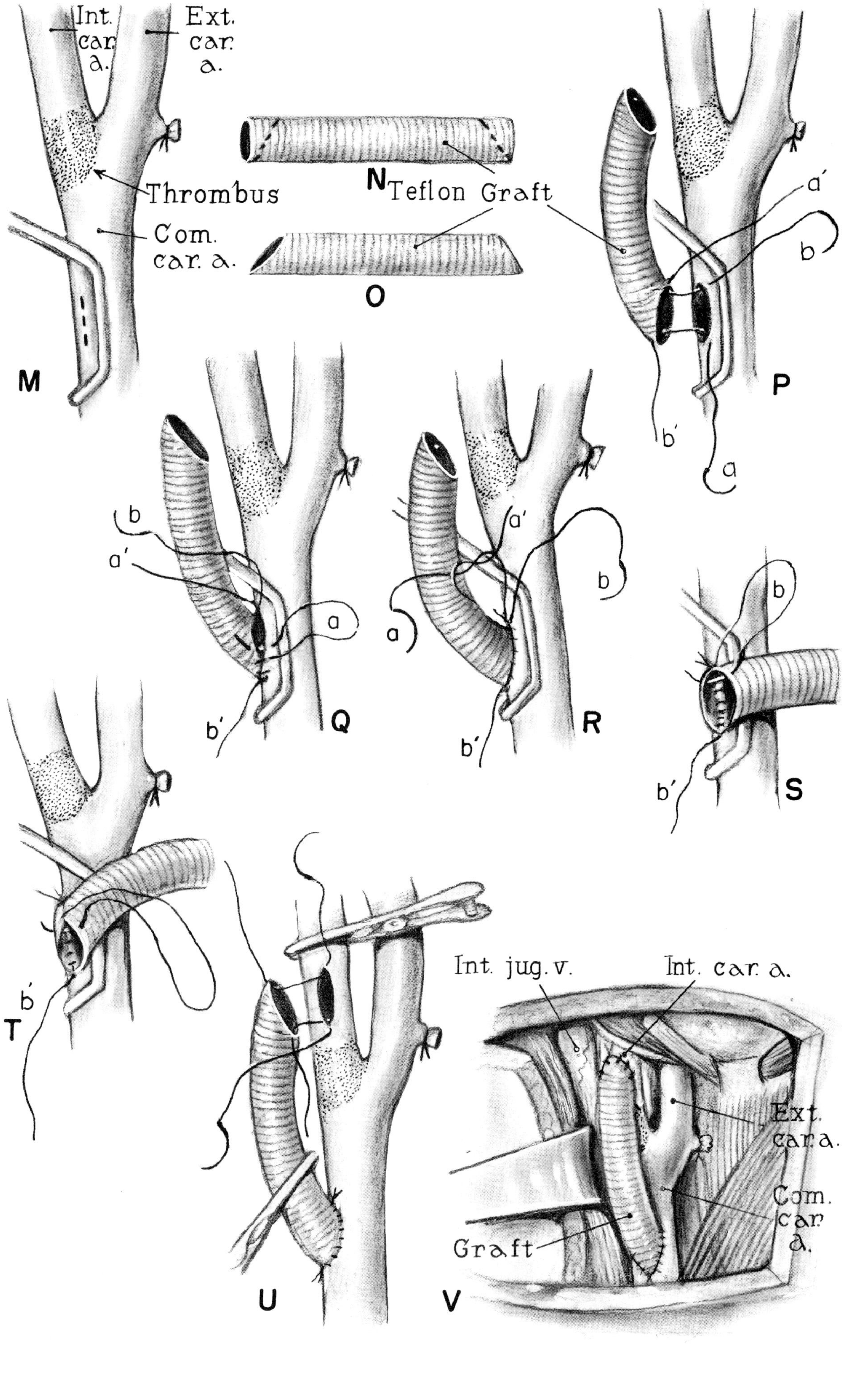
Int. car. a.
Ext. car. a.
Thrombus
Com. car. a.
M
N
Teflon Graft
O
a'
b
b'
a
P
Q
R
S
T
U
V
Int. jug. v.
Int. car. a.
Ext. car. a.
Com. car. a.
Graft

CAROTID GLOMECTOMY

A. The skin incision (broken line), which begins at the angle of the mandible and parallels the anterior border of the sternomastoid muscle, extends obliquely caudad for one-third the distance from the angle of the mandible to the sternoclavicular junction.

B. The incision is deepened through the subcutaneous fatty tissue layer, and the underlying platysma muscle is shown being severed with a scalpel.

C. The sternomastoid muscle is retracted laterally, and one of a group of cervical lymph nodes, held in a clamp (Babcock), is being mobilized by scissor dissection. Although not commonly a problem in the exposure of the carotid bulb, in this particular patient there was an unusually large group of lymph nodes, the removal of which was necessary before continuing the dissection.

D. The common facial vein, doubly ligated in continuity, is being severed between the ligatures with scissors. This vein, formed by the junction of the anterior and posterior facial veins, is a tributary of the internal jugular vein. A second tributary, the superior thyroid vein, is also visible.

E. The dissection is completed to expose the carotid bulb and related structures. The ligated stumps of the internal jugular vein tributaries previously described are visible. The common carotid artery and the superior thyroid artery are encircled with cotton tapes preparatory to dissection of the carotid bifurcation. The superior thyroid artery, usually described as the first branch of the external carotid artery, not uncommonly arises from the common carotid artery proximal to its bifurcation, as illustrated. The hypoglossal nerve is seen to cross the external carotid artery just cephalad to its occipital and lingual branches. The descending branch of the hypoglossal nerve is visible in relation to the internal jugular vein and the internal and common carotid arteries.

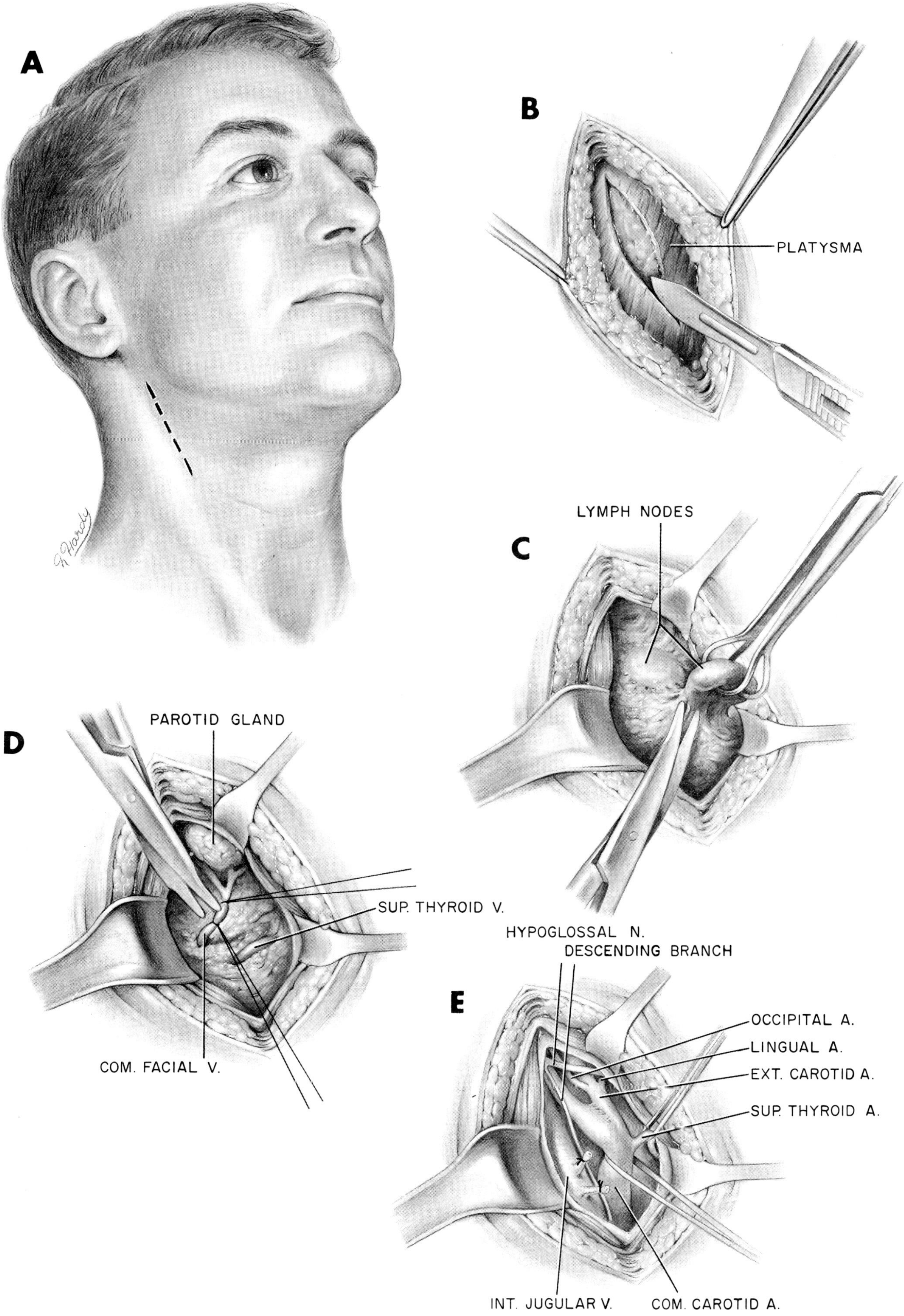
A
B
PLATYSMA
LYMPH NODES
C
D
PAROTID GLAND
SUP. THYROID V.
COM. FACIAL V.
HYPOGLOSSAL N.
DESCENDING BRANCH
E
OCCIPITAL A.
LINGUAL A.
EXT. CAROTID A.
SUP. THYROID A.
INT. JUGULAR V.
COM. CAROTID A.

F. The carotid artery and its branches are encircled by cotton tapes for traction as the adventitia at the carotid bifurcation is removed by scissor dissection. As the dissection proceeds posteriorly, it will include the small flattened carotid body, the glomus.

G. The dissection posteriorly may be facilitated by traction on the ligated stump of the superior thyroid artery and rotation (arrow) of the carotid bulb about a 180° axis.

H, I. After the glomectomy has been completed, the traction tapes are removed, and a soft rubber tissue drain is inserted down to the operative area. The platysma muscle layer is being closed about the drain using interrupted sutures of 000 silk (H). Similarly, the skin is next closed with interrupted sutures of 000 silk (I).

J. The completed closure of the incision with the drain anchored in its lower portion by one of the skin sutures is shown. A thyroid dressing is subsequently applied to complete the operation. The drain is removed in 48 hours. Alternate skin sutures are removed on the third postoperative day and the remainder of the sutures on the following (fourth) day.

Discussion—Dr. Richard H. Overholt. There is growing clinical evidence that a substantial majority of asthmatics can be helped by a cervical glomectomy. Large groups of patients so treated in Japan, Poland, Germany, and in this country have been reported. The mechanism of benefit is not clearly understood. In the asthmatic subject carotid reflexes may be hypersensitive, so that minor disturbances induced by irritants, allergens, emotions, or exertion may trigger bronchospasm on slight provocation. The removal of a carotid body dampens this reflex.

The operation has been advised for cases of intractable asthma that constitute medical failures or for cases of controlled asthma when the drug program has become an intolerable burden.

The illustrations are clear and will guide a surgeon experienced in neck procedures to the area of the carotid body. They reveal the relationship of contiguous structures and indicate that the procedure can be consummated without injury to them.

I prefer a slightly more transverse incision, paralleling the lower angle of the mandible and placed two finger breadths below it. If the incision precisely follows a natural crease line of the skin, the resulting scar will be completely or nearly invisible. Fibers of the platysma need not be divided but can be split and retracted.

A drain is shown in the last three illustrations. Careful hemostasis will eliminate with advantage the necessity for a drain in such a small wound.

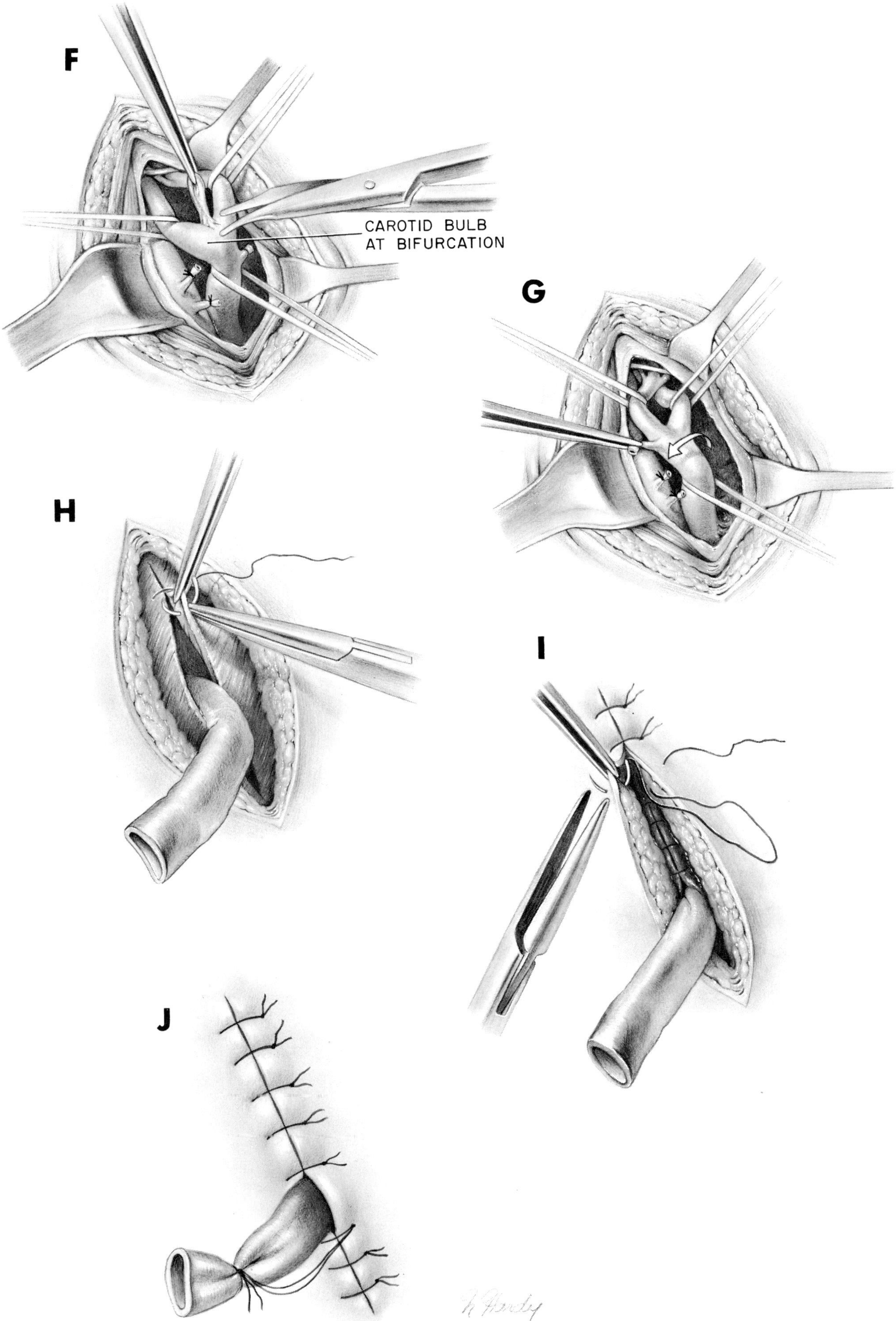
F
CAROTID BULB
AT BIFURCATION
G
H
I
J

RESTORATION OF PERIPHERAL ARTERIAL CONTINUITY BY RESECTION AND GRAFT (VEIN) REPLACEMENT OR A SHUNT BYPASS

A. The anterior thigh incision employed (solid line) and its abdominal extension (dotted line) are depicted.

B, C, D. The long saphenous vein is mobilized by sharp dissection from the subcutaneous fatty tissue layer medially (B, C), and a 16-cm. length of the vein is removed as indicated (D). Either a suture knot is placed in the adventitia coat of the vein or the ligated stumps of the tributary veins are used as landmarks to determine the cephalad and caudad ends of the vein. The vein is then immersed in a solution of heparin and saline (100 mg. of heparin in 250 ml. of saline) until ready for use. The direction of the vein is always reversed prior to insertion to prevent the possibility of an obstruction to the flow of blood caused by competent valves within its lumen.

E. The long length of the constricted and obliterated arterial segment involving the distal portion of the external iliac artery, the common femoral artery, and the proximal two-thirds of the superficial femoral artery is visible. The patent arterial segments cephalad and caudad are occluded with clamps, and the intervening segment is transected at the sites indicated (dotted lines).

F. Preparatory to the performance of the blood vessel anastomosis, 10 ml. of the heparin-saline solution is injected into the lumen of the artery caudad. The direction of the vein graft is reversed, and the caudad end is now cephalad. Two of the three equidistantly placed cardinal guy sutures which are used to approximate the ends of the vessels are inserted but not tied. The vein graft shown anterior to the inguinal ligament is subsequently withdrawn beneath it immediately after the completion of the cephalad end of the anastomosis.

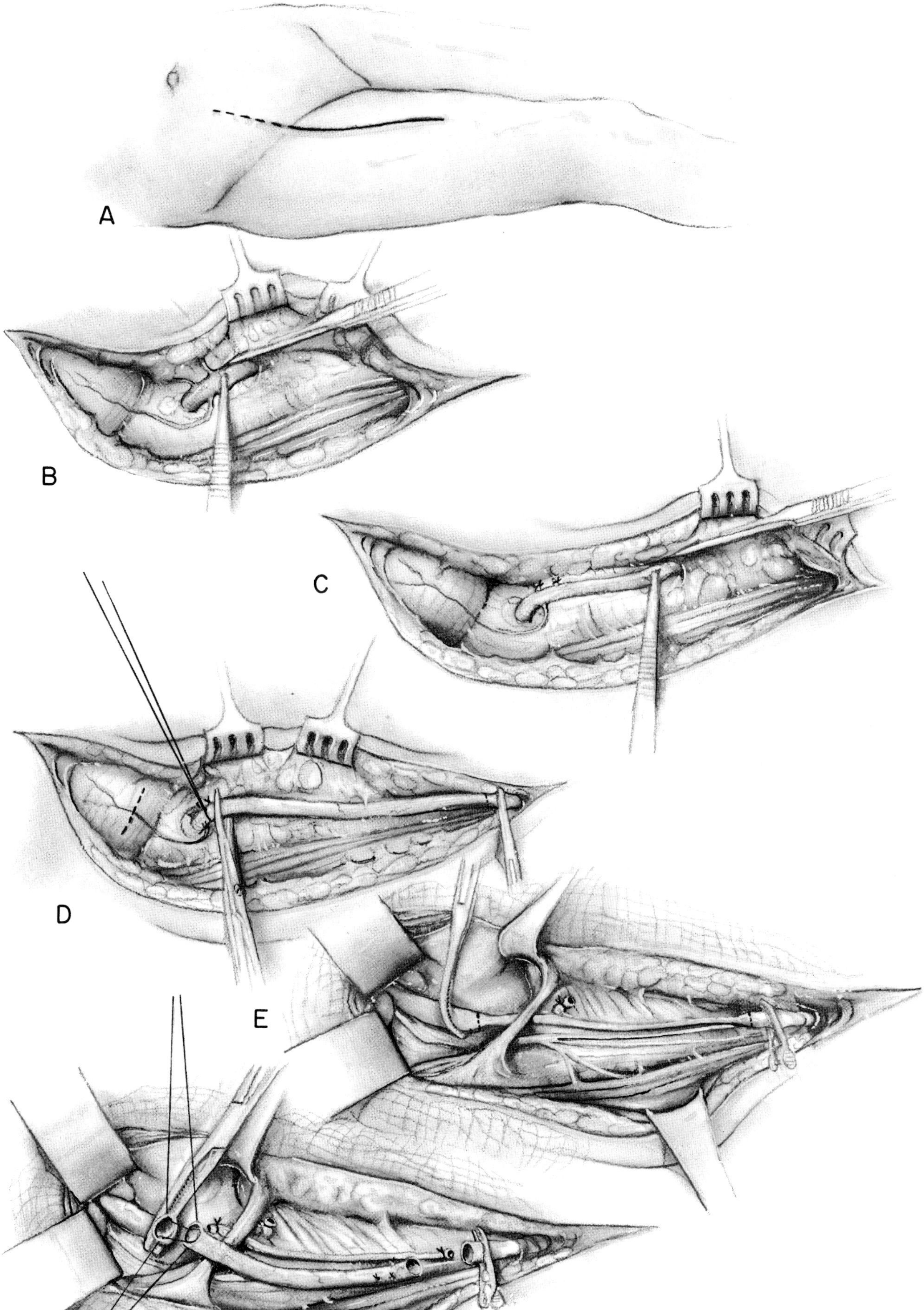
A
B
C
D
E
F

G, H, I, J, K. These are close-up views to show the details of the anastomosis. The free end of the vein graft is turned upward, and the three cardinal guy sutures are inserted but not tied (G). One of the guy sutures is inserted in the midline posteriorly, and each of the remaining two are inserted at either lateral angle (G). The cardinal guy sutures are tied (H), and the ends of the vessels are approximated posteriorly with everting mattress sutures of 00000 silk swedged on minimum trauma needles (H, I, J). The free end of the vein graft is then turned downward, and, in like manner, the anterior layer of the anastomosis is being completed (K).

L. The insertion of the autogenous vein (saphenous) graft is completed, and its relation to the occluded segment of the femoral artery and to the inguinal ligament are demonstrable.

M, M^1, M^2, M^3, M^4, M^5. These close-up views demonstrate an alternate method of performing a blood vessel anastomosis by the use of a continuous over and over suture of arterial (00000) silk. The suture is started posteriorly (M) with the needle strand of one of the lateral guy sutures and is continued to the midline where it is tied to the free strand of the posterior guy suture (M^1). The needle strand of this suture is continued (M^2) toward the opposing lateral guy suture and tied to its free strand (M^3). The vein graft is then turned downward, and the needle strand of the second lateral guy suture is continued anteriorly toward the opposing lateral angle suture (M^4) where the anastomosis was originally started. The completion of the insertion of the vein graft using a simple over and over suture is shown (M^5). This particular technic, the more desirable, is a simple, rapid, and effective method of anastomosis.

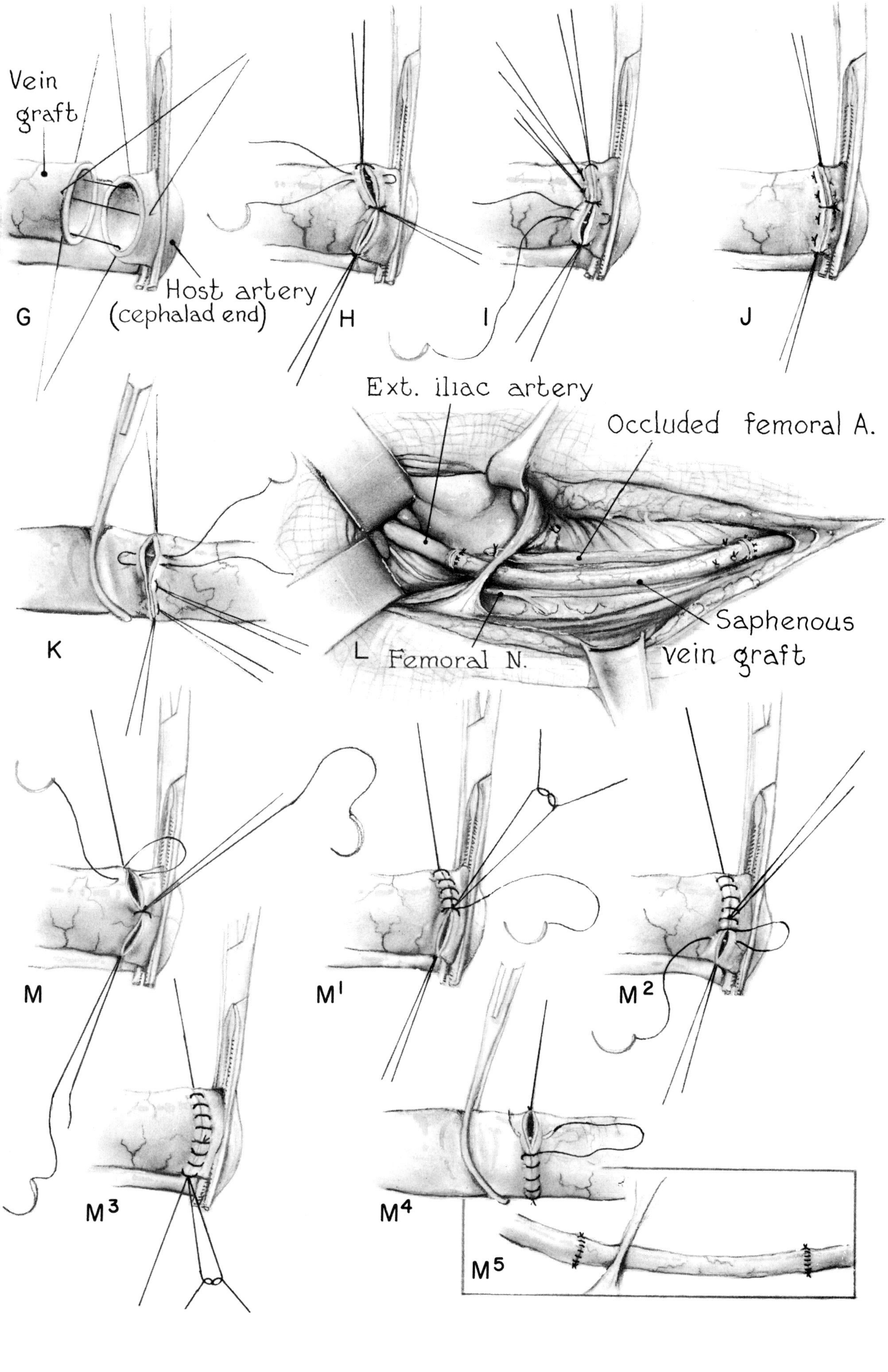
Vein graft
Host artery
(cephalad end)
G
H
I
J
Ext. iliac artery
Occluded femoral A.
K
L
Femoral N.
Saphenous
vein graft
M
M1
M2
M3
M4
M5

N, N^1, N^2, N^3, N^4, N^5. The technic of performing the anastomosis illustrated is the same as that previously described (M, M , M^2, M^3, M^4, M^5) with the exception that a continuous everting mattress rather than an over and over suture is employed. This technic, included for completeness, is the least desirable.

O, O^1, O^2, O^3, O^4. These illustrations depict the technic for the performance of an end-to-side bypass of an occluded arterial segment. The artery cephalad is cross-clamped, and, just below the clamp, a lateral opening is made into the arterial lumen (O). The end of the vein graft is cut on a bias (dotted outline) to obtain a flat approximation to the side of the artery (O). The angle guy sutures (00000 silk) are inserted but not tied (O^1). The needle strand of the lower guy suture is inserted from below upward as an over and over suture toward the upper angle guy suture (O^2), where it is tied to its free end. The needle strand of the upper angle guy suture is then inserted on the opposite side from above downward as an over and over suture toward its starting point at the lower angle (O^3), where it is tied to the free strand of the lower angle guy suture. The inset (O^4) shows the completion of the end-to-side bypass shunt utilizing an autogenous vein (long saphenous) graft.

P. This inset shows a modified bypass shunt in which an end-to-end anastomosis is performed cephalad and an end-to-side anastomosis caudad. This method was used in one patient in whom a thrombus formed in the lumen of an end-to-side bypass shunt vein within 8 to 10 minutes after its insertion. The cephalad end of the anastomosis was disconnected, the thrombus evacuated, and the lumen of the vein was irrigated with heparin–saline solution. The reanastomosis cephalad was performed end-to-end rather than end-to-side, with a satisfactory result.

In the restoration of continuity in the lower iliac and femoral arteries either by resection and graft or a shunt bypass, the use of an autogenous vein (long saphenous) as illustrated (A to L), rather than an arterial homograft or cloth prosthesis, is preferred. The illustrations (A to L) depicting the insertion of the autogenous vein graft were from sketches made at the time of operation upon a 65-year-old man. This patient was admitted to the hospital because of severe pain secondary to an ischemic ulcer (4 by 3 cm.) of two years duration overlying the anterior aspect of the midportion of the right leg. A lumbar sympathetic ganglionectomy performed 18 months previously had no beneficial effect. In fact, because of the severity of the pain, the patient requested that the leg be amputated. Following the insertion of the vein graft as depicted (A to L), pulsations in the dorsalis pedis and posterior tibial arteries were restored. Postoperatively, the relief of pain was immediate, and the ulceration of the leg healed completely in 11 days. At the end of a follow-up period of two and one-half years, the patient was still asymptomatic and the peripheral arterial pulsations were easily palpable.

Discussion—Dr. John P. West. With experience and skill, a surgeon can expect to restore circulation about an occluded femoral artery with the various technics so clearly shown in these drawings. The recorded experience to date indicates that a higher percentage of good results are obtained by end-to-side anastomosis as shown in Plate 154O^4. The anastomotic orifices need to be wide, and better results follow the use of large caliber grafts.

When well supported by muscle, an autogenous vein graft may be the ideal arterial substitute. However, the removal of the vein adds to the operative trauma, and at times the saphenous vein is not of ideal caliber. Further experience is needed to determine the relative merits of homologous arteries and cloth prostheses.

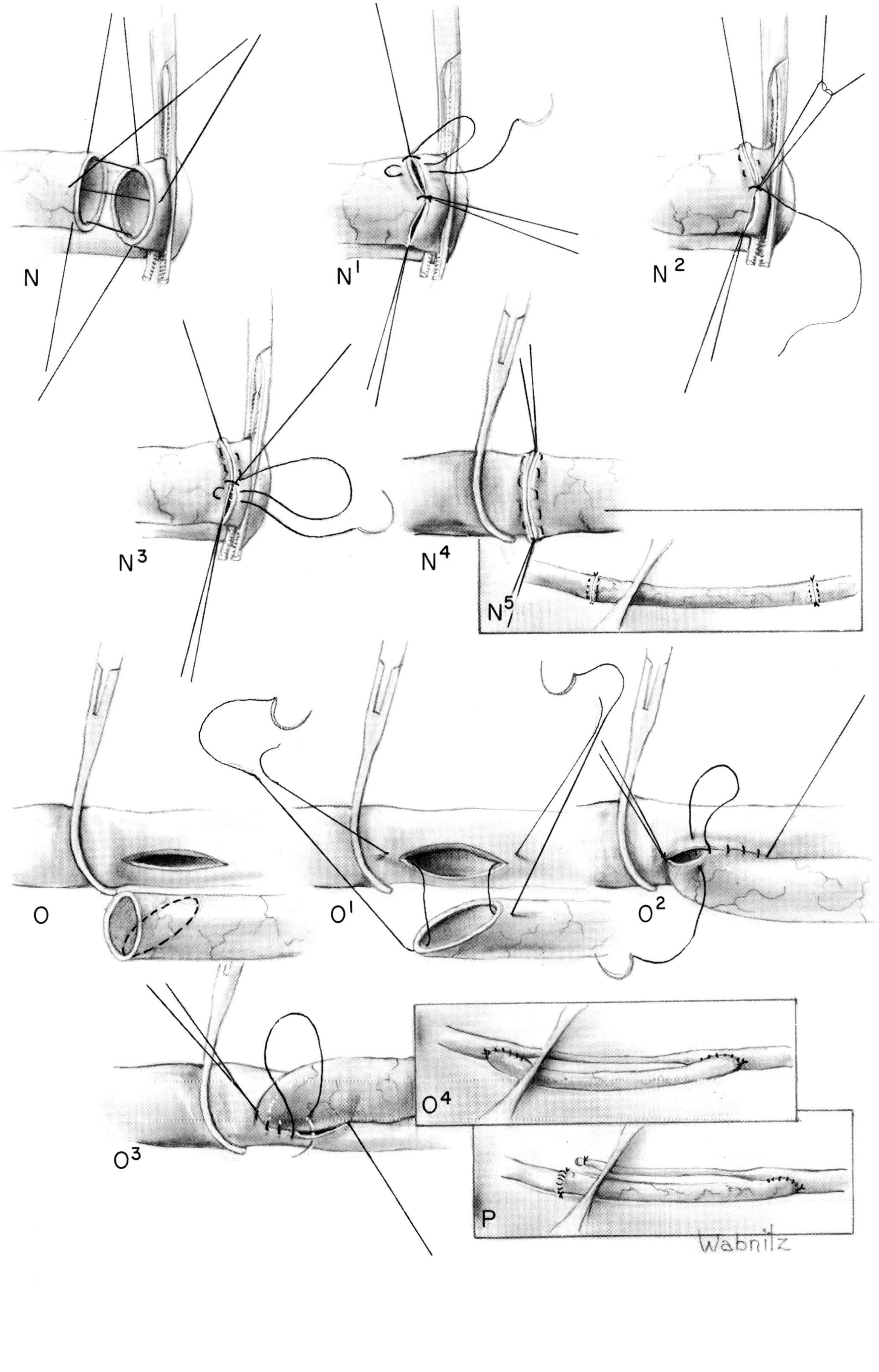
N
N1
N2
N3
N4
N5
O
O1
O2
O3
O4
P
Wabnitz

SURGICAL EXPOSURE OF THE POPLITEAL VESSELS AND POSTERIOR TIBIAL NERVE IN THE UPPER THIRD OF THE LEG

A. The two exploratory incisions in the thigh are packed loosely with moist gauze sponges, and the incision in the anteromedial aspect of the proximal third of the leg is indicated by the solid black line.

B. The incision is deepened through the subcutaneous fatty tissue layer and the crural fascia is being incised (broken line). The saphenous vein and the ligated stumps of its tributaries are visible.

C. The cut margins of the crural fascia are retracted to expose a broad expanse of the gastrocnemius muscle. A small segment of vein in the central portion of the muscle is visible.

D. The gastrocnemius muscle is retracted to show the fascial attachment of the soleus muscle to the tibia being incised. This is necessary to obtain adequate exposure of the underlying neurovascular bundle. The relation of the plantaris muscle to the operative field is depicted.

E. The fascial incision is completed and a good exposure of the structures that comprise the neurovascular bundle is obtained.

E_1. This close-up view shows the usual relation of the nerve, vein, and artery. The artery is posterior in relation to the vein and nerve, each of which is encircled by a cotton tape and retracted to obtain the necessary exposure of the artery that is required. The anterior tibial artery, not depicted, arises from the popliteal artery immediately proximal to the arterial segment that is visible.

In explorations of the femoral artery in the thigh for a bypass graft, thromboendarterectomy, or excision and graft replacement, the peripheral arterial run-off may prove unsatisfactory. Under such circumstances it is considered advisable to explore the popliteal artery in the leg, utilizing the approach as illustrated.* It is believed by many that the extension of the disease process to this level would preclude a satisfactory operative result. In such circumstances, however, the excellent results not infrequently obtained are believed to justify the continued use of this operation.

* This approach was originally described by Szilagyi in 1959. See references on Reconstructive Arterial Surgery.

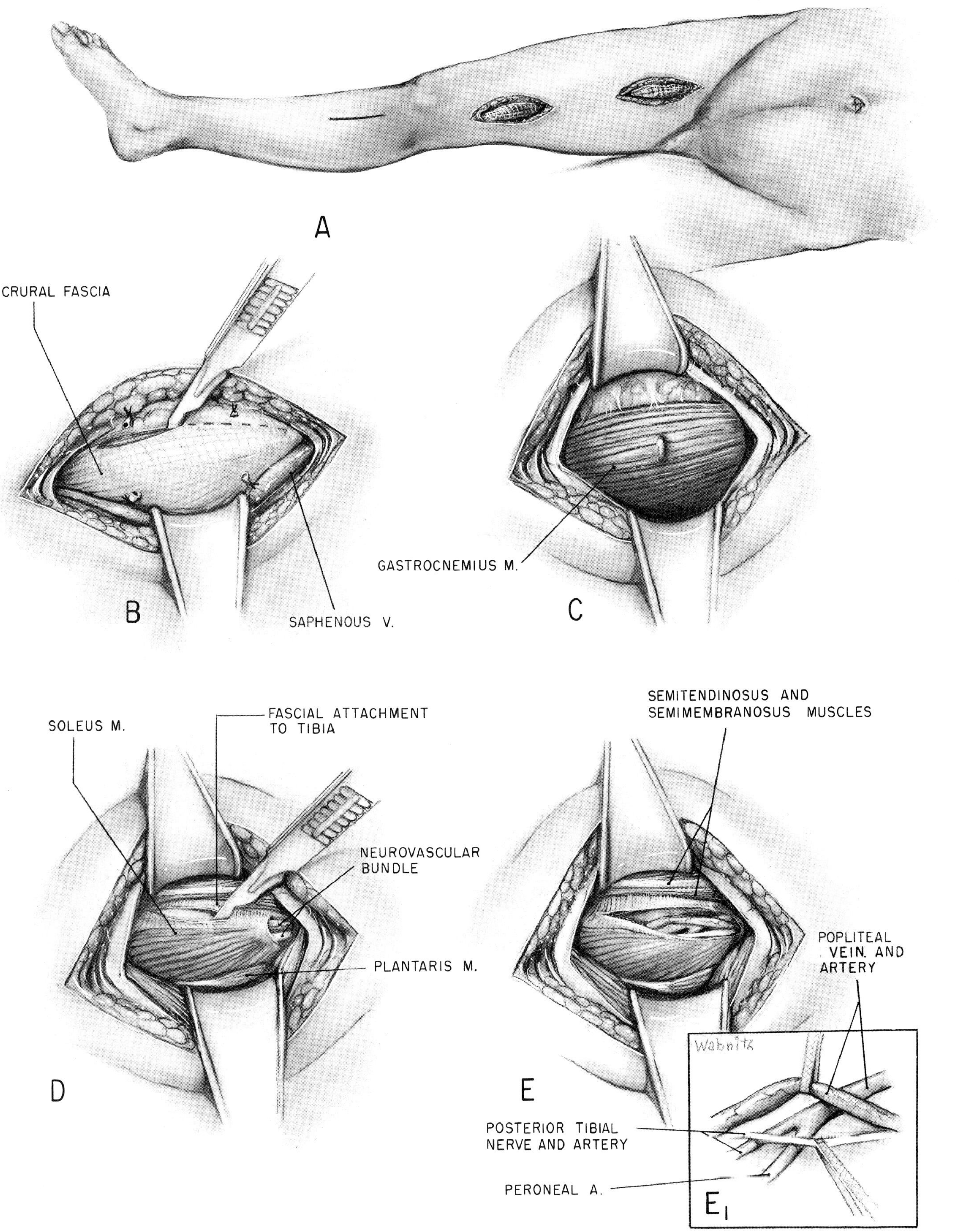
A
CRURAL FASCIA
B
SAPHENOUS V.
GASTROCNEMIUS M.
C
SOLEUS M.
FASCIAL ATTACHMENT
TO TIBIA
NEUROVASCULAR
BUNDLE
PLANTARIS M.
D
SEMITENDINOSUS AND
SEMIMEMBRANOSUS MUSCLES
POPLITEAL
VEIN AND
ARTERY
E
Wabnitz
POSTERIOR TIBIAL
NERVE AND ARTERY
PERONEAL A.
E_1

FEMORAL THROMBOENDARTERECTOMY

A. The incision overlying the femoral triangle (solid line) and its subsequent extension caudad (dotted line) are indicated. If desired, separate cephalad and caudad incisions may be employed. However, in the experience of the author, the single long incision has proved the more satisfactory. It is not associated with an increase in the operative morbidity, and the objection to the length of the incision based on cosmetic reasoning is believed not of practical significance.

B, C. The femoral artery is incised (B), and, after the insertion of guy sutures of silk (00000) in either incised margin, the underlying thrombus is mobilized with a dissecting instrument of special design* (C). In making the incision in the artery (B), the thinness of its wall overlying the thrombus should be emphasized. Otherwise the thrombus itself may be incised and the improper cleavage plane entered. Characteristically, the inner lining of the wall of the artery surrounding the thrombus has a glistening sheen which is indicative of the proper plane for dissection.

* Manufactured by Edward Weck & Co., Brooklyn, New York.

D. The mobilized portion of the thrombus, which occludes the lumen of the femoral artery, is elevated on a clamp (Mixter), and a small segment is excised (dotted line).

E, F. The transected end of the caudad portion of the thrombus is secured in a curved clamp, and, with the use of the dissecting instrument, the thrombus is separated from the arterial wall.

G, H, I. In like manner, a second separate incision is made in the lower portion of the femoral artery within Hunter's canal (G), and the underlying thrombus is mobilized (H, I) as previously described. If need be, three rather than two femoral arteriotomies may be made.

J, K. A catheter (No. 14 F) is inserted into the lumen of the femoral artery distally, and through it a solution of heparin (100 mg. of heparin in 250 ml. of normal saline) is intermittently instilled (J). Through the lower femoral arteriotomy, the thrombus is mobilized cephalad (J) to the level of the completed dissection previously made in a caudad direction through the upper femoral arteriotomy, and the intervening thrombotic segment is withdrawn (K).

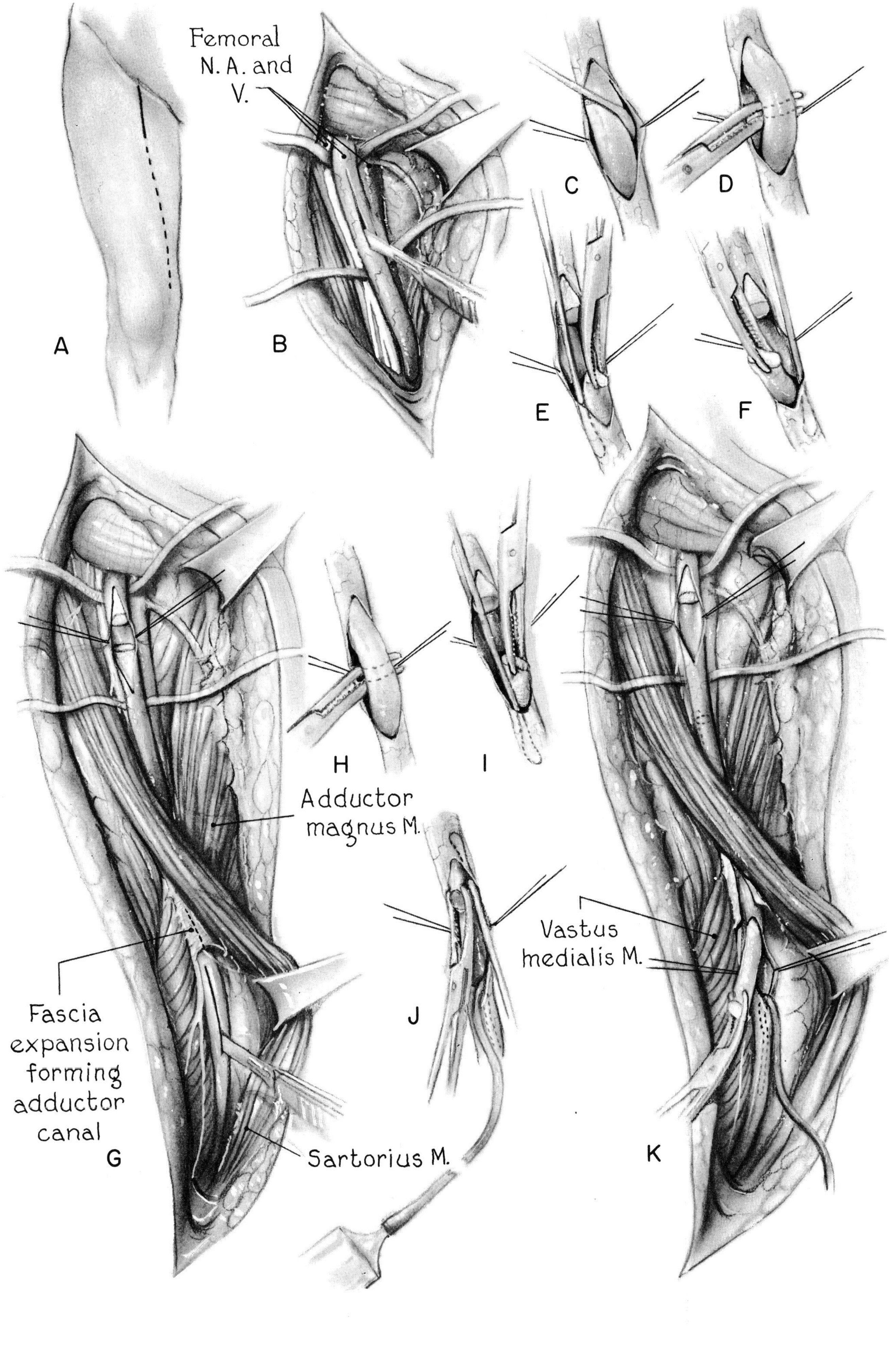
Femoral
N. A. and
V.
A
B
C
D
E
F
H
I
Adductor
magnus M.
J
Vastus
medialis M.
Fascia
expansion
forming
adductor
canal
G
Sartorius M.
K

L. The lower arteriotomy is closed with a continuous suture of 00000 arterial silk swedged on a minimum trauma needle. Similarly, the caudad portion of the upper arteriotomy is closed, and the dissection of the cephalad portion of the thrombus within the femoral artery is begun. A catheter (No. 14 F), through which a solution of heparin is intermittently instilled, is inserted within the cleared lumen of the femoral artery distally.

M, N, O. The dissection of the thrombus is continued (M), and, when it is completed, bleeding is controlled by gentle digital compression (N). A kidney-stone-grasping forceps is inserted cephalad in the lumen of the femoral artery to remove any remaining thrombotic debris (N). Upon completion of the thromboendarterectomy, bleeding is controlled by digital compression rather than clamp occlusion of the femoral artery cephalad as the closure of the upper arteriotomy is being completed (O). In this patient, a 74-year-old man, an excellent pulsation throughout the whole length of the femoral artery was restored.

P, Q. In patients in whom the femoral arterial pulsations are present, and the popliteal, dorsalis pedis, and posterior tibial pulsations are absent, exploration of the femoral artery in Hunter's canal is performed. The patient is placed in the lateral recumbent position, and the lower extremity that is uppermost is supported on pillows (P). The linear incision overlying Hunter's canal (solid line) and its subsequent S-shaped extension (dotted line) to expose the popliteal artery are depicted (P). Upon exploration of the femoral artery in Hunter's canal (Q), adequate arterial pulsations were present. Accordingly an S-shaped extension, depicted by the dotted line (Q), was made for exposure of the popliteal artery.

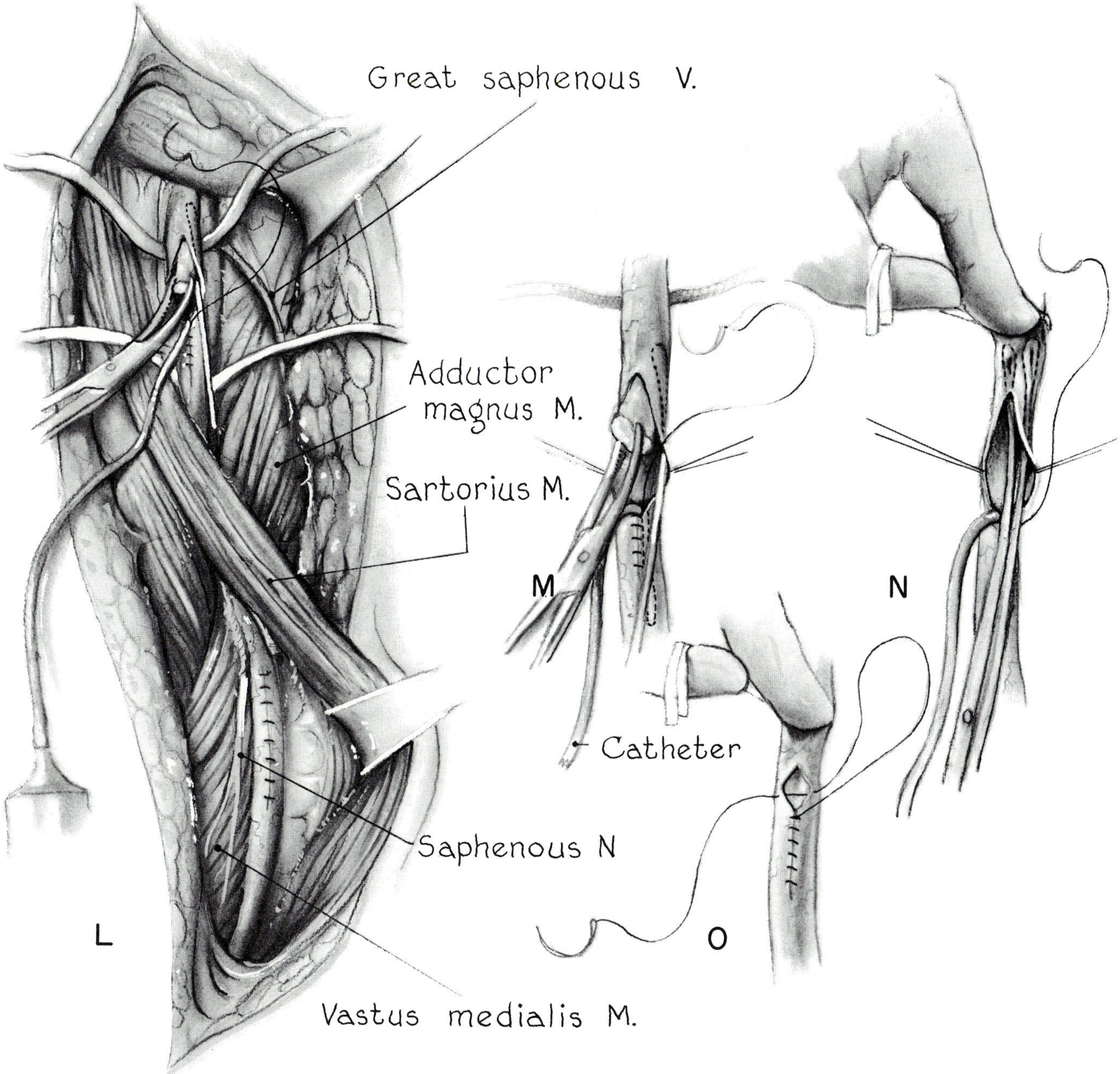
Great saphenous V.
Adductor magnus M.
Sartorius M.
Saphenous N
Vastus medialis M.
Catheter

L M N O

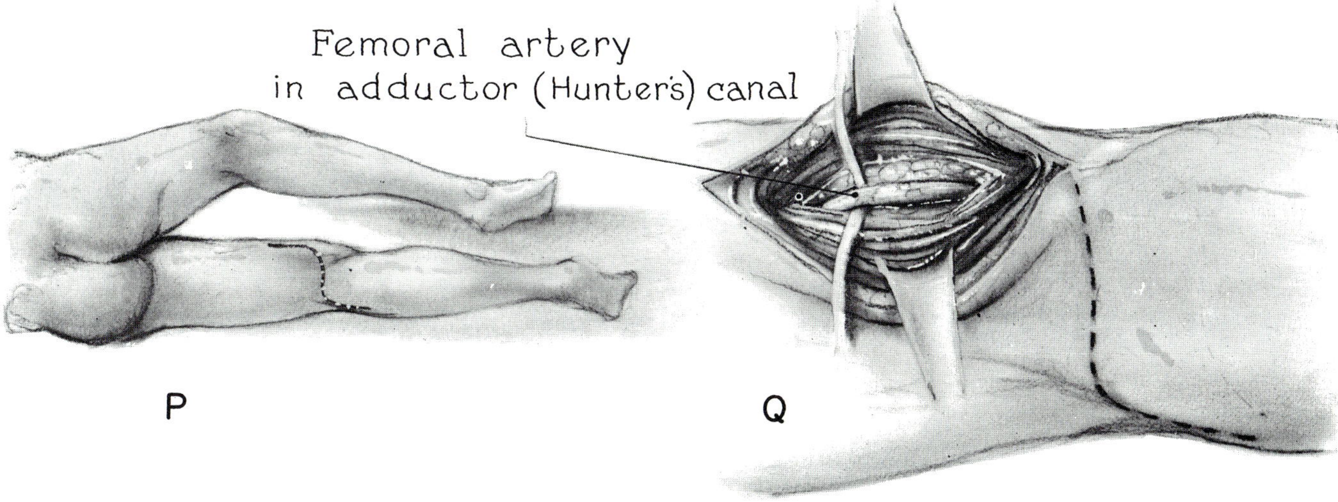
Femoral artery in adductor (Hunter's) canal

P Q

R. The S-shaped incision in the popliteal space is completed, the flaps are mobilized, and the incision in the posterior crural fascia is shown in dotted outline.

S. The incision in the posterior crural fascia is completed, and the neurovascular contents of the popliteal fossa are exposed.

T. The tibial nerve is encircled by a guy suture of silk (00) and retracted to show the subjacent popliteal vein and artery. The branch of the tibial nerve which bifurcates before its entrance into the medial head of the gastrocnemius muscle is shown. Similarly, the collateral tributary and branch of the popliteal vein and artery, respectively, are depicted. Although an excellent pulsation in the collateral arterial vessel was present, the lumen of the popliteal artery immediately caudad was occluded with a thrombus.

U, V, W, X, Y. The incision in the popliteal artery and the mobilization of the thrombus is the same as previously described (B, C, D, E, F). Similarly, heparin solution is instilled intermittently through a catheter (No. 12 F) into the cleared lumen of the popliteal artery caudad as the thrombus is being dissected cephalad (X). Upon completion of the removal of the thrombus, bleeding is controlled by proximal digital compression as the arteriotomy is closed, using a continuous over and over suture of 00000 arterial silk swedged on a minimum trauma needle. In this patient, a 53-year-old man with a serpiginous ulceration overlying the lateral aspect and lower third of the left leg, an excellent pulsation was restored in the popliteal artery.

Z. Inset to show the completion of the closure of the S-shaped incision in the popliteal fossa.

Discussion—Dr. John P. West. The illustrated technic of thromboendarterectomy is a most satisfactory one. However, it has been our experience that, in general, attempts to clear the lumen of long segments of small vessels, such as the superficial femoral and popliteal arteries, are often unsuccessful. The incidence of prompt recurrent occlusion has been high. For this reason, we favor a bypass operation when a good and patent artery can be found at either end of the obstruction. The ideal case for thromboendarterectomy is one in which there is a short segmental occlusion. Such obstructions are often found at the bifurcation of the common femoral artery. In some cases, removal of a segment of thrombus facilitates the insertion of a graft, and, in such cases, a judicious combination of thrombectomy and grafting is likely to give the best result.

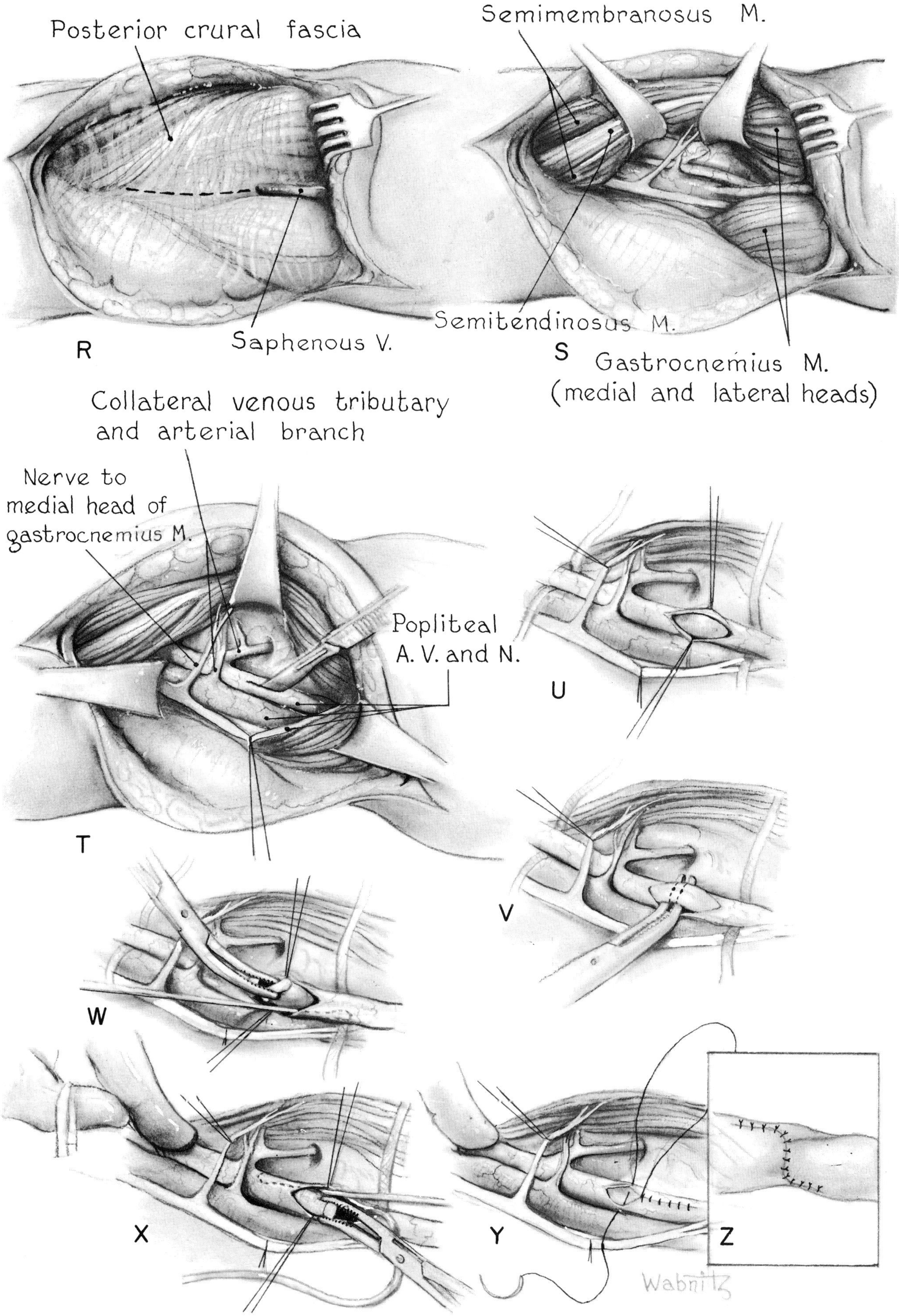
Posterior crural fascia
Semimembranosus M.
R
Saphenous V.
Semitendinosus M.
S
Gastrocnemius M.
(medial and lateral heads)
Collateral venous tributary
and arterial branch
Nerve to
medial head of
gastrocnemius M.
Popliteal
A. V. and N.
U
T
V
W
X
Y
Z
Wabnitz

RENAL THROMBOENDARTERECTOMY

The patient, a 46-year-old white man, was admitted to the hospital because of severe and persistent headache, pain in the cervical region posteriorly, and numbness in the left upper extremity. These symptoms had been present for the preceding 10 days. The blood pressure was 240/120. One year previously the diagnosis of essential hypertension was made.

A selective renal function study was done. On the left side the urinary volume and sodium excretion were normal. There was no excretion of urine on the right side. A translumbar aortogram showed opacification of the left renal artery but not the right. Accordingly, the right renal artery was explored and the operation as illustrated was performed.

The right renal artery was occluded for a distance of 2 cm. by an atherosclerotic thrombus which extended partly into the lumen of the aorta. The artery distal to the thrombus was soft, pliable, and patent but had no pulsatile flow of blood.

Postoperatively the patient had an uneventful convalescence. The day after operation the blood pressure was 130/90. The decrease in the blood pressure was concomitant with complete relief of the headache. It is now 4 years since the operation was performed and the patient is asymptomatic. The blood pressure is 130/80.

A. The patient is placed in the supine position, and the right paramedian abdominal incision is indicated by the solid line.

B. The peritoneal cavity is entered, and the right side of the colon and its hepatic flexure are mobilized by scissor dissection along the "white line" and subsequent transection (broken line) of the phrenocolic ligament.

C. The mobilized right side of the colon is retracted toward the midline, and several of the retroperitoneal structures are depicted. The broken line indicates the incision for the mobilization of the duodenum.

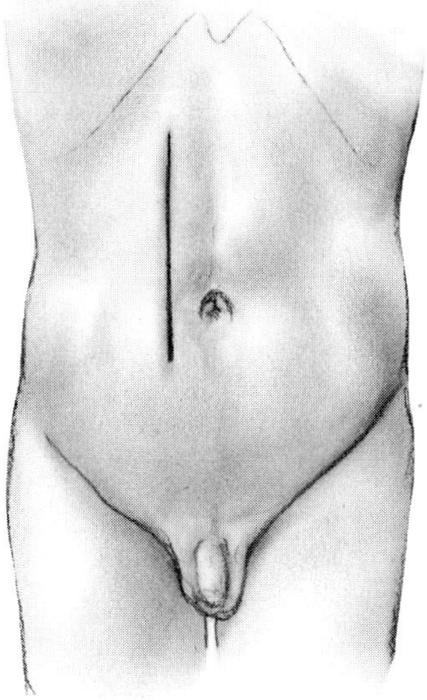

A

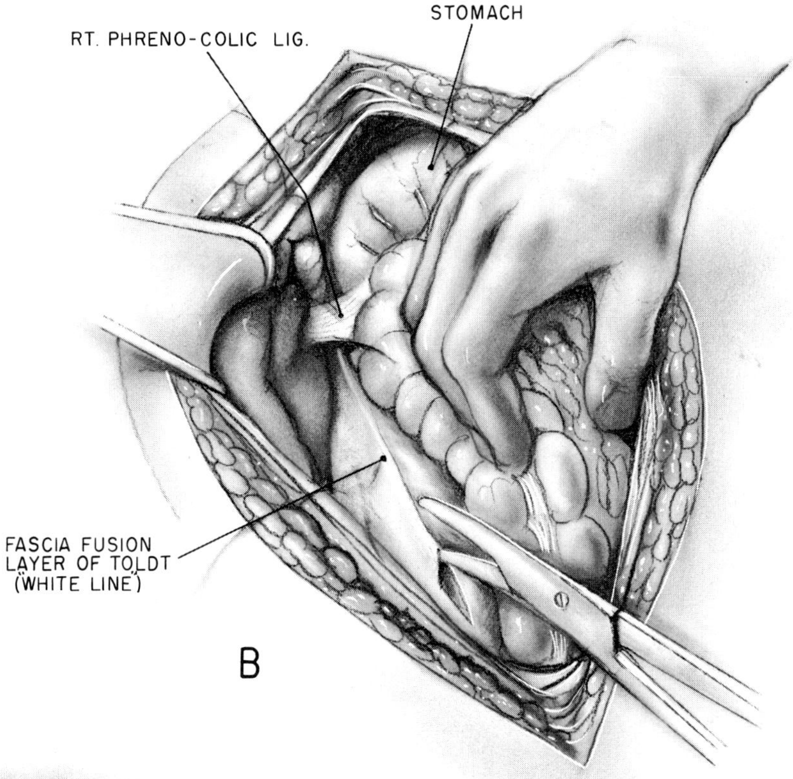
STOMACH
RT. PHRENO-COLIC LIG.
FASCIA FUSION
LAYER OF TOLDT
(WHITE LINE)

B

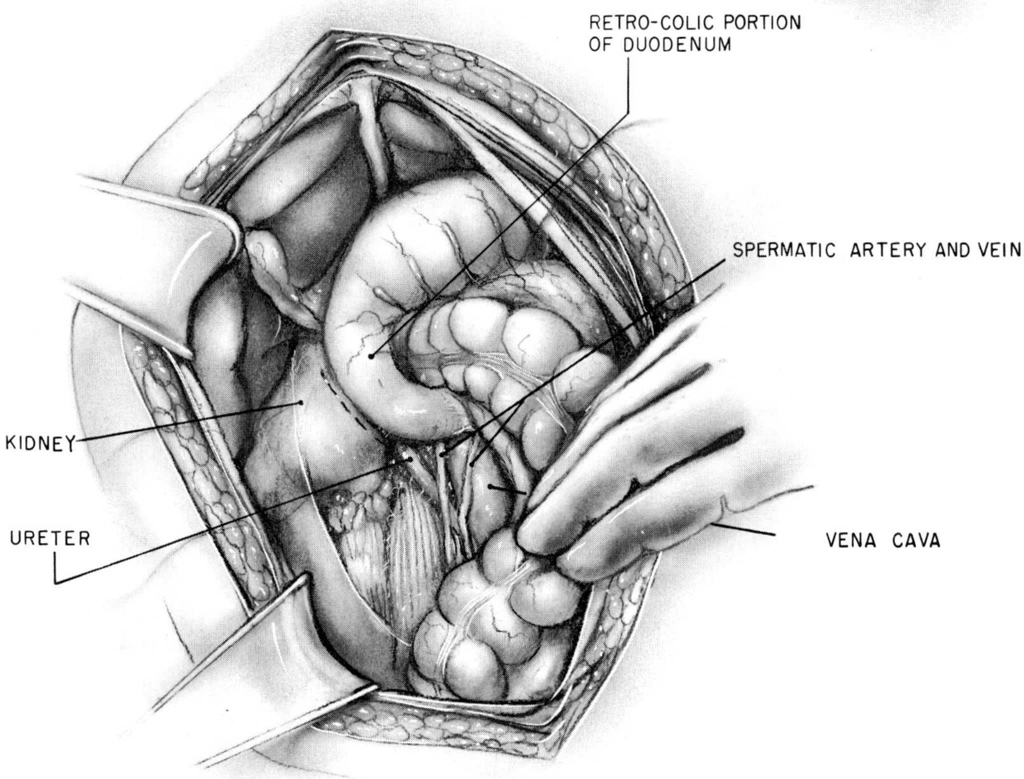
RETRO-COLIC PORTION
OF DUODENUM
SPERMATIC ARTERY AND VEIN
KIDNEY
URETER
VENA CAVA

C

D. The mobilized duodenum is rotated and retracted medially to expose the operative field. The mobilized right renal artery, cephalad and posterior to the renal vein, is being encircled by a cotton tape, as was the renal vein previously.

E, F. Close-up views to show the clearance of the abdominal aorta and its spermatic and inferior mesenteric arterial branches (F) by scissor dissection of the preaortic lymph nodal tissue mass (E). The superior mesenteric artery branch and its relation to the left renal vein, over which it arches, are clearly visible (E, F).

G, H. The inferior vena cava cephalad is retracted medialward to expose a segment of the aorta and its right renal arterial branch. The pressure distal to the block is first measured (G); later it will be measured proximally to determine the pressure gradient across the block. The site of the block is indicated by the stippling (H). The right adrenal gland and its vein, a tributary of the inferior vena cava, may also be seen.

I. A segment of the abdominal aorta in juxtaposition to the origin of the renal artery is occluded tangentially with a Beck-Potts clamp, and the renal artery, tensed by traction on the encircling tape, is incised longitudinally.

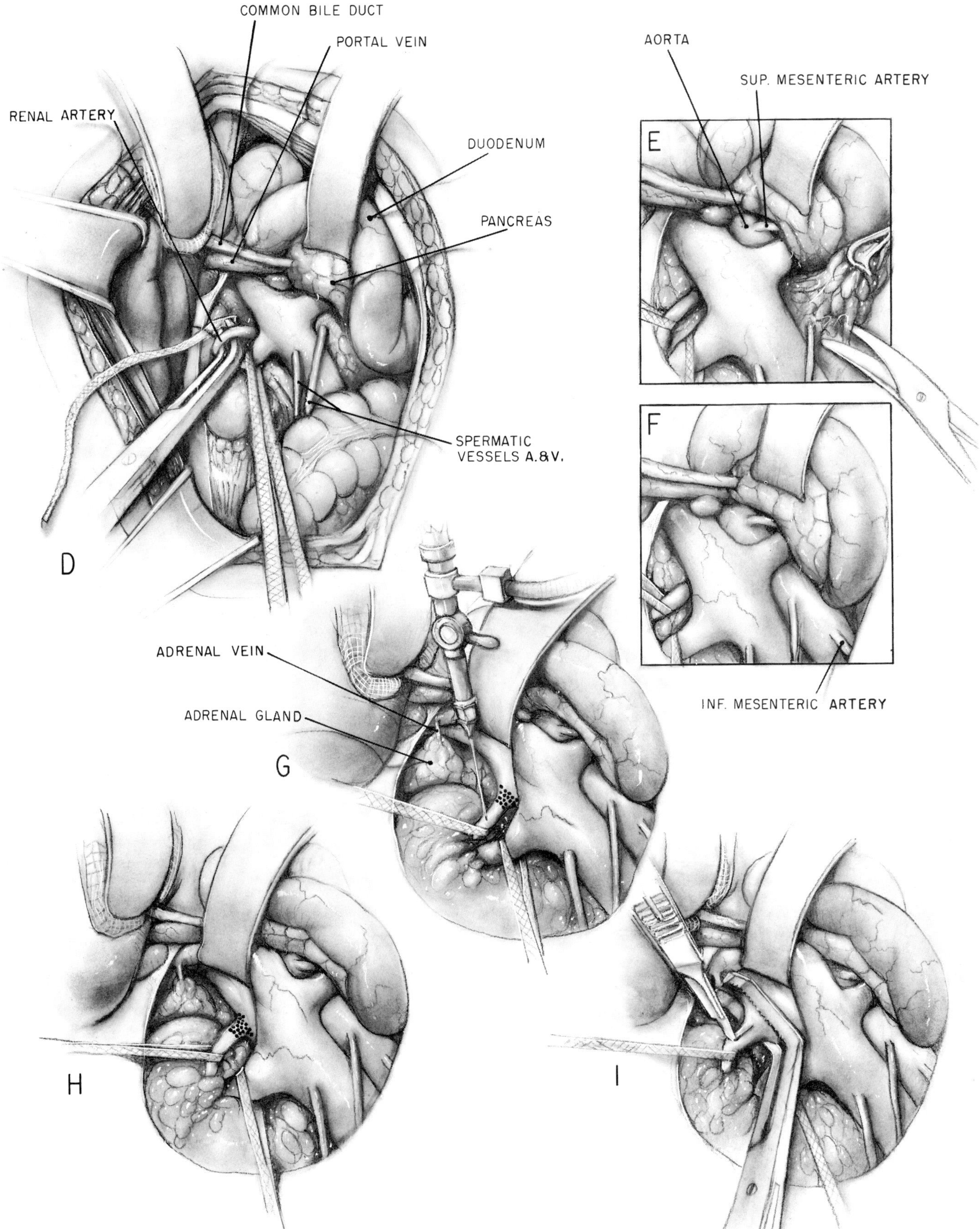
COMMON BILE DUCT
PORTAL VEIN
RENAL ARTERY
DUODENUM
PANCREAS
SPERMATIC VESSELS A.&V.
D
AORTA
SUP. MESENTERIC ARTERY
E
F
INF. MESENTERIC ARTERY
ADRENAL VEIN
ADRENAL GLAND
G
H
I

J. The incision in the renal artery is deepened to the surface of the thrombus, and the thrombus is mobilized throughout its circumference, using a specifically designed instrument.* The mobilized segment of the thrombus is elevated on the instrument, and its site of transection is indicated by the broken line.

K. The distal segment of the thrombus is removed and the proximal segment is being dissected. During this dissection, the clamp on the aorta is temporarily released to permit the extraction of the intra-aortic projection of the thrombus. Subsequent to the extraction of the thrombus the aorta is again occluded as previously (J).

L. Upon completion of the thromboendarterectomy the opening in the artery is closed with interrupted sutures of a 00000 arterial silk swedged on a minimum trauma needle. Prior to completion of the closure, the clamp on the aorta is again temporarily released to determine the patency of the arterial lumen and to wash out any existing clots. The angulated Potts clamp distally remains occluded.

M. The operative field on completion of the operation is shown. The renal arterial pressure was again recorded and the pressure gradient (80 mm. Hg.) was observed to have been eliminated.

* Manufactured by Edward Weck & Co., Long Island City, N.Y.

DISCUSSION—DR. PAUL T. DE CAMP. The inferior vena cava creates a problem in approaching the right renal artery because it lies across the major portion of the artery. From the lateral approach the vena cava can be retracted to the left, as illustrated in D. From the midline approach it may be retracted either to the right or to the left, whichever will give the best exposure to the involved portion of the artery. A bypass graft should be placed behind the vena cava.

The important observation of the intrarenal arterial pressure is illustrated in G. In my opinion and experience in true cases of renovascular hypertension the distal pressure will be found significantly lower than the proximal. In 89 per cent of the cases the mean pressure difference has been greater than 50 mm. of mercury.

The superior mesenteric artery may be so close to the renal that it interferes with the placement of the exclusion clamp to partially occlude the aorta and may compromise the exposure of the orifice of the renal artery. It may be necessary to cross clamp the aorta, but if this is done, the contralateral renal artery must not be occluded fo too long a period. The opposite kidney, unlike the kidney served by a severely stenosed renal artery, is not protected by a collateral circulation.

Endarterectomy of an arteriosclerotic renal artery (I-K) must be effected with extreme caution, as the renal artery is often friable and may be torn to bits. My arterial incision extends onto the aorta where it curves caudad. This permits easier endarterectomy of the aortic orifice of the artery. I always employ a vein patch for closure; with its use I am insured of a most adequate lumen and am not tempted to "push" the endarterectomy and possibly tear up the vessel.

The renal artery may be small, and closure must be meticulous. Interrupted sutures are preferable in small vessels or at critical angles of suture to minimize the production of strictures or kinks.

Alternatively, renal endarterectomy may be performed through an obliquely placed transecting incision in the artery just distal to the occlusion plaque. Proximal dissection is performed, and the vessel is reanastomosed with interrupted sutures.

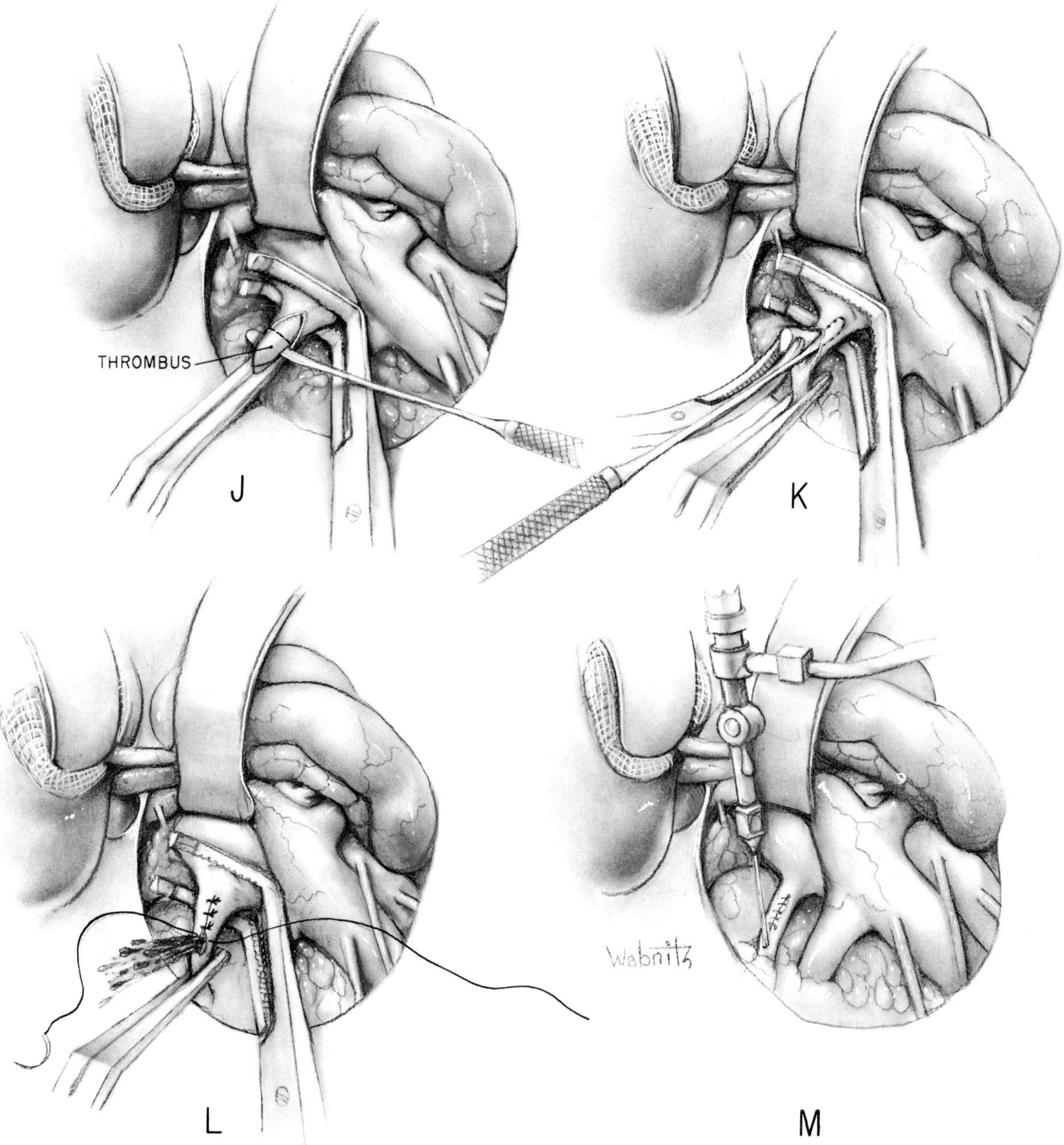
THROMBUS
J
K
L
Wabnitz
M

AORTORENAL BYPASS GRAFT

A. The patient is placed in the supine position, and the left paraumbilical incision is indicated by the solid black line.

B. The peritoneal cavity is entered, and the proximal portion of the descending colon is mobilized by scissor dissection along the "white line," as depicted. This dissection is extended to sever the phrenocolic, the lienocolic, and the gastrocolic ligaments in order to facilitate the mobilization of the splenic flexure, the distal half of the transverse colon, and the related portion of the greater curvature of the stomach.

C. The mobilized portion of the colon is retracted to the right, and the retroperitoneal structures are exposed. The left renal vein is anterior to and obscures almost completely the left renal artery. Its relation to the kidney and the adrenal gland is clearly visible. In this patient there was a multiplicity of renal vein tributaries, which were too numerous to name. Superiorly there were two adrenal veins; inferiorly, instead of one internal spermatic vein, there were four tributaries. The posterior location of the renal artery and the multiplicity of the renal tributaries made the exposure of the artery somewhat difficult.

D. The adrenal tributary vein (or veins) is routinely preserved. Three of the tributaries inferiorly were doubly ligated in continuity and severed. The mobilized segments of both the vein and artery have been encircled by cotton tapes and elevated by upward traction on the tapes. The one tributary inferiorly that was not ligated was particularly large and had a branch tributary that coursed cephalad beneath the renal artery. The site of origin and name of this vein and its tributary were both undetermined.

E. Inset shows the dacron prosthesis preparatory to its insertion. The extremity of the graft that is to be anastomosed to the aorta is cut at a 45° angle to facilitate its proper alignment between the aorta and the renal artery.

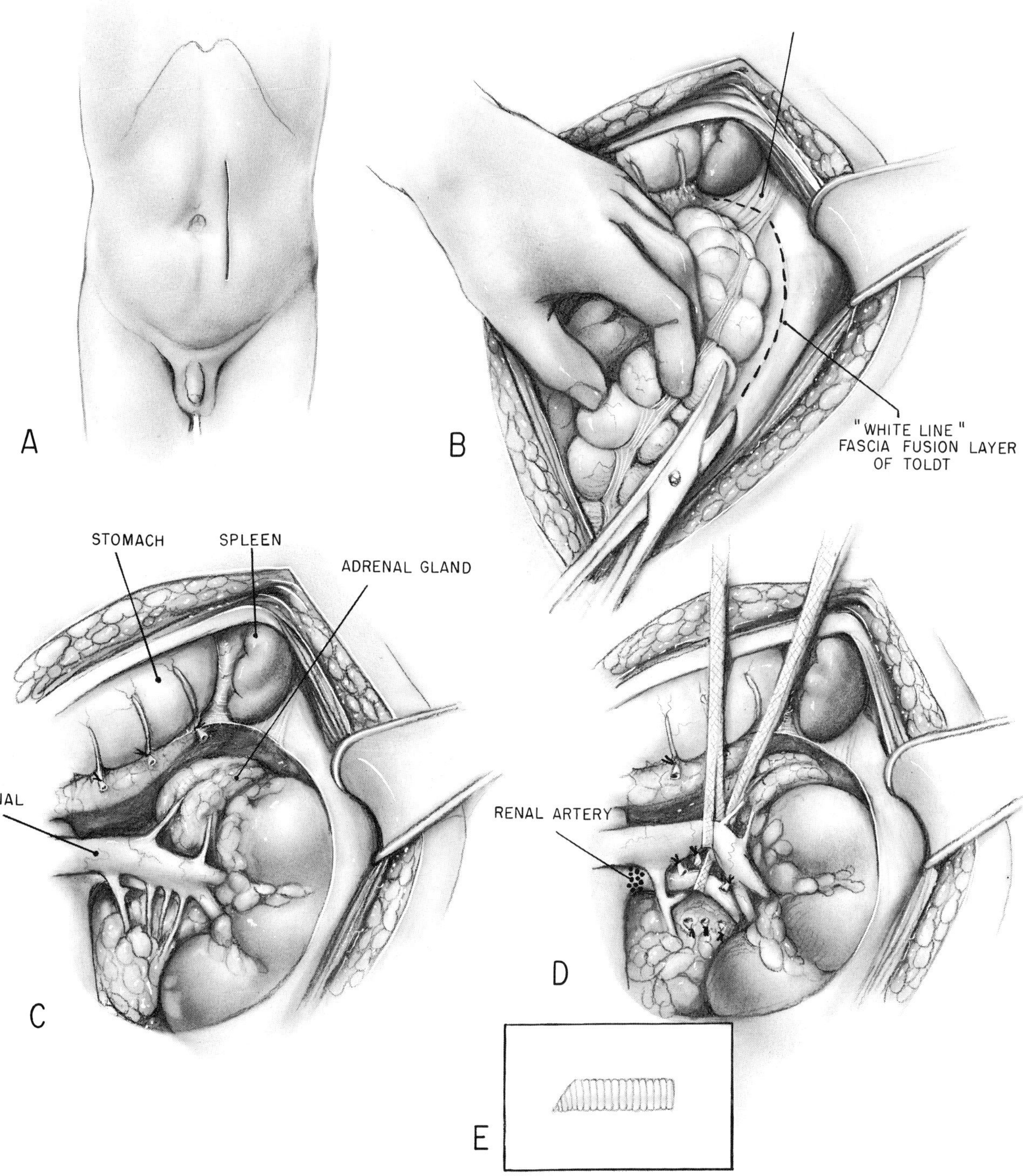
A
B
"WHITE LINE"
FASCIA FUSION LAYER
OF TOLDT
STOMACH
SPLEEN
ADRENAL GLAND
LT. RENAL
VEIN
C
RENAL ARTERY
D
E

F. The branch tributary beneath the renal artery is ligated and severed, and the left renal vein is elevated by upward traction on the cotton tape. A segment of the aorta is occluded in a Beck-Potts clamp, which is applied tangentially to its longitudinal axis. An opening is made into the lumen of the occluded segment, and a suture of 00000 silk is inserted in each angle of the graft and the host aorta, respectively. The lowermost angle suture is tied, and the uppermost suture is inserted but untied.

G, H. The needle strand segment of the suture cephalad (a) is continued caudad as a simple over-and-over suture (G), and at its termination at the lower angle it is tied to the needle free strand (b′) of the opposing suture (H). The needle strand of the suture in the lower angle (b) is similarly inserted as an over-and-over suture, which is to be tied to the needle free strand (a′) at the upper angle. The suture strands may be seen within the lumen of the anastomosis. The purported disadvantage of this has proved more theoretical than real.

I. The insertion of the graft between the side of the aorta and the side of the left renal artery is completed, and the relation of the graft to the surrounding structures may be clearly seen.

Discussion—Dr. Paul T. De Camp. The dissection (C, D) illustrates numerous inferior branches of the left renal vein. Branches are common in this area and dissection must be meticulous to avoid annoying hemorrhage.

In view of the relatively poor long-term results from plastic prostheses used in the reconstruction of the arteries in the thigh that are of a size comparable to the renal artery, I prefer autogenous saphenous vein grafts for aortorenal bypass. Only time will tell whether the slight additional effort involved is worthwhile. Vein grafts have the additional advantages of flexibility and adaptability so that kinking is less likely to occur, which is a matter of some importance in such a vital area and to an organ as mobile as the kidney.

The technic of graft insertion is well illustrated (F-I). I prefer to make the more critical, and to me technically more difficult, renal arterial anastomosis first. Circulation is then permitted to resume through the renal artery while the aortic anastomosis is performed. This preference may be dictated by my use of the anterior approach. If a vein graft is used, it is technically easier to place the sutures through the arterial wall rather than through the graft first, which is the preferred technic with a plastic prosthesis.

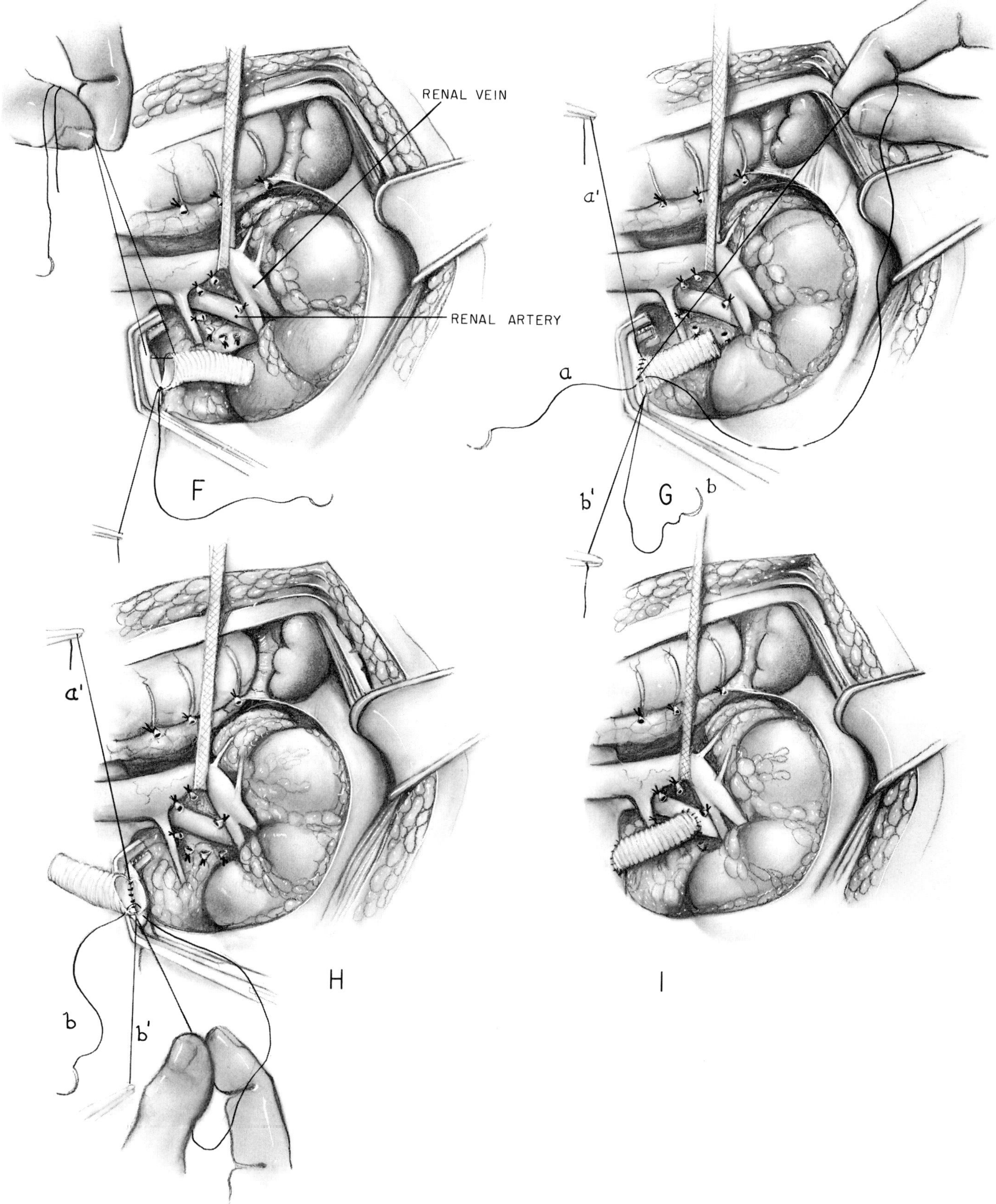
RENAL VEIN
RENAL ARTERY
F
a'
a
b'
G
b
a'
b
b'
H
I

SEGMENTAL RESECTION OF THE RENAL ARTERY AND PRIMARY ANASTOMOSIS; SPLENORENAL ARTERIAL ANASTOMOSIS

J. The left renal vein, encircled by a cotton tape, is elevated to show the site of segmental blockage of the renal artery. The broken lines indicate the boundaries for transection of the renal artery.

K. On completion of the segmental resection of the renal artery, continuity is restored by end-to-end anastomosis using two continuous sutures of 00000 silk swedged on small minimum trauma needles.

L. This illustration depicts the use of a dacron patch graft (angioplasty) following segmental renal thromboendarterectomy. This has proved a most useful technic in the smaller artery as a prophylaxis to a decrease in the size of the lumen.

M. The splenic artery is used to revascularize the kidney. The use of this technic, first described by Hurwitt and subsequently employed by others, is particularly adapted to renal arterial obstruction (stippled area) to the left kidney. The left renal vein is retracted downward and the mobilized greater curvature of the stomach upward to show the site of the end-to-end splenorenal arterial anastomosis in relation to the surrounding structures.

Discussion—Dr. Paul T. De Camp. In this condition certain operative diagnostic procedures are as much the responsibility of the surgeon as are therapeutic maneuvers. It is not as yet clear what renal hemodynamic changes are essential to renal arterial insufficiency (or renovascular hypertension), but one must at least determine whether significant hemodynamic changes are present. The simplest, and most reliable, observation is the intra-arterial pressure proximal and distal to the stenosis. Provided reliable equipment is available, the renal arterial blood flow is also significant. One or both of these parameters should be determined in every case.

Furthermore, the surgeon must determine whether *other* lesions are present which may cause hypertension or affect renal function. With routine bilateral wedge renal biopsies in proved cases of renal arterial insufficiency, I have found nephrosclerosis in 79 per cent of the cases, while in 43 per cent of all cases the grade has been moderately severe to severe. Pyelonephritis, generally of lesser severity, has been found in 50 per cent of the cases. Findings of this type may significantly affect the prognosis and permit a more intelligent appraisal of the subsequent course of the patient.

Operative diagnostic observations should include careful palpation of both kidneys and adrenals, careful palpation, inspection and pressure determinations in both renal arteries, and open wedge biopsies of representative areas of both kidneys.

It is chiefly for these reasons that my approach differs from that described, and is the same regardless of the side of the primary lesion. My incision is midline extending to the xyphoid. The transverse colon is lifted out at the upper angle of the wound, and the small bowel is eviscerated into a plastic bag. The ligament of Treitz is divided and the distal duodenum freely mobilized, which provides access to both renal arteries. The kidneys may be biopsied directly through this approach or through a more lateral short posterior peritoneal incision.

Alternatively, a curved transverse abdominal incision may be employed. With either the midline or the transverse abdominal incision either kidney and its vessels may be approached by a paracolic dissection as illustrated.

Discussion of Segmental Resection of Renal Artery and Primary Anastomosis, Renal Arterial Patch Angioplasty, Splenorenal Arterial Anastomosis. Occasionally areas of stenosis may be excised with direct reanastomosis of the artery. This is a very satisfactory procedure when possible. Stenosis of the suture line is avoided by oblique incisions and interrupted sutures.

In cases of left renal arterial stenosis the splenic artery may be employed as a bypass graft if it is not itself diseased. It is more useful in younger individuals without arteriosclerosis. With the transverse colon lifted up out of the wound, the body of the pancreas rotates forward in the transverse mesocolon, and the splenic vessels may be readily exposed posterior to the cephalad margin of the pancreas. A segment of the artery is cleared, and the vessel is divided. An end-to-side splenorenal anastomosis is performed. The spleen is not disturbed. I have experienced no difficulty with stenosis of this suture line and see no need to perform the technically more difficult side-to-side anastomosis.

I have been unfavorably impressed by attempts to reimplant renal arteries into the aorta. This procedure may be complicated by sclerosis of the aortic wall and/or by tension incident to a short remaining renal arterial segment.

Although bypass grafts may be satisfactorily inserted into the primary bifurcation of the renal artery, a word of caution is expressed concerning overly extending the indications for reconstruction to small reduplicated or to segmental arteries, as the danger of technical failure is great.

Sometimes the distal arterial "runoff" is inadequate and preoperative arteriographic evidence of this may be lacking because of inadequate visualization of these vessels. Careful operative evaluation of the "runoff" vessels is then imperative. There is, furthermore, no point in arterial reconstruction if the renal tissue served is destroyed. The renal biopsy may assist in making this decision.

Under marginal circumstances it is wiser not to attempt arterial reconstruction, but to remove the renal tissue served by the diseased vessel, provided that sufficient renal function may be maintained.

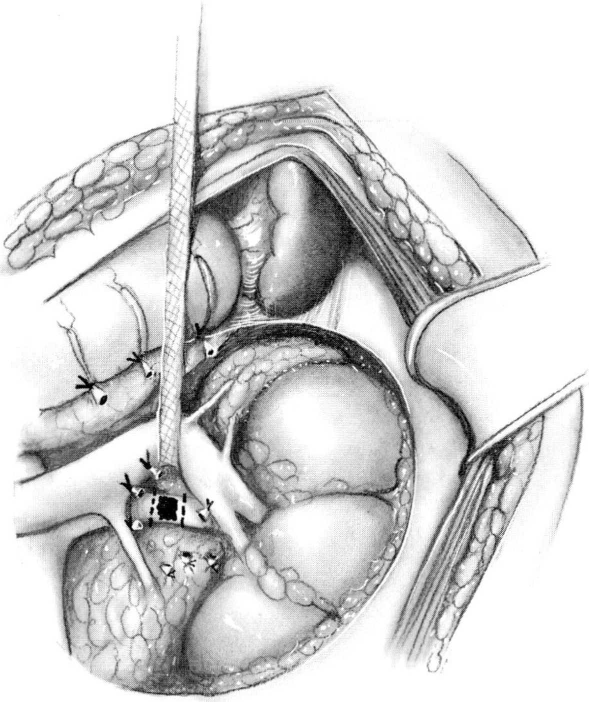

J

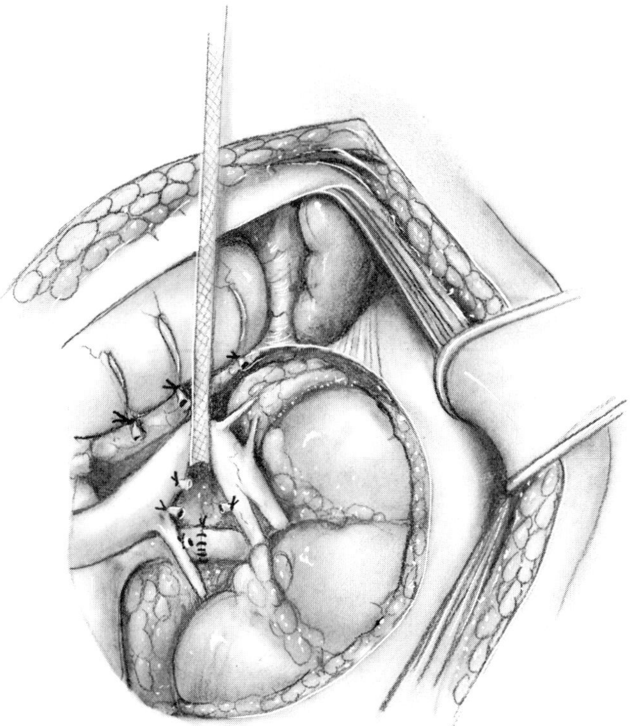

K

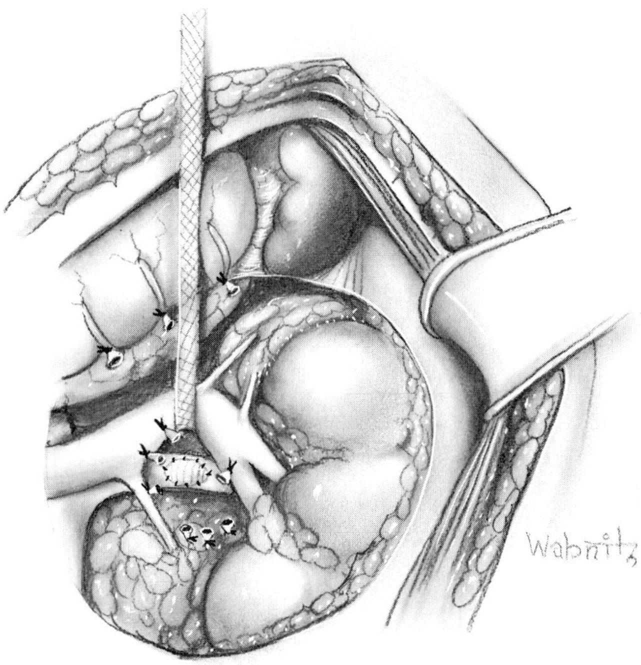

L

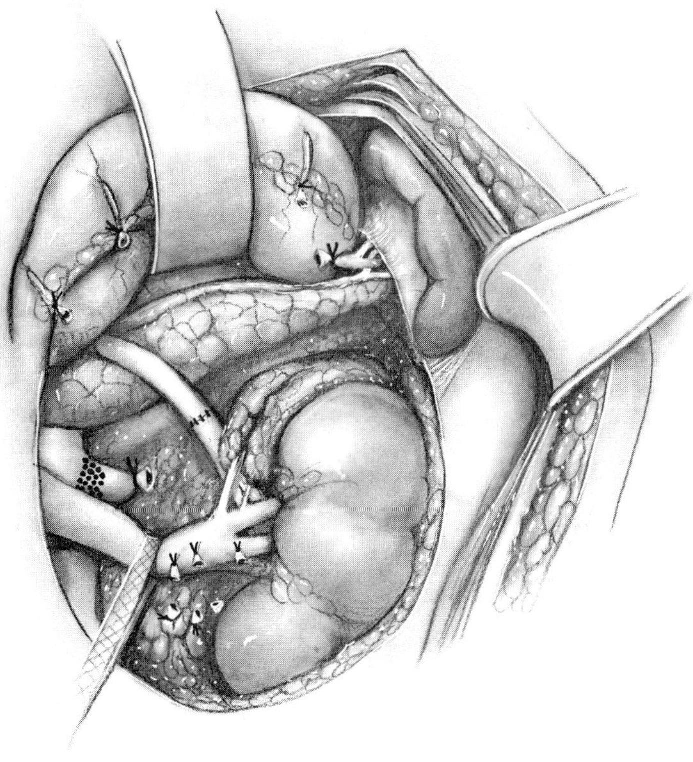

M

LIGATION OF THE SUPERFICIAL FEMORAL VEIN

A, B. The patient is placed in a 10- to 15-degree semi-Fowler's position (A). The site of the incision in the upper third of the thigh overlying Scarpa's triangle is indicated in dotted outline (B).

C, D. The incision is deepened through the underlying subcutaneous fat and deep fascia (C) to expose the medial border of the sartorius muscle, which is retracted laterally to demonstrate the proximal portion of the femoral sheath and the enclosed femoral artery and vein (D). The characteristic anatomic feature of the common femoral sheath is that the encased vessels are each enclosed by their own respective sheaths, which are demonstrable in the succeeding illustrations (E, F).

E. The common femoral sheath is opened, and the mobilized portion of the femoral artery is encircled with a cotton tape and retracted laterally. The separate sheath encasing the femoral vein is incised, and the lateral cut margin is secured in a guy suture (000 silk) for traction preparatory to the mobilization of the underlying femoral vein.

F. The femoral artery is encircled by two cotton tapes and retracted laterally. In this regard, caution must be observed to avoid excessive tension and angulation of the artery because of the danger of producing arterial spasm and secondary stasis thrombosis. In fact, the traction force and angulation of the artery depicted in the illustration is unwarranted and should not be practiced. The superficial femoral vein is mobilized and partially encircled by two ligatures of silk (00). The dotted line between the ligatures indicates the site of the opening to be made in the anterior wall of the vein by scissor dissection. The clot within the lumen of the vein is depicted by the dark shadow extending cephalad to the level of entrance of the profunda femoris tributary.

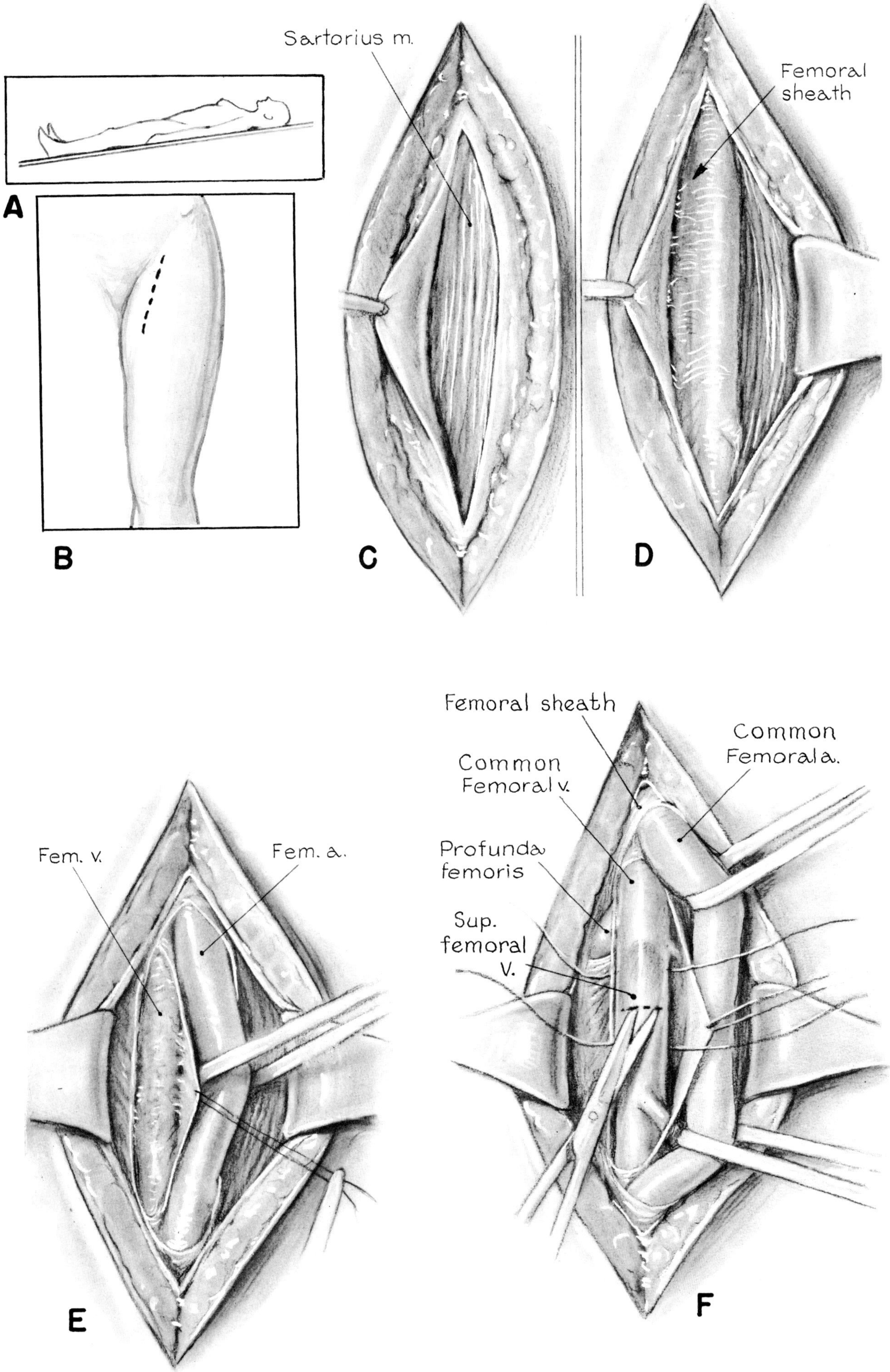
A
B
Sartorius m.
C
Femoral sheath
D
Fem. v.
Fem. a.
E
Femoral sheath
Common Femoral a.
Common Femoral v.
Profunda femoris
Sup. femoral V.
F

G. The incision in the superficial femoral vein is completed, and the partially extruded clot is being aspirated by suction.

H, I, J. By digital retrograde "milking," more of the clot is extruded through the phlebotomy site (H), and, when the cephalad evacuation of the clot is completed, the upper encircling ligature of silk (00) is tied (I). Similarly by digital "milking," the clot, caudad in the lumen of the vessel, is evacuated (I), and the lower encircling ligature is tied (J). The superficial femoral vein is doubly clamped between the ligatures, and the transection of the vein at the site of the phlebotomy is completed as indicated by the dotted line (J).

K. The distal transected end of the superficial femoral vein is further occluded with a suture ligature of silk (000), and its proximal transected end is being similarly occluded. For clarity, the clamp has been removed from the proximal transected end as the suture ligature is being inserted.

L, M. The deep fascia (L) and skin (M) are closed with interrupted sutures of 000 silk to complete the operation.

DISCUSSION—DR. W. G. ANLYAN. First and foremost I do not believe in interrupting the superficial femoral vein following thrombectomy. Instead, at our clinic we have closed the venotomy incision and repaired the vein, leaving its continuity intact.

The position we have used has been the supine position rather than the reverse Trendelenberg, and no embolic phenomena that have been recognized have occurred in the course of this procedure.

In the exposure of the vessel the artery may be left completely intact and should not be retracted. The saphenofemoral junction has been the principal site of selection for our venotomy incision.

To aid in the evacuation of a clot after opening the venotomy incision, we have milked the extremity starting just above the malleoli and working upward with a snug circumferential roll of stockinette. While this is being done, care must be taken to ensure that the proximal femoral vein is completely occluded by the cotton tape. At times this milking maneuver has produced a very long clot, which has been a cast of the deep venous system.

After completing the milking procedure a soft plastic catheter is introduced proximally and connected to gentle suction while it is being advanced proximally to suction out all the clot in the proximal common femoral vein and external iliac vein. After securing brisk bleeding both proximally and distally, the vein is irrigated with heparinized saline and the venotomy incision closed with 00000 arterial silk. We prefer to do this procedure under unilateral spinal anesthesia, but it can be done equally readily under local anesthesia.

Usually 50 mg. of heparin is administered intravenously immediately following the induction of the spinal anesthetic and before the skin incision is made. The patient is maintained on heparin postoperatively by the subcutaneous route.

Following the operation the patient is kept in the Trendelenburg position.

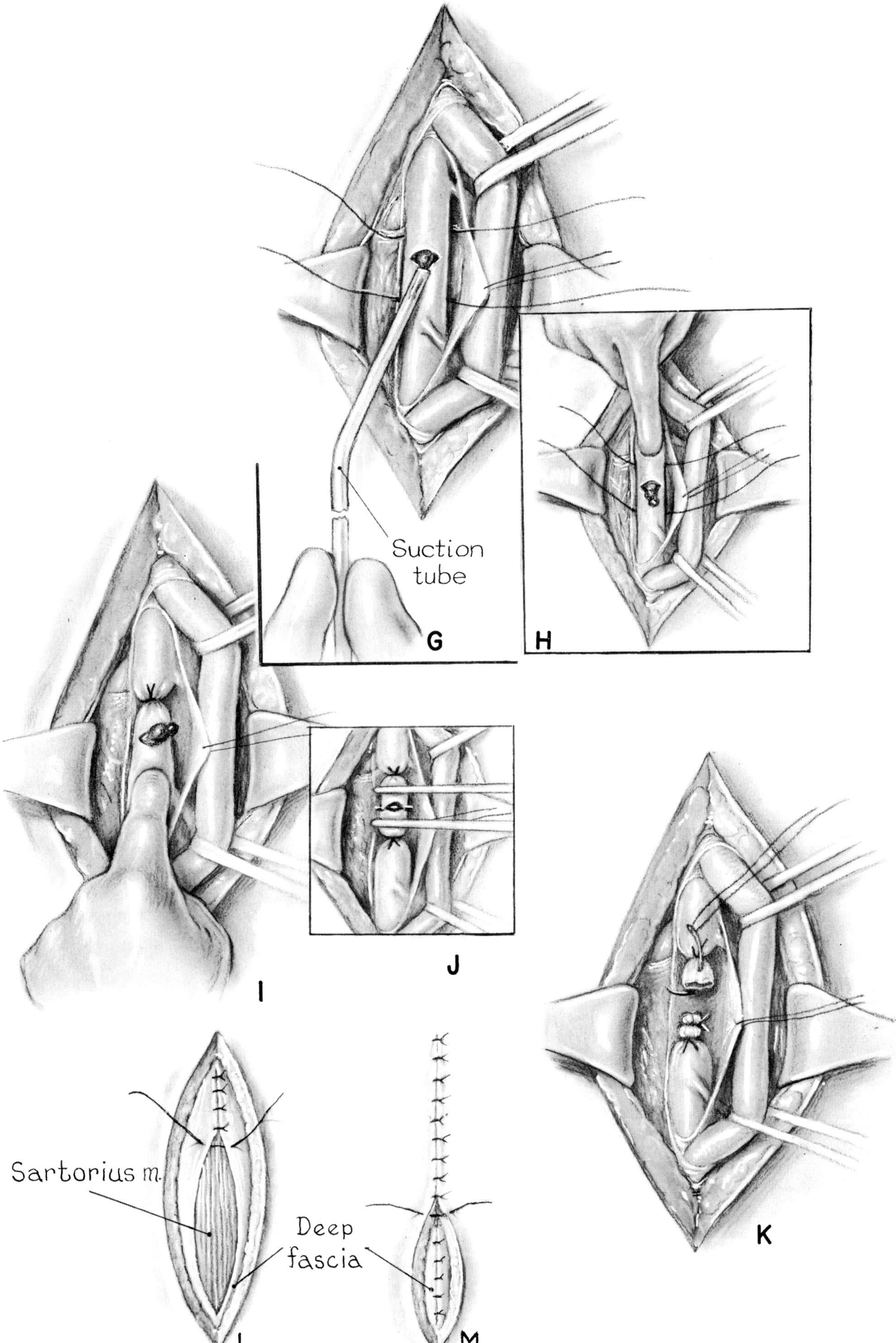
Suction tube
G
H
I
J
K
Sartorius m.
Deep fascia
L
M

LIGATION OF THE INFERIOR VENA CAVA

A. The patient is placed in the supine position, and the right side is elevated to approximately a 25 degree angle from the horizontal. The incision extends transversely from the lateral border of the rectus muscle at the level of the umbilicus outward to the midaxillary line just beneath the costal margin, as indicated in dotted outline.

B. The upper and lower skin flaps are dissected immediately beneath the subcutaneous tissue plane and retracted to expose a large surface area of the external oblique muscle and the line of separation of its fibers. A portion of the rectus sheath is also visible.

C. The separated margins of the external oblique muscle are retracted to expose the fibers of the internal oblique, which is the thickest of the three muscles to be separated. Through the line of separation of the fibers of the internal oblique, the underlying transversus abdominis muscle and one of the intercostal nerves are visible.

D. The transversus abdominis muscle is separated in the direction of its fibers, and the irregular line of apposition of the retroperitoneal fat with the peritoneum is visible. The dissection of this muscle, the thinnest of the group, is begun laterally and continued medially to lessen the possibility of opening into the peritoneal cavity.

E. The muscles of the anterolateral abdominal wall are separated, and the line of apposition of the retroperitoneal fat and peritoneum may now be clearly seen. The dotted line indicates the site of incision in the transversalis fascia overlying the retroperitoneal fat.

F. The transversalis fascia is incised by scissor dissection, and a portion of the retroperitoneal fat is seen to herniate through the opening.

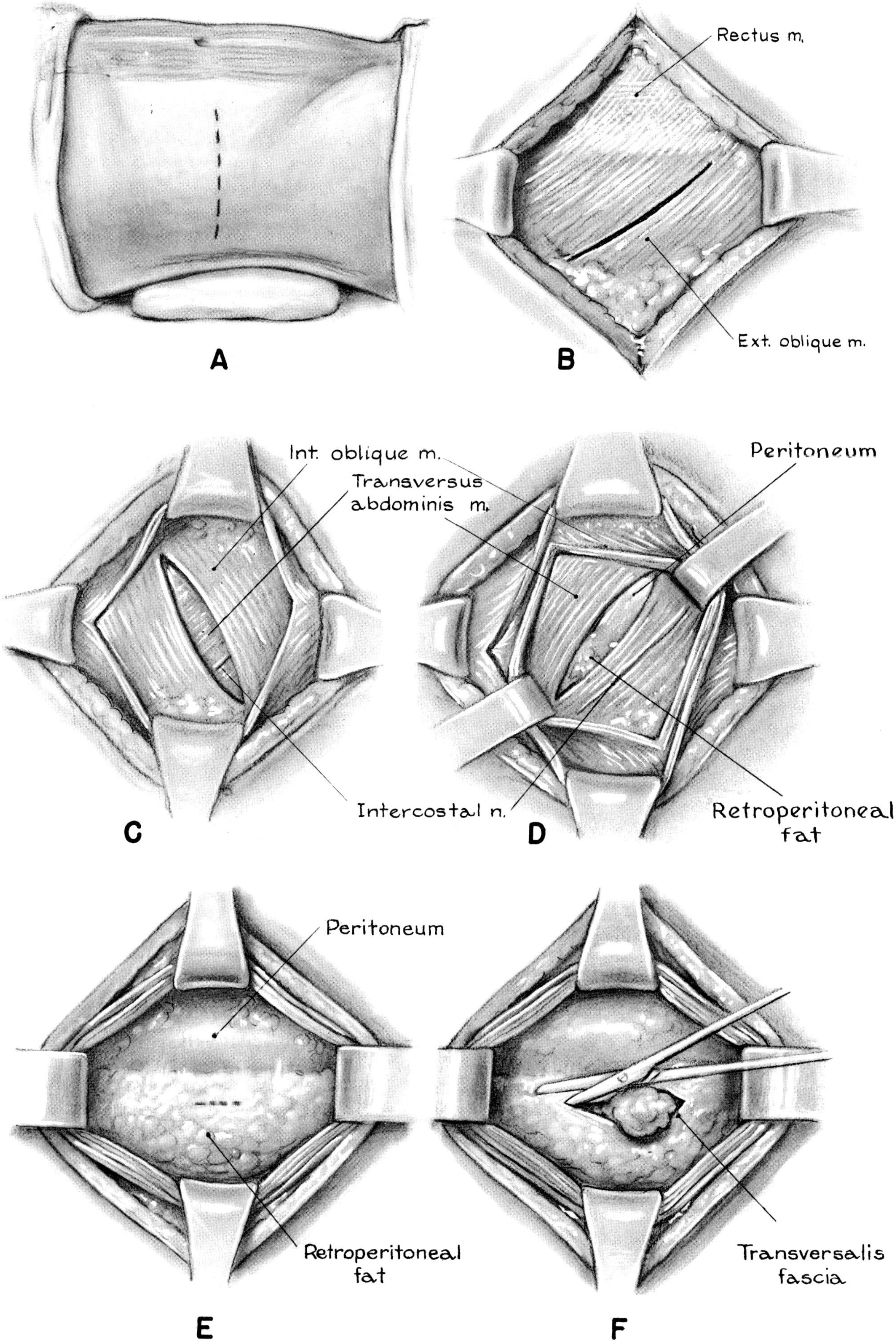
A
Rectus m.
Ext. oblique m.
B
Int. oblique m.
Transversus
abdominis m.
Peritoneum
Intercostal n.
Retroperitoneal
fat
C
D
Peritoneum
Retroperitoneal
fat
Transversalis
fascia
E
F

G, H. By blunt digital dissection in the retroperitoneal fatty tissue plane, the peritoneum and the intraperitoneal viscera adjacent are displaced toward the midline. During this dissection, an important landmark is the psoas major muscle, which is located more anteriorly than one generally assumes. The tissue dissection is continued anterior and medial to this muscle; otherwise, troublesome technical difficulties may ensue. When the dissection is completed to the vertebral column, blunt digital dissection is continued, first cephalad and then caudad in the same plane. A wide-type Harrington retractor is used to maintain retraction of the peritoneum and the encased adjacent viscera. The right ureter is then identified as it courses along in the fatty tissue plane on the anterior surface of the inferior vena cava.

I. The right ureter is retracted from the anterior surface of the vena cava, and the line of incision in the overlying fibroareolar tissue layer (fascia of Gerota) is depicted.

J. The inferior vena cava is exposed preliminary to the completion of the mobilization of its circumference at the level selected for ligation. In the isolation and mobilization of the inferior vena cava, a medium sized "kidney pedicle" clamp and a malleable ligature carrier* with a ball-point protected tip are the instruments that have proved the most useful. Medially, the vena cava is intimately adherent to the adjacent tissues, and the lumbar veins enter posteromedially. Accordingly, during the dissection and mobilization posteriorly and medially, one must be careful to avoid either an avulsion tear of one of the lumbar veins or an inadvertent perforation of the vena cava. Should either occur, bleeding is best controlled by immediate compression of the vena cava with "stick" sponges both proximal and distal to the site of hemorrhage. Hemostasis may then be obtained by closure of the opening with sutures of fine silk (00000) swedged on a minimum trauma needle.

K, L. The mobilized segment of the vena cava is encircled with two ligatures of braided silk (No. 1), using a malleable ligature carrier, and a double ligation in continuity is performed.

* Manufactured by Edward Weck & Co., Inc., Brooklyn, N. Y.

Discussion—Dr. Jere W. Lord. During the decade from January 1, 1948, through December 31, 1957, on the surgical services of the Fourth Division, Bellevue Hospital, the University Hospital, and in this commentator's private practice, only two patients were subjected to ligation of the inferior vena cava. The vast majority of the patients with thromboemboli were treated with anticoagulants. In fact, only 10 patients were operated upon. In six of these, ligation of the superficial femoral vein was performed. In two of the remaining four, one had a ligation of the superficial femoral vein and the other had a ligation of the right common iliac vein. In the remaining two, ligation of the inferior vena cava was done. At operation, when palpation revealed thrombotic material, the vein was opened, aspirated both proximally and distally, and then doubly ligated in continuity.

Although the author's personal experience has been most favorable with ligation of the inferior vena cava, several papers in the literature have emphasized the serious late sequelae of ulceration, edema, and recurrent phlebitis. We have observed these complications in three patients in whom ligation of the inferior vena cava was performed on the Fourth Surgical Division of Bellevue Hospital between 1944 and 1948.

In the postoperative management of the patient following ligation of the superficial femoral vein or ligation of the inferior vena cava, the important factors which should be stressed are: (1) the wearing of custom-made elastic stockings for prolonged periods to control the edema of the legs; (2) elevation of the foot of the bed on blocks (10 inches); and (3) the adherence to strict hygienic measures in the care of the feet to avoid a fungus infection. In some patients the wearing of an elastic support may be discontinued within six to eight months, whereas, in others, it may be necessary to continue the use of elastic supports for the remainder of their lives.

In regard to surgical technic, the artist's illustrations are clear and the accompanying text is entirely adequate. The use of "stick" sponges for the control of bleeding from torn lumbar veins is considered the best method for hemostasis. The sponges are held in place for 8 to 10 minutes to allow the formation of a blood clot to block the bleeding point. The venous pressure in the inferior vena cava is usually low and may be lowered still further by depressing the head of the table (Trendelenburg position). Clamps should rarely be applied to the vena cava. If bleeding persists, it should be controlled either by the use of silver (dural or Cushing) clips or transfixion sutures of fine silk (00000) swedged on a minimum trauma needle.

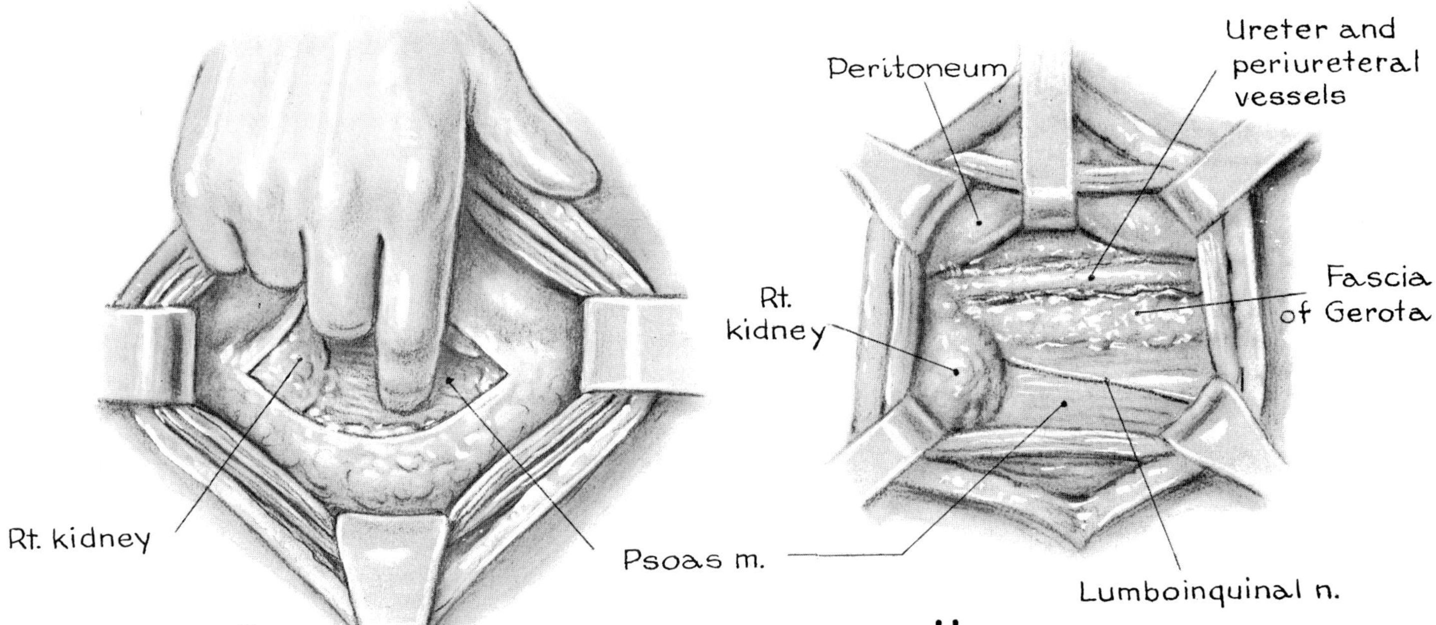
Rt. kidney
Psoas m.
Peritoneum
Ureter and periureteral vessels
Fascia of Gerota
Rt. kidney
Lumboinquinal n.

G H

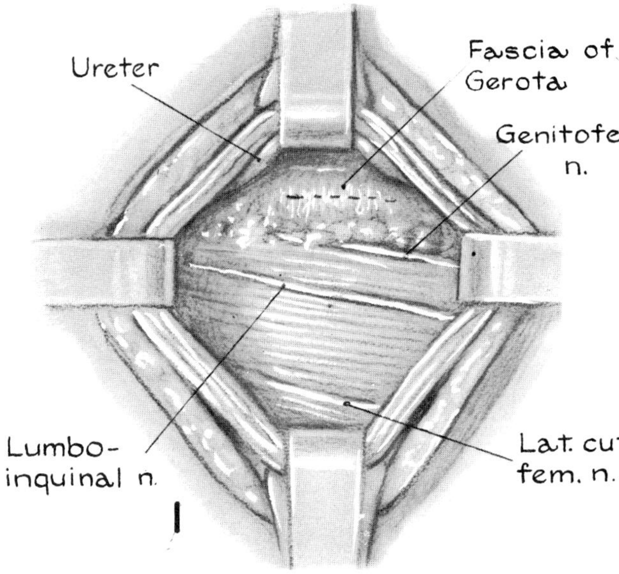
Ureter
Fascia of Gerota
Genitofem. n.
Lumbo-inquinal n.
Lat. cut. fem. n.

I

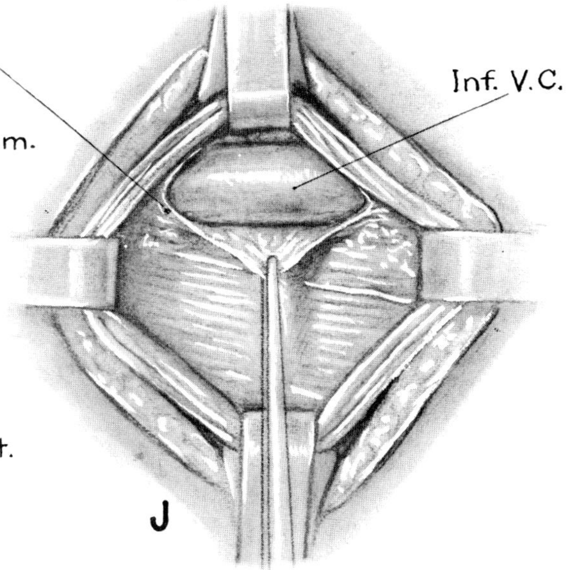
Inf. V.C.

J

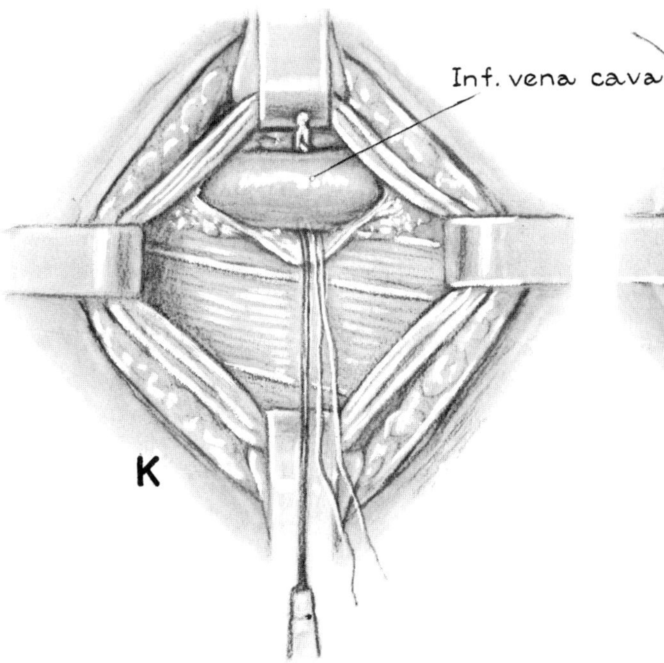
Inf. vena cava

K

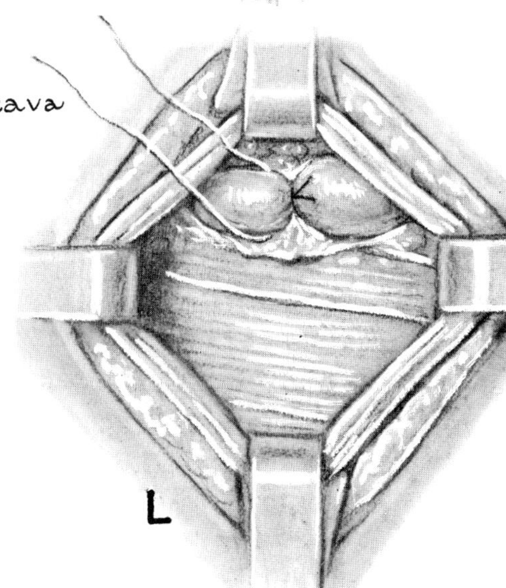

L

M. The operative field after completion of the double ligation in continuity of the inferior vena cava is shown.

N, O, P, Q. These illustrations depict the technic that is employed when a thrombotic occlusion of the lumen of the inferior vena cava, commonly associated with phlegmasia cerulea dolens, is present. The vena cava is incised between the encircling but untied ligatures of silk (No. 1), and the thrombus is evacuated (O). This is done by digital compression, first from above downward until free retrograde bleeding from the renal veins occurs. The proximal ligature is then tied (P). The thrombus is next evacuated from below upward, and the distal ligature is tied (P). If desired, an additional suture of the transfixion type may be inserted between the ligatures as indicated (Q).

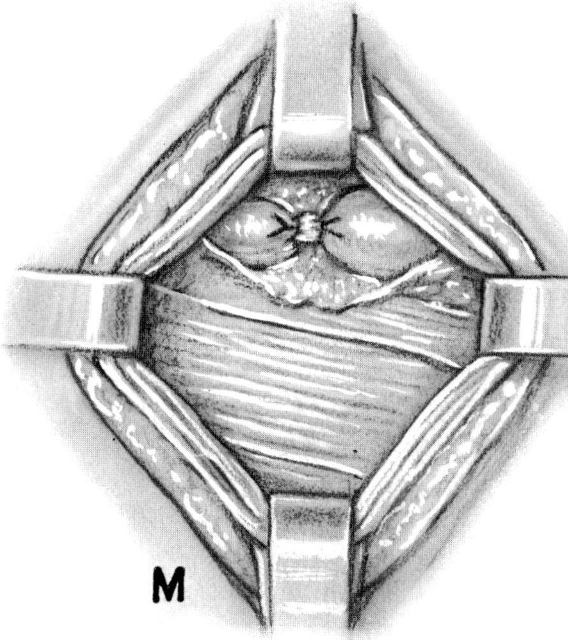

M

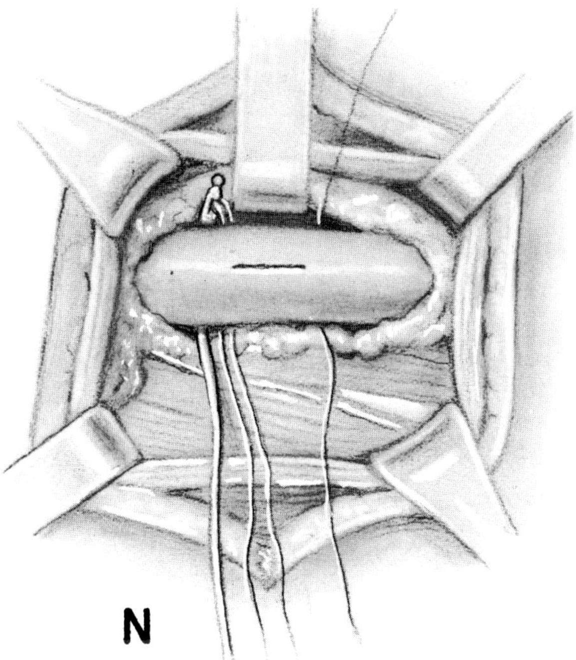

N

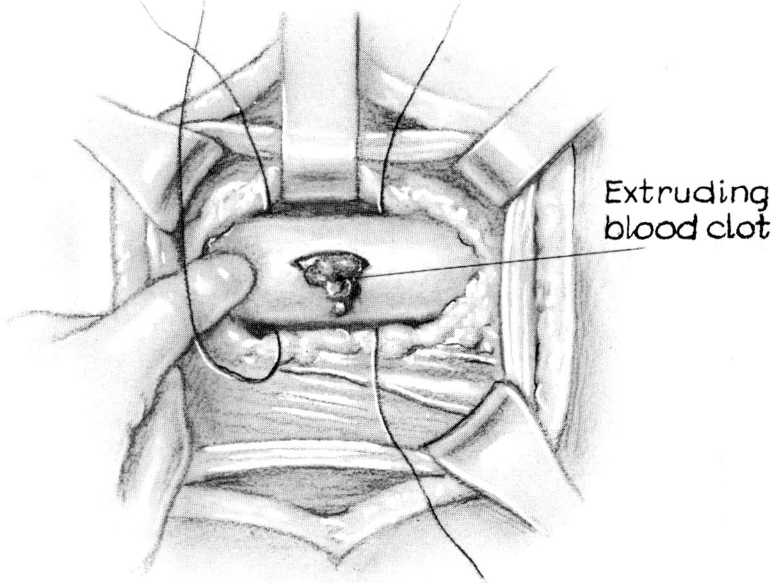

O

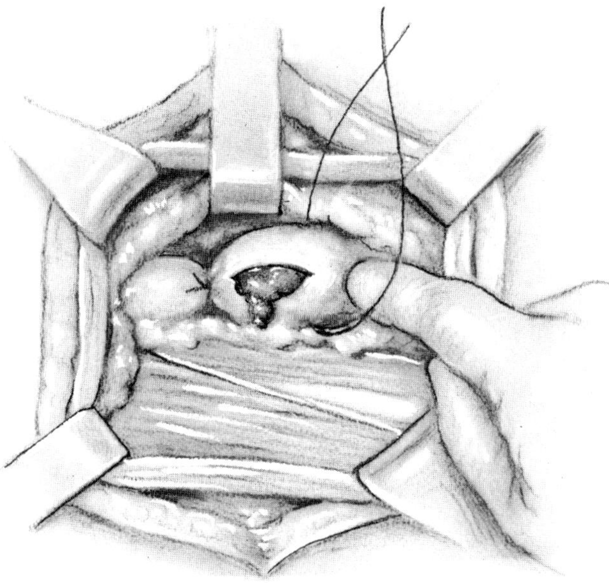

P

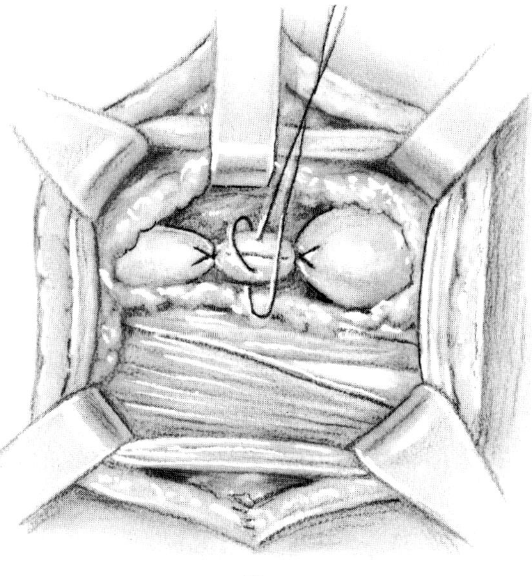

Q

R, S. These illustrations depict an alternate but less desirable method of transection of the vena cava. This is done between clamps following double ligation in continuity. The severed ends are occluded with transfixion sutures of silk as the clamps are removed.

T. The retractors in the retroperitoneal tissue plane have been removed, and the overlying muscle layers of the anterolateral abdominal wall tend to approximate themselves. The line of apposition of the retroperitoneal fat and peritoneum is visible beneath the incompletely approximated fibers of the transversus abdominis muscle. The adjacent intercostal nerve may also be seen.

U, V, W. The closure of the remainder of the muscle layers and the skin, using interrupted sutures of silk (000), is depicted.

Discussion—Dr. W. G. Anlyan. I prefer a slightly more oblique skin incision more in line with the direction of the fibers of the external oblique muscle and fascia, since it is less vascular and tends to be more in the direction of the superficial nerves. The usual landmarks used by us are from the tip of the eleventh rib to the lateral border of the rectus muscle at a point midway between the umbilicus and the symphysis pubis. There are three instances in which a midline or pararectus incision should be used instead of the muscle-splitting incision: (1) in patients who have visible in the flank area large collaterals that would be disrupted by the flank incision; (2) in patients requiring venal caval ligation who have had a previous right lumbar sympathectomy, where the amount of scar tissue in the retroperitoneal area would make this approach difficult; and (3) in female patients who are either post partum or who have septic pelvic thrombophlebitis, where a concomitant ligation of the ovarian veins is necessary. Otherwise, the flank incision as outlined above is certainly to be favored.

We prefer to tie the vena cava at the most convenient level above the highest point of thrombus formation that is palpable, and we do not routinely try to go up to the level just below the renal veins. We have not attempted any plication occlusions of the vena cava, since most of our patients have repeated small pulmonary emboli as the main indication for ligation rather than a single massive one. Division of the vena cava is unnecessary and complicates the procedure.

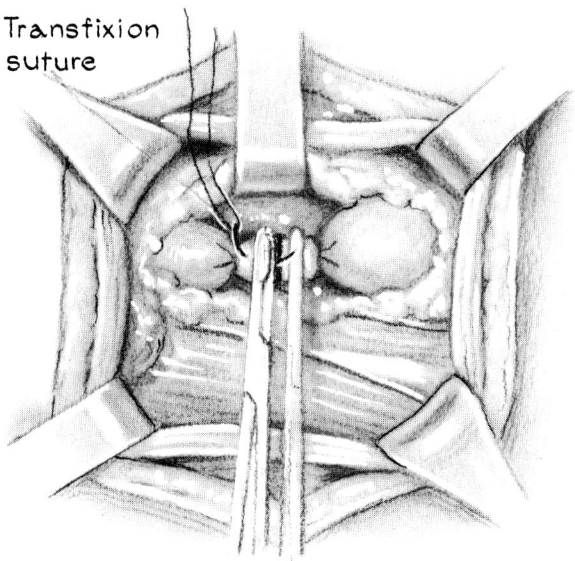
Transfixion
suture

R

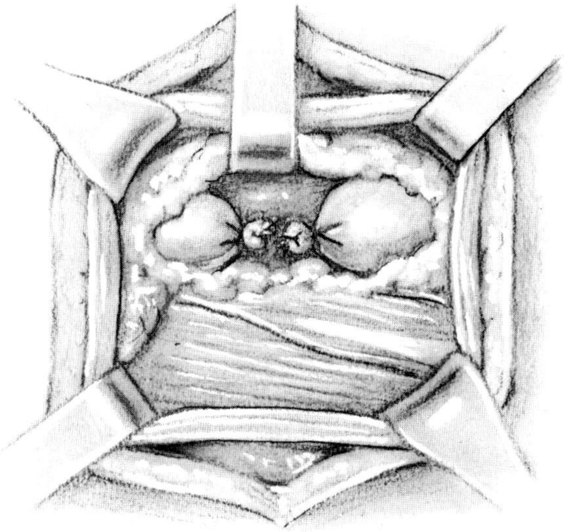

S

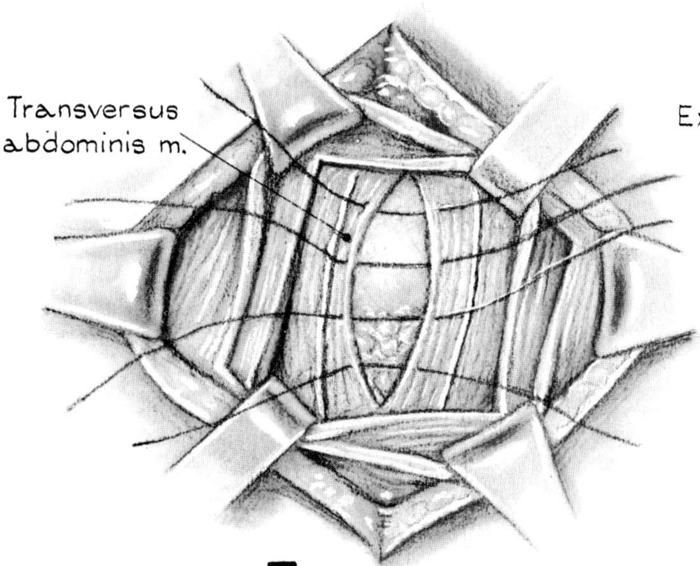
Transversus
abdominis m.

T

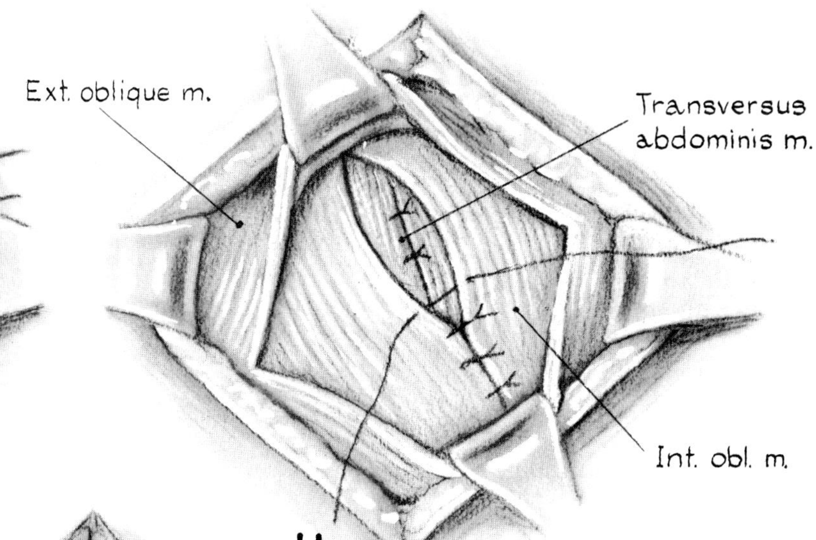
Ext. oblique m.
Transversus
abdominis m.
Int. obl. m.

U

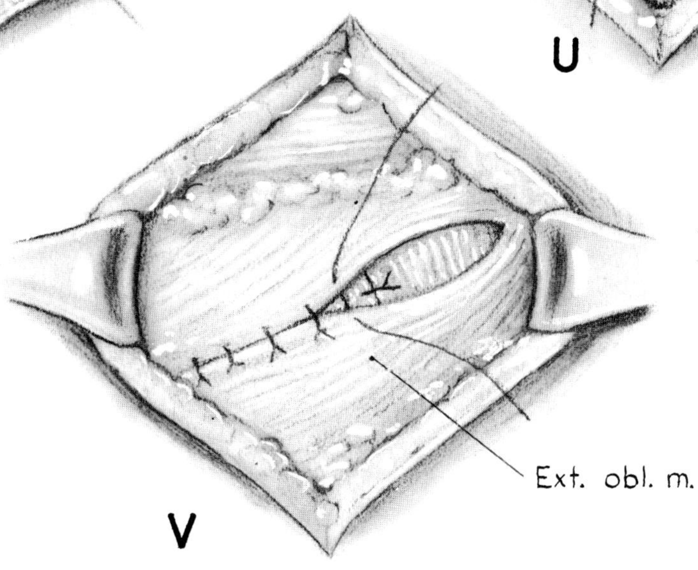
Ext. obl. m.

V

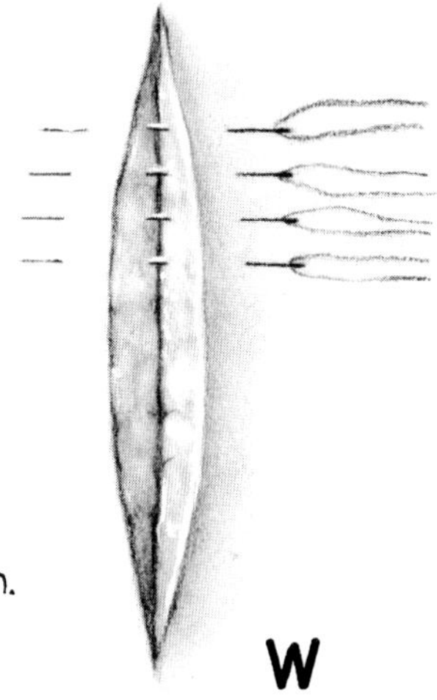

W

REPAIR OF TRAUMATIC LACERATION OF THE INFERIOR VENA CAVA

The patient, a 39-year-old police officer shot by an assailant, was admitted to the hospital in shock. Examination revealed a bullet wound of entrance below and to the right of the umbilicus and a wound of exit in the right loin. Replacement of blood loss and operation were done concomitantly. There were two perforations in the small bowel and a large retroperitoneal hematoma on the right side. The perforations were temporarily occluded with clamps, and the large retroperitoneal hematoma was evacuated. The lacerated wound of the inferior vena cava was repaired as illustrated, and the intestinal wounds were closed in layers (2). The postoperative convalescence of the patient was uneventful.

A. The patient is in the supine position, and the right paraumbilical incision is outlined. The bullet wound of entrance is indicated by the black circle.

B. The peritoneal cavity is entered, and the bulging retroperitoneal hematoma is visible. Mobilization of the right colon is begun by scissor dissection along the fascia fusion layer of Toldt, the "white line."

C. Mobilization of the right colon is continued by digital dissection. The subsequent severance of the phrenocolic ligament to free the hepatic flexure is indicated by the broken line cephalad. The clotted blood retroperitoneally (caudad) is also visible.

D, E, F. Following decompression of the retroperitoneal space by the evacuation of large quantities of clotted blood, active bleeding from the traumatic laceration in the inferior vena cava ensued (D). The bleeding was immediately controlled by digital compression (E). The "blind" application of clamps for hemostasis is dangerous and should be judiciously avoided. Large pledgets of dry gauze, secured in clamps, are used to compress the inferior vena cava both cephalad and caudad to the site of digital compression. The fingers are removed, and the margins of the laceration in the inferior vena cava are approximated with clamps * (Babcock) modified on the Potts principle (F).

G, H. Gauze compression of the inferior vena cava is maintained as the clamps are removed (G), and the lacerated wound is closed using interrupted sutures of 00000 arterial silk (G, H).

* Manufactured by Edward Weck & Co., Long Island City, N.Y.

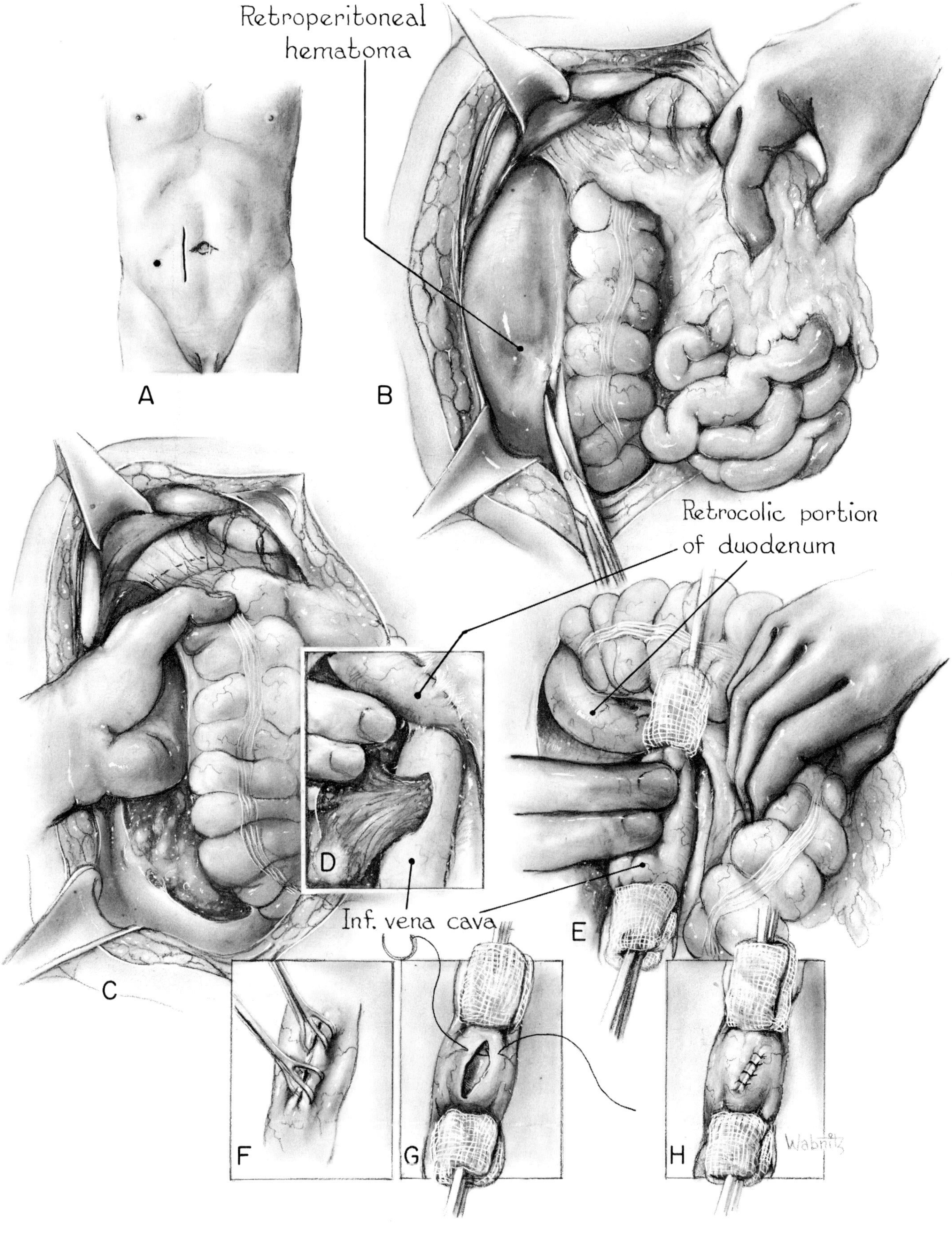
Retroperitoneal hematoma
Retrocolic portion of duodenum
Inf. vena cava
A
B
C
D
E
F
G
H
Wabnitz

CIRCUMFERENTIAL VENOUS LIGATION FOR POSTPHLEBITIC ULCER

A. Palpation of a "feeder" vein subjacent to the ulcer.

B. The incisions in relation to the ulcer are shown and the lowermost is being deepened through the underlying indurated tissue.

C. The "feeder" vein is isolated.

D. It is doubly ligated in continuity and severed.

E. The operation is completed. The wounds, rather than being sutured, are packed loosely with sterile dry gauze and a compression dressing is applied.

Discussion—Dr. John L. Keeley. The operation described by Dr. Madden appears to offer a promising solution for a very troublesome lesion. His results justify its further trial, as it is a procedure that in the past has not been as helpful in the hands of others. If an ulcer such as that illustrated is dependent upon venous stasis alone, interruptions of the neighboring veins as described should be beneficial. However, many will be associated with postphlebitic induration in the surrounding blood-poor tissues, such as fat, ligaments, tendons, and periosteum. In patients with normal tissues healing is slower in the region of the ankle than at higher levels. This is well illustrated in the healing of incisions at the ankle level compared to those which take place at higher levels in the ligation and stripping of varicose veins uncomplicated by previous cellulitis. The ankle is near the end of the "blood supply line." If arteriosclerosis is also present, one hesitates to cut off blood supply coming to an ulcerated area through vessels in the skin or immediately under it by partially surrounding the ulcer with incisions. Patients with either ulcer or postphlebitic induration should be warned of the vulnerable status of tissues in the areas so characteristically involved. Trauma to the region, whether surgical or accidental, may be followed by ulceration or slow healing.

One wonders if the postoperative care following circumferential venous ligation is more carefully planned and executed than that ordinarily accorded the patient with an ulcer not subjected to a surgical procedure. Attention paid to cleanliness and asepsis and to effective support for the area may contribute significantly to the good results the author has attained.

It seems reasonable that the patient with an ulcer about which "feeder" veins may be demonstrated and with minimal evidence of postphlebitic cellulitis might be treated by this procedure on a trial basis. In some patients it may suffice. If it fails, the more formidable operations of fasciectomy and individual ligation of perforating communicating veins, with or without skin grafting, may be needed.

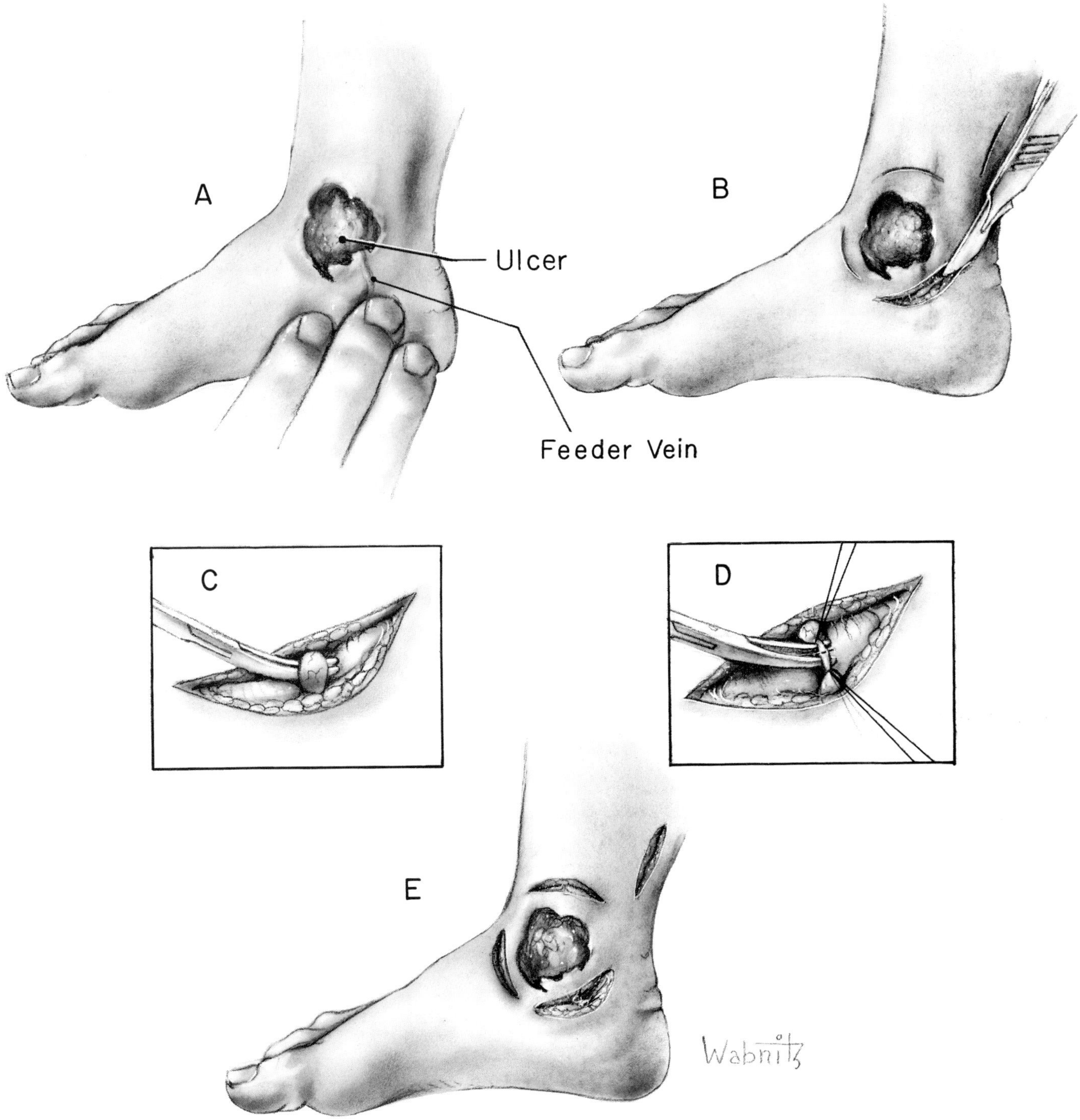
A
Ulcer
B
Feeder Vein
C
D
E
Wabnitz

SPLENECTOMY AND END-TO-SIDE SPLENORENAL SHUNT

A. The patient is placed in the supine position, and the left side is elevated on a pillow support to approximately a 30 degree angle from the horizontal. The incisions of choice, a long curvilinear subcostal incision solid line), that extends from the left costophrenic angle to the posterior axillary line, and an abdominothoracic incision (dotted outline), that enters the left pleural cavity through the eighth interspace, are shown. In this particular patient, the subcostal incision was used.

B, C. The incision is deepened through the rectus sheath, the underlying fibers of the rectus abdominis, the external oblique, and the internal oblique muscles to expose the transversus abdominis muscle and its aponeurosis.

D. The peritoneal cavity is entered, and the relation of the enlarged spleen to the surrounding structures is depicted. An opening is made in an avascular segment of the gastrocolic ligament preliminary to the serial clamping and severance of its proximal extension, the anterior layer of the gastrosplenic ligament.

E. The mobilization of the spleen is continued by doubly clamping and cutting (dotted line) the anterior layer of the gastrosplenic ligament and its contained vasa brevia.

F. The superior border of the pancreas is exposed, and the splenic artery is encircled by a ligature of silk (00) for traction as mobilization of the artery is completed by scissor dissection. A second ligature of silk (00) is subsequently inserted, and double ligation, in continuity, of the splenic artery is performed.

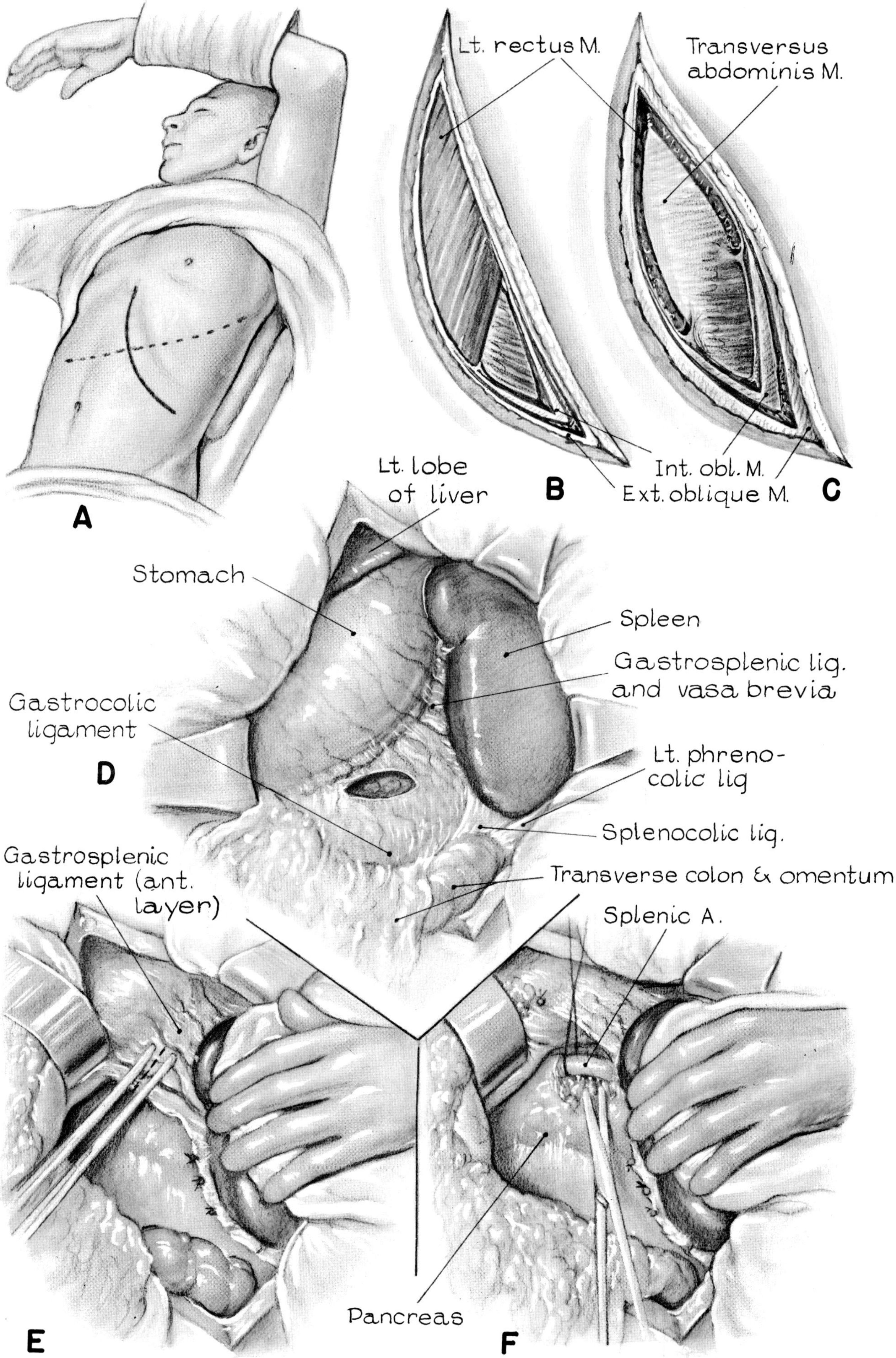
Lt. rectus M.
Transversus abdominis M.
Int. obl. M.
Ext. oblique M.
A
B
C
Lt. lobe of liver
Stomach
Spleen
Gastrosplenic lig. and vasa brevia
Gastrocolic ligament
D
Lt. phreno-colic lig
Splenocolic lig.
Transverse colon & omentum
Gastrosplenic ligament (ant. layer)
Splenic A.
Pancreas
E
F

G. The spleen is manually rotated and displaced toward the midline, and the reflection of the posterior parietal peritoneum forming the posterior layer of the lienorenal ligament is severed under direct vision by scissor dissection. Normally this ligament is avascular. However, in the presence of portal hypertension, the application of clamps to this ligament is frequently required to prevent excessive blood loss from the extensive collateral vascular bed.

H. The spleen is reposited laterally, and the superior segment of the gastrocolic ligament is doubly clamped and severed (dotted line). This segment is the narrowest portion of the gastrosplenic ligament, and particular care should be observed in the application of clamps to prevent injury to the greater curvature of the stomach. Furthermore, one of the largest of the vasa brevia is contained in this narrow uppermost portion of the gastrosplenic ligament in relation to the superior pole of the spleen. Accordingly, in the mobilization of the superior pole of the spleen, one should proceed with caution to avoid an avulsion laceration of this vessel and resulting hemorrhage.

I. Following the completion of the severance of the anterior layer of the gastrosplenic ligament, the spleen is again rotated toward the midline, and the pad of vascular areolar tissue, in relation to the inferior pole of the spleen and the tail of the pancreas, is doubly clamped prior to its severance.

J. The splenic vein in the hilum of the spleen is encircled with a traction ligature of silk (00), and the vein is mobilized by clamping and dividing the pancreatic tributary veins as indicated.

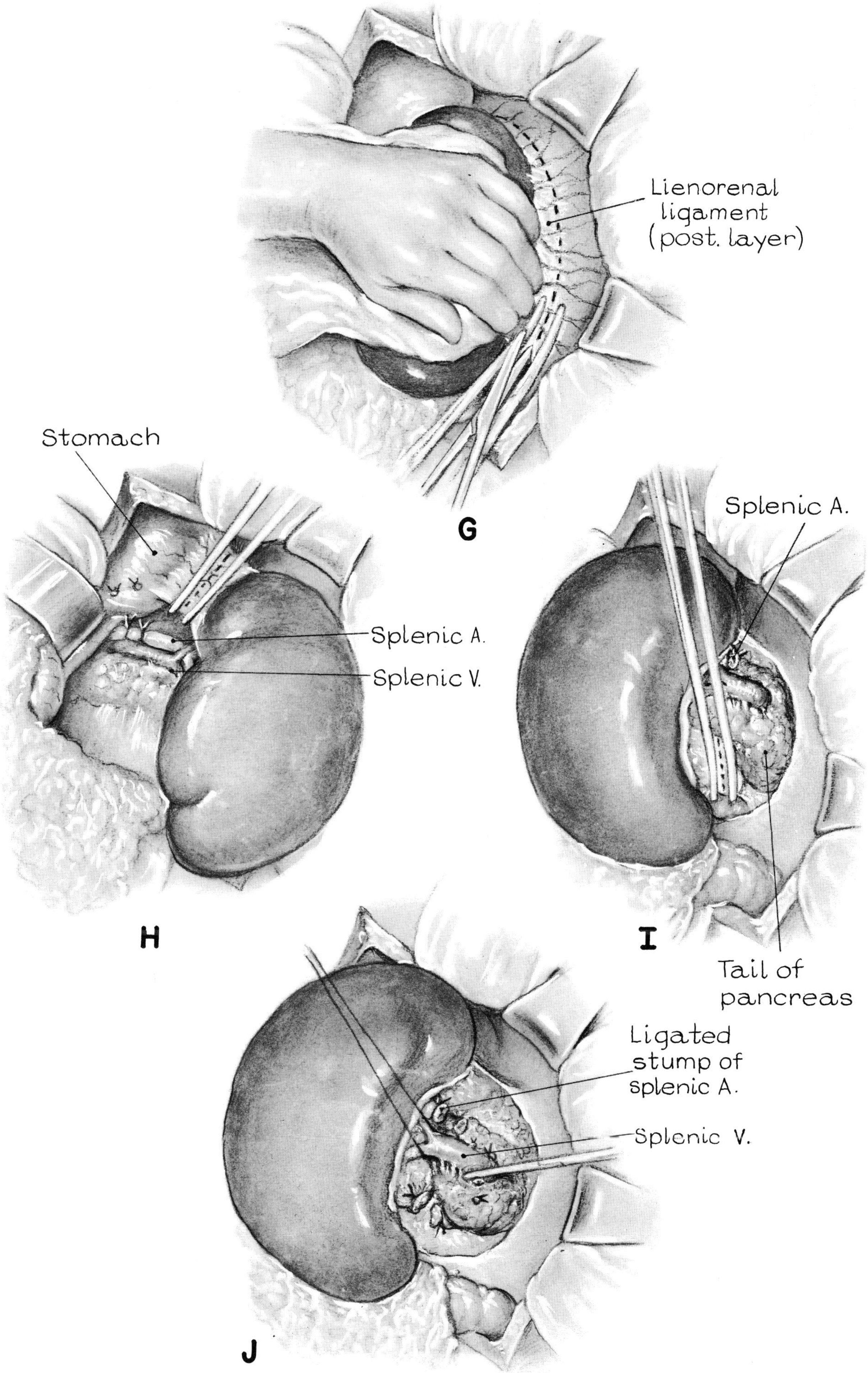
Lienorenal ligament (post. layer)
G
Stomach
Splenic A.
Splenic V.
H
Splenic A.
I
Tail of pancreas
Ligated stump of splenic A.
Splenic V.
J

K. The mobilized segment of the splenic vein is doubly clamped using both angulated and straight Potts ductus clamps. The site for transection of the vein, in juxtaposition to its bifurcation at the hilum of the spleen, is indicated by dotted lines. The incision in the anterior layer of the renal fascia for the exposure and subsequent mobilization of the kidney is also indicated in dotted outline.

L. The left kidney is mobilized from its surrounding adipose capsule and rotated toward the midline. The relation of the kidney to the left adrenal gland and the surrounding structures is visible.

M. The mobilized kidney is rotated laterally and posteriorly, and the distal segments of the renal artery and vein are mobilized by a combination of blunt and sharp dissection. The renal vein is encircled by cotton traction tapes to facilitate its manipulation.

N. The lumen of the renal vein is partially occluded by a Potts–Smith clamp, and the proximal cut end of the splenic vein is turned down toward the incised opening in the renal vein preparatory to the anastomosis.

DISCUSSION—DRS. ARTHUR H. BLAKEMORE AND ARTHUR B. VOORHEES, JR. The position of the patient on the operating table, the location and technic of the incision are similar to those described in *Portal vein-to-vena cava anastomosis,* with the exception that all takes place on the left rather than the right side of the patient (Fig. 1).

When the operative incision and general abdominal examination have been completed, manometric pressures in the portal system are recorded by the described technic. A liver biopsy is obtained in the described fashion; however, in this case it is usually obtained from the left lobe rather than the right lobe of the liver.

At this point the operation can be divided into three steps for sake of convenience of description. The first step is the mobilization and subsequent resection of the spleen. The second step is the identification and mobilization of the splenic vein, and the third step is the performance of an end-to-side anastomosis between the splenic vein and the left renal vein.

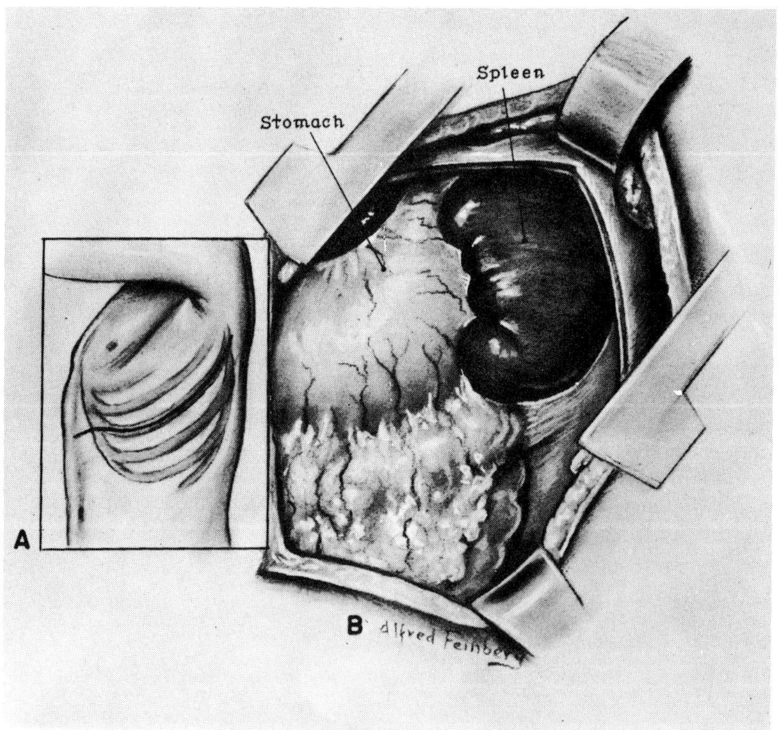

Fig. 1. A, line of incision; B, illustrating exposure following completion of a thoracoabdominal approach. Note that splitting the diaphragm affords direct access to control of hemorrhage in separating an adherent spleen from the diaphragm.

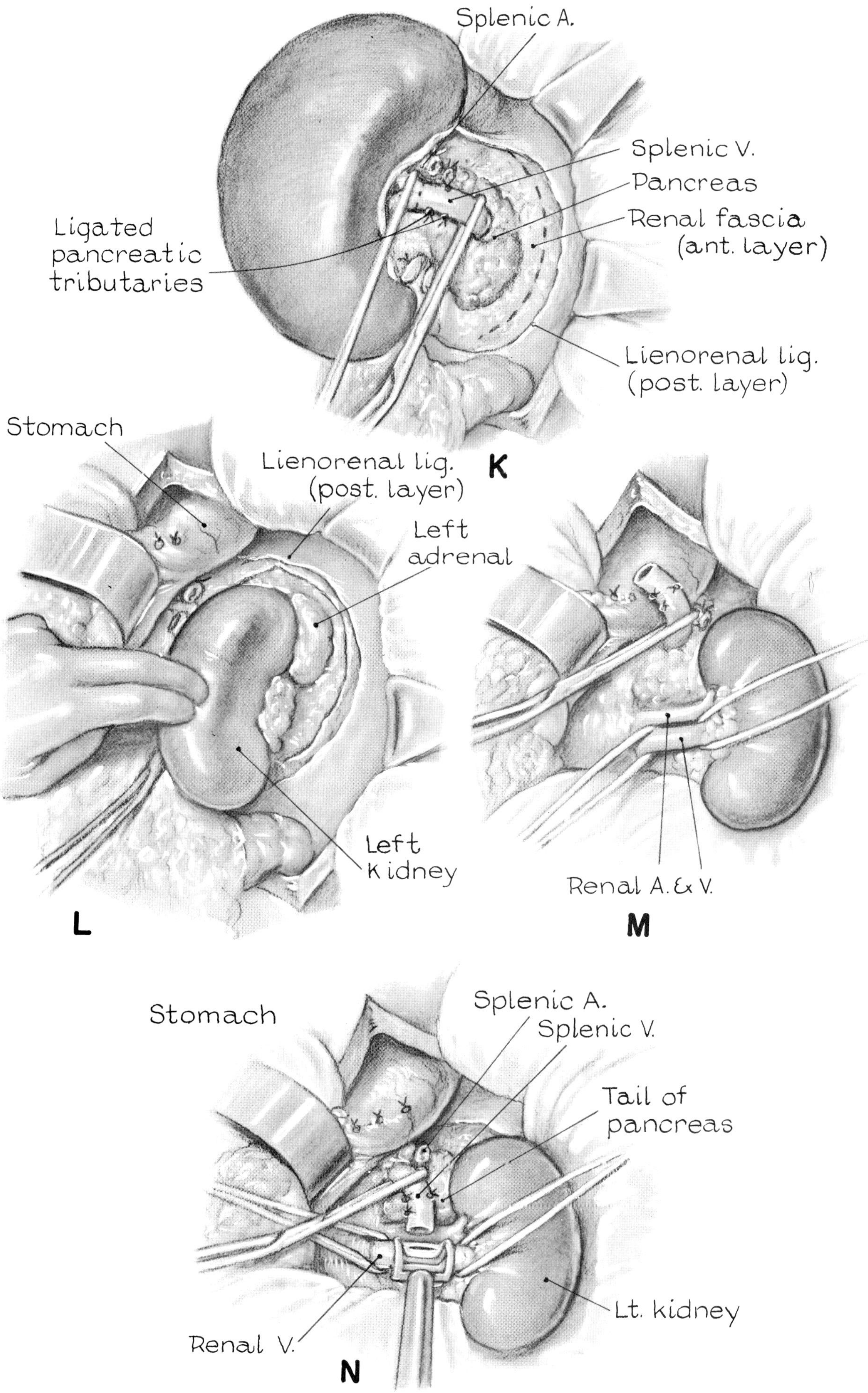
Splenic A.
Splenic V.
Pancreas
Renal fascia (ant. layer)
Ligated pancreatic tributaries
Lienorenal lig. (post. layer)
K
Stomach
Lienorenal lig. (post. layer)
Left adrenal
Left kidney
L
Renal A. & V.
M
Stomach
Splenic A.
Splenic V.
Tail of pancreas
Lt. kidney
Renal V.
N

O, P, Q, R. Close-up illustrations to show more clearly the technic of the anastomosis of the proximal cut end of the splenic vein to the longitudinal opening in the side of the left renal vein.

O, P. The posterior suture layer is inserted. This is a continuous eversion suture of 00000 arterial silk on a swedged-on minimum trauma needle. The suture is commenced from the "outside in" on the splenic vein and terminates from the "inside out" on the same vein. Between its commencement and termination, the suture is inserted alternately from the "inside out" to the "outside in" on the renal and splenic veins respectively. Accordingly, the loop is on the outside of the lumen, and, when the suture is drawn taut, it causes an eversion of the tissues with intima to intima approximation.

Q. The anterior layer of the anastomosis consists of a series of interrupted everting mattress sutures of silk (00000). These sutures are all inserted, and the end sutures are tied. One of the strands of each of the end mattress sutures is then tied to either end of the continuous everting posterior suture (a–a).

R. The completed anterior layer of the anastomosis prior to the release of the Potts–Smith clamp is shown.

S. The completed end-to-side splenorenal shunt and its relation to the surrounding structures is illustrated.

DISCUSSION—DRS. BLAKEMORE AND VOORHEES (cont.)

Step 1 (Figs. 2 and 3). The gastrolienal and lienocolic ligaments are divided. The anterior rim of the spleen is rotated laterally in order to expose the hilar structures. The splenic artery is identified and doubly ligated proximal to its subdivision. The splenic vein is identified and gradually mobilized by sharp dissection to the hilus of the spleen. A rubbershod noncrushing clamp is applied as the splenic vein goes beneath the tail of the pancreas, and a crushing clamp is applied to the splenic vein as it emerges from the hilum. The vein is transected, and the spleen is removed after division of its diaphragmatic attachments.

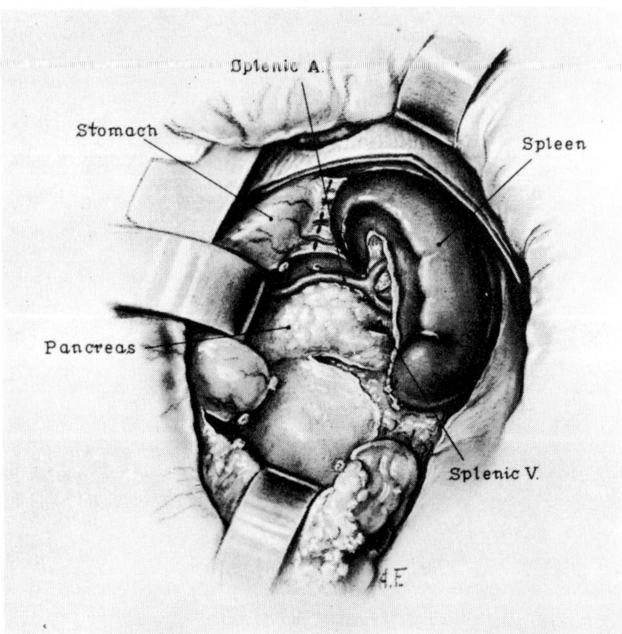

Fig. 2. Exposure of short gastric vessels, splenic artery, and splenic vein.

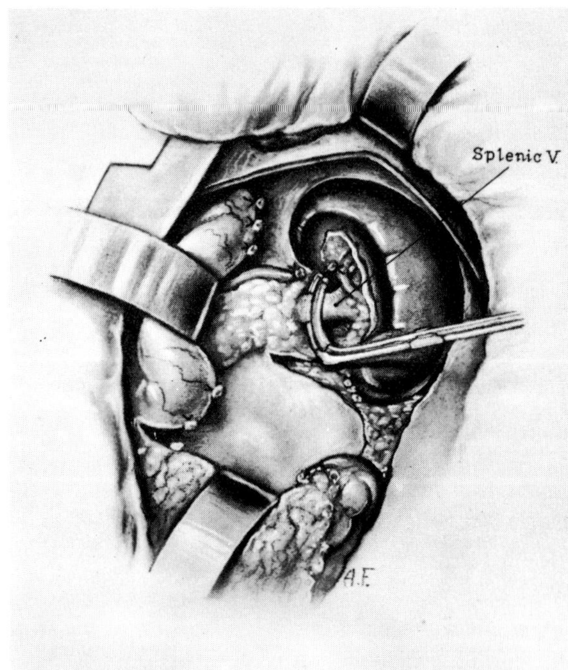

Fig. 3. A rubbershod clamp has been placed on the splenic vein, and it is ready for section well distal to the clamp.

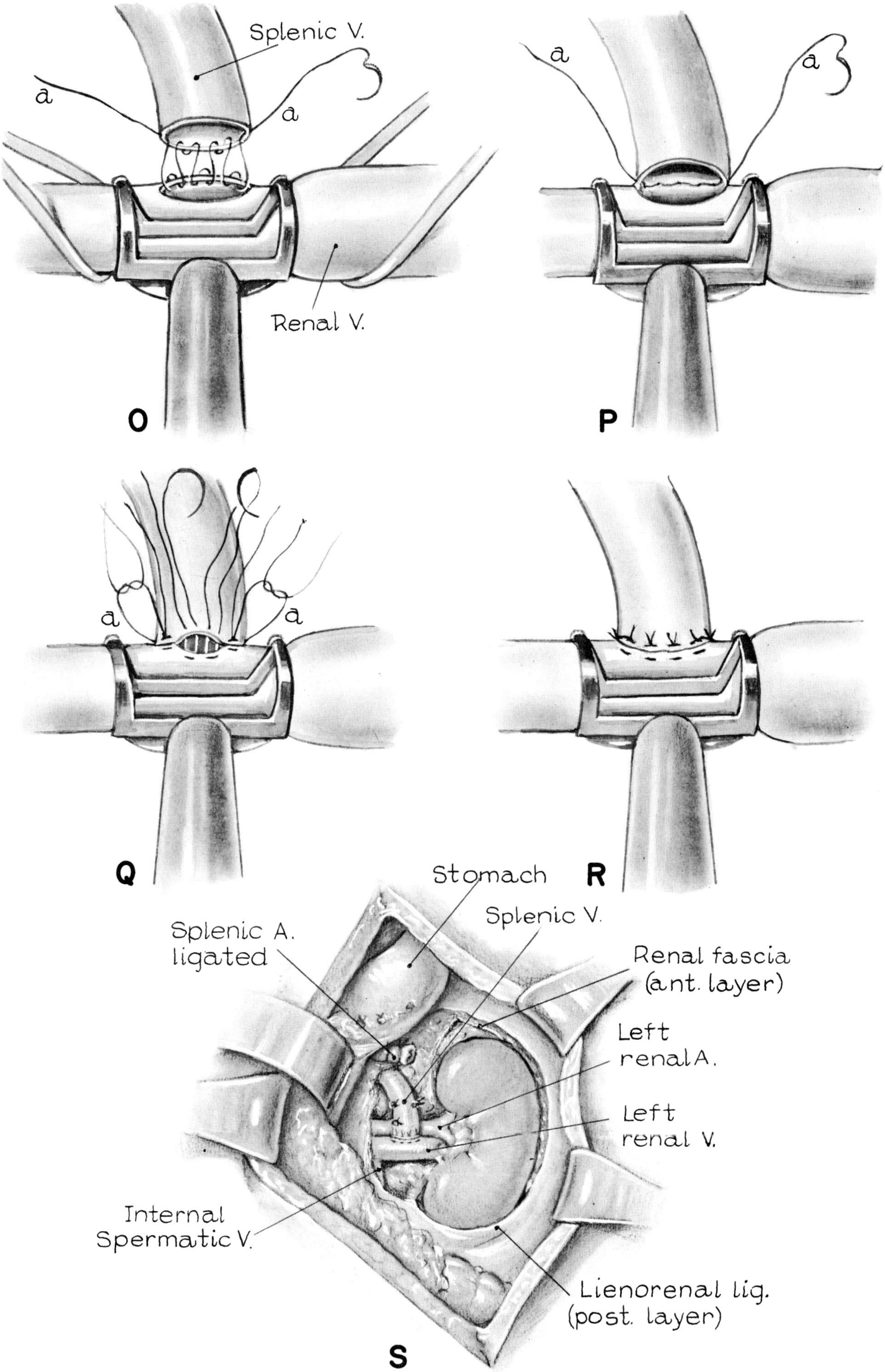
Splenic V.
a
a
a
Renal V.
O
a
a
P
a
a
Q
R
Stomach
Splenic V.
Splenic A. ligated
Renal fascia (ant. layer)
Left renal A.
Left renal V.
Internal Spermatic V.
Lienorenal lig. (post. layer)
S

DISCUSSION—DRS. BLAKEMORE AND VOORHEES (cont.)

Step 2 (Figs. 4 and 5). The noncrushing rubbershod clamp compressing the stump of the splenic vein is released for an instant to allow a rush of venous blood through the splenic vein stump to carry away any clot which may have formed in the splenic vein during the course of the splenectomy. Following this, the rubbershod clamp is reapplied, and 20 ml. of a dilute heparin–saline solution are injected into the splenic vein stump proximal to the point of compression by the clamp. The vein is retracted forward, and a usually incomplete collar of pancreatic tissue is divided between clamps along the posterior aspect of the splenic vein stump. Following the division of this areolar and pancreatic tissue for a distance of approximately 3 cm. parallel to the posterior aspect of the splenic vein stump, the tail of the pancreas is drawn forward, and the splenic vein is drawn laterally. The splenic vein is gradually dissected free from the overlying tail of the pancreas. During this last maneuver, it is exceedingly important to identify and to transfix with 00000 braided arterial silk the numerous, tenuous, venous tributaries entering the splenic vein from the tail of the pancreas. If these veins are placed under too much traction, they will tear at their juncture with the splenic vein, and the subsequent repair of the tear in the splenic vein will compromise the lumen and subsequently jeopardize the efficiency of the shunt. The mobilization of the splenic vein stump is carried medially to the point where the inferior mesenteric vein joins the splenic vein.

Step 3 (Fig. 6). The peritoneum overlying the left kidney is incised over the hilus of the kidney. This initial line of incision is bisected by a similar peritoneal incision running parallel to the left renal vein. The renal vein is gradually mobilized over a distance of approximately 3 cm. midway between the hilus of the kidney and the vena cava. Two major venous

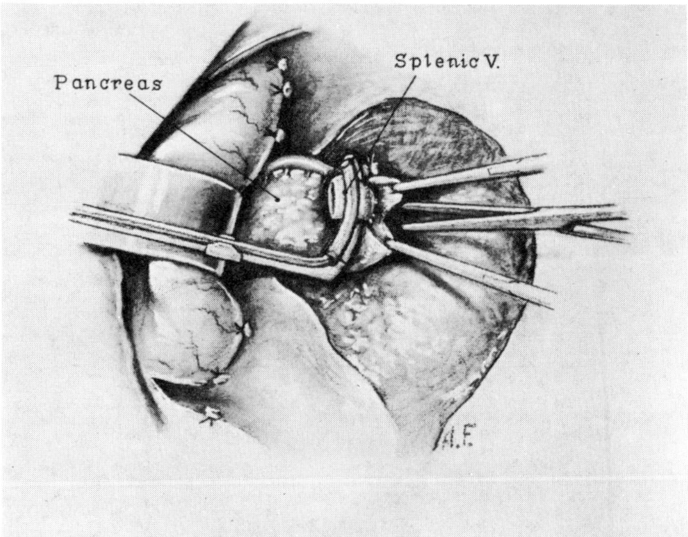

Fig. 4. Illustrates beginning mobilization of splenic vein.

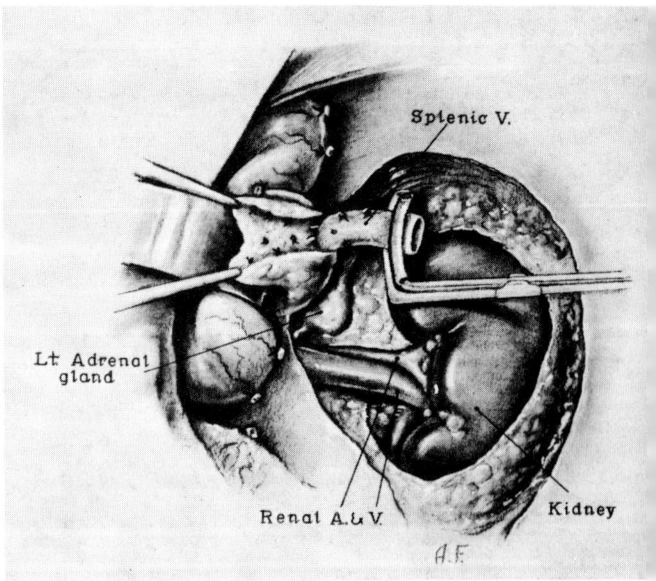

Fig. 5. Displays the mobilized stump of the splenic vein. Note the tunnel between the left adrenal gland and the upper pole of the left kidney, the result of removing retroperitoneal fat.

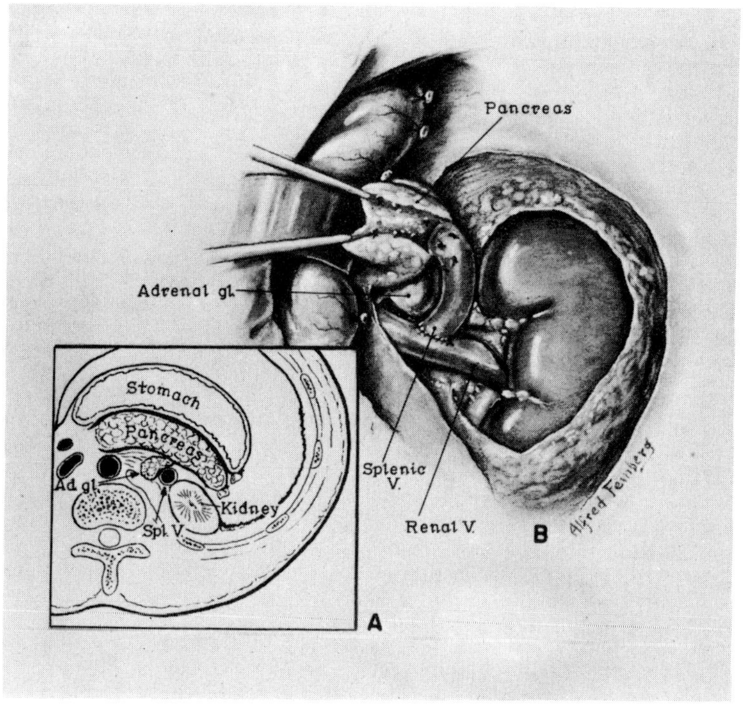

Fig. 6. B, an illustration of the completed splenorenal shunt. Note in cross-section illustration A that the splenic vein rests in a deep sulcus between the left adrenal gland and the upper pole of the kidney, out of harm's way from compression by the pancreas.

DISCUSSION—DRS. BLAKEMORE AND VOORHEES (cont.)

tributaries, the left spermatic (or ovarian) vein and the adrenal vein, should be identified and preserved where possible. However, if the preservation hampers subsequent anastomosis, both may be ligated with impunity. After clearing the renal vein, the left adrenal gland and its vascular supply are identified, and the adrenal gland is pushed medially by dividing its adventitial attachment to the kidney capsule. By pushing the adrenal gland medially, a sulcus can be developed between the adrenal gland and the upper pole of the left kidney, which will subsequently accommodate the splenic vein and offer it protection from subsequent compression by the overlying pancreas. We feel that the development of this protected channel is of utmost importance. By trial placements of the splenic vein stump, a suitable site for end-to-side anastomosis with the renal vein is selected so that an anastomosis of maximum obliquity between the splenic vein and the renal vein can be achieved. It is desirable that the splenic vein and the renal vein form an acute angle of roughly 60 degrees. After selection of the site of anastomosis, marking stay sutures are placed in the renal vein, and the vein is tented and grasped by a Beck–Potts clamp. An end-to-side anastomosis is achieved in precisely the same fashion as that described for the portacaval shunt, with the exception that, in children where growth is expected, interrupted horizontal mattress sutures are employed in the anterior row of the anastomosis instead of the continuous over and over everting suture. Following completion of the anastomosis, the clamps are removed, and the shunt is carefully examined for deformities which may compromise the efficiency of the shunt. The pancreatic tail is allowed to resume its natural position. Portal pressures are again taken, with and without splenic vein compression, to test the efficiency of the shunt. The splenic flexure of the colon is allowed to fall into place, and no effort is made to reperitonize the operative area. The abdominal and thoracic wounds are closed in similar manner to that described for the portal vein-to-vena cava shunt.

Discussion—Dr. C. Stuart Welch. The indications for the use of an anastomosis from splenic vein to renal vein instead of a direct portacaval shunt have diminished greatly in the past ten years. In our hospital today we seldom perform splenectomy and splenorenal shunt. Splenorenal shunt had its vogue because technically it seemed to be a less dangerous procedure than portacaval shunt. That is to say, it avoided dissection in the hepatic pedicle, where injury to the common bile duct, hepatic artery, and indeed the portal vein itself might occur. With increasing experience with the right-sided operation (portal vein to vena cava shunt), it became apparent that splenorenal anastomosis was more difficult and time-consuming than was a portacaval anastomosis. But, most important, the rate of recurrent bleeding from esophageal varices directly caused by thrombosis or closure of the splenorenal shunt was found to be high—much higher than in portacaval shunts when late results were evaluated (30 per cent for the former as contrasted to 2 per cent or less for the latter).

The reason for the high rate of splenorenal shunt failures is technical. The splenic vein is smaller than the portal vein. Furthermore, angulation and slowing of the current of shunted blood can occur, encouraging clotting. Splenorenal anastomosis is a rather awkward shunt.

As an indication for the use of splenectomy and splenorenal shunt, most surgeons accept the absence of a useful portal vein, as is found in extrahepatic portal hypertension due to congenital or acquired obliteration of the portal vein as a prime indication. The one difficulty with using splenorenal anastomosis in such cases is that variceal bleeding occurs in very young patients with extrahepatic bed block. In these patients the splenic vein is often so small as to invite anastomosis failure if it is used. Experience has shown that splenorenal anastomosis is doomed to failure in the very young. It is only when the child passes 10 years of age that a good sized splenic vein can be a reasonable hope. Even then the site for splenic vein anastomosis must be as near the portal vein as possible to secure a good lumen. Bleeding from varices in the very young can be temporarily controlled by such expediencies as small esophagogastric resection and jejunal or colonic interposition. This operation has more success than simple ligation of esophageal varices. By employing methods for the temporary control of bleeding, the child grows in the meantime and there is hope that a large splenic vein will be found and a satisfactory splenic renal vein decompression can be fashioned.

The remark made above about the indications for splenorenal shunt must be taken with some reservation now that another alternative shunt has been found to be useful in the very young. This is the Marion Shunt, which is performed by anastomosis of the cephalad cut end of the vena cava below the renal veins to the side of the superior mesenteric vein. The technic of this shunt is not part of the present discussion. Suffice it to say that its employment as thus far reported indicates that a more substantial shunt can be performed by the Marion technic than by the splenorenal method and that, therefore, the indications for splenorenal shunts are again lessened.

Another indication for splenectomy and splenorenal shunt is said to exist when a large spleen with a blood dyscrasia exists. Such blood dyscrasias are usually mild pancytopenias when found in patients with cirrhosis of the liver and congestive splenomegaly. Unless the dyscrasia is severe (and it is rarely so), a direct portacaval shunt should be the procedure of choice because of its greater efficiency in controlling portal hypertension. In 80 per cent of patients with pancytopenia, portacaval shunts result in shrinking of the size of the spleen and return of the cellular elements of the blood to normal or near normal. In the other 20 per cent only mild dyscrasias of no clinical importance persist. If splenectomy is needed because of a persistent dyscrasia, it can be done later. I have never had to do a secondary splenectomy.

In short, while it can be said that the above indications (blood dyscrasias) for splenectomy and splenorenal shunt exist, seldom need this procedure be applied. Since the hematologist may demand it, however, it must be done occasionally.

In regard to the technic of splenectomy and splenorenal anastomosis depicted in the illustrations, there is some area for disagreement although the variation which I will point out may be personal.

At any rate, in reference to A, B, and C, I offer the following comments. I believe that the thoracoabdominal incision is the best choice for this procedure, and I normally use it. I hold the opposite view for portacaval shunt (abdominal exposure only). Exposure is much more adequate with a left thoracoabdominal incision than a subcostal incision, both for the performance of the dissection and the shunt. There may be very troublesome bleeding to control during the operation of splenectomy and splenorenal shunt in the following instances. Vascular adhesions of the spleen to the diaphragm are often troublesome. Large and multiple retroperitoneal collaterals from the spleen, particularly laterally, may be difficult to manage without a large exposure. Pancreatic tributaries of the splenic vein must be carefully dissected and ligated to prevent abnormal blood loss. Finally, dissection in and about the kidney pedicle is facilitated by the thoracoabdominal exposure. Therefore, I always make a thoracoabdominal incision when I perform a splenorenal shunt.

In reference to D, E, and F, I would like to comment on the matter of preliminary ligation of the splenic artery. It is true that splenic artery ligation helps control bleeding from the spleen and its collaterals during its mobilization and removal but I believe that it is not a necessary preliminary step. I prefer to perform step G (lateral mobilization of the spleen) first and do not ligate the splenic artery unless bleeding is excessive. My reason for doing so is that a large full splenic vein is more easily dissected.

As Dr. Madden points out, injury to the stomach in detaching it from the spleen is possible, particularly high on the greater curvature at the superior pole of the spleen, where the stomach is in contact with the spleen and the false application of a clamp or ligature on the greater curvature of the stomach can result in necrosis and subsequent gastric fistula with peritonitis.

I, J, and K, would indicate that dissection of the

Discussion—Dr. Welch (cont.)

splenic vein is done posteriorly after mobilization of the spleen and rotating it medially. I do not believe that this technic can be carried out satisfactorily. Mobilization of the splenic vein is best done anteriorly with the spleen in nearly its usual position. The splenic vein is actually partially imbedded in the pancreas. Securing all of the small intrapancreatic tributaries is the important feature of this step.

L, M, N, O, P, Q, R, and S deal with mobilization of the kidney and the actual anastomosis of the end of the splenic vein to the side of the renal vein partially occluded in a Potts-Smith clamp. This would seem to be a good technique employing the everting suture anastomosis. If the renal vein is large, an oval opening can be made in the occluded segment. This is said to make the anastomosis less "slitlike" and less likely to close. A transverse opening in the renal vein may also be made. It tends to gape and stay open, which lessens the likelihood of anastomotic thrombosis. Such an incision requires that the blood supply to the kidney be occluded during the anastomosis. This is done by putting a bull dog clamp on the renal artery to occlude temporarily its blood supply. The actual time needed to complete a splenorenal anastomosis is approximately 20 minutes, which is readily tolerated by the kidney. I have used temporary renal artery occlusion during splenorenal anastomosis in many patients without permanent damage to the kidney as judged by postoperative intravenous pyleograms. This technique is particularly useful when the application of a clamp to partially occlude the renal vein is difficult and awkward.

Discussion—Dr. Louis M. Rousselot. Portasystemic shunts are primarily indicated for the relief of gastroesophageal hemorrhage, by lowering the portal tension in the syndrome of portal hypertension. Dr. Madden's preference is a direct end-to-side portocaval shunt rather than a splenorenal shunt. It is my opinion that a splenorenal shunt be reserved for those cases in which the former is not feasible—i.e., an extrahepatic portal vein block, either congenital or acquired.

The incisions illustrated in A represent standard approaches. The combined thoracoabdominal incision (broken line) gives the optimal exposure. With the combined approach, the abdominal component should be initially opened to confirm the diagnosis and establish operability. An unsuspected hepatoma or a secondary malignant disease that obstructs the portal bed may be established, a biopsy taken, and the operation terminated forthwith.

In the presence of inflammatory pulmonary disease, the incision should be limited to the abdomen. Besides the subcostal incision shown in A, a long transverse incision from the midline well out to the flank may be substituted.

The operative steps in A through S are clearly illustrated with exactitude. Certain admonitions and variations are presented. Rarely should blunt dissection be attempted in any operation for portal hypertension. The relatively avascular organ attachments found in other disease states are not present in portal hypertension. Extensive collateralization is regularly found in the splenocolic ligament (D), the gastrosplenic ligament (E), and the lienorenal ligament (G). Furthermore, highly vascular adhesions usually envelop the spleen and fix it to the diaphragm and the lateral parietal peritoneum. These should be serially clamped, severed, and ligated. Blunt dissection is extremely hazardous and may be accompanied by severe blood loss (G).

D through J represent the exposure of the true pedicle from its lateral and posterior aspects. An alternate method is to expose the pedicle from its anterior surface, medial to the splenic hilum. The steps depicted in D through H are followed as shown. At this juncture, several moist laparotomy pads are inserted into the splenic "bed" in the subphrenic space, and the spleen is displaced downward and forward. The arterial ligation is completed as shown in H. However, the mobilization of the splenic vein proceeds from the anterior surface of the pedicle as in H, rather than rotating the spleen and continuing the dissection as demonstrated in I, J, and K.

Upon completion of the exposure of the pedicle of the left kidney, I find it desirable to identify early the ureter and to "tab" it with cotton tape, similar to the manner in which the renal vein is "tabbed" in M. Occasionally limitations of exposure make the use of short, spring "bulldog" clamps preferable to the long handle Potts' ductus clamps shown in K. Individual preference may again call for a modification in technic. The Glover auricular clamp or Satinsky clamp is in my opinion a more versatile instrument than the Potts-Smith clamp used in N. A greater surface area of the renal vein may be occluded, which permits the surgeon a wider clearance between the edge of the new stoma and the margin of the occlusive clamp. The cutting of an oval opening in the side wall of the renal vein rather than making a linear incised wound as indicated (N) is again an alternative step. This facilitates the suture anastomoses and minimizes late stenosis or closure of the stoma site.

In O through S, several modifications are permissible. Instead of using interrupted sutures in the anterior layer (Q) a continuous suture may be used, like that shown for the posterior layer (O). In children interrupted sutures are probably preferable for both the posterior and the anterior layers, to compensate for the increase in the size of the vessels during growth and, accordingly, to prevent decrease in size of the stoma. Instead of the "everting" type of sutures depicted (O, Q), a continuous noneverting suture, interrupted only at the angles of the anastomosis, may be used both anteriorly and posteriorly. Furthermore, if desired, additional "stay" sutures may be inserted at each angle prior to the insertion of the continuous sutures forming the anterior and posterior layers of the anastomosis.

END-TO-SIDE PORTACAVAL SHUNT

A. The patient is placed in the supine position, and the right side is elevated to an angle of 40 to 45 degrees from the horizontal. The thoracoabdominal incision overlying the ninth intercostal space is in dotted outline.

A′. Inset to show the long oblique subcostal incision (broken line) which is the one of preference. The use of this incision provides adequate exposure and lessens the high incidence of postoperative morbidity that is associated with the thoracoabdominal approach (A).

B, C, D. The incision is deepened through the subjacent musculature, the costal arch, the diaphragm, the pleura, and the peritoneum to expose the underlying intraperitoneal and intrapleural viscera.

E. The liver is displaced downward and then rotated and retracted upward into the adjacent right pleural cavity. The hepatic flexure of the colon is mobilized by severance of the right phrenocolic ligament, as indicated in dotted outline.

DISCUSSION—DRS. ARTHUR H. BLAKEMORE AND ARTHUR B. VOORHEES, JR. The key to a successful portacaval shunt is a rapidly moving stream of blood. The precise mechanism by which the process of thrombosis is accelerated in a slow-moving stream or retarded in a fast-moving stream is not known, but, for practical purposes, this observation may be accepted for fact. A high rate of flow can be achieved where the pressure within the portal system is high and the pressure within the vena cava or renal vein is low, thereby establishing a satisfactory pressure gradient. A high rate of flow can be further assured by minimizing peripheral resistance, particularly in the portal or the splenic vein. Angulation and constriction of the vein along its course or at the site of anastomosis, or turbulence in the vena cava or renal vein in close proximity to the stoma of the shunt, may spell disaster. In the gradual evolution of the portacaval shunt as a surgical procedure, we hold the foregoing facts in a position of paramount importance in the planning and execution of the operation.

As a result of animal experimentation and observation derived from 350 portacaval shunts in the human, we are convinced that the end-to-side portal vein-to-vena cava anastomosis is the most efficient and that the side-to-side portal vein-to-vena cava anastomosis and the end-to-side splenic vein-to-renal vein anastomosis are less efficient. These differences in efficiency are reflections of the rates of flow that can be usually achieved by the three major shunt configurations.

In addition to these broad considerations, scrupulous attention must be paid to the gentle handling of the veins and to the maintenance of aseptic conditions. A crushing forceps or insignificant infection may represent the initial nidus of a subsequently occluding thrombus.

General considerations. Strict aseptic technic in the operating room is imperative. In addition to the usually accepted methods of skin sterilization and sterile draping, the use of helmets rather than caps, double masks rather than single masks, double glove technic during the skin incision, and skin towels carefully applied by Michel's clips spaced approximately 2 cm. apart serve two useful functions. First, this technic minimizes possible contamination of the operative site by bacteria from the skin, nasal and oral pharynx, and the hair. Second, if one insists on such a technic, which is somewhat variant from the routine, the operating room personnel is constantly alerted to the need for extraordinary precautions. As a further precaution, 300,000 units of fortified procaine penicillin and 1 gm. of streptomycin are administered intramuscularly to the patient immediately prior to the skin incision. This will provide an adequate therapeutic level of antibiotics within the body during the course of the operative procedure.

Technic of portal vein-to-vena cava shunt. The patient is placed in a supine position on the operating table so that the break in the table or kidney elevator is at the approximate level of the third lumbar vertebra (Fig. 1). A flat sandbag is then placed under the right shoulder, and another similar sandbag is placed under the right hip. Side braces, suitably padded, are placed along the left lateral chest wall and at the level of the left hip, thereby permitting subsequent tilting of the table to the left approximately 15 degrees. The right arm can either be suspended from the ether screen or allowed to rest at the patient's side. By breaking the table and elevating the kidney elevator, the patient is placed in a hyperextended position. After careful skin preparation and sterile draping, the skin incision is made for the thoracoabdominal approach. The line of incision commences at the anterior axillary line over the ninth rib and is carried obliquely, medially across the costal margin to a point approximately 2 to 3 cm. above the umbilicus in the midline of the abdomen. The skin incision is deepened through the subcutaneous tissue to the level of the deep fascia, and, at this point, skin towels are applied with the use of Michel's clips spaced approximately 2 cm. apart. The incision is then deepened through the muscle layers to the level of the periosteum of the ninth rib. The periosteum is stripped from the ninth rib, and the rib is transected at the midaxillary line. The rib and its costal cartilage are then resected. Medially, the incision is deepened through the oblique musculature, anterior and posterior rectus sheaths, and peritoneum. After entry into the peritoneal cavity, the remainder of the thoracic portion of the incision is completed by entering the chest cavity through

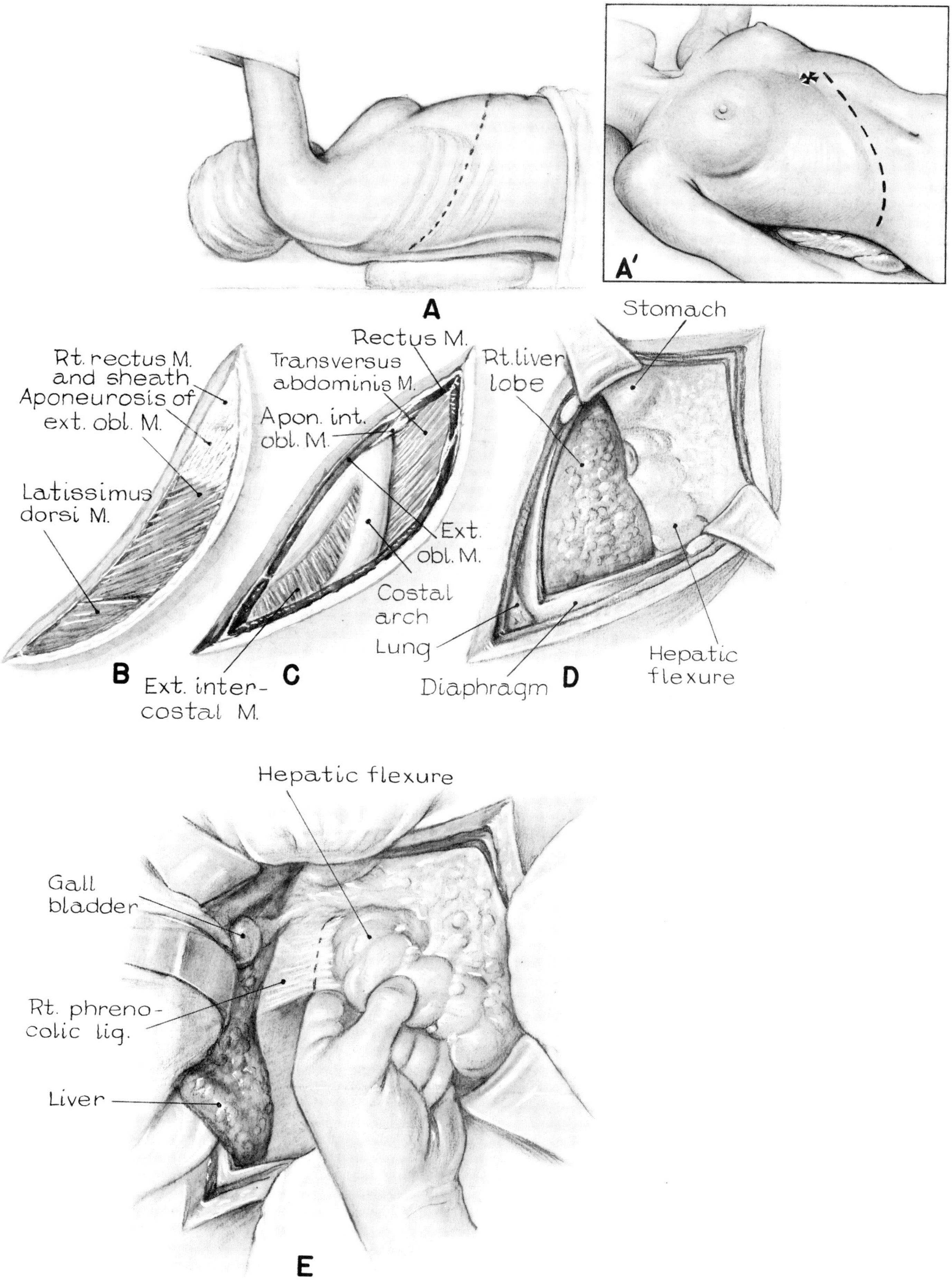
A'
A
Stomach
Rectus M.
Rt. rectus M. and sheath
Transversus abdominis M.
Rt. liver lobe
Aponeurosis of ext. obl. M.
Apon. int. obl. M.
Latissimus dorsi M.
Ext. obl. M.
Costal arch
Lung
Hepatic flexure
B
Ext. inter-costal M.
C
Diaphragm
D
Hepatic flexure
Gall bladder
Rt. phreno-colic lig.
Liver
E

F. The mobilized hepatic flexure of the colon is displaced downward toward the left lower quadrant of the peritoneal cavity and the foramen of Winslow; the pylorus, the head of the pancreas, and the retrocolic portion of the duodenum are exposed. Mobilization of the descending portion of the duodenum is commenced by scissor dissection of the posterior parietal peritoneal layer along its lateral border (Kocher maneuver). Normally, this peritoneal layer, like the posterior layer of the lienorenal ligament, is avascular and may be severed with impunity. However, in the presence of portal hypertension, the application of clamps to prevent excessive blood loss may be required.

The mobilization of the duodenum as depicted is no longer practiced. This maneuver was often associated with unnecessary blood loss and prolongation of the operation. Instead, dissection of the portal vein is immediately commenced and is then followed by mobilization of the inferior vena cava.

G. The mobilized segment of the duodenum and the head of the pancreas are retracted toward the midline to expose the related structures as depicted.

H. The dissection is continued, and the structures are now more clearly visualized. The dissection and isolation of the structures shown is both tedious and difficult because of the edema and increased vascularity of the tissues. The mobilized segment of the inferior vena cava is encircled by a traction tape of rubber tissue and partially retracted to expose clearly the group of lymph nodes between the aorta and the inferior vena cava.

I. The portal vein is occluded, first proximally with an angulated Potts ductus clamp, and then distally with a ligature and a suture ligature of silk (00) respectively. The site for transection of the portal vein is indicated in dotted outline. The convergence cephalad of the portal vein and the inferior vena cava and their separation by the caudate process of the liver may be readily seen. In some instances, partial resection of an enlarged caudate process, as suggested by Blakemore, may be required to permit the performance of a portacaval shunt.

DISCUSSION—DRS. BLAKEMORE AND VOORHEES (cont.) the bed of the ninth rib, incising the diaphragmatic pleura and peritoneum, and splitting the diaphragm in the course of its muscle fibers for approximately 12 to 15 cm. After general abdominal examination and confirmation of the diagnosis, a specimen for biopsy is obtained from the right lobe of the liver by making a cruciate incision through the liver capsule on the anterior margin and inserting a cork borer, of approximately 5 mm. in diameter, to the depth of 4 cm. The plug of liver tissue thus obtained is immediately given to the pathologist for early fixation. Bleeding from the biopsy site is controlled by suitably placed mattress sutures tied over a plug of skeletal muscle.

For the sake of convenience, the subsequent operative procedure can be divided into three parts. The first step is that of mobilization of the duodenum and

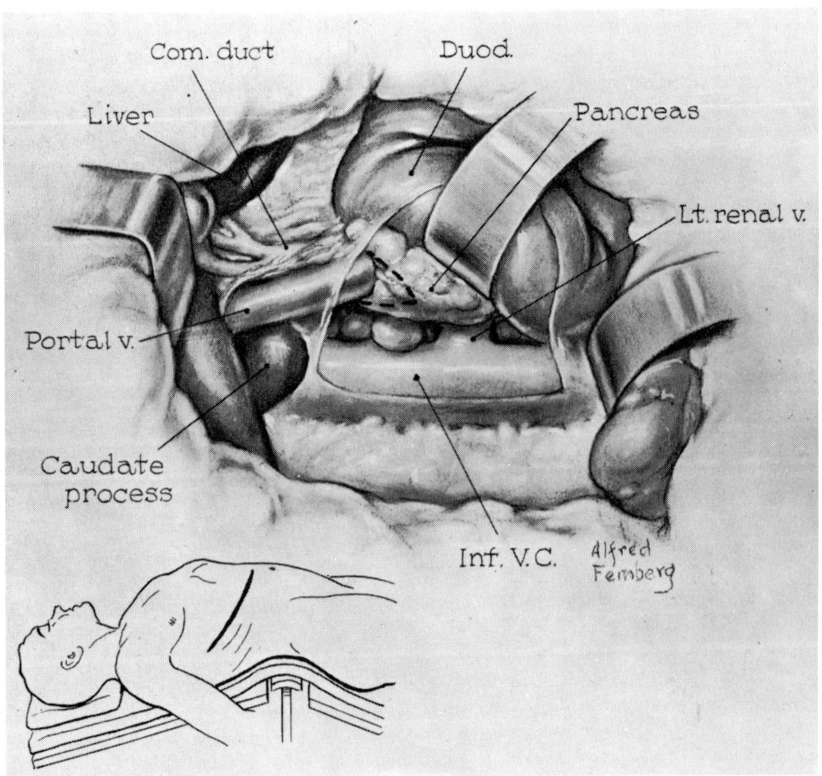

Fig. 1.

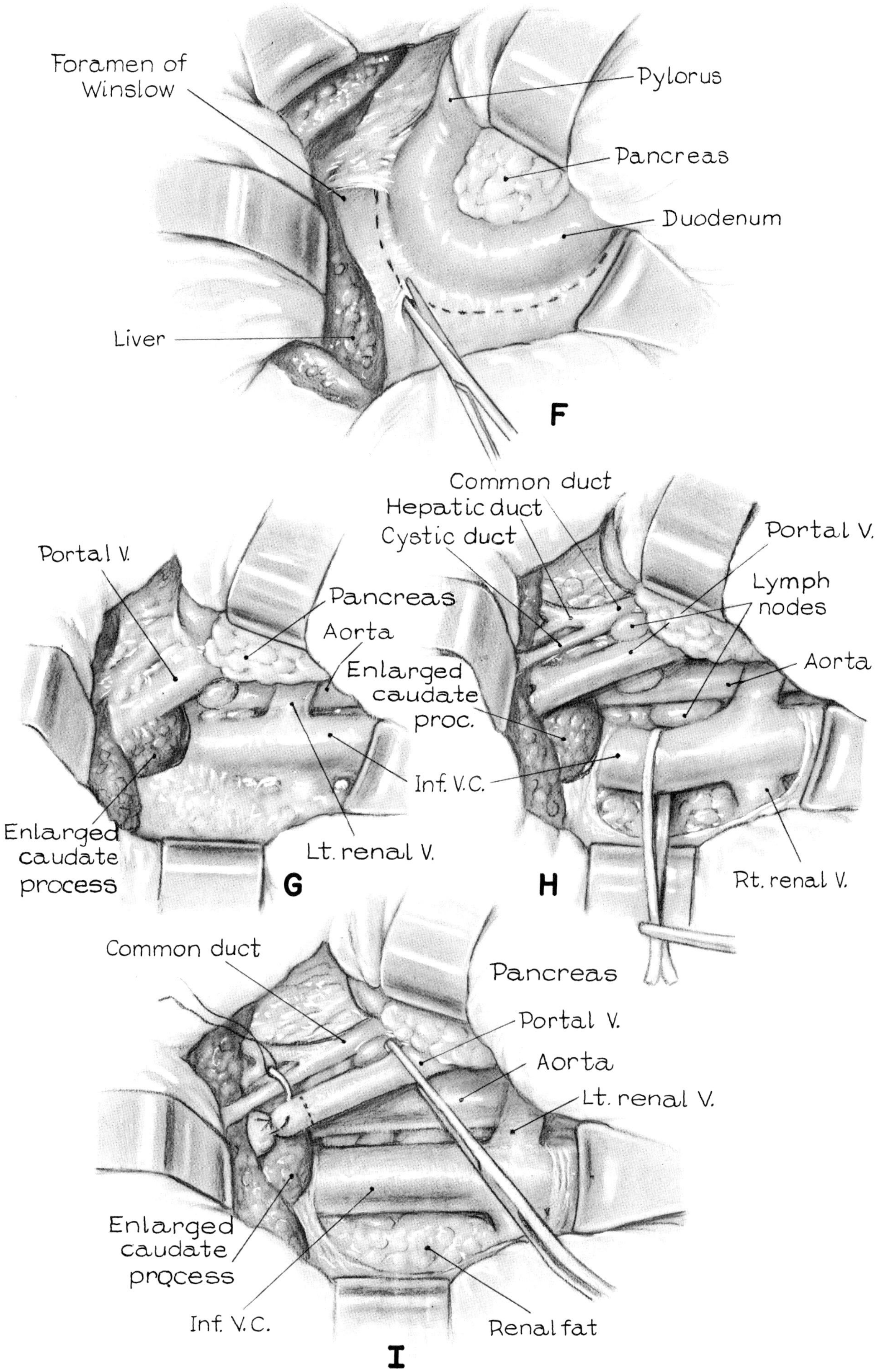
Foramen of Winslow
Pylorus
Pancreas
Duodenum
Liver
F
Common duct
Hepatic duct
Cystic duct
Portal V.
Pancreas
Aorta
Enlarged caudate proc.
Portal V.
Lymph nodes
Aorta
Inf. V.C.
Enlarged caudate process
Lt. renal V.
G
H
Rt. renal V.
Common duct
Pancreas
Portal V.
Aorta
Lt. renal V.
Enlarged caudate process
Inf. V.C.
Renal fat
I

J. The whole of the circumference of the inferior vena cava superior to the renal veins is completely mobilized, and its lumen is partially occluded by a Potts–Smith clamp. However, if desired, a Potts curved portacaval clamp may be used. The advantage of this type of clamp is that a longitudinal segment of the inferior vena cava may be occluded without the necessity of mobilizing the whole of the circumference of the inferior vena cava. The proximal transected end of the portal vein is turned downward toward the inferior vena cava preliminary to the performance of the venovenous shunt. The dotted line in the occluded segment of the inferior vena cava indicates the site of the incision for the anastomosis.

This type of clamp or one of the Beck-Potts type is now preferred.

K. The posterior suture layer of the anastomosis is inserted. This is a continuous eversion type of suture (silk, 00000) with intima to intima approximation. The suture is commenced from the "outside in" on the portal vein and terminates from the "inside out" also on the portal vein. Between its commencement and termination, the suture proceeds from the "inside out" to the "outside in" relative to the lumens of the portal vein and the inferior vena cava. Accordingly, the loops formed by the suture are always on the outside of the lumen of the vessel.

L. The posterior suture, a–a, is drawn taut, and the intimal surfaces of the portal vein and the vena cava are in close approximation. None of the silk suture is exposed within the lumen.

M. A series of interrupted everting mattress sutures of silk (00000) is employed for the anterior layer of the anastomosis. All of these sutures are first inserted and then tied. The mattress sutures at either end are tied first, and one of the long ends of each of these sutures is in turn tied to either end, a–a, of the continuous everting suture of silk used for the posterior layer.

N. The intervening mattress sutures are tied to complete the anterior layer of the anastomosis.

A single continuous over-and-over suture is now used routinely instead of the everting sutures as illustrated. However, the mattress stay sutures at each angle are still employed. The needle strand of each mattress suture is continued as an over-and-over suture to terminate in the center of the anastomosis anteriorly.

O. The operative field upon completion of the end-to-side portacaval shunt is shown.

DISCUSSION—DRS. BLAKEMORE AND VOORHEES (cont.)
identification and partial mobilization of the inferior vena cava. The second step is identification and mobilization of the portal vein. The third step is the anastomosis of the portal vein to the vena cava.

Step 1 (Fig. 1). The peritoneal reflection overlying the first and the second portions of the duodenum is incised along the greater curvature of the first and second portions of the duodenum. By blunt and sharp dissection, the first and second portions of the duodenum are rolled toward the midline. When the undersurface of the pancreas can be identified along the lesser curvature of the duodenum, the medial mobilization of the duodenum has been sufficient. With the duodenum in its medial reflected position, the vena cava lies immediately posterior to the area from which the second portion of the duodenum was reflected. The overlying strands of areolar tissue can be divided with safety along the anterior midline of the vena cava. If the right spermatic or ovarian vein is visible, the anterior mobilization of the vena cava has been begun too far caudad. For the purposes of the operation, it is usually sufficient to mobilize only the anterior and medial aspects of the vena cava from the level of the left renal vein to the caudate isthmus of the liver. Mobilizing the right lateral aspect of the vena cava in this region is unnecessary and extremely hazardous because of the numerous veins coming from the adrenal gland and entering the vena cava directly. It is also important to identify with precision the left renal vein since it will subsequently represent a landmark in selection of the site of anastomosis. In certain patients, hypertrophy of the caudate process may encroach upon the subsequent site of anastomosis, and, in these instances, the caudate process must be resected (Fig. 2). When this is the case, it is necessary to ligate two or more pairs of minute veins running from the caudate process to the vena cava. These are frequently unrecognized during manipulation of the process and may be torn, giving rise to troublesome hemorrhage in an area difficult to control. Once the caudate process has been freed from the underlying vena cava, it can be cross-clamped and resected. Hemostasis is achieved by multiple vertical mattress sutures placed approximately 1 cm. from the cut margins.

Step 2. It must be remembered that, with the patient in a hyperextended left semilateral position, the operator is usually looking at the right lateral aspect of the hepatoduodenal ligament, and, in this position, the common duct lies in an anterior location and the portal vein in a posterior location in the ligament (Fig. 1). The peritoneal investment of the hepatoduodenal ligament is incised in the posterior right lateral aspect of the hepatoduodenal ligament from the porta hepatis to the greater curvature of the duodenum. In making this incision, care should be exercised to avoid cutting unnecessarily any recognizable lymphatic channels. Once the peritoneum is incised, the vein can usually be identified by finger dissection and palpation. Upon identification, the

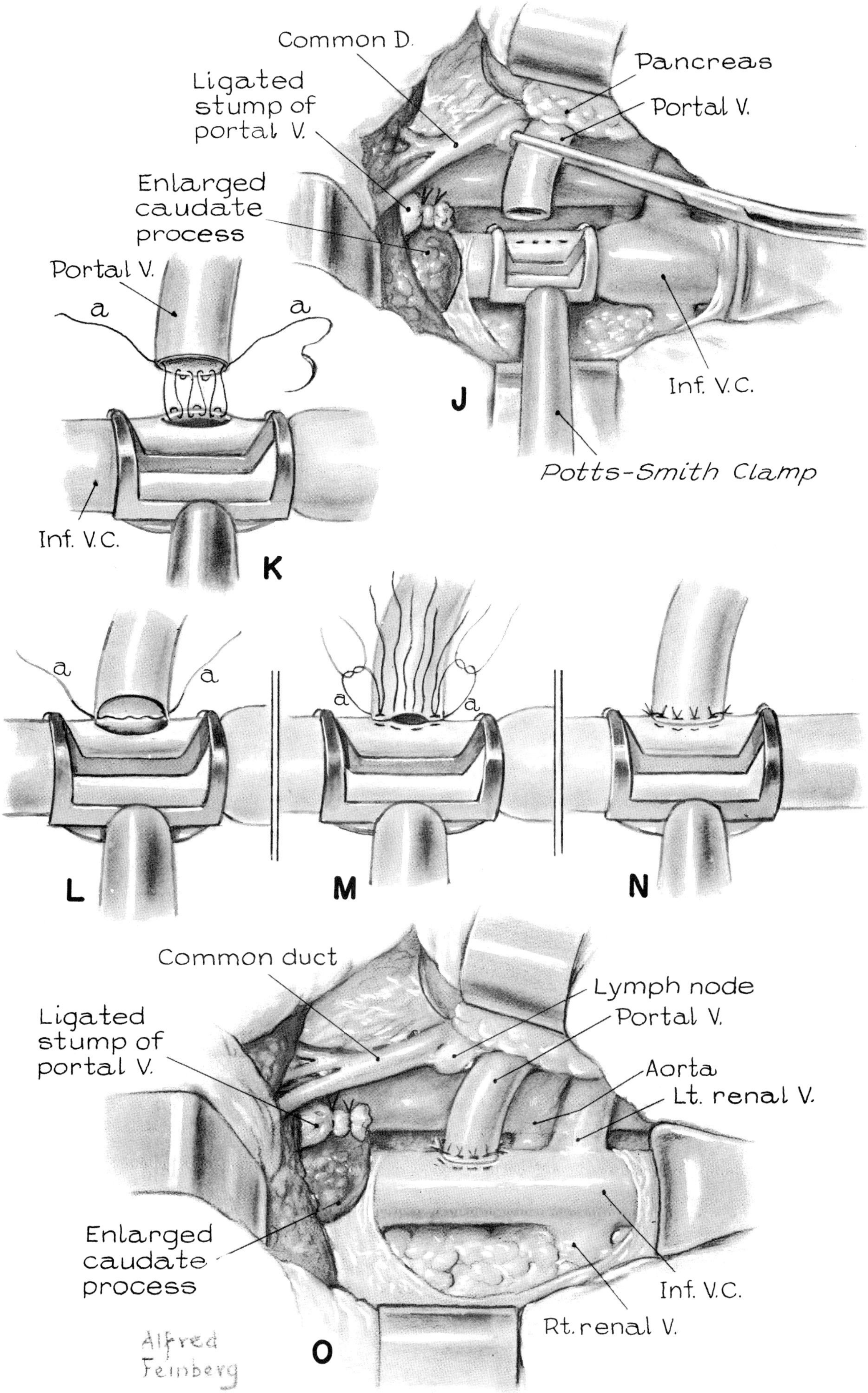
Common D.
Pancreas
Ligated stump of portal V.
Portal V.
Enlarged caudate process
Portal V.
a
a
J
Inf. V.C.
Potts-Smith Clamp
Inf. V.C.
K
a
a
a
a
L
M
N
Common duct
Lymph node
Ligated stump of portal V.
Portal V.
Aorta
Lt. renal V.
Enlarged caudate process
Inf. V.C.
Rt. renal V.
Alfred Feinberg
O

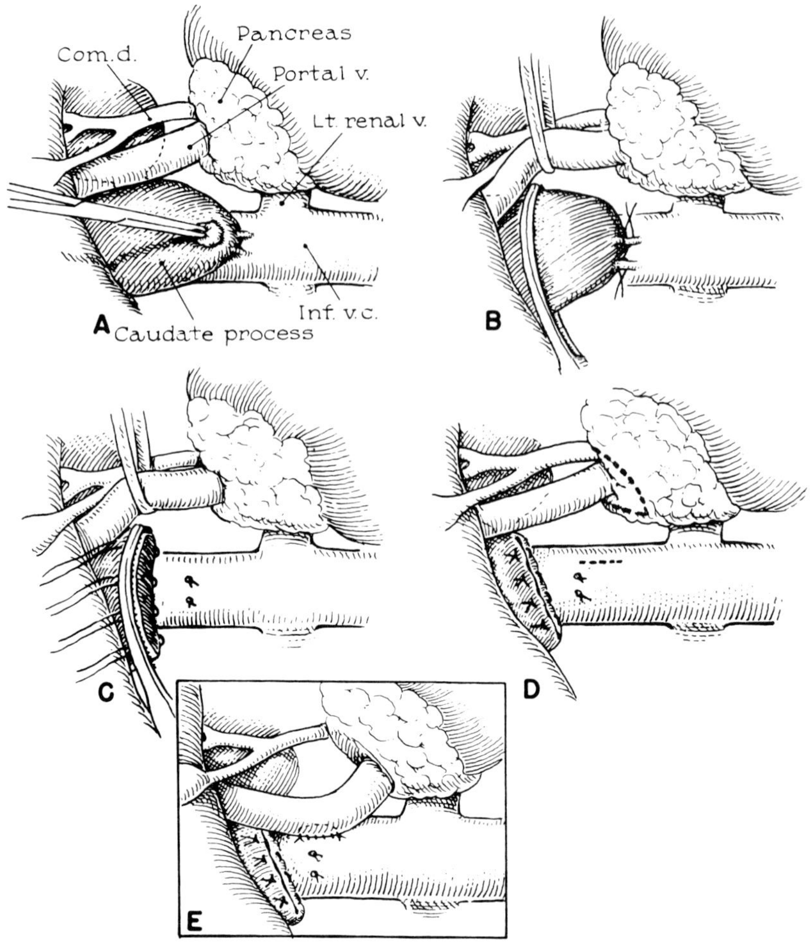
Pancreas
Com.d.
Portal v.
Lt. renal v.
Inf. v.c.
A
Caudate process
B
C
D
E

Fig. 2.

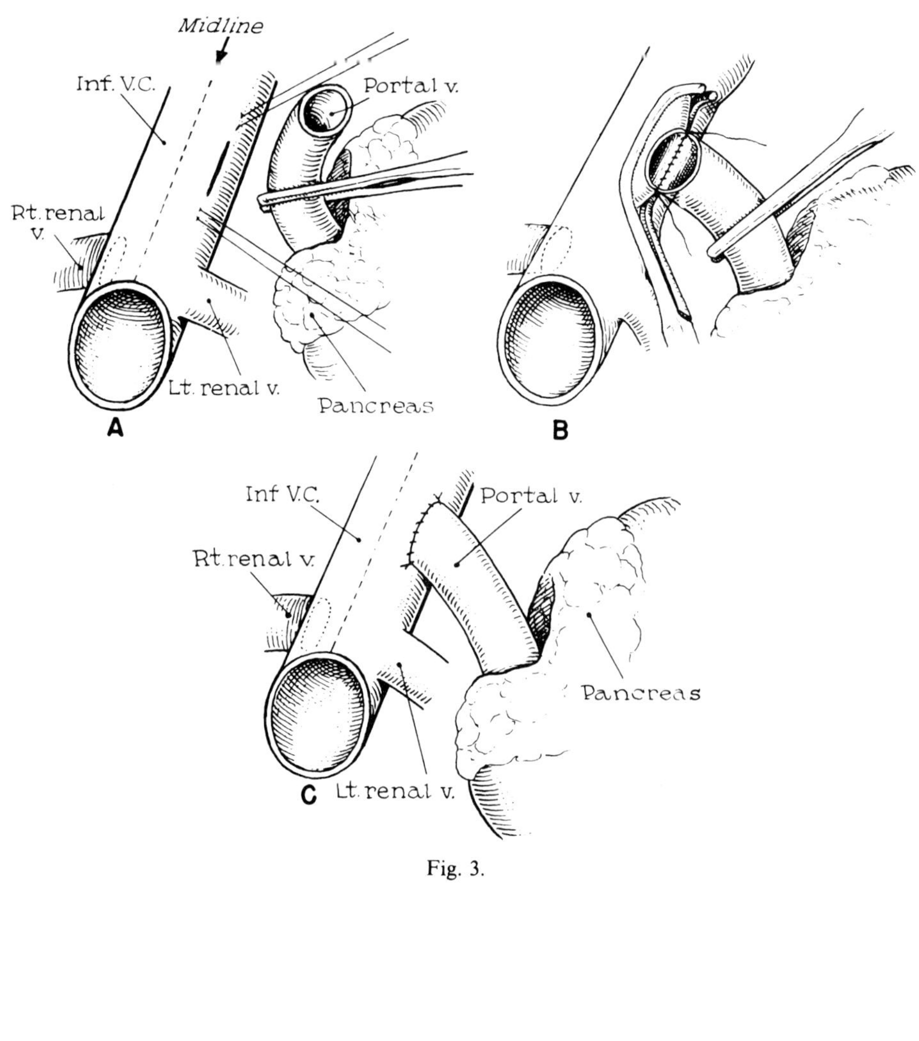
Midline
Inf. V.C.
Portal v.
Rt. renal v.
Lt. renal v.
Pancreas
A
B
Inf V.C.
Portal v.
Rt. renal v.
Pancreas
C
Lt. renal v.

Fig. 3.

vein should be dissected bluntly in the adventitial plane at roughly its midportion between the porta hepatis and the head of the pancreas. Following local circumferential dissection of the vein, a short piece of umbilical tape can be passed about the vein for the purpose of gentle traction. This serves as a useful method for avoiding unnecessary instrumentation of a vein subsequently to be used as a shunt. The dissection is carried cephalad to the porta hepatis. The bifurcation of the portal vein into the right and left hepatic veins should be identified. This represents the highest point of dissection, and at this time there are usually no significant venous tributaries which must be dealt with. The portal vein is mobilized caudad by sharp and blunt dissection to the level of the head of the pancreas. Two major tributaries to the portal vein, if unrecognized, may tear and cause troublesome hemorrhage. The first tributary is on the medial aspect of the portal vein and enters directly into the head of the pancreas. The second tributary is on the lateral inferior aspect of the portal vein, just beneath a collar of pancreatic tissue where the portal vein emerges from the head of the pancreas. Both tributaries should be identified and individually ligated by transfixion ligatures of 00000 braided silk. After mobilization of the portal vein, it is appropriate to make initial pressure readings in the portal system from a large branch of the gastroepiploic vein. Simple manometric readings, using the manubrial notch as the reference point, should be made with the portal vein open and then with the portal vein compressed. If the pressure rise following compression of the portal vein is in excess of 150 mm. of saline, then a side-to-side portal vein-to-vena cava anastomosis is advised. As the last portion of this second step in preparation for an end-to-side anastomosis, a ligature of heavy silk is passed about the portal vein at the level of the bifurcation into the right and left hepatic veins. The ligature is tied, and a second transfixion suture employing 00 braided silk is placed approximately 3 mm. from the primary tie. A rubbershod clamp that will occlude, but not crush, the vein is placed around the vein as it emerges from the head of the pancreas, and the vein is transected immediately proximal to the transfixion suture. Twenty to thirty millimeters of a solution of heparin containing 10 mg. of heparin in 100 ml. of saline is instilled in the portal vein proximal to the rubbershod clamp.

Step 3. An imaginary line coursing parallel to the vena cava on its anterior medial aspect, equidistant from the true anterior aspect of the vena cava and the true left lateral aspect of the vena cava, which may be indentified by the juncture of the left renal vein, is defined and marked by two arterial silk sutures as the future axis of the anastomosis (Fig. 3). The vena cava is tended and grasped by a Beck–Potts clamp. An oval "window" is then cut in the vena cava, corresponding in diameter to the fully distended portal vein. The anastomosis is placed as near to the liver as practical so that the angle formed between the portal vein and the vena cava will be an acute angle, 45 to 60 degrees. A single layer anastomosis is achieved by a simple over and over suture of 00000 braided silk. It is desirable to exert some tension on the angle stay sutures during the anastomosis to avoid pursestringing the stoma. In the posterior suture line, care must be exercised to avoid dragging small strands of adventitial tissue into the suture line by the suture material. After completion of the anastomosis, the vena cava clamp is released first, and the portal vein clamp released second. Anastomoses in a low pressure system rarely leak seriously, and minimal suture line leaks occurring shortly after the removal of the clamps should be controlled by simple finger pressure over the area. Unless the suture line leak is a serious one, reinforcing sutures should not be taken since they may cause distortion or constriction of the stoma. Once flow has been established in the newly formed shunt, the point of emergence of the portal vein from the region of the head of the pancreas should be carefully examined. Frequently, a collar of pancreatic tissue will cause angulation or actual compression of the portal vein in its newly established course. If this collar exists, a wedge of pancreatic tissue should be excised (Fig. 4). This compression feature is an exceedingly important one

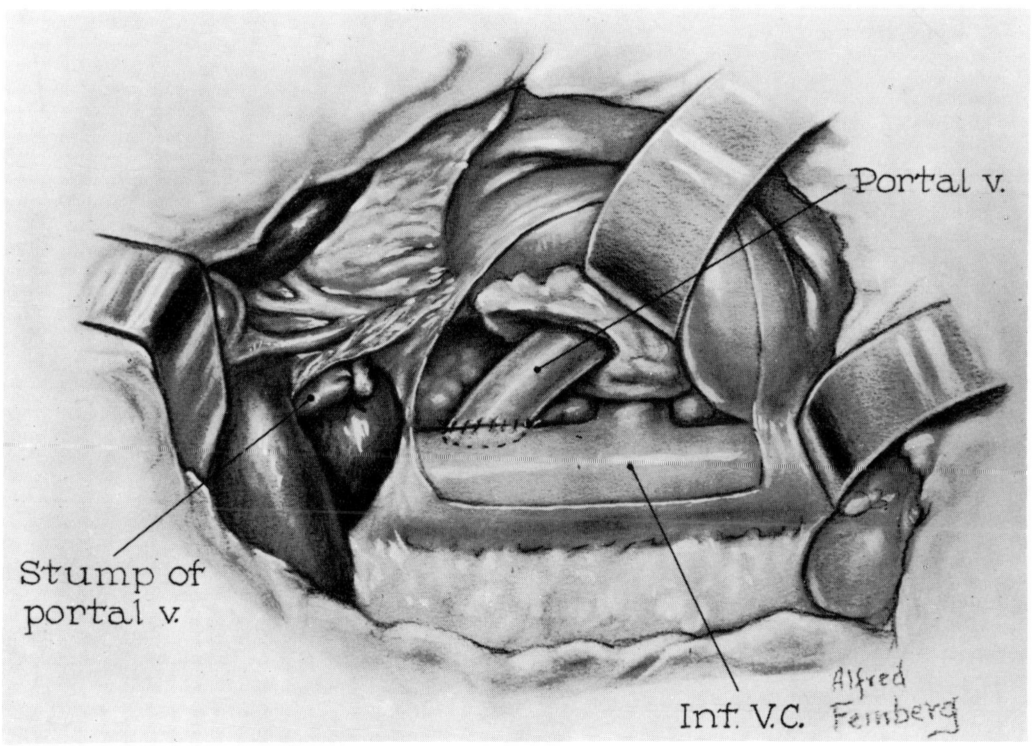

Fig. 4.

and may not be recognized by a cursory examination; it must be actively looked for.

In those instances where side-to-side anastomoses between the portal vein and the vena cava are deemed advisable because of a pressure rise in the portal system in excess of 150 mm. of saline following compression of the portal vein, the portal vein is not divided. Contiguous surfaces of the vena cava and portal vein are marked by arterial sutures, the vena cava is grasped by a Beck–Potts clamp in a fashion similar to that previously described, and a 15 mm. diameter oval "window" is cut (Fig. 2). The portal vein is temporarily occluded above and below the site of anastomosis by a simple double turn of umbilical tape, and a corresponding 15 mm. diameter oval "window" is cut in the previously marked site. The anastomosis is accomplished in precisely the same manner as that described for the end-to-side anastomosis.

After completion of the portal vein-to-vena cava shunt, manometric pressures are again recorded in the portal system, with and without portal vein compression. In ideal circumstances, the pressure in the portal system should be less than 200 mm. of water pressure. If this pressure has not been achieved, the possibility of mechanical impediment to flow by distortion of the portal vein, or at the site of anastomosis, should be excluded by inspection. In the closure of the operative wound, no attempt is made at reperitonization or closing the retroperitoneal tissues over the site of anastomosis. The abdominal and thoracic portions of the wound are anatomically reconstituted. The abdomen is closed without drainage, and the chest cavity is closed over a large caliber catheter, which is withdrawn at the conclusion of the chest closure after residual air and fluid have been evacuated from the cavity.

DISCUSSION—DR. C. STUART WELCH. The illustrations show a technic for end-to-side portacaval shunt that deals with the incision, a minor part of the dissection, and the anastomosis. I shall deal with each of these items separately.

First, the right thoracoabdominal incision shown is unnecessary for 90 or 95 per cent of portacaval shunts. Thoracoabdominal incisions consume time in opening and closing and also result in greater blood loss and thus greater need for replacement. Patients with liver cirrhosis should have the least number of blood transfusions possible. It also is a fact that opening the pleural cavity invites pulmonary complications and morbidity. I use a subcostal abdominal incision, as depicted in A′. The right side of the patient is elevated 30° off the table, and the incision is begun halfway between the xiphoid process and the umbilicus. It is then directed to the right under the rib cage extending beneath the twelfth rib in the costovertebral angle. One indication for a thoracoabdominal incision is a very large liver.

It is, of course, impossible for the author to depict the dissection because of the variability of the disease, but this is the most important and difficult part of the operation. I first expose the inferior vena cava, because this maneuver is quite easy and establishes an important landmark.

Next I dissect the portal vein. The important point in this dissection is to know where this vein is. It is posterior and medial in the hepatic pedicle. In most cases there is no need to make a formal Kocher mobilization of the duodenum. There is also no need to first expose the common duct or hepatic artery. The portal vein can be approached directly by putting the right hand to the left of the hepatic pedicle and exerting pressure posteriorly and to the right at the same time that the left hand dissects out the portal vein. The most annoying part of the dissection is encountered in dealing with the large vascular lymph glands that surround the portal vein and lie between it and the vena cava. All of the tributaries of the portal vein are medial, and they vary in number from none to three or four. They must be accurately secured. Once the vein is free it remains only to decide whether or not a nick should be made in the pancreas to allow a freer right-angle swing of the portal vein to meet the vena cava. The next step is a high severance of the portal vein at its bifurcation. Here I recommend a free tie of 00 silk, distal to which I place a suture ligature.

Relative to the anastomosis, there is little of importance to say. An ellipse should be cut out of the vena cava. I prefer an everting type of suture anastomosis. The clamp shown in the drawings is an awkward one and would seem to require unneeded mobilization of the cava. A Satinsky clamp or Thomas Smith intestinal clamp is much easier to use. Mobilization of the cava posteriorly and medially is unnecessary and may result in bleeding from lumbar tributaries. The posterior row of sutures need not be laid and then drawn; the suture line can be made with continuous approximation. Most surgeons believe that an everting anastomosis is unnecessary, and if they are correct, the anastomosis is that much easier. At any rate, the anastomosis is the least difficult part of the operation.

SIDE-TO-SIDE PORTACAVAL SHUNT

A, B. The portal vein is cross-clamped caudad and cephalad by angulated Potts' clamps. Next, a tented segment of the inferior vena cava, cephalad to the renal vein tributaries, is occluded in a Beck-Potts' clamp. Openings (2.5-3 cm.) are then made into the lumen of the portal vein and the lumen of the occluded segment of the inferior vena cava preparatory to their anastomosis. A continuous suture of 00000 silk swedged on a small curved needle is used for the posterior layer. This suture is started from the outside-in at the caudad angle of the opening in the inferior vena cava (A). It is then continued as a simple over-and-over suture to terminate from the inside-out at the cephalad angle of the opening in the portal vein (B). To facilitate its insertion, guy sutures (00000 silk) for traction are inserted in the anterior margins of the openings in the inferior vena cava and portal vein (A, B).

The use of a continuous over-and-over suture, though theoretically objectionable because of the silk strands within the lumen, has proved most satisfactory in practice and is preferred to the continuous everting mattress suture.

C. The posterior suture is drawn taut, and the respective cut margins of the portal vein and vena cava are firmly approximated.

D. Interrupted everting mattress sutures are inserted at either angle of the anastomosis. The mattress suture at the caudad angle is tied, and its needle-free strand is being tied to the caudad end of the posterior suture. The insertion of the mattress suture at the cephalad angle is completed, and its needle-free strand will be tied to the cephalad end of the posterior suture.

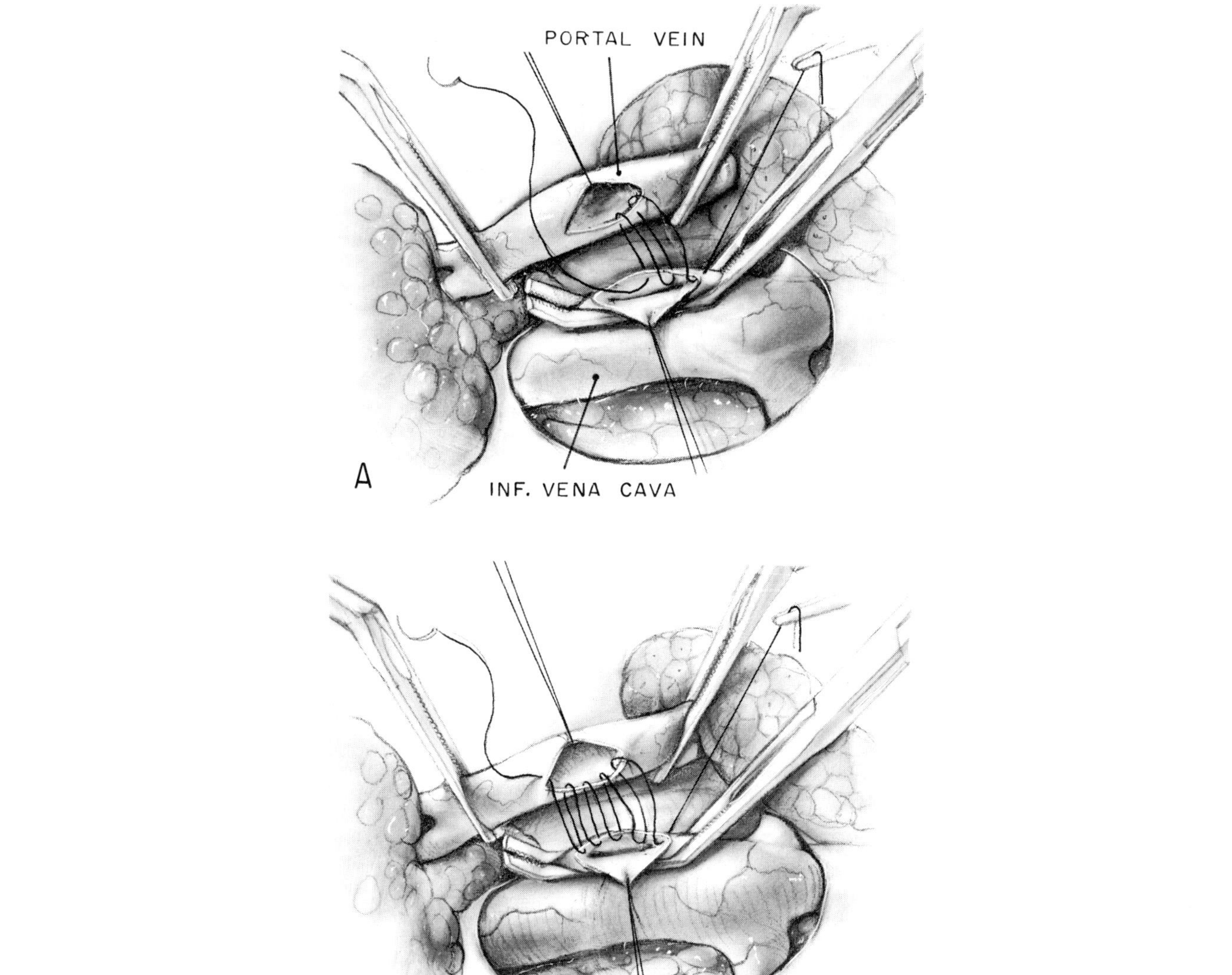
PORTAL VEIN
A
INF. VENA CAVA
B
C
D

E, F. The needle strands of the everting mattress sutures at either angle are continued as simple over-and-over sutures (E) to terminate in the center of the anastomosis anteriorly, where they are tied to each other and the strands cut to complete the anastomosis (F). Just prior to completion of the anastomosis, the traction guy sutures, visible in E, are withdrawn.

G, G_1. A completed direct side-to-side shunt, using interrupted everting mattress sutures, is shown (G_1). In some instances when a direct side-to-side shunt is not feasible technically, it may be effected by the interposition of an autogenous vein (superficial femoral) graft, the so called H graft (G).

Discussion—Dr. C. Stuart Welch. Anastomosis of the portal vein to the vena cava done by a tangenital technic is the original Eck fistula and can be done instead of end-to-side portacaval shunt for the prevention of bleeding from esophageal varices. It also has, I believe, a preferential place in the surgical treatment of certain cases of ascites. Some discussion of the indications for this shunt is apropos, because there are some surgeons who never use it and admit of no indication for its use.

If the problem before the surgeon is simply to reduce splanchnic portal pressure in a patient who has survived a hemorrhage from esophageal varices, a simple end-to-side shunt with interruption of the portal vein suffices. I say this because there is no question that end-to-side anastomosis is much more easily performed. However, a side-to-side shunt, if well made, is equally good functionally and is not harmful provided the anastomosis is not too large. If too large it predisposes to ammonia intoxication. A shunt of 2 or 2.5 cm. is of sufficient size and need not be exceeded.

The special indication for a side-to-side portacaval shunt is persistent and intractable ascites. The rationale of the use of this type of shunt in the treatment of ascites is based on the supposition that decompression of the liver may be obtained by retrograde portal blood flow. Time does not permit a complete discussion of the cause of ascites. Suffice it to say there is evidence of outflow block in the liver and evidence that reverse or retrograde portal blood flow in a side-to-side portacaval shunt *can* prove beneficial. From the practical standpoint, the use of this type of shunt has cured patients with ascites. Although it should not be applied to all patients with ascites, it is difficult to lay down rules for its application. However, in the surgical management of patients with ascites, a side-to-side shunt is believed superior to an end-to-side shunt.

From the technical standpoint, several features bear comment. Nothing is said about the incision in the illustrations. The right side of the patient should be elevated about 30° from the horizontal and a large subcostal abdominal incision employed. A thoracoabdominal incision should not be used routinely. It is time-consuming and the morbidity is high. It is only when one is dealing with a very large liver that a planned thoracoabdominal incision is needed. The subcostal incision begins at the linea alba halfway between the xiphoid process and the umbilicus and extends under the twelfth rib to the costovertebral angle.

A side-to-side shunt is not technically feasible in all patients because of the distance between these two veins and the interposition of the caudate lobe. I would estimate that it can be done in 75 per cent of the patients. Two technical maneuvers are especially helpful in making a good side-to-side shunt: (1) resection of the caudate lobe and (2) mobilization of the vena cava. "If the mountain will not go to Mahomet, Mahomet must go to the mountain." To effect this mobilization, the right renal vein must be loosened. If a side-to-side shunt adequate in size and without tension or angulation is not possible it should not be done. An end-to-side is a good alternative. I mention this because a poorly made side-to-side shunt is doomed to failure by thrombosis.

The illustrations depict a side-to-side shunt that is very easy to do, and I would warn that the technical difficulties described previously bear consideration. It is good to take ellipses out of both the portal vein and the vena cava as a preliminary to the anastomosis. I also favor an everting stitch because it leaves so little suture material exposed within the lumen.

In some instances a side-to-side shunt can be done by using a high transverse incision in the inferior vena cava when it would be impossible with a longitudinal incision as shown in the drawings. Then Satinsky clamps are applied a right angles to the cava.

Finally, I would never recommend an H shunt using an autogenous femoral vein. In such grafts the incidence of thrombosis is high. It is better to do an end-to-side anastomosis even though a side-to-side would be more desirable if the former seems too difficult. In some instances, ascites has been relieved by an end-to-side portacaval shunt.

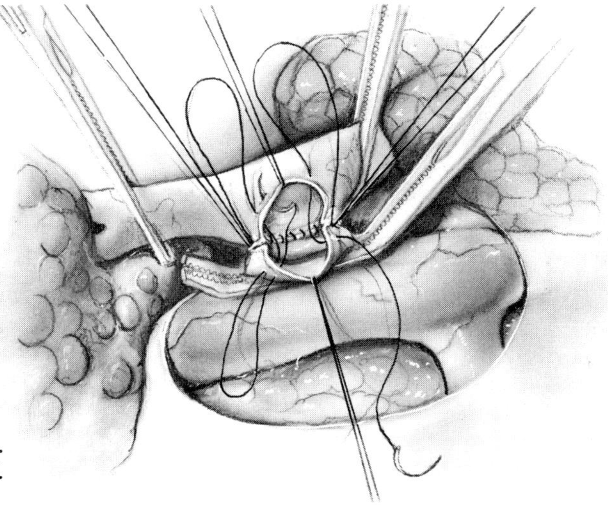

E

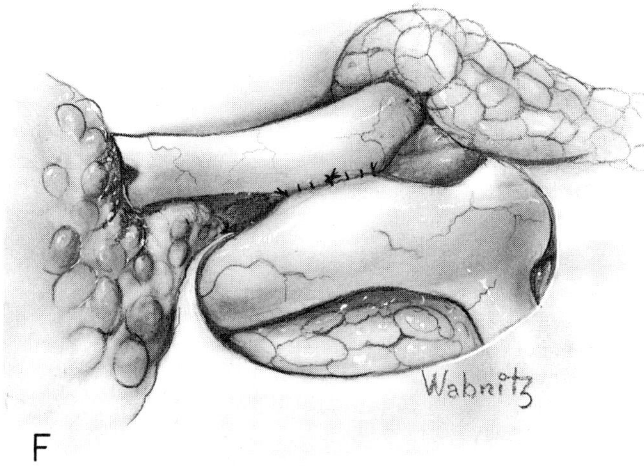
Wabnitz

F

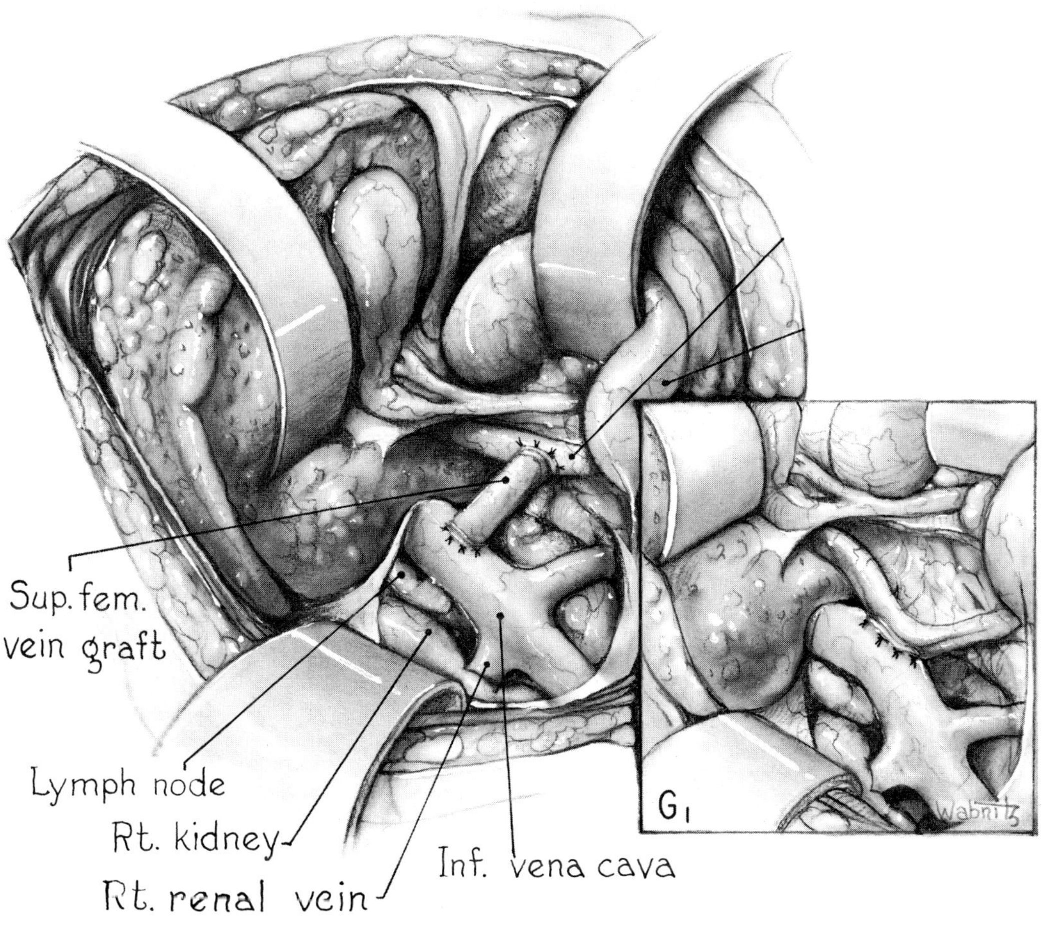
Sup. fem.
vein graft
Lymph node
Rt. kidney
Rt. renal vein
Inf. vena cava
G₁
Wabnitz

G

RIGHT TRANSAXILLARY, TRANSPLEURAL THORACIC SYMPATHETIC GANGLIONECTOMY

A. The patient is placed in the direct left lateral prone position, and the flexed right upper extremity is elevated and supported above the head. The transverse skin incision (broken line) overlies the third intercostal space and extends from the lateral border of the pectoralis major muscle to the anterior border of the latissimus dorsi muscle.

B. The incision is deepened through the subcutaneous fatty tissue layer to expose the line of incision (broken line) in the axillary fascia.

C. The transected tissue layers are retracted, and the lateral cutaneous branch (intercostohumeral) of the second thoracic nerve with an accompanying vein are shown within the surrounding fatty areolar tissue. A lymph node between the nerve and vein is faintly outlined.

D. The fatty areolar tissue is cleared to show clearly the lymph node and the intercostohumeral nerve in relation to the anterior serratus muscle. The ligated ends of the severed vein are also visible.

E. The nerve is retracted anteriorly, and the incision in the anterior serratus muscle is indicated (broken line).

F. The cut margins of the muscle are retracted, and the periosteum overlying the third rib is incised (broken line). The blood vessels arching upward from below the fourth rib may be seen.

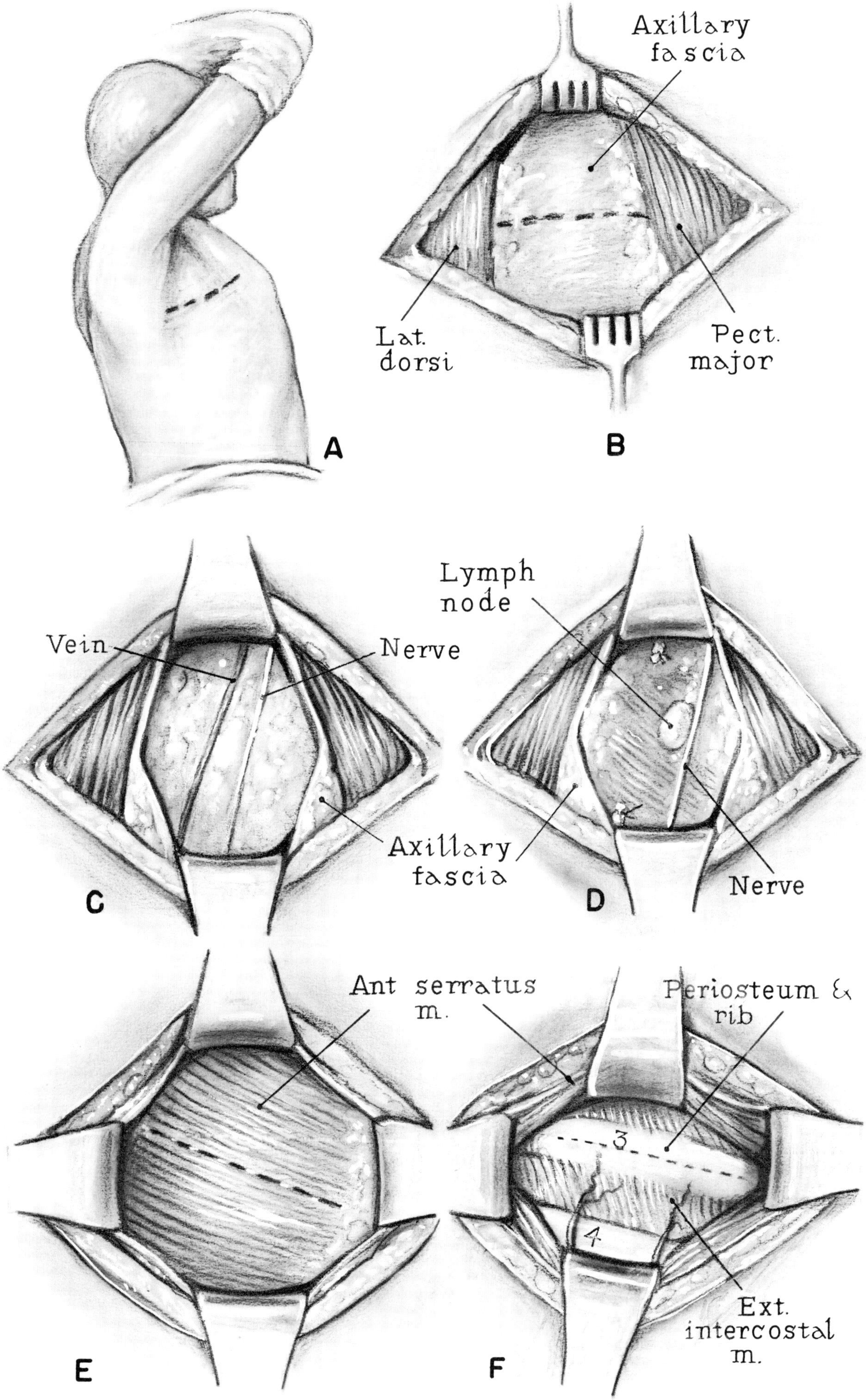
Axillary fascia
Lat. dorsi
Pect. major
A
B
Vein
Nerve
Lymph node
Axillary fascia
Nerve
C
D
Ant serratus m.
Periosteum & rib
3
4
Ext. intercostal m.
E
F

G, H. The lower half of the periosteum is separated from the third rib (G), and the left index finger is inserted between the separated periosteum and the rib (H) to mobilize it by blunt dissection from the underlying endothoracic fascia and parietal pleura (Brock technic).

I, J, K. An opening previously made into the pleural cavity is extended by scissor dissection (I), and the adjacent ribs (third and fourth) are retracted (J). The cut margins of the posterior parietal pleura are retracted with guy sutures of silk (0000), and the thoracic sympathetic chain and ganglia in relation to the adjacent structures are visible (J, K).

L. The thoracic sympathetic chain is transected between a silver clip (Cushing) and clamp caudad to the fourth ganglion and is then mobilized cephalad by sharp dissection using a curved knife blade (No. 12).

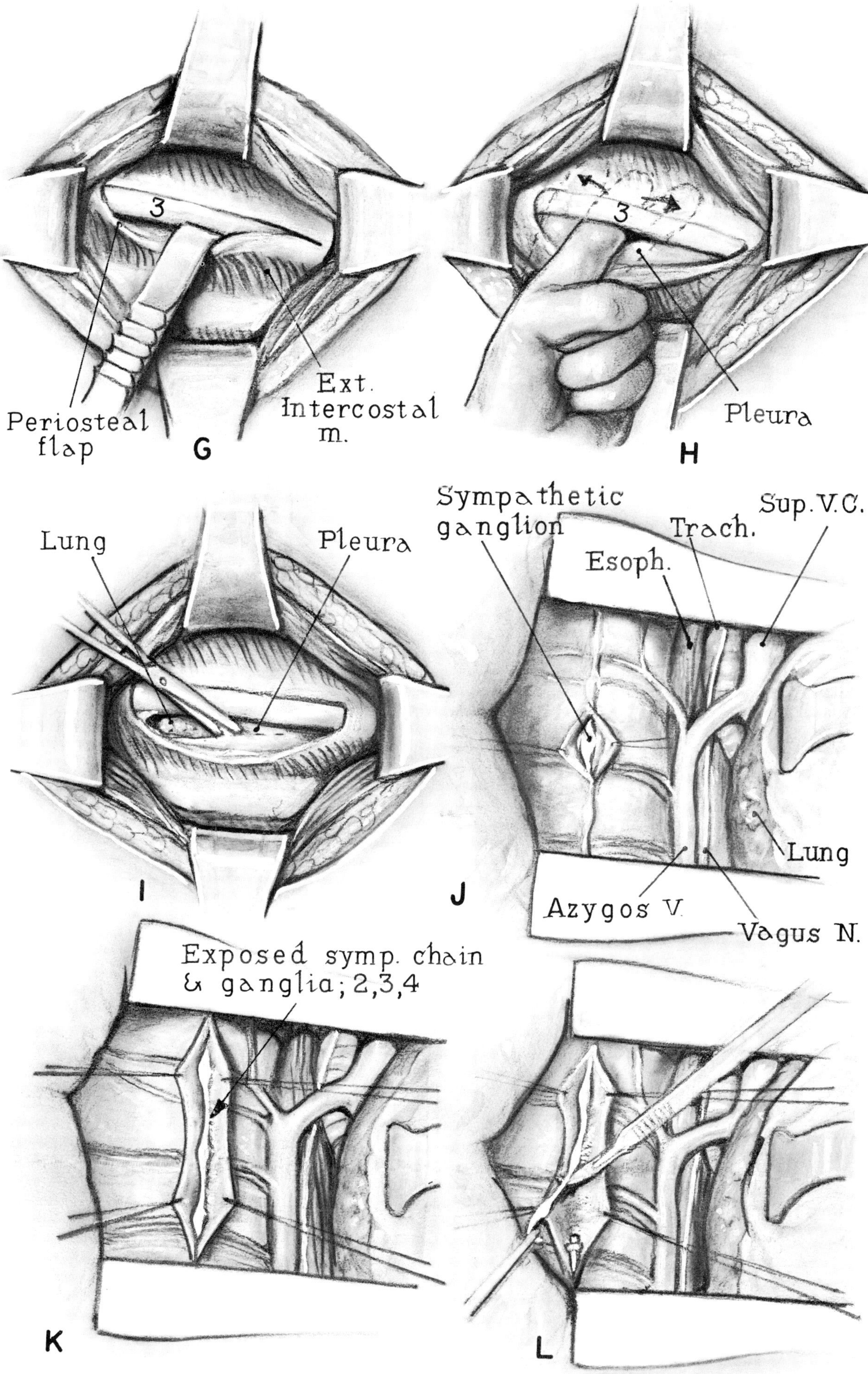
3
Periosteal flap
Ext. Intercostal m.
G
3
Pleura
H
Lung
Pleura
I
Sympathetic ganglion
Esoph.
Trach.
Sup. V.C.
Lung
Azygos V.
Vagus N.
J
Exposed symp. chain & ganglia; 2,3,4
K
L

M. The mobilized sympathetic chain is being severed with scissors proximal to a silver clip (Cushing), which was previously placed on the chain just caudad to the stellate ganglion.

N, O. The rib cage is approximated with two pericostal double strand sutures of chromic catgut (No. 2) about a catheter (18 F) that is used for temporary water seal drainage of the pleural cavity. To possibly obviate post-thoracotomy pain, periosteal "windows" are formed to avoid impingement of the sutures on either the periosteum or subjacent intercostal nerve.

P, Q. The anterior serratus muscle and axillary fascia are closed with interrupted silk (000) sutures about the catheter (P), which is subsequently withdrawn on completion of the skin closure (Q), using interrupted sutures of silk (000).

DISCUSSION—DR. CHARLES A. HUFNAGEL. Thoracic sympathectomy for the sympathetic denervation of the upper extremity has long been a subject of considerable controversy. Without discussing in detail the evidence for a ganglionectomy as opposed to preganglionic types, I should state that I believe that a ganglionectomy type of sympathectomy is preferable and that its results are not altered to a significant degree with the passage of time.

Transaxillary thoracic ganglionectomy offers a relatively simple approach to the sympathetic chain in the upper thorax. It can be performed rapidly. It is cosmetically more acceptable than either thoracotomy or a posterolateral thoracotomy. This approach brings the surgeon much closer to the sympathetic chain than does the anterior approach. It is quite obvious, then, that I do favor the procedure.

There are other considerations, however, which are not, in my opinion, so preferable. The exposure through this incision is relatively limited. When one rib is resected, the opening through which one works makes the control of bleeding difficult, particularly at the upper aspect of the chain. The intercostal artery and vein are frequently closely adherent to the chain and require careful dissection to avoid injuring them. This is particularly true in the region of the stellate ganglion. For a complete sympathetic denervation of the upper extremity, I have found it extremely useful to include the inferior half of the stellate ganglion in the ganglionectomy. If one carefully dissects the stellate ganglion, one can isolate the fibers which pass superiorly to the ganglion and preserve them. The inferior half of the ganglion can then be removed with the second, third, fourth, and fifth ganglia. Using this maneuver, one can achieve a more complete sympathectomy of the upper extremity, and at the same time avoid the production of a Horner's syndrome that accompanies total excision of the stellate ganglion. This exposure of the stellate ganglion is sometimes difficult to achieve through the transaxillary approach. The posterolateral approach through the fourth interspace gives one a sufficiently wide exposure that this dissection becomes quite simple.

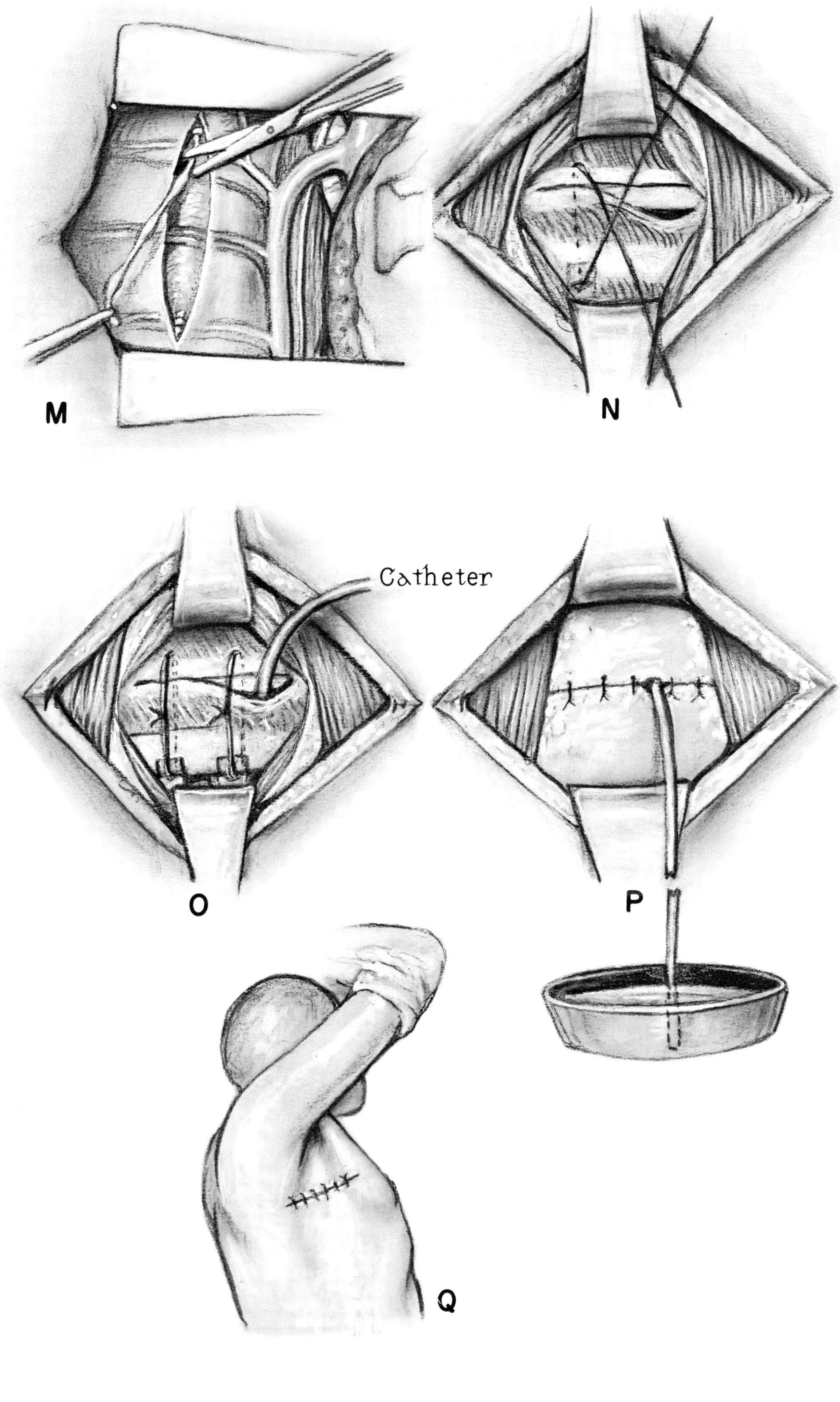
M
N
Catheter
O
P
Q

LEFT TRANSAXILLARY, TRANSPLEURAL THORACIC SYMPATHETIC GANGLIONECTOMY

A. The patient is placed in the direct right lateral prone position and the transaxillary incision is indicated (broken line).

B. The left pleural cavity is entered, and the rib cage retracted to expose the opening in the posterior parietal pleura and the start of the mobilization of the sympathetic chain and ganglia. The neighboring intrathoracic structures are visible. The broken lines in relation to the lower borders of the second and third ribs indicate the incisions to be made in the parietal pleura for the exposure of the second and third thoracic nerves.

C. The segmental resection of the sympathetic chain and ganglia (D2, D3, and D4) and the third intercostal nerve is completed. The second intercostal nerve is transected, and its clamped posterior segment is being mobilized to expose its anterior (motor) and posterior (sensory) roots.

D. The anterior root is transected, and the posterior root is being severed with scissors just distal to its sensory ganglion. In this dissection the subarachnoid space may be entered and cause a leakage of spinal fluid. In the experience of the author, the inclusion of the segmental resection of the somatic nerves (T2 and T3) has not been associated with an improvement when compared with the clinical results obtained when this is not done.

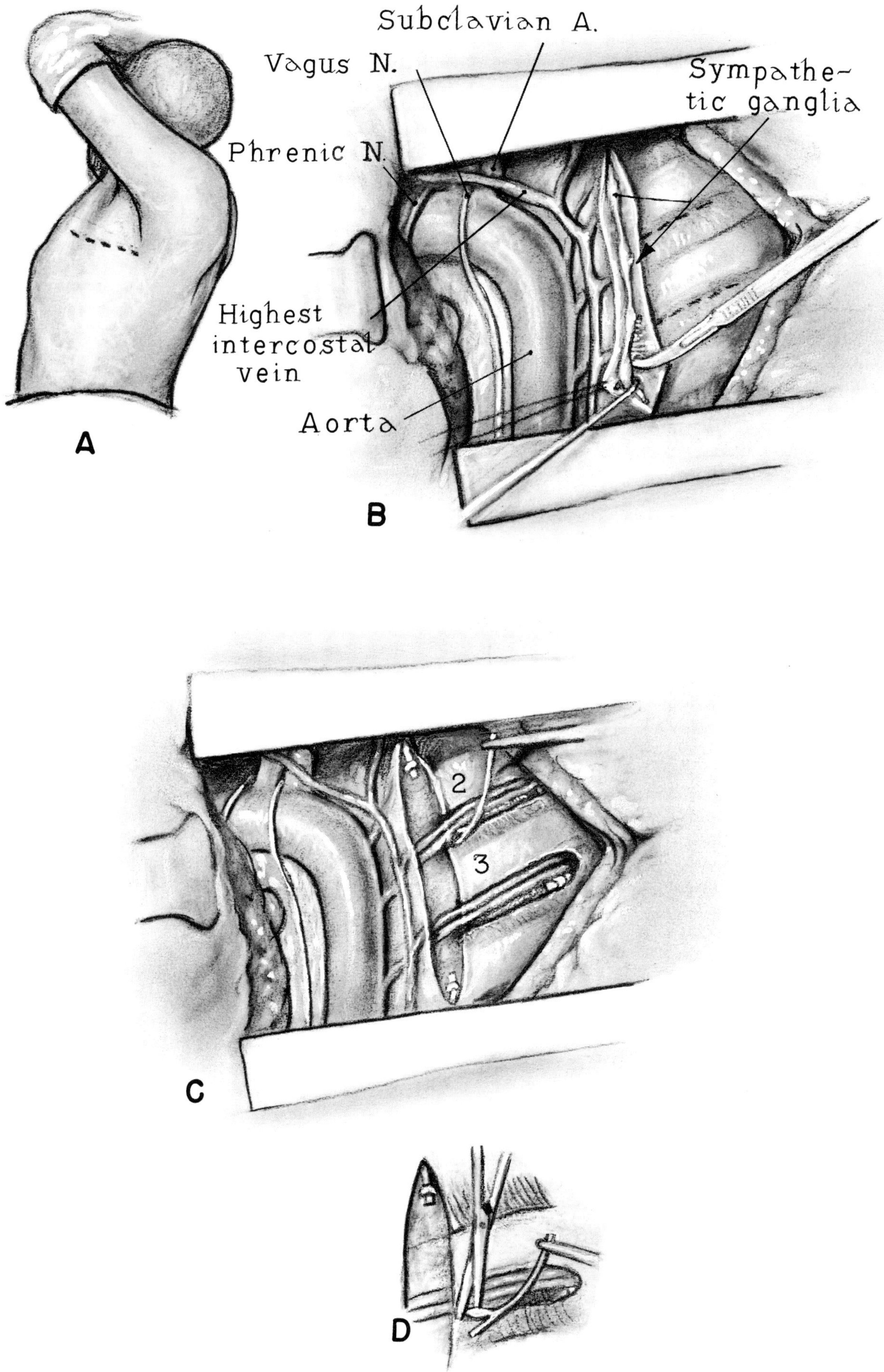
A
Subclavian A.
Vagus N.
Sympathetic ganglia
Phrenic N.
Highest intercostal vein
Aorta
B
2
3
C
D

LEFT LUMBAR SYMPATHETIC GANGLIONECTOMY

A. The patient is placed in the supine position, and the left side is elevated on a pillow support to approximately a 25 degree angle to the horizontal.

B. Traction with a multipronged (rake) retractor is maintained upward on the upper flap as its mobilization is completed by scalpel dissection. The lower flap was previously mobilized in like manner.

C. The outer angle of the incision is also mobilized by scalpel dissection until the musculature of the lateral abdominal wall is readily visible.

D. The mobilized skin margins are retracted, and the incision in the external oblique muscle in the direction of its fibers is visible. This incision is always made through the muscle fibers and never through the aponeurosis, which is located medially.

E. The separated fibers of the external oblique muscle are retracted to expose the opening in the internal oblique muscle layer through which the underlying fibers of the transversus abdominis muscle are visible. The internal oblique is the thickest and the transversus abdominis is the thinnest of the three muscle layers that are to be separated.

F. The muscle fibers of the internal oblique are separated by finger dissection, and care is observed to avoid avulsion of the underlying intercostal nerves between which an opening is made through the fibers of the transversus abdominis muscle. The dissection of this muscle is begun laterally and continued medially to lessen the possibility of opening into the peritoneal cavity. The opening in this muscle layer exposes a portion of the irregular line of overlap of the retroperitoneal fat on the lateral parietal peritoneum.

G. The muscle layers are retracted, and the transversalis fascia overlying the retroperitoneal fat is severed by scissor dissection. A herniation of a portion of the retroperitoneal fat through the opening made in the transversalis fascia is visible.

Discussion—Dr. Gerald H. Pratt. We have found spinal anesthesia not only safe, but one which, by its muscle relaxation, makes the operation technically easier. The level of anesthesia must be to the fourth or fifth dorsal nerves. A hypobaric solution permits the operative area to be elevated at once. The patient is placed on the table at a 45 degree angle to the operator by placing a sandbag underneath the hip and shoulder. The table is then broken, and the hand on the operator's side is raised high above the patient's head to pull the lower ribs out of the way. In this position, the space between the last ribs and the crest of the ilium, which is normally only about 2 inches, can be widened to 4 or 5 inches, and the lumbar spine is brought quite close underneath the operative incision.

We use approximately the same incision for lumbar sympathectomy as the author, a transverse one made in the line of the skin cleavage at the level of L-2. If the separation of the external oblique muscle, the most restricting of the muscles, is extended longer than that through the other lateral abdominal muscles, the wound can be moved to excise a ganglion found anatomically higher or lower than usual.

On the transversalis muscle and fascia lie the intercostal nerves and blood vessels. These nerves and vessels can be protected by making the transversalis incision between them, thus preserving the nerve supply to the muscles and also reducing the incidence of a painful neuritis. If the level of spinal anesthesia is slightly lower than desired, these nerves can be injected with procaine to avoid the addition of a general anesthesia, which we consider to be an added danger.

Mounted damp sponge sticks are adequate dissectors for moving the peritoneum and its contents forward without injury to the peritoneum. One must avoid dissecting behind the iliacus or between the iliacus and the psoas muscles.

Any dissection of the vena cava must be gentle since its lumbar branches are thin and easily torn. We dissect the upper part of the chain first follow-

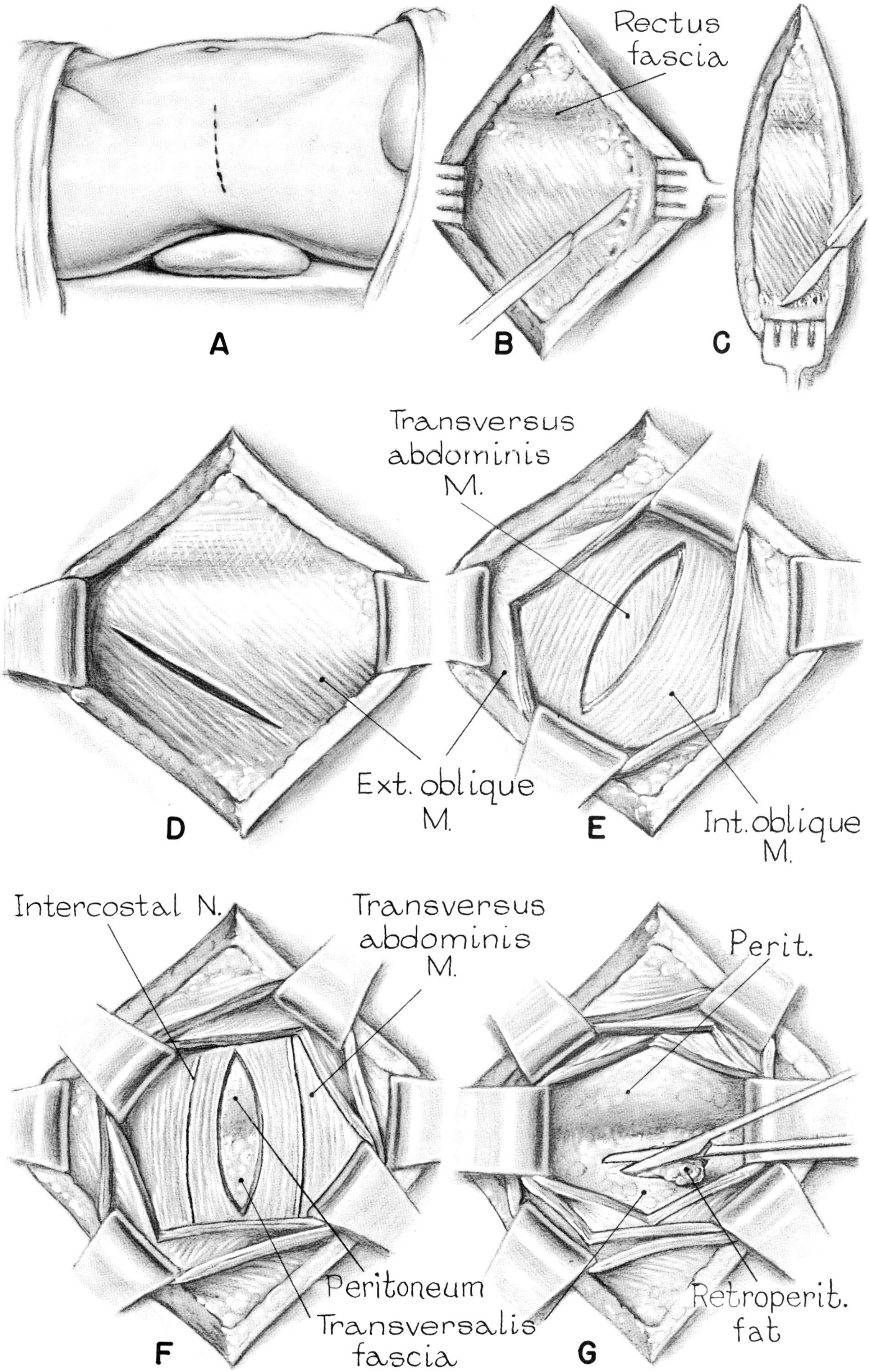
Rectus
fascia
A
B
C
Transversus
abdominis
M.
Ext. oblique
M.
D
E
Int. oblique
M.
Intercostal N.
Transversus
abdominis
M.
Perit.
Peritoneum
Transversalis
fascia
Retroperit.
fat
F
G

H. By blunt digital dissection in the retroperitoneal fat, the peritoneum and the adjacent intraperitoneal viscera are displaced toward the midline. During this dissection, the important landmark is the psoas major muscle, which is located more anteriorly than one generally assumes. The tissue dissection is continued anteriorly and medial to this muscle; otherwise, troublesome technical difficulty may ensue.

I. The peritoneum and the related intraperitoneal viscera are retracted toward the midline to expose the left ureter which overlies Gerota's fascia. The ureter is always first identified before being retracted from the operative field. The adjacent related structures are readily demonstrable.

J. The ureter is retracted medially. The line of the incision to be made in the fascia of Gerota is indicated by the dotted line.

K. The incision in Gerota's fascia is completed, and, by blunt dissection with a long tissue forceps (deleted for clarity) in the underlying fatty areolar tissue, the lumbar sympathetic trunk and the lumbar vessels are exposed along the anterolateral surface of the vertebral column. Further identification of the sympathetic trunk may be obtained by digital palpation against the sides of the lumbar vertebrae. The genitofemoral nerve, frequently mistaken for the sympathetic trunk, may be seen coursing downward and lateralward along the medial aspect of the psoas muscle. This nerve is white in color, nonganglionated, easily mobile, always on muscle (psoas), and directed downward and lateralward. Contrariwise, the lumbar sympathetic trunk is yellowish-white in color, ganglionated, and located on the anterolateral aspect of the bodies of the lumbar vertebrae and never on muscle. Furthermore, it is taut and relatively fixed in position by the attachment of the rami communicantes to their respective ganglia and is the most posteriorly situated structure along the vertebral column. Finally, its direction is downward and slightly medialward. These anatomic differences should serve to differentiate the genitofemoral nerve from the lumbar sympathetic trunk.

L. The sympathetic trunk is mobilized on a nerve hook, and, with upward traction maintained, the anchoring rami communicantes are severed with a curved knife blade (No. 12).

Discussion—Dr. Pratt (cont.)

ing it as high as possible, usually to the diaphragm. To increase the extent of sympathectomy, we avulse or exerese it from its surrounding tissue, and, if the pull on the chain is directly in the line of its fibers, the maneuver does not tend to lacerate any vessels.

The so-called fool's sympathetic, the genitofemoral nerve, is seen lying on the muscle in contradistinction to the chain which is in close approximation to the periosteum of the vertebrae with its enlargements (ganglia). The chain has a characteristic feeling to the palpating finger. We do not remove any structure as a chain until it is further identified manually by rubbing it against the vertebrae and feeling its cord, not unlike the vas deferens.

The artist's drawing depicts the sympathetic chain as a single nerve with ganglia. More often it is found as a plexus of nerve fibers with several communicating branches entering the main trunk above and below the ganglia. We feel it is important to remove all such fibers, even those that cross to the other side. Thus the lumbar sympathetic nerves are a plexus and not just a nerve with ganglia. There can be from two to eight ganglia in the lumbar area, and all the fibers should be removed in order to do a complete operation. In many instances, a repeat lumbar sympathectomy has been effective, the preceding operation having only removed one or two ganglia with a continuation of sympathetic effect by collateral sympathetic nerves. Identification of the upper and lower ends of the resected sympathetic chain by a silver clip is practical, as the author has pointed out, and also prevents an annoying hemorrhage from an accompanying vessel. The author brings attention to the variations of the anatomy in the right and left sides and the danger of injuring vertebral veins. The removal of the underlying chain by dividing it at the overlying vein and teasing it under the vein is a safe measure, if done carefully. While these lumbar veins can be clamped and divided, an attempt at their ligation is fraught with danger. Serious complications have developed from trying to ligate small lumbar veins. Silver clips are best used at this stage for hemostasis. These veins in themselves are small, but they open directly into the vena cava. If these veins tear, one has a laceration in the wall of the vena cava, and the small vein stump retracts and is a hole in the cava. In cases of serious hemorrhage, packing is advisable, at least until blood for transfusion is available. This venous bleeding can be controlled by a hemostatic pack, while a laceration from traumatic tearing of a hastily applied clamp on the vena cava might be serious or even fatal.

In closing the wound, one should again be careful to prevent inclusion of the nerves on the transver-

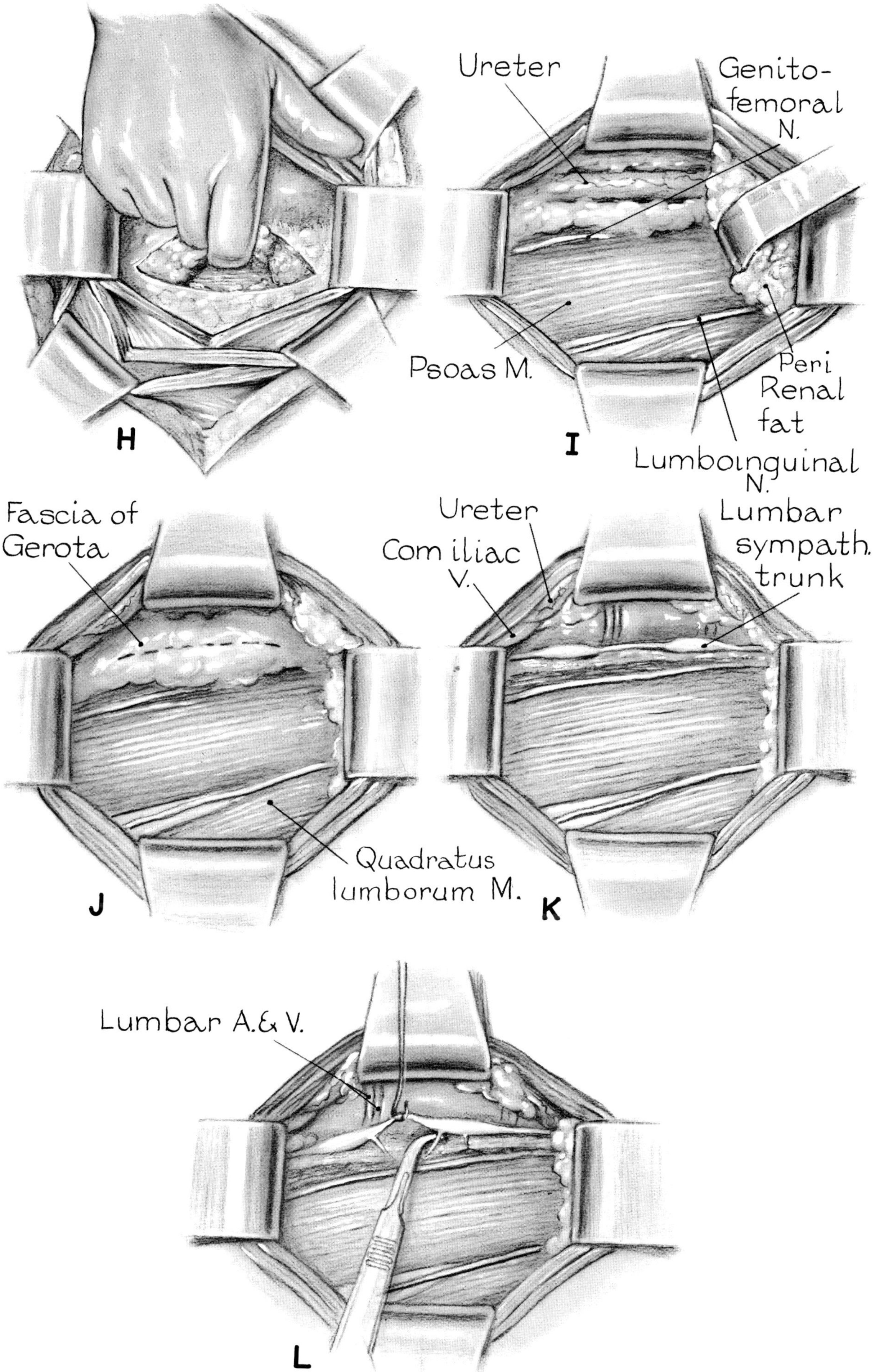
H
Ureter
Genito-
femoral
N.
Psoas M.
Peri
Renal
fat
I
Lumboinguinal
N.
Fascia of
Gerota
Ureter
Com iliac
V.
Lumbar
sympath.
trunk
Quadratus
lumborum M.
J
K
Lumbar A.& V.
L

M. Upon completion of the mobilization of the lumbar sympathetic trunk, a Cushing silver brain clip is applied proximally, and, immediately below the clip, the trunk is severed by scissor dissection.

N. Similarly, a silver clip is applied distally, immediately above which the trunk is severed.

O, P, Q, R. On removal of the retractors, the separated fibers of the various muscle layers tend to approximate themselves. The wound closure is in layers using interrupted sutures of silk (000) for the transversus abdominis muscle (O), the internal oblique muscle (P), the external oblique muscle (Q), and the skin (R). The relation of the intercostal nerves to the line of closure of the transversus abdominis muscle is visible (O).

DISCUSSION—DR. PRATT (cont.)

salis muscle in the sutures because of the subsequent annoying neuritis. We close the transversalis with chromic catgut and the rest of the layers with No. 32 stainless steel wire. We believe this technic has removed the wound reaction that some elderly patients evince.

The use of spinal anesthesia, good operative position, a careful study of the anatomy, light hands on the retractors, and care in avoiding laceration of lumbar veins will prevent most of the usual complications. We know of four ureters removed as sympathetic chains, and nearly every type of fascia, muscle, nerve, blood vessel, and lymphatic vessel has been removed and sent to the pathologist as a sympathetic ganglia.

It is our Clinic's teaching that many of the poor results attributed to sympathectomy are due either to inadequate sympathectic denervation or too long delay in the use of this operative intervention.

The author's technic is fundamentally excellent, and the results when it is followed correctly will be good.

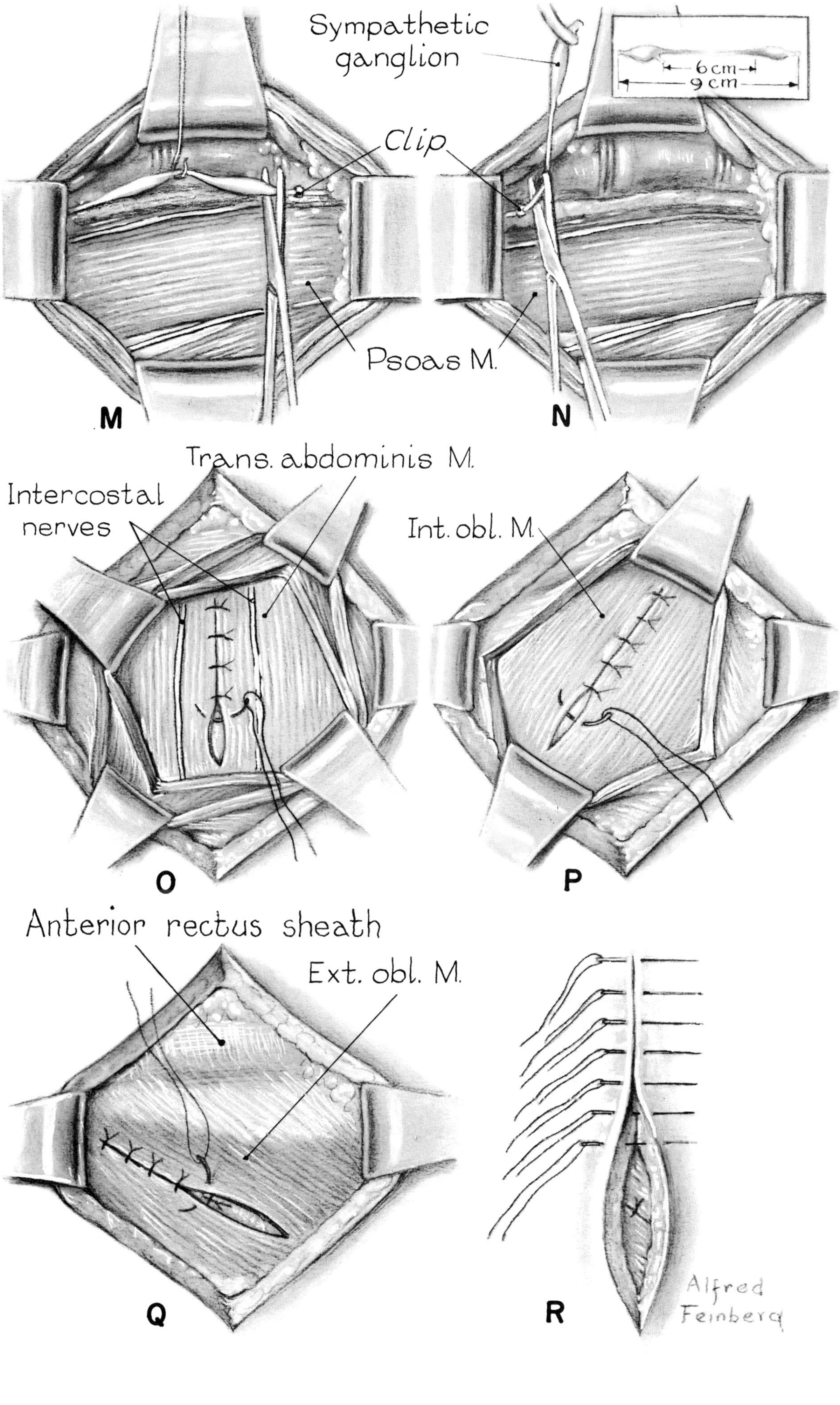
Sympathetic ganglion
6 cm
9 cm
Clip
Psoas M.
M
N
Trans. abdominis M.
Intercostal nerves
Int. obl. M.
O
P
Anterior rectus sheath
Ext. obl. M.
Q
R
Alfred Feinberg

RIGHT LUMBAR SYMPATHETIC GANGLIONECTOMY

A. The incision on the right side is similar to the one employed in the performance of a left lumbar sympathetic ganglionectomy. It extends laterally from the outer border of the right rectus at the level of the umbilicus to the midaxillary line at a point midway between the costal arch and the iliac crest.

B. The muscles of the anterolateral abdominal wall are split in the direction of their fibers and retracted. The beginning of the blunt digital dissection in the retroperitoneal space is shown, and the lower pole of the right kidney, enveloped in the perirenal fat, may be seen.

C. The dissection in the plane of the retroperitoneal fat is completed, and the ureter is visible along the anterior surface of the inferior vena cava, which is covered by the fascia of Gerota and underlying fatty areolar tissue.

D. The ureter is retracted. The line of incision in Gerota's fascia is represented by the dotted line.

E. Gerota's fascia is opened, and the inferior vena cava is retracted medially. The lumbar sympathetic trunk is secured on a curved nerve hook, and upward traction is maintained as the chain is mobilized by severing the rami communicantes using a curved knife blade (No. 12). The silver clip shown on the distal portion of the chain is applied immediately below the site of election for transection after this portion of the chain is completely mobilized.

F. The sympathetic trunk, severed distally, is mobilized proximally, and a silver clip is applied to the trunk just cephalad to the site of its transection. The relation of the adjacent genitofemoral nerve (nonganglionated) to the underlying psoas muscle and its downward and lateral direction are visible.

G. In this illustration, an alternate relation of the lumbar sympathetic trunk to the vertebral vessels is demonstrable. One may note in particular that the distal portion of the sympathetic trunk is posterior to the vertebral vessels. This is not uncommon on the right side, but it is infrequent on the left. Accordingly, on the right side, caution should be observed in the mobilization of the lower portion of the trunk. It should not be mobilized by avulsion because of the possibility of injury to the lumbar vessels. When the vessels are anterior, in order to remove the trunk completely, it is necessary either to sever the chain above and, by traction below, deliver it from behind the vessels, or to doubly clamp, sever, and ligate the overlying vessels. When severance of the vessels is indicated, preferably they are severed between hemostatic brain clips (Cushing).

H. Following the sympathectomy, the wound is irrigated with saline solution, and complete hemostasis is obtained. The retractors are then removed, and the wound closure is performed in layers, using interrupted sutures of 000 silk as previously described in the closure of the left side.

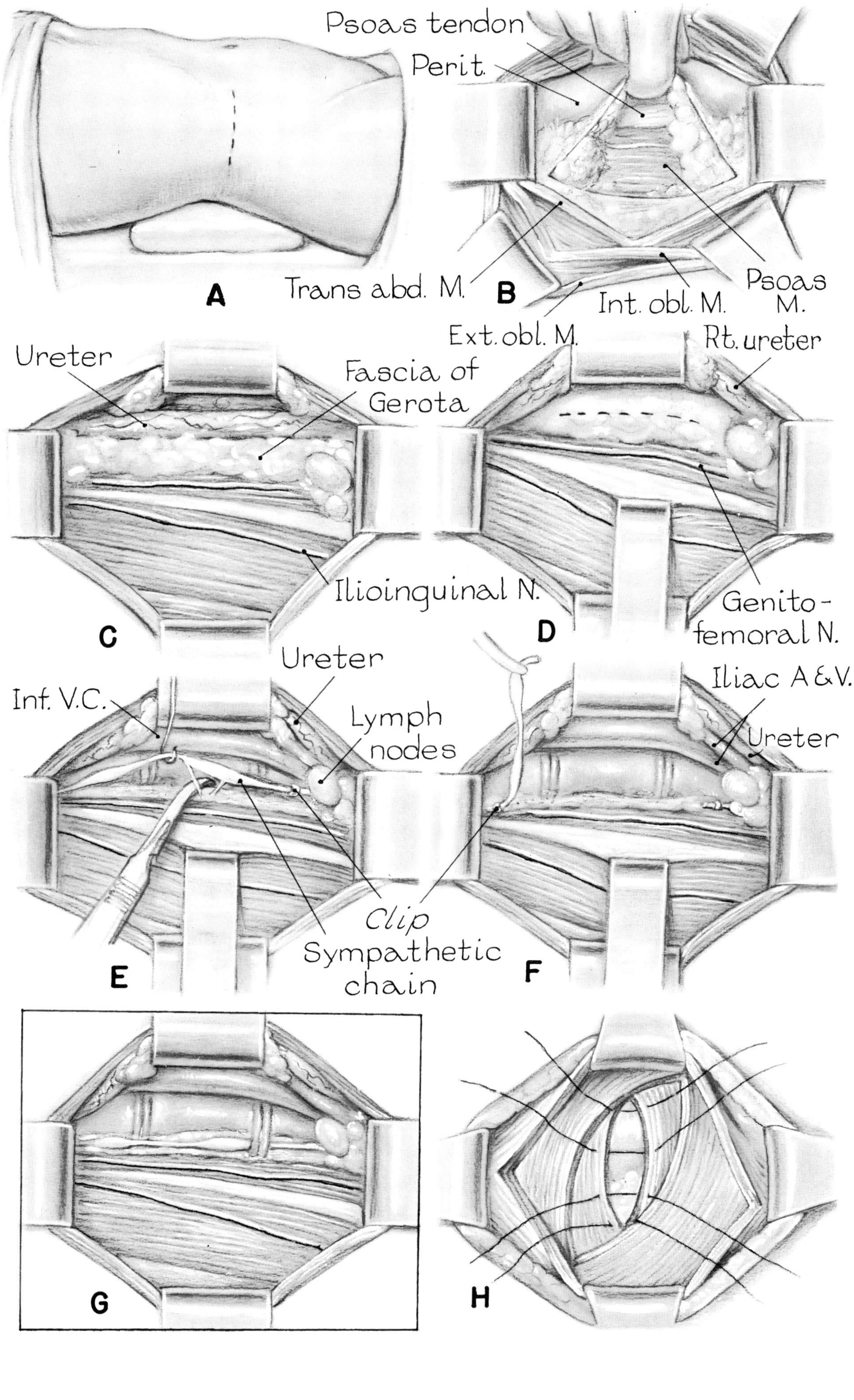
Psoas tendon
Perit.
Trans abd. M.
Psoas M.
Int. obl. M.
Ext. obl. M.
A
B
Ureter
Fascia of Gerota
Rt. ureter
Ilioinguinal N.
Genito-femoral N.
C
D
Ureter
Inf. V.C.
Lymph nodes
Iliac A & V.
Ureter
Clip
Sympathetic chain
E
F
G
H

MODIFIED KONDOLÉON OPERATION

A. The skin incision (solid line) on the medial aspect of the left leg and foot is deepened by scalpel dissection into the superficial subcutaneous fatty tissue plane.

B. Folded moist towels are secured to the skin margins of the incision by towel clamps, and, with upward traction maintained first through the clamps and subsequently by multipronged (rake) retractors, the skin flaps are mobilized from the surface of the lymphedematous tissue to the midline both anteriorly and posteriorly.

C. The mobilization of the skin flaps is completed, and the mass of lymphedematous tissue and underlying deep fascia is removed by scalpel dissection from the surface of the subjacent muscles.

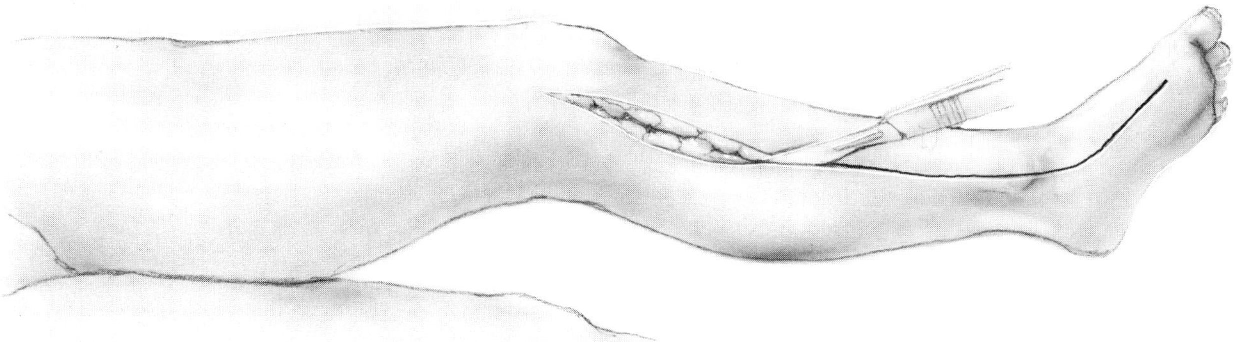

A

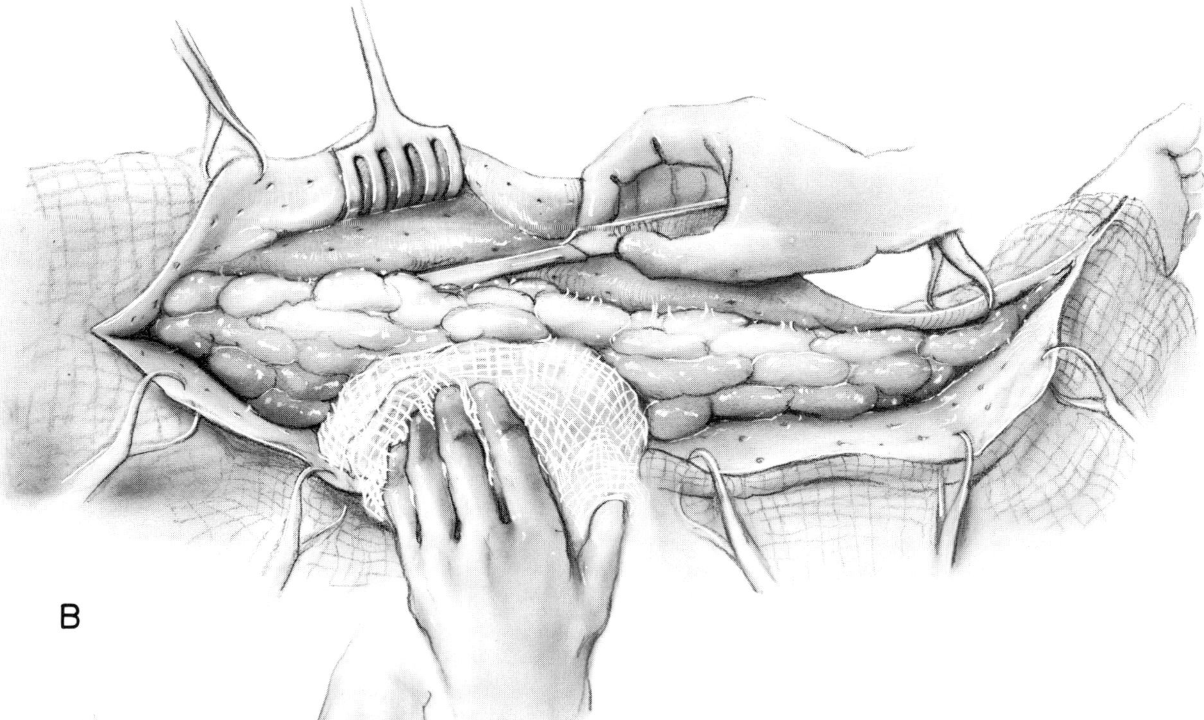

B

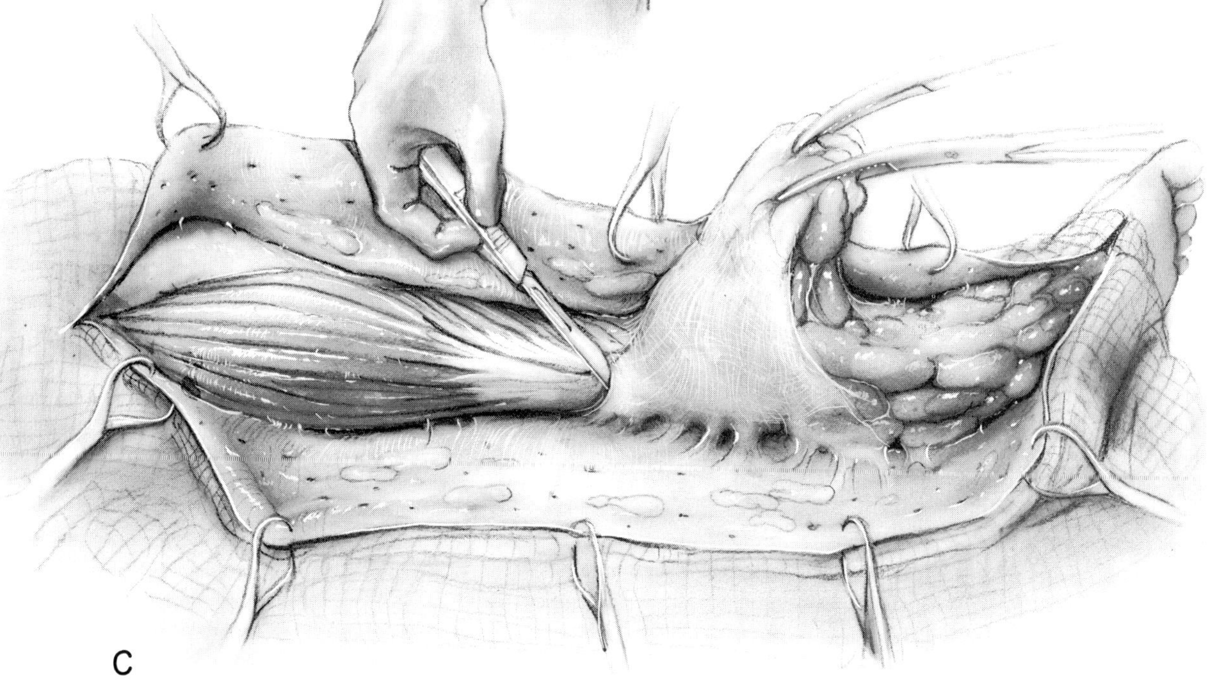

C

D. The excision of the lymphedematous tissue and deep fascia is completed, and the muscle structures of the medial aspects of the leg and foot are exposed. Small islands of fat may be seen adherent to the undersurface of the skin flaps. A catheter (12 F) with multiple openings in its tip is partially withdrawn through a stab wound opening in the lower skin flap for continuous suction drainage.

E. The skin flaps are approximated from either end of the incision toward the center with continuous interlocking sutures of 00 silk. The application of a compressive bandage completes the operation. Approximately four to six weeks later, a similar operation is performed on the lateral side of the leg and foot.

DISCUSSION—DR. HERBERT CONWAY. The surgical approaches to the control of persistent lymphedema have been many. Handley (1908) attempted to overcome the postulated lymphatic block in chronic lymphedema by implanting silk threads across the barrier. Ransohoff (1945) has more recently employed the same principle but substituted nylon. Kondoleon (1912), believing the superficial lymphatics to be obstructed proximally, excised long strips of deep fascia to permit escape of lymph from the abnormal superficial compartment into the deeper and presumably normal lymphatics. Gillies and Fraser (1935) attempted to bridge the lymphatic barrier by implanting across it normal tissue in the form of pedicled flaps of skin and subcutaneous tissue; Conway and Neumann (1949), Mowlem (1948), and Pratt and Wright (1941) further explored this technic. Homans (1940), Gibson and Tough (1954), Watson (1953), and others have attempted to control the process by ablating the diseased tissue. Although all of these approaches to the surgical treatment of lymphedema are now being employed, their results are often disappointing.

The work which I did with Neumann (1949) related to a postmastectomy lymphedema of the upper extremity. Neumann and I had planned flaps over the scapula area, to be rotated to the axilla and upper arm in the hope that these would carry the burden of lymphatic drainage from the upper extremity. Unfortunately, kinking of the flap due to the weight of the arm in adduction prevented any effective drainage through these pedicled tissues. In the management of unilateral edema of the lower extremity, large thoracoepigastric tubes were built, then stretched, and subsequently set into the upper thigh—across the inguinal ligament. After these procedures, dye tests showed that the lymph was being transported across the region of inguinal blockage. However, insufficient fluid was transported to effectively relieve the difficulty.

Following these experimental cases, the procedure of Gibson and Tough, in which ablation of the weighty, waterlogged tissue is carried out, the extremity being covered in annular fashion with split grafts of skin, was performed. This is perhaps the most commonly used operation at the present time. All of the follow-up examinations I have made on cases in which the Kondoleon operations were performed showed that they did little more than to reduce the size of the extremity by the amount of tissue which was actually removed. In other words, the re-establishment of lymphatic drainage through the deeper channels of the leg, as espoused by Kondoleon, did not succeed practically. In 1962 my associate Dr. James W. Smith and I reported on a new type of pedicled flap that was turned over as a hinge into the axilla for cases of lymphedema and elephantiasis of the upper extremity. This operation is described in detail in the medical literature. It has continued to show promise.

Noel Thompson of England reported upon a very ingenious surgical procedure in which a large section of lymphedematous fat is removed. A split graft is taken from the skin flap overlying the area of excision of adipose tissue, and the denuded flap is then curled down so that its cut margin is im-

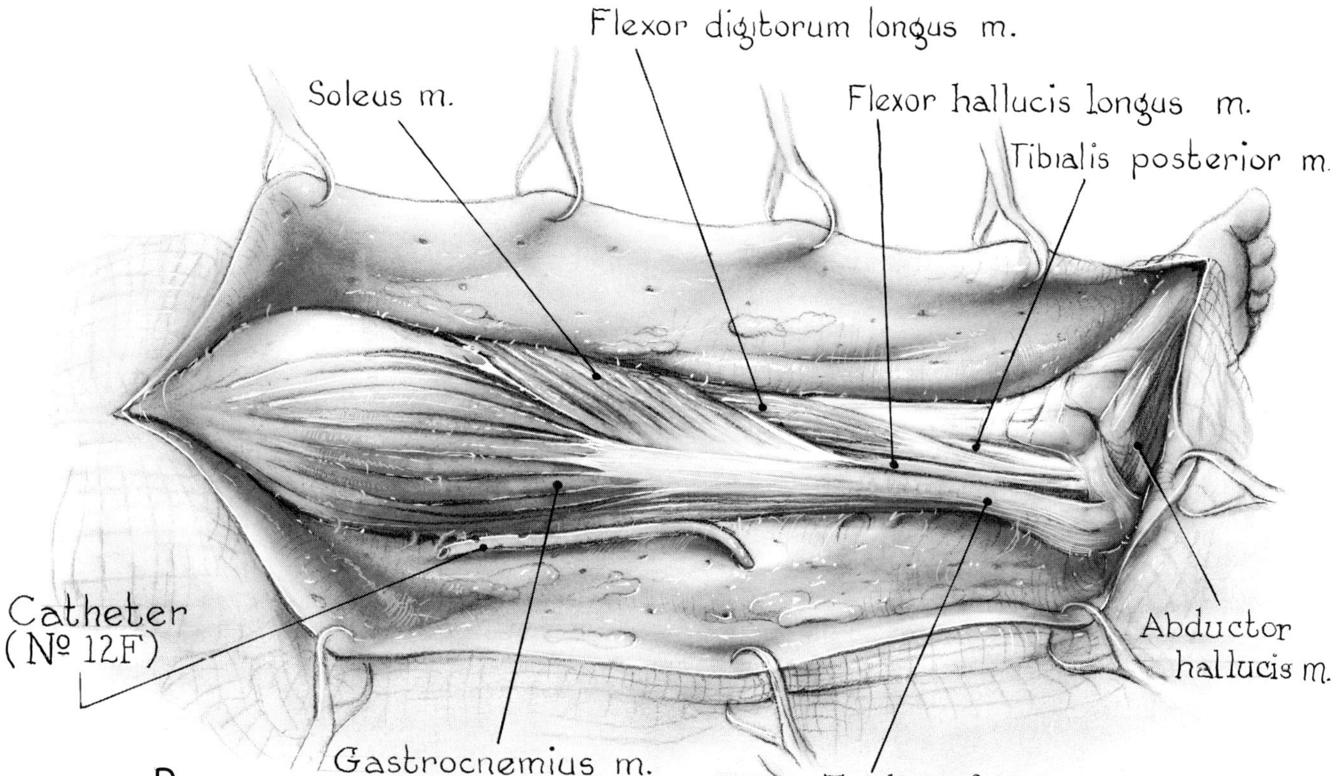
Flexor digitorum longus m.
Soleus m.
Flexor hallucis longus m.
Tibialis posterior m.
Catheter (Nº 12F)
Abductor hallucis m.
Gastrocnemius m.
Tendon of achilles

D

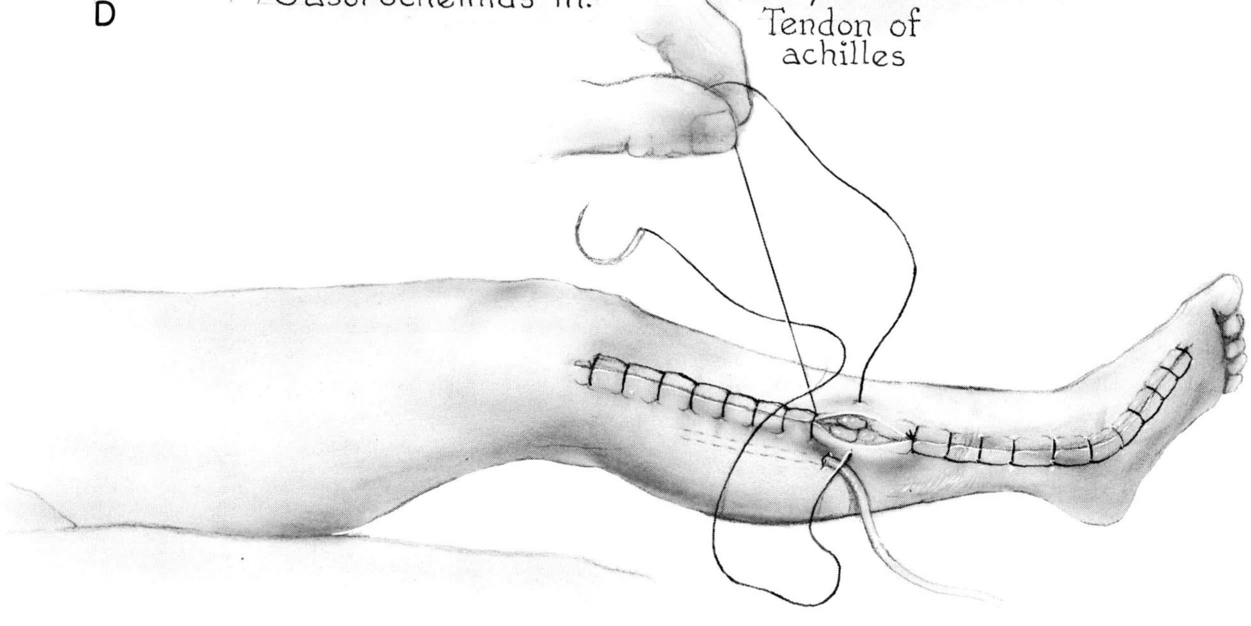

E

Wabnitz

A. The first and second stage operations on the medial and lateral aspects of the leg and foot respectively are completed, and, four to six weeks after the second stage operation on the leg, the third stage operation on the inner aspect of the thigh is performed. The incision on the medial aspect of the thigh (solid line) midway between its anterior and posterior surfaces is being deepened by scalpel dissection into the superficial subcutaneous fatty tissue plane.

B, C. Similarly as in the leg, moist folded towels are secured to the skin margins with towel clamps. Traction is maintained upward on the clamps as scalpel dissection is continued in the tissue planes between the skin flaps and the lymphedematous subcutaneous fatty tissue.

Discussion—Dr. Conway (cont.)

bedded deeply between the muscular layers. This operation has been used on three cases in this clinic, but, unhappily, clinical results do not measure up to the high hopes that the ingenuity of this surgical procedure naturally engenders.

The important point is that the surgeon must differentiate between those cases in which there is diffuse lymphatic damage and those in which there is obstruction or destruction of major lymphatic trunks.

I believe that there is a distinct relationship between the etiology and pathology of chronic lymphedema and its treatment. The several causes of this disorder are well known, but they seem to have been seriously disregarded in the selection of surgical procedures appropriate for its control. If greater emphasis were placed on these factors, results might be improved.

Lymphedema, by definition, is a swelling of skin and subcutaneous tissue resulting from imperfect lymphatic drainage. This definition, however, describes the end result of any one of a number of processes that can affect the lymphatic system. It fails to indicate whether or not the alteration is congenital or acquired, or whether the condition is due to a localized block or a generalized lymphatic disorder. It does not consider the several causative roles; namely, infection, previous surgery, radiation therapy, or malignancy. These are the factors responsible for the disorder, and treatment should be based upon consideration of the *cause* of the lymphedema.

The lymphatic disorders most frequently causing lymphedema are of two types.

Primary lymphedemas include developmental or function abnormalities of congenital origin, congenital lymphedema, lymphedema praecox, and Milroy's disease. Secondary lymphedemas include acquired functional abnormalities, infection, filariasis, surgery, radiation therapy, and metastatic disease.

In the primary lymphedemas there is no lymphatic block at one or more specific levels. The lymphedema is the result of a disorder involving the entire lymphatic system of the extremity. If surgery is to be considered in these cases, ablation of the diseased tissue is the only procedure that will prove effective.

Acquired *diffuse* lymphatic damage is usually the sequela of infection or filarial infestation. The site of the infection, its severity, and its chronicity are some of the factors determining the degree of resultant lymphatic damage. The localized lymphedema accompanying a chronic varicose ulcer and the generalized lymphedema following thrombophlebitis are examples of this type of disorder. In some of these patients lymphatic damage may be primarily at the capillary level; in others it may be confined to major lymphatic trunks involving all levels of the lymphatic tree. When surgery is contemplated for these patients, the underlying cause should be given prime consideration in the selection of the appropriate procedure.

Acquired *obstruction* or *destruction* of major lymphatic trunks usually results from operation, radiation therapy, or lymphatic blockage by metastases. In these cases the lymphatic distal to the site of obstruction are intact and potentially func-

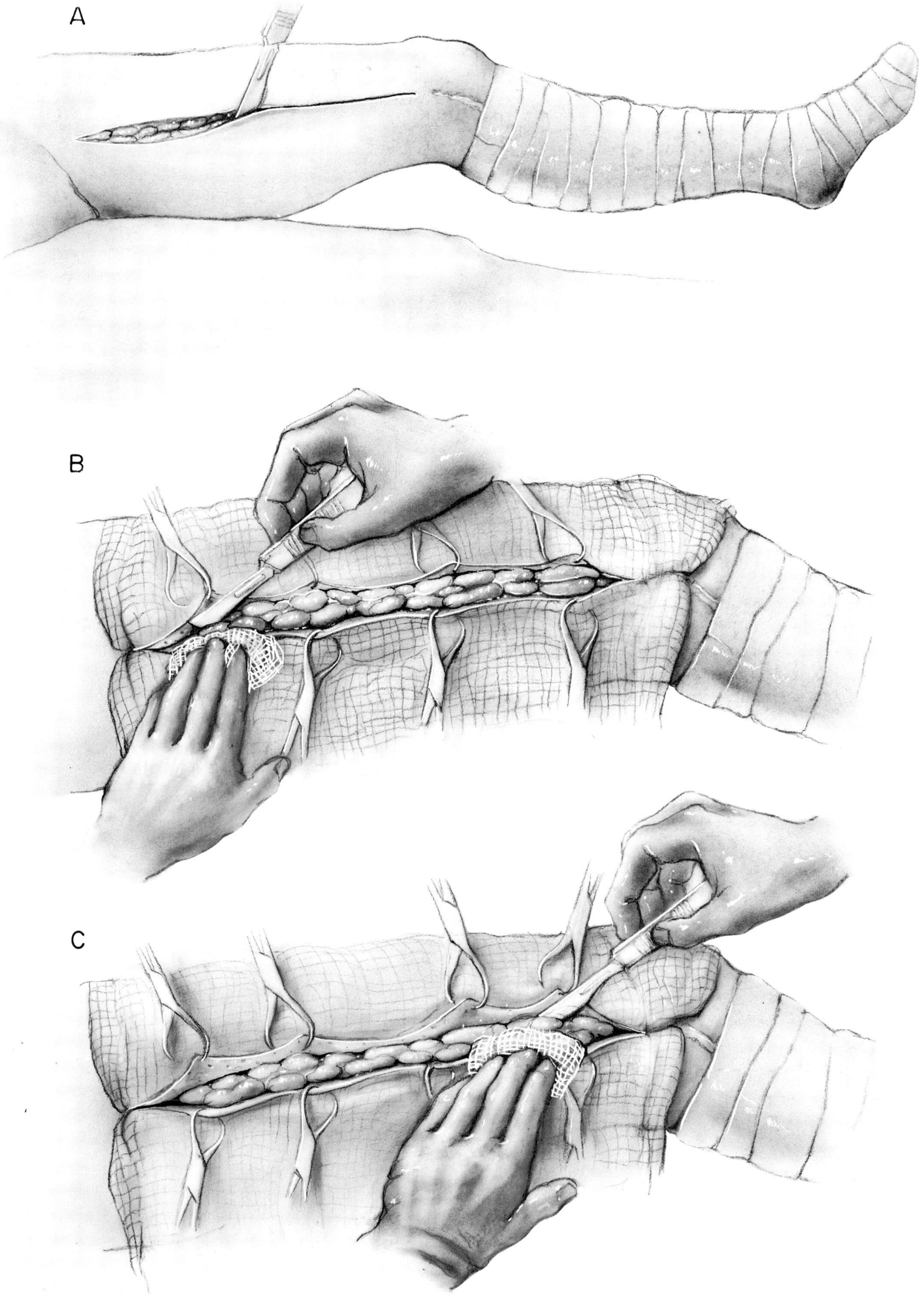
A
B
C

D, E. The scalpel dissection immediately subjacent to the skin flaps is progressively deepened (D), and as the dissection progresses, multipronged (rake) retractors are used to elevate the partially mobilized skin flaps (E). The dissection of the skin flaps is continued to the midline on the anterior and posterior surfaces of the thigh.

F, F_1. The mobilization of the skin flaps is completed, and a segment of the saphenous vein in the upper medial aspect of the thigh is visible (F). An untied ligature is applied to the caudad portion of the exposed proximal segment of the saphenous vein, and the vein is doubly clamped and severed as indicated by the dotted line (F_1). The severed ends of the vein are doubly occluded with ligatures and suture ligatures respectively of 000 silk. Each suture ligature is inserted between the occluding silk ligature and the clamp, which is removed as the suture ligature is tied.

DISCUSSION—DR. CONWAY (cont.)

tional, and in some, adequate drainage can be restored if the obstruction is eliminated or bypassed. Ablation, in contrast, may increase the severity of the disorder distal to the site of operation through further lymphatic destruction.

Finally, it is my feeling that the important matter in the treatment of lymphedema or elephantiasis of the extremities is selection of the proper type of procedure. Ablative operations, as espoused by Homans, and Gibson and Tough, are of use in those patients in whom there is generalized lymphangiectasis. This approach is also indicated when the weight of the extremity is such that the individual is handicapped. Stripped grafts over denuded muscle fascia are permanently effective, though often hypertrophic scars develop at lines of suture. These may be quite troublesome. In patients where the lymphedema or elephantiasis is due to direct obstruction, the transposition by one of the many technics for the use of pedicled flaps seems to be indicated. In my opinion, the Kondoleon operation as classically described is not of value. It is partially effective only in those patients in whom the operation emphasizes excision of tissue and accomplishes that step in a significant manner. On the other hand, the Gibson-Tough procedure, in which the leg or arm is covered with split grafts, has been practically effective as have many of the varied applications of pedicled flaps.

REFERENCES

Conway, H., and Neumann, C. G. Unpublished work.

Gibson, T. and Tough, J. S. The surgical correction of chronic lymphedema of the legs. Brit. J. Plast. Surg., 7:195, 1954.

Gillies, H., and Fraser, F. R. Treatment of lymphedema by plastic operation (a preliminary report). Brit. M. J., 1:96, 1935.

Handley, W. S. Lymphangioplasty. Lancet, 1:783, 1908.

Homans, J. Lymphedema of the limbs, Arch. Surg., 40:232, 1940.

Kondoleon, E. Die operative Behandlung der elephantiastischen Odeme, Zentralbl. Chir., 39:1022, 1912.

Mowlem, R. The treatment of lymphedema, Brit. J. Plast. Surg., 1:48, 1948.

Pratt, G. H., and Wright, I. S. Surgical treatment of chronic lymphedema (elephantiasis), Surg., Gynec. & Obst., 72:244, 1941.

Ransohoff, J. L. Surgical treatment of lymphedema, Arch. Surg., 50:269, 1945.

Smith, J. W., and Conway, H. Selection of Appropriate Surgical Procedures in Lymphedema, Plast. & Reconst. Surg. 30:10, 1962.

Thompson, Noel. Surgical treatment of chronic lymphedema of the lower limb, Brit. Med. J., 11:1566, 1962.

Watson, J. Chronic lymphedema of the extremities and its management, Brit. J. Surg., 41:31, 1953.

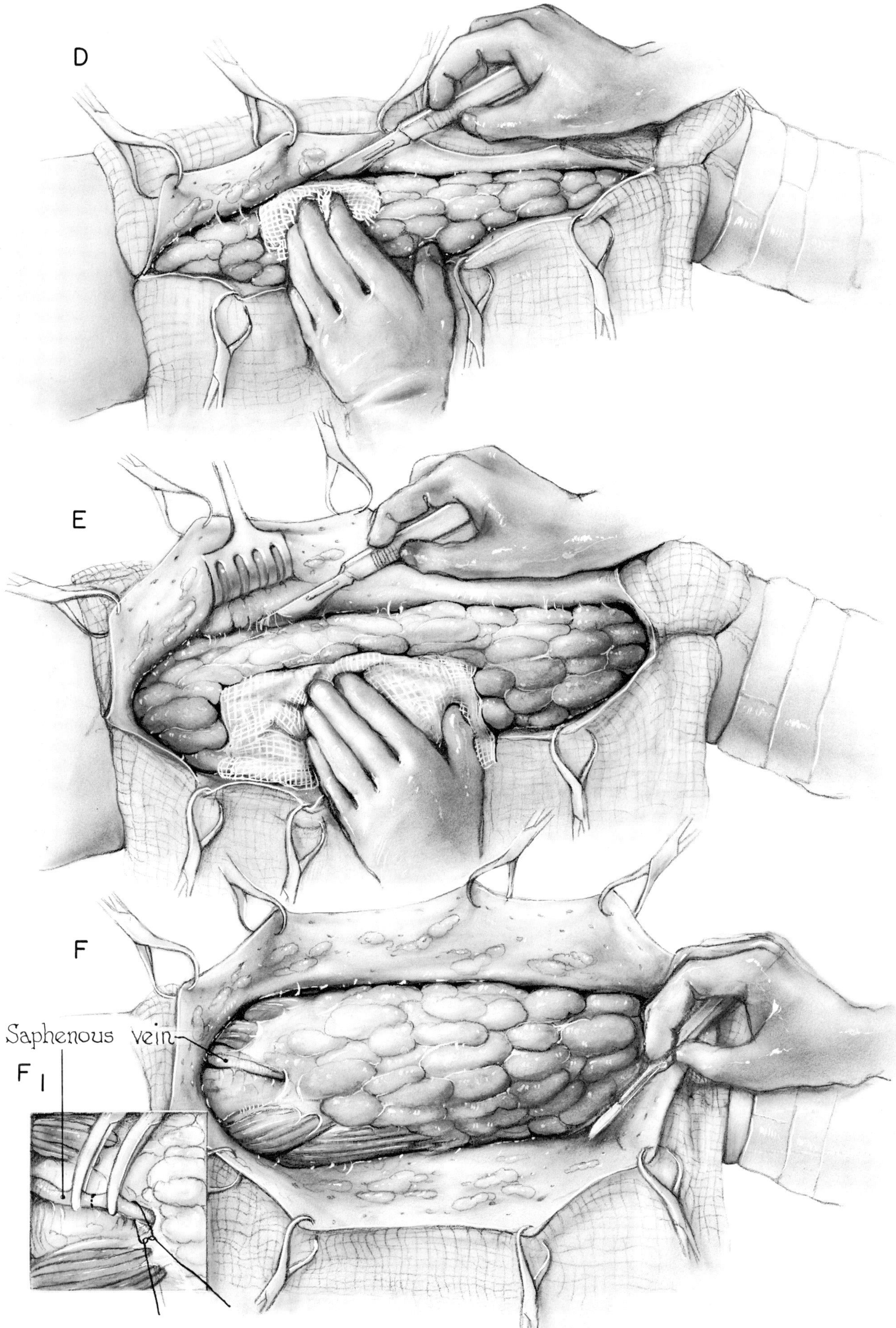
D
E
F
Saphenous vein
F 1

G, H. The cephalad margin of the lymphedematous tissue is grasped in clamps, and, as downward traction is maintained, it is removed en bloc with the underlying fascia from the subjacent muscles by scalpel dissection.

Discussion—Dr. Gerald H. Pratt. The author's incision, as shown in Plate 192A, is in the classic medial position. At times, we have placed this incision directly in the midline of the back of the leg to correspond to the suture line of a stocking. This also permits equal sized flaps to be raised medially and laterally around to the tibia. Plate 192B shows the raising of these flaps with the typical "pigskin" appearance of the denuded skin, indicating that all possible fat and fascia have been removed from the skin flap itself. The removal of all of the superficial and deep fascia en bloc is then shown. In B, one can see some fat and tissue globules still left on the elevated skin flaps which we feel should be removed subsequently. Many fat collections are found in the layers between and under the muscles, and, in our experience, any fat retained will cause lymphedema to recur. Plate 191D demonstrates well all the muscles which can be seen at this operative intervention. Sometimes we retain the saphenous vein as a help in subsequent drainage. Phisohex whirlpool baths will help clean the first operative area between stages.

In the thigh, the removal of the fascia is not nearly as difficult as it is below the knee, where the fascia itself also becomes muscle fascia. It is extremely important that all of this fascia and fat be excised. The muscle demonstration in Plate 192 I is excellent. We remove all the fat on the skin and all the fat between those muscle bundles. The excessive skin must be removed prior to approximating the skin edges.

Individual variations exist in surgeons' technics. We leave small strips of fascia over the tendon Achilles and the peroneus muscles at the ankle to prevent the tendons from bowing out. We use no drains, feeling that a drain may be a portal of entry for infection in these limbs already depleted of their lymphatic defenses by their disease. The utilization of interrupted fine steel wire sutures (No. 36) inserted loosely reduces, we feel, secondary tissue reaction to suture material. This is an individual variation in technic. We bevel the remaining tissue at the incision margin so there is not a sudden change in the size of the leg from the nonoperative to the operative area.

Some years ago, after performing a large number of these operations by the technic described, we found the recurrence rate quite high. The recurring attacks of cellulitis continued, and the overall results were not satisfactory. A much more radical procedure was then performed and described. By biopsy, we found that lymph did not accumulate in the epithelium of the skin until a depth of 1/50 of an inch was reached. Therefore, with an electric dermatome, the epithelium was removed at only 15/1000 of an inch in depth. The second finding was that all fat and all fascia accumulate lymph in lymphedema. We removed all such tissue down to the denuded red muscles. The operation, then, consists of removing all of the skin with an electric dermatome set at 15/1000 of an inch thickness and then removing all of the rest of the skin, superficial and deep fascia, as well as all the fat. The *same* thin epithelial covering is then replaced directly on the denuded red muscle. Other technics retained either deep or muscle fascia.

While this operation resulted in some keloiding and occasional dermatitis, due to the fact that the skin was of poor texture, the reduction in size was satisfactorily maintained if all of the fat and fascia were removed. Lymphangitis attacks often continue to occur after any operation due to the fact that the lymphatic defense in these limbs is inadequate. This complication can be relieved by use of long term antibiotic therapy, giving the drugs just before cellulitis should develop, as determined by a fever bout calendar. We reserve this more radical technic, however, for those patients who have tremendous lymphedemas and those in whom recurrence has resulted after the method described by the author. Only in the mild lymphedemas have we been able to effectively do away with the grotesque enlargement by the method described. Elevation and support continue to be necessary in most patients for an indefinite time.

G

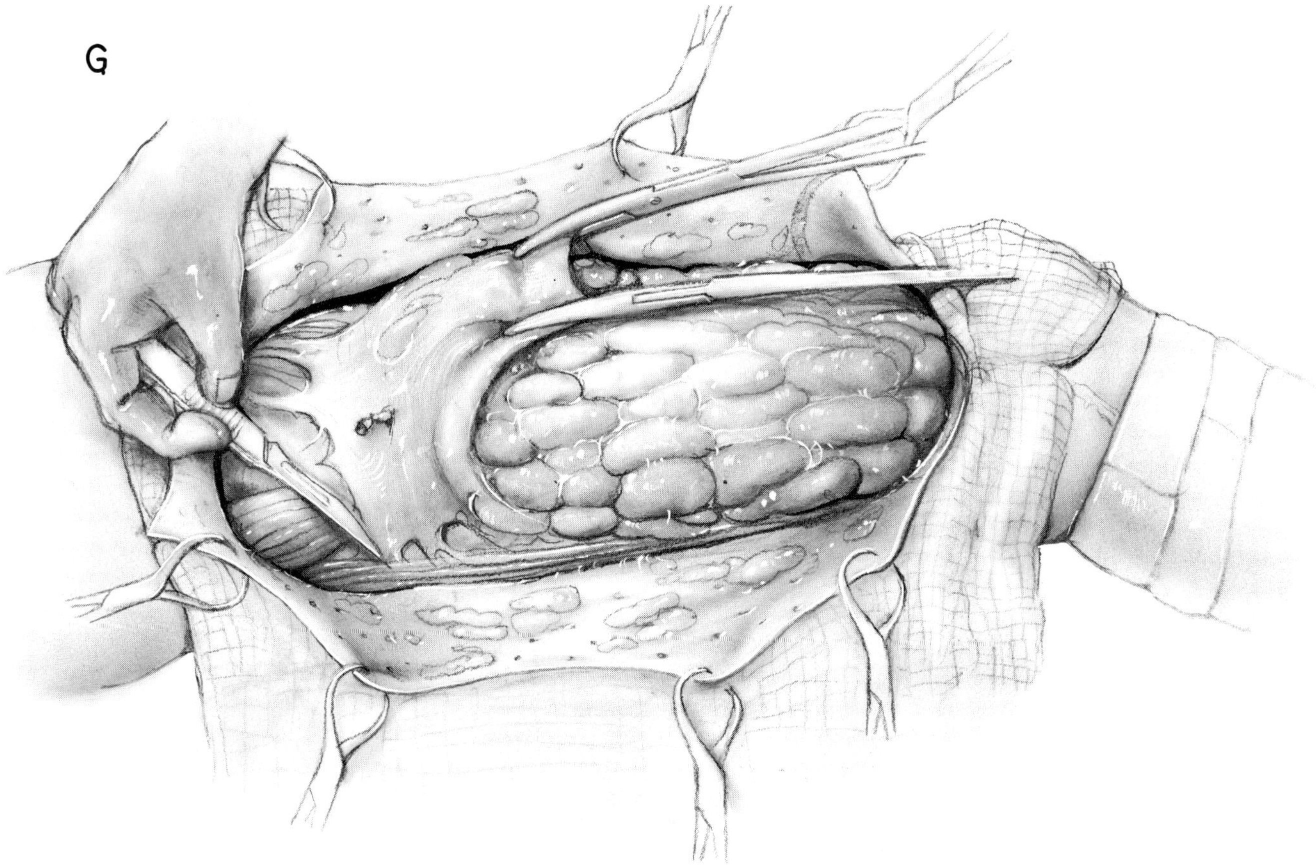

H

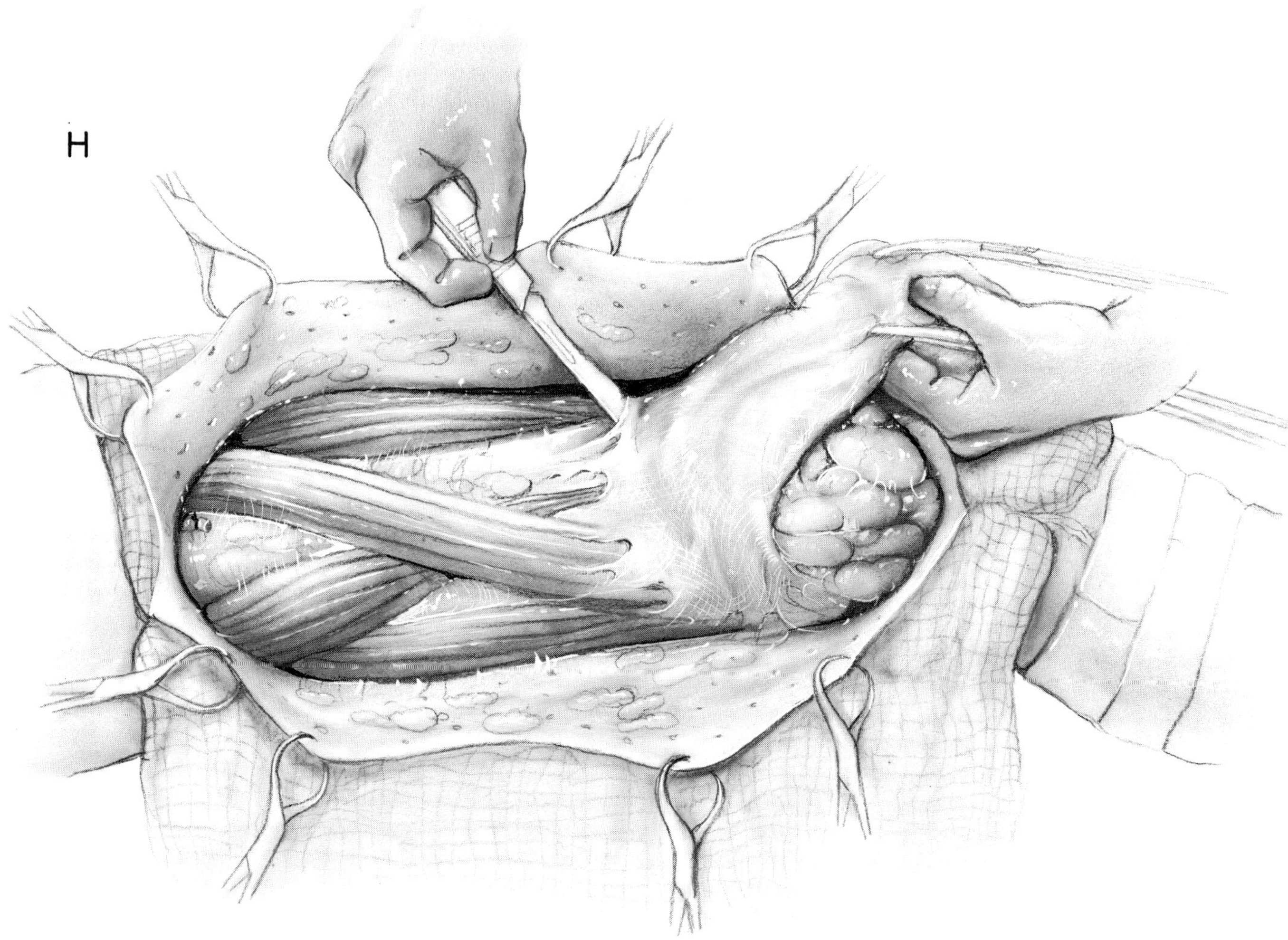

I. The excision of the lymphedematous tissue and underlying fascia is completed to expose the subjacent muscle structures on the medial aspect of the thigh. A catheter (No. 12 F) for continuous suction drainage is inserted through a stab wound in the lower flap.

J. The skin incision is closed, using a continuous interlocking suture of 00 silk. Upon completion of the closure of the skin incision, a compressive bandage is applied. The fourth and last stage of the operation is performed on the lateral aspect of the thigh four to six weeks later.

The technic illustrated is preferred to the removal of split thickness (0.020 inches) skin grafts which are applied directly to the subjacent muscle structures after excision of the lymphedematous tissue and underlying fascia. The postoperative results following this operation have proved unsatisfactory because of the high incidence of recurrent attacks of cellulitis, excessive keloid formation, prolonged disability, and persistent enlargement of the extremities.

In the elevation of the skin flaps as depicted in the illustrations, areas of necrosis of varying sizes frequently occur along the line of the incision. However, subsequent skin grafting to cover the resulting tissue defects is only occasionally required. In general, the overall results with the use of the illustrated modification of the Kondoléon operation have proved most satisfactory.

I

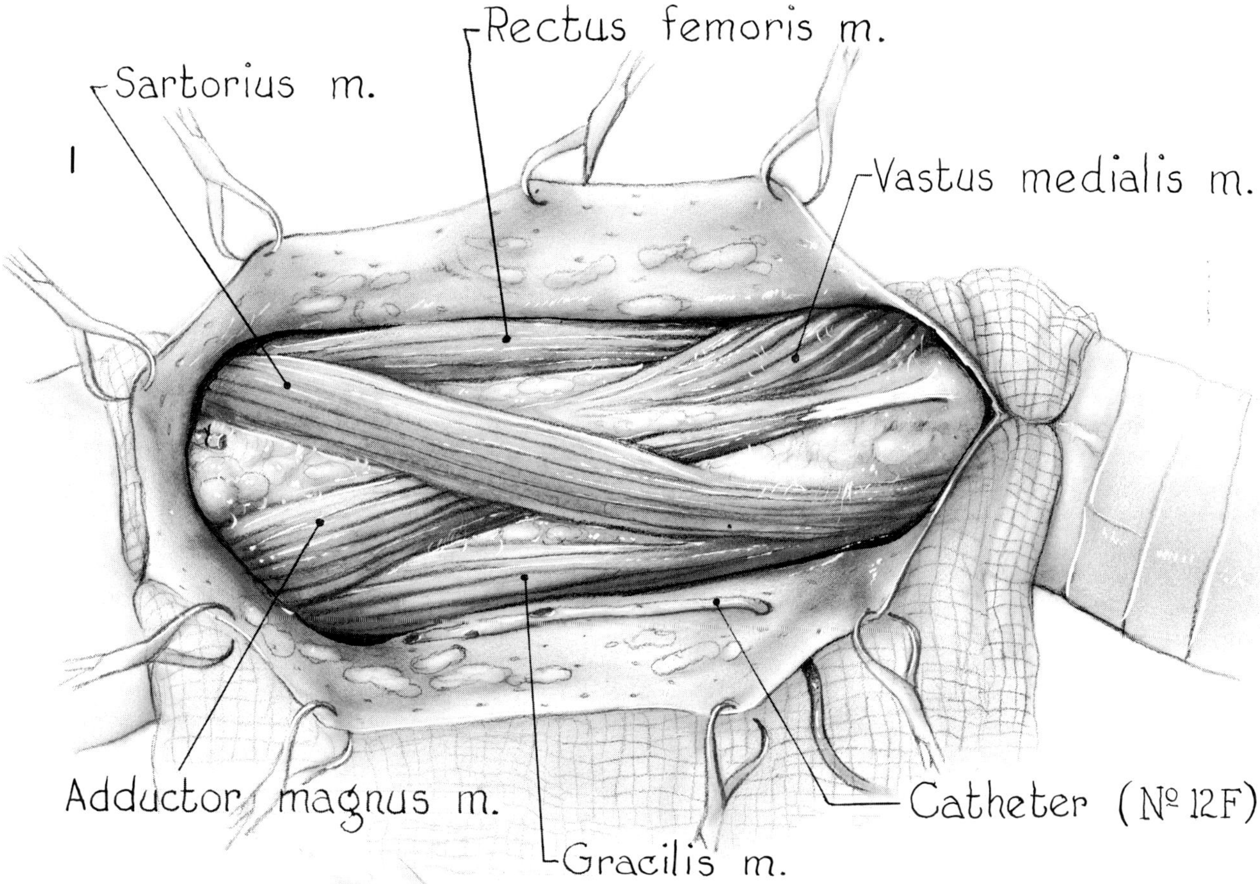
Rectus femoris m.
Sartorius m.
Vastus medialis m.
Adductor magnus m.
Catheter (№ 12F)
Gracilis m.

J

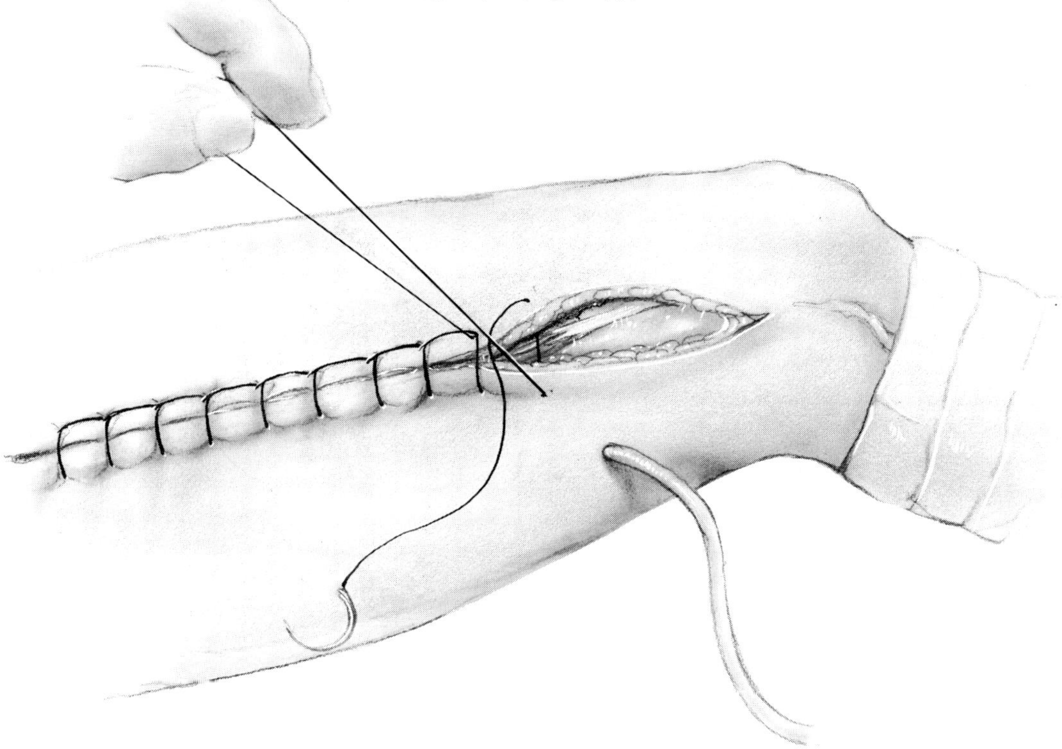

TRANSTHORACIC, SUPRADIAPHRAGMATIC RESECTION OF THE VAGUS NERVES

A. The patient is placed in the direct right lateral prone position, and a relatively short incision in the eighth interspace, extending from the anterior to the posterior axillary lines, is outlined.

B, C. The incision is deepened through the underlying muscle layers and the left pleural cavity is entered (D).

D. The adjacent rib margins are retracted and the entrance into the posterior mediastinal space through an incision in the reflection of the pleura forming the inferior pulmonary ligament is shown.

d′. An inset to demonstrate an alternate method of incising the inferior pulmonary ligament between suture ligatures of silk (000).

E. The cut margins of the posterior mediastinal pleura are reflected by guy sutures of silk (0000), and by blunt scissor dissection, an opening is made in the avascular fatty areolar tissue overlying the esophagus.

F. The esophagus is displaced posteriorly, and the left or anterior vagus nerve is mobilized on a nerve hook. This nerve, smaller than the right, is always in close approximation to the anterior surface of the esophagus.

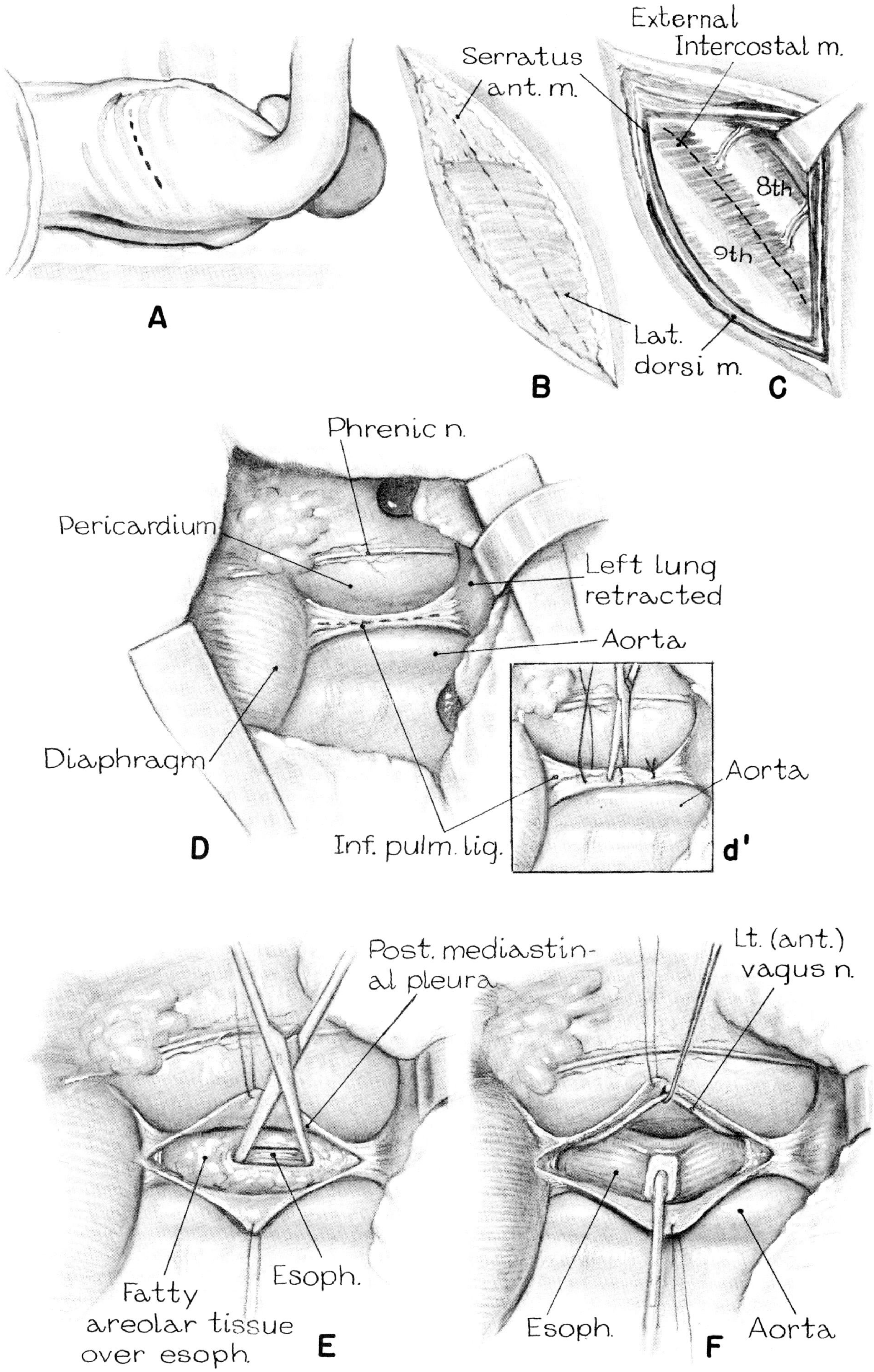
A
Serratus
ant. m.
Lat.
dorsi m.
B
External
Intercostal m.
8th
9th
C
Phrenic n.
Pericardium
Left lung
retracted
Aorta
Diaphragm
D
Inf. pulm. lig.
Aorta
d'
Post. mediastin-
al pleura
Fatty
areolar tissue
over esoph.
Esoph.
E
Lt. (ant.)
vagus n.
Esoph.
F
Aorta

G, H. A segment of the left (anterior) vagus nerve is removed between demarcating silver clips. A communicating branch of the vagus nerve is visible.

I, J, K. The esophagus is displaced anteriorly to visualize the right (posterior) vagus nerve which lies in the fatty areolar tissue plane posterior and medial to the esophagus. Similarly, as previously demonstrated, a segment of this nerve is resected.

L. The communicating branch is mobilized on a nerve hook preliminary to its severance. Subsequently careful digital exploration of the complete circumference of the esophagus is performed to detect and sever all of the additional nerve fibers which may be present. The importance of this maneuver cannot be overemphasized since the success of the operation is dependent upon the completeness of the vagal denervation of the stomach.

M, N, O. The layer closure of the incision is illustrated. Just prior to the completion of the closure the water-seal drainage catheter is removed. Two periosteal flaps are raised at the lower border of the ninth rib to permit the insertion of the pericostal sutures (No. 2 silk) without impingement upon the subjacent intercostal nerve. It is believed that the use of this technic may lessen the incidence of post-thoracotomy pain. If preferred, heavy sutures of chromic catgut may be used for the pericostal sutures.

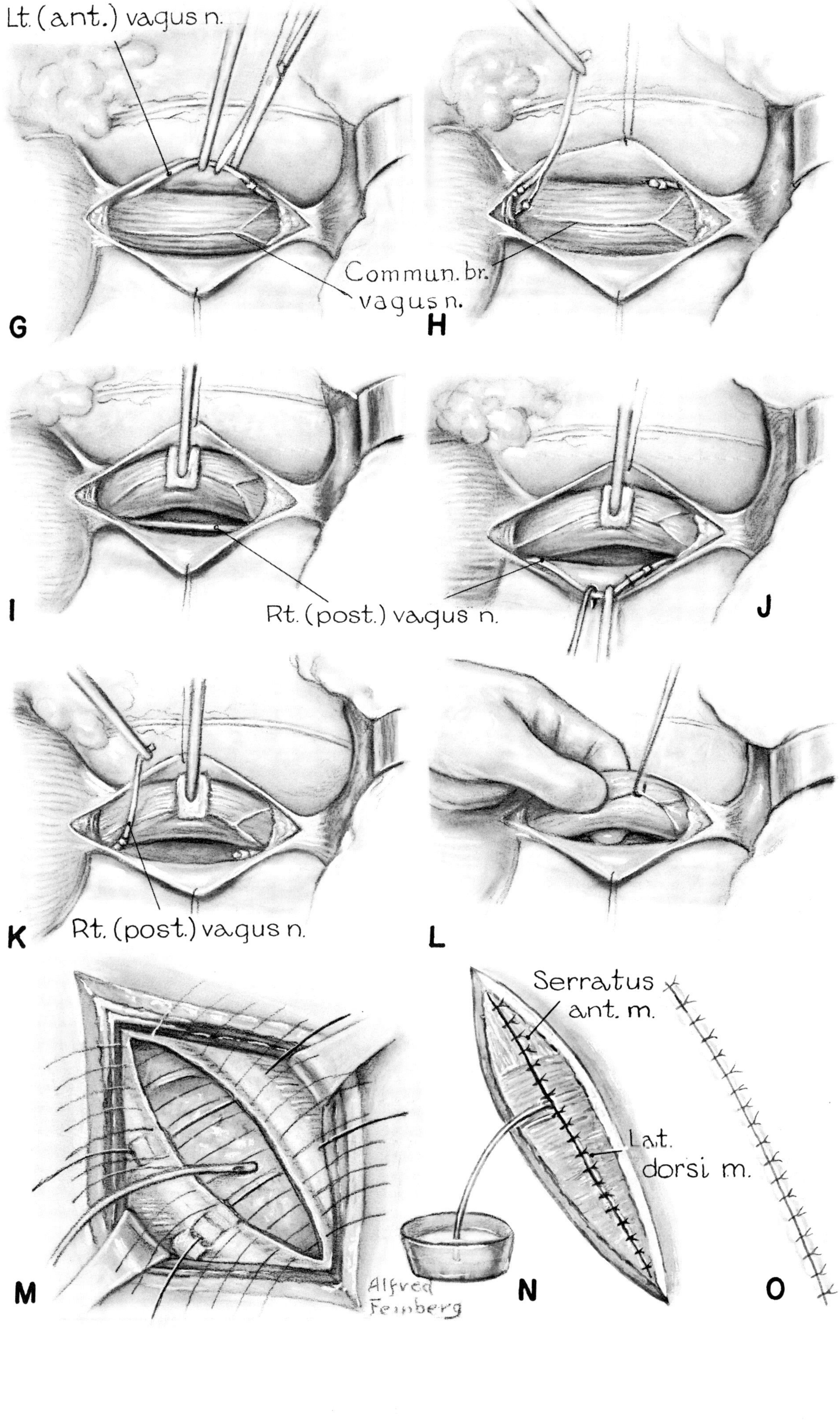
Lt. (ant.) vagus n.
Commun. br. vagus n.
G
H
Rt. (post.) vagus n.
I
J
Rt. (post.) vagus n.
K
L
Serratus ant. m.
Lat. dorsi m.
M
N
O
Alfred Feinberg

REFERENCES

Thoracic Incisions

Carter, N. B. The combined thoraco-abdominal approach with particular reference to its employment in splenectomy, Surg., Gynec. & Obst., 84:1019, 1947.

Chamberlain, J. M., and Finnerty, J. J. Modern techniques in thoracic surgery, S. Clin. North America, 29:557, 1949.

Crafoord, C. On the technique of pneumonectomy in man, Acta. Chir. Scandinav., Supp. 54, 81:1, 1938.

Hart, R. H. Thoracoabdominal incisions; a review, Surgery, 34:733, 1953.

Heaney, J. P., and Humphreys, G. H., II. The right thoraco-abdominal approach, Ann. Surg., 128:948, 1948.

Humphreys, G. H., II. An approach to resection of the esophagus and gastric cardia, Ann. Surg., 124:288, 1946.

Johnson, J., and Kirby, C. K. Surgery of the Chest; A Handbook of Operative Surgery, Chicago, The Year Book Publishers, Inc., 1952.

Overholt, R. H., and Langer, L. The Technic of Pulmonary Resection, Springfield, Illinois, Charles C Thomas, 1949.

Rienhoff, W. F., Jr. Present status of the surgical treatment of carcinoma of the lung, Ann. Surg., 125:541, 1947.

——— Pneumonectomy: a preliminary report of the operative technique in two successful cases, Bull. Johns Hopkins Hosp., 43:300, 1933.

Sweet, R. H. Thoracic Surgery, Philadelphia, W. B. Saunders Co., 1950.

Scalenotomy

Adson, A. W., and Coffey, J. R. Cervical rib; a method of anterior approach for the relief of symptoms by division of the scalenus anticus, Ann. Surg., 85:839, 1927.

——— Surgical treatment for symptoms produced by cervical ribs and the scalenus anticus muscle, Surg., Gynec. & Obst., 85:687, 1947.

Craig, W., and Knepper, P. A. Cervical rib and the scalenus anticus syndrome, Ann. Surg., 105:556, 1937.

Donald, J. M., and Morton, B. F. The scalenus anticus syndrome with and without cervical rib, Ann. Surg., 111:709, 1940.

McGowan, J. M. Cervical rib: the role of the clavicle in occlusion of the subclavian artery, Ann. Surg., 124:71, 1946.

Naffziger, H. C. The scalenus syndrome, Surg., Gynec. & Obst., 64:119, 1937.

——— and Grant, W. T. Neuritis of the brachial plexus mechanical in origin, the scalenus syndrome, Surg., Gynec. & Obst., 67:722, 1938.

Ochsner, A., Gage, M., and DeBakey, M. Scalenus anticus (Naffziger) syndrome, Am. J. Surg., 28:669, 1935.

Patterson, R. H. Cervical ribs and the scalenus muscle syndrome, Ann. Surg., 111:531, 1940.

Spurling, R. G., and Bradford, F. K. Scalenus neurocirculatory compression, Ann. Surg., 107: 708, 1938.

Telford, E. D., and Stofford, J. S. B. The vascular complications of cervical rib, Brit. J. Surg., 18:557, 1930–1931.

——— Cervical rib and hyperhidrosis, Brit. M. J., 2:96, 1942.

White, J. C., Poppel, M. H., and Adams, R. Congenital malformation of the first thoracic rib, Surg., Gynec. & Obst., 81:643, 1945.

Tracheostomy

Abbey, P. Laryngostomy in acute laryngeal obstruction, Lancet, 1:573, 1963.

Carter, B. N., and Giuseffi, J. The use of tracheotomy in the treatment of crushing injuries of the chest, Surg., Gynec. & Obst., 96:55, 1953.

Cawthorne, T. Tracheotomy, Surg., Gynec. & Obst., 68:782, 1939.

Colvin, E. M., and Morrison, W. M. The value of tracheotomy in acutely ill surgical patients, Surg., Gynec. & Obst., 96:338, 1953.

Conley, J. J. Diagnosis and treatment of encrustations in trachea, J.A.M.A., 154:829, 1954.

Davis, H. S., Kretchmer, H. E., and Bryce-Smith, R. Advantages and complications of tracheotomy, J.A.M.A., 153:1156, 1953.

Dickman, M. D., and Baronofsky, I. D. Tracheotomy—one solution for pulmonary problems in the critically ill patient, Journal Lancet, 71:43, 1951.

Jackson, C., and Jackson, C. L. Tracheotomy, Am. J. Surg., 46:519, 1939.

Kofman, S., Lepper, M. H., Jackson, G. G., and Dowling, H. F. Effect of proteolytic enzymes on physical and chemical characteristics of tracheobronchial secretion of patients with poliomyelitis, Am. J. M. Sc., 228:426, 1954.

Lahey, F. H., and Hoover, W. B. Tracheotomy after thyroidectomy, Ann. Surg., 133:65, 1951.

Lepper, M. H., Kofman, S., Blatt, N., Dowling, H. F., and Jackson, G. G. Effect of eight antibiotics used singly and in combination on tracheal flora following tracheotomy in poliomyelitis, Antibiotics & Chemother., 4:829, 1954.

TRACHEOSTOMY (cont.)

Lichtenstein, M. E. Acute injuries to the neck involving the food and air passages, Surg., Gynec. & Obst., 85:734, 1947.

Negus, V. E. Some disorders of the larynx. Hunterian Lecture, Lancet, 2:581 (Sept. 19), 1925.

Nelson, T. G. Tracheotomy: a clinical and experimental study: part I, The American Surgeon, Vol. 23, No. 7, July, 1957; part II, The American Surgeon, Vol. 23, No. 8, August, 1957; part III, The American Surgeon, Vol. 23, No. 9, September, 1957.

Plum, F., and Dunning, M. F. Technics for minimizing trauma to the tracheobronchial tree after tracheotomy, New England J. Med., 254:193, 1956.

Steigman, A. J., and Scott, C. H. Trypsin in poliomyelitis patients with tracheotomy, J.A.M.A., 150:1403, 1952.

Thompson, St. Clair. Tranquil tracheotomy by injecting cocaine within the windpipe, Brit. M. J., 2:460 (Oct. 11), 1919.

——— and Negus, V. E. Diseases of the Nose and Throat, New York, D. Appleton-Century Co., 1937, pp. 868–885.

Ulin, A. W., Olsen, A. K., and Martin, W. L. Factors determining mortality in patients with acute head injury, J.A.M.A., 157:496, 1955.

Waitaker, H. T., and Lee, S. S. Indications for tracheotomy, Ann. Surg., 145:974, 1957.

Waldapfel, R. The opening of the anterior tracheal wall in tracheotomy, Surg., Gynec. & Obst., 71:191, 1940.

Watts, J. McK. Tracheotomy in modern practice, Brit. J. Surg., 50:954, 1963.

Wilhelm, D. L. Regeneration of tracheal epithelium, J. Path. & Bact., 65:543, 1953.

Williams, M. H. Multiple rib fractures: an indication for tracheotomy, Surgery, 30:664, 1951.

PULMONARY LOBECTOMY AND PNEUMONECTOMY

Archibald, E. Technic of total unilateral pneumonectomy, Ann. Surg., 100:796, 1934.

Alexander, J. Observations on total pulmonary lobectomy and pneumonectomy, Ann. Surg., 101:393, 1935.

Allison, P. R. Intrapericardial approach to lung root in treatment of bronchial carcinoma by dissection pneumonectomy, J. Thoracic Surg., 15:99, 1946.

Björk, V. O. Lobectomy for pulmonary tuberculosis; an analysis of 301 cases, J. Thoracic Surg., 33:754, 1957.

——— Partial resection of the only remaining lung with the aid of respirator treatment, J. Thoracic & Cardiovasc. Surg., 39:179, 1960.

Blades, B., and Kent, E. M. Individual ligation technique for lower lobectomy, J. Thoracic Surg., 10:84, 1940.

——— and Kent, E. M. The surgical anatomy of the pulmonary lobes, J. Thoracic Surg., 12:18, 1942–43.

——— Conservation of lung tissue by partial lobectomy, Ann. Surg., 118:353, 1943.

Boyd, D. P., Smedal, M. I., Kirtland, H. B., Jr., Kelley, G. E., and Trump, J. G. Carcinoma of the lung: a report of 403 cases, J. Thoracic Surg., 28:392, 1954.

——— Adenoma of the bronchus, S. Clin. North America, 41:747, 1961.

Boyden, E. A. The interhilar and related segmental anatomy of the lung, Surgery, 18:706, 1945.

Brock, R., and Whytehead, L. L. Radical pneumonectomy for bronchial carcinoma, Brit. J. Surg., 43:8, 1955.

Brunn, H. Surgical principles underlying one-stage lobectomy, Arch. Surg., 18:490, 1929.

——— and Goldman, A. Bronchial adenoma, Am. J. Surg., 54:179, 1941.

Burford, T. H., Center, S., Ferguson, T. B., and Spjut, H. J. Results in the treatment of bronchogenic carcinoma: an analysis of 1,008 cases, J. Thoracic Surg., 36:316, 1958.

Chamberlain, J. M., and Ryan, T. C. Segmental resection in pulmonary diseases, J. Thoracic Surg., 19:199, 1950.

——— and Klopstock, R. Segmental resection for pulmonary tuberculosis, S. Clin. North America, 36:913, 1956.

Christiansen, K. H., and Smith, D. E. Bronchogenic carcinoma: A sixteen-year study, J. Thoracic & Cardiovasc. Surg., 43:267, 1962.

Churchill, E. D. Lobectomy and pneumonectomy in bronchiectasis and cystic disease, J. Thoracic Surg., 6:286, 1937.

——— and Belsey, R. Segmental pneumonectomy in bronchiectasis, Ann. Surg., 109:481, 1939.

——— Sweet, R. H., Scannell, J. G., and Wilkins, E. W. Further studies in the surgical management of carcinoma of the lung, J. Thoracic Surg., 36:301, 1958.

Clagett, O. T., and Brindley, G. V., Jr. Bronchogenic carcinoma, S. Clin. North America, 24:839, 1944.

Collier, F. C., Blakemore, W. S., Kyle, R. H., Enterline, H. T., Kirby, C. K., and Johnson, J. Carcinoma of the lung: Factors which influence five-year survival with special reference to blood vessel invasion, Ann. Surg., 146:417, 1957.

Crafoord, C. On technique of pneumonectomy in man, Acta. chir. Scandinav. (supp. 54) 81:1, 1938.

Davis, E. W., Peabody, J. W., Jr., and Katz, S. The solitary pulmonary nodule; a ten-year study based on 215 cases, J. Thoracic Surg., 32:728, 1956.

Gebauer, P. W. Bronchial resection and anastomosis, J. Thoracic Surg., 26:241, 1953.

Gibbons, J. H., Templeton, J. Y., and Nealon, T. F. Factors which influence the long term survival of patients with cancer of the lung, Ann. Surg., 145:637, 1957.

Ginsberg, R. L., Cooley, J. C., Olsen, A. M., Kirklin, J. W., and Clagett, O. T. Prognosis of bronchiectasis after surgical resection, Surg., Gynec. & Obst., 101:99, 1955.

Graham, E. A., and Singer, J. F. Successful re-

PULMONARY LOBECTOMY AND PNEUMONECTOMY (cont.)

moval of an entire lung for carcinoma of the bronchus, J.A.M.A., 101:1371, 1933.

——— Burford, T. H., and Mayer, J. H. Middle lobe syndrome, Med. 4:29, 1948.

Gronquist, Y. K., Clagett, O. T., and McDonald, J. R. Involvement of the thoracic wall in bronchogenic carcinoma; study of 16 cases in which pneumonectomy or lobectomy and simultaneous resection of the thoracic wall were done, J. Thoracic Surg., 33:487, 1957.

Halasz, N. A., Lindskog, G. E., and Liebow, A. A. Esophagobronchial fistula and bronchopulmonary sequestration. Report of a case and review of the literature, Ann. Surg., 155:215, 1962.

Heuer, G. J. Development of lobectomy and pneumonectomy in man, J. Thoracic Surg., 3:560, 1934.

Hood, R. T., Jr., McBurney, R. P., and Clagett, O. T. Metastatic malignant lesions of lungs treated by pulmonary resection; report of 43 cases, J. Thoracic Surg., 30:81, 1955.

Jackson, C. L., and Huber, J. F. Correlated applied anatomy of the bronchial tree and lungs with a system of nomenclature, Dis. Chest, 9:1, 1943.

Johnson, J., Kirby, C. K., and Blakemore, W. S. Should we insist on "Radical Pneumonectomy" as a routine procedure in the treatment of carcinoma of the lung? J. Thoracic Surg., 36:309, 1958.

Kent, E. M., and Blades, B. Anatomic approach to pulmonary resection, Ann. Surg., 116:782, 1942.

Kirklin, J. W., McDonald, J. R., Clagett, O. T., Moersch, H. J., and Gage, R. R. Bronchogenic carcinoma: cell type and other factors relating to prognosis, Surg., Gynec. & Obst., 100:429, 1955.

Koletsky, S. Primary carcinoma of the lung: a clinical and pathologic study of 100 cases, Arch. Int. Med., 62:636, 1938.

Lindskog, G. E. Bronchiogenic carcinoma, Ann. Surg., 124:667, 1946.

——— and Hubbell, D. S. Analysis of 215 cases of bronchiectasis, Surg., Gynec. & Obst., 100: 643, 1955.

Longacre, J. J. Experimental total pneumonectomy, J. Thoracic Surg., 4:587, 1935.

Maier, H. C., and Grace, E. J. Putrid empyema, Surg., Gynec. & Obst., 74:69, 1942.

Mason, G. A. Extirpation of lung (Hunterian Lecture Abridged), Lancet, 1:1047, 1936.

Meyer, W. Pneumonectomy with the aid of differential air pressure: an experimental study, J.A.M.A., 53:1978, 1909.

Milloy, F. J., Wragg, L. E., and Anson, B. J. The pulmonary arterial supply to the right upper lobe of the lung based upon a study of 300 laboratory and surgical specimens, Surg., Gynec. & Obst., 116:34, 1963.

Miscall, L., and Cornell, C. M. Surgical anatomy of the bronchi and vessels, J. Thoracic Surg., 12:526, 1942–43.

Murphy, J. B. Surgery of the lung, J.A.M.A., 31: 34, 1898.

Nelson, H. P. Postural drainage of lungs, Brit. M. J., 2:251, 1934.

Neuhof, H., and Touroff, A. S. W. Acute putrid abscess of the lung; principles of operative treatment, Surg., Gynec. & Obst., 63:353, 1936.

Nicholson, M. J., and Crehan, J. P. Anesthesia for thoracic surgery, S. Clin. North America, 41: 591, 1961.

Ochsner, A., and DeBakey, M. Surgical considerations of primary carcinoma of the lung: review of literature and report of 19 cases, Surgery, 8: 992, 1940.

——— Dixon, J. L., and DeBakey, M. Primary bronchiogenic carcinoma: An analysis of 190 cases, 58 of which were successfully treated by pneumonectomy: a review of literature, Clinics, 3:1187, 1945.

——— DeBakey, M. E., and Dixon, L. Primary pulmonary malignancy treated by resection, Ann. Surg., 125:522, 1947.

——— Clemmens, E. F., and Mitchell, W. T., Jr. Treatment of metastatic pulmonary malignant lesions, Journal-Lancet, 83:16, 1963.

Overholt, R. H. Surgical treatment of carcinoma of lung: technique of lobectomy and pneumonectomy, Surg., Gynec. & Obst., 64:209, 1937.

——— and Langer, L. A new technique for pulmonary segmental resection: its application in the treatment of bronchiectasis, Surg., Gynec. & Obst., 84:257, 1947.

——— Woods, F. M., and Ramsay, B. H. Segmental pulmonary resection. Details of technique and results, J. Thoracic Surg., 19:207, 1950.

——— and Bougas, J. A. Fifty-one cases of lung cancer with five-year survival, J.A.M.A., 161: 961, 1956.

——— and Bougas, J. A. Common factors in lung cancer survivors, J. Thoracic Surg., 32:508, 1956.

Pancoast, H. K. Superior pulmonary sulcus tumor, J.A.M.A., 99:1391, 1932.

Paulson, D. L. Survival rates following resection for bronchogenic carcinoma, Ann. Surg., 146: 997, 1957.

——— Shaw, R. R., Kee, J. L., Mallams, J. T., and Collier, R. E. Combined preoperative irradiation and resection for bronchogenic carcinoma, J. Thoracic & Cardiovasc. Surg., 44:281, 1962.

Pellett, J. R., and Gale, J. W. The solitary pulmonary lesion, Arch. Surg., 83:81, 1961.

Reinhoff, W. F., Jr. Pneumonectomy: a preliminary report of the operative technique in two successful cases, Bull. Johns Hopkins Hosp., 53:390, 1933.

——— Present status of surgical treatment of carcinoma of lung, Ann. Surg., 125:541–565, 1947.

——— A clinical analysis and follow-up study of

PULMONARY LOBECTOMY AND PNEUMONECTOMY (cont.)

five hundred and two cases of carcinoma of the lung, Dis. Chest., 17:33, 1950.

Robinson, J. L., Jones, J. C., and Meyer, B. W. Indications for lobectomy in the treatment of carcinoma of the lung, J. Thoracic Surg., 32: 500, 1956.

Robinson, S. Pneumonectomy: its possibilities, Ann. Surg., 55:513, 1912.

Sanger, P. W. Decortication in acute empyema thoracis, Surg., Gynec. & Obst., 82:71, 1946.

Sarot, I. A. Extrapleural pneumonectomy and pleurectomy in pulmonary tuberculosis, Thorax, 4:173, 1949.

Shaw, R. R., Paulson, D. L., and Kee, J. L. Treatment of the superior sulcus by irradiation followed by resection, Ann. Surg., 154:29, 1961.

Shimkin, B., Connelly, R. R., Marcus, C. S., and Cutler, S. J. Pneumonectomy and lobectomy in bronchogenic carcinoma: A comparison of end results of the Overholt and Ochsner Clinics, J. Thoracic & Cardiovasc. Surg., 44:503, 1962.

Siebens, A. A., Grant, A. R., Kent, D. C., Klopstock, R., and Cincotti, J. J. Pulmonary cystic disease; physiologic studies and results of resection, J. Thoracic Surg., 33:185, 1957.

Spear, H. C., Daughtry, D. C., Chesney, J. G., and Marks, A. The surgical management of large pulmonary blebs and bullae, Am. Rev. Resp. Dis., 84:186, 1961.

Strieder, J. W., and Lynch, J. P. Putrid empyema, New England J. Med., 234:1, 1946.

Touroff, A. S. W., Nabatoff, R. A., and Neyhoff, H. Acute putrid abscess of lung; late results of surgical treatment, J. Thoracic Surg., 20:266, 1950.

Wall, C. A., and Lucide, J. L. Intralobar bronchopulmonary sequestration, Surg., Gynec. & Obst., 103:701, 1956.

Watson, W. L. Radical surgery for lung cancer: evaluation of the operation of radical pneumonectomy and five years' end results, Cancer, 9:1167, 1956.

Webb, W. R. Clinical evaluation of a new mucolytic agent, acetylcysteine, J. Thoracic & Cardiovasc. Surg., 44:330, 1962.

Witten, D. N., Clagett, O. T., and Woolner, L. B. Intralobar bronchopulmonary sequestration involving the upper lobes, J. Thoracic & Cardiovasc. Surg., 43:523, 1962.

Young, G. A., Ellis, F. W., and Reingold, I. M. One thousand and eleven cases of bronchogenic carcinoma with results of treatment, Dis. Chest, 42:257, 1962.

THYMECTOMY

Andrus, W. DeWitt, and Foot, N. C. Report of a large thymic tumor successfully removed by operation, J. Thoracic Surg., 6:648, 1937.

Bayrd, E. D., and Bernatz, P. E. Benign thymona and agenesis of erythrocytes, J.A.M.A., 163: 723, 1957.

Blalock, A. Thymectomy in the treatment of myasthenia gravis; Report of twenty cases, J. Thoracic Surg., 13:316, 1944.

——— Mason, M. F., Morgan, H. J., and Riven, S. S. Myasthenia gravis and tumors of thymic region; report of a case in which the tumor was removed, Ann. Surg., 110:544, 1939.

Boyd, P. E. Weight of the thymus and component parts and the number of Hassell corpuscles in health and diseases, Am. J. Dis. Child., 51:313, 1936.

Castleman, B. Tumors of the thymus gland, Atlas of Tumor Pathology, Sect. V, Fasc. 19, 1955.

——— and Norris, E. H. Pathology of the thymus in myasthenia gravis, Medicine, 28:27, 1949.

Eaton, L. M., and Clagett, O. T. Thymectomy in treatment of myasthenia gravis, J.A.M.A., 142: 963, 1950.

——— Present status of thymectomy in treatment of myasthenia gravis, Am. J. Med., 19:703, 1955.

Effler, D. B., and McCormack, L. J. Thymic neoplasma, J. Thoracic Surg., 31:60, 1956.

Ehrenreich, T., and Allen, A. C. Myasthenia gravis following extirpation of an asymptomatic thymoma, Cancer, 11:173, 1958.

Genkins, G., Kreel, I., Jacobson, E., Osserman, K. S., and Baronofsky, I. D. Studies in myasthenia gravis: technical care of the thymectomy patient, Bull. New York Acad. Med., 36:826, 1956.

Hermann, C., Jr., Mulder, D. G., and Fonkalsrud, W. Thymectomy for myasthenia gravis, Ann. Surg., 158:85, 1963.

Humphreys, G. H. II, and Southworth, H. Aplastic anemia terminated by removal of a mediastinal tumor, Am. J. M. Sc., 210:501, 1945.

Jolly, F. Üeber Myasthenia Gravis Pseudoparalytica, Berl. Klin. Wchnschr, 32:1, 1895.

Josse, J. W., and Zacks, S. I. Thymoma and pancytopenia, New England J. Med., 259:113, 1958.

Kane, C. A. Effect of certain endocrine glands on myasthenia gravis, Am. J. Med., 19:729, 1955.

Keynes, G. The results of thymectomy in myasthenia gravis, Brit. M. J., 2:611, 1949.

——— Surgery of the thymus gland: second (and third) thoughts, Lancet, 1:1197, 1954.

Lange, M. J. The preparation for and the results of surgery in myasthenia gravis, Brit. J. Surg., 48:285, 1960.

Lattes, R. Thymoma and other tumors of the thymus; Analysis of 107 cases, Cancer, 15:1224, 1962.

MacLean, B., and Wilson, J. A. C. See-saw relationship between hyperthyroidism and myasthenia gravis, Lancet, 1:950, 1954.

Matras, A., and Priesel, A. Üeber einige gewächse des thymus, Bietr.z path. Anat., u.z. Allgpath., 80:270, 1928.

Musselman, M. M., and Porter, J. W. Thymectomy for myasthenia gravis, Am. J. Surg., 99: 404, 1960.

THYMECTOMY (cont.)

Osserman, K. E. Studies in myasthenia gravis, New York State J. Med., 56:2512, 1956.

——— Myasthenia Gravis. New York and London, Grune & Stratton, 1958.

Pennington, G. W., and Edwards, F. R. Respiratory crisis after thymectomy in patients with myasthenia gravis, Thorax, 15:26–65, 1960.

Root, G. T., Jernigan, S. K., Waller E., and Christensen, B. H. Problems of thyroidectomy in patients with hyperthyroidism associated myasthenia gravis, Arch. Surg., 85:324, 1962.

Ross, J. F., Finch, S. C., Street, R. B., Jr., and Strieder, J. W. The simultaneous occurrence of benign thymoma and refractory anemia, Blood, 9:915, 1954.

Rowland, L. P., Hoefer, P. F. A., Aranow, H., Jr., and Merritt, H. H. Fatalities in myasthenia gravis, Neurology, 6:307, 1956.

——— Aranow, H., Jr., and Hoefer, P. F. A. Myasthenia gravis appearing after removal of thymoma, Neurology, 7:584, 1957.

Schumacher, and Roth. Thymektomie bei einen Fall zon Morbus Basedowi mit myasthenie, Mitt. a. d. Grenzgeb. d. med. u. Chir., 25:746, 1913.

Schwab, R. S., and Leland, C. C. Sex and age in myasthenia gravis as critical factors in incidence and remission, J.A.M.A., 153:1270, 1953.

Seybold, W. D., McDonald, J. R., Clagett, O. T., and Good, C. A. Tumors of the thymus, J. Thoracic Surg., 20:195, 1950.

Simpson, J. A. Evaluation of thymectomy in myasthenia gravis, Blood, 81:112, 1958.

Soffer, L. J., Gabrilove, J. L., Laquer, H. P., Volterra, M., Jacobs, M. D., and Sussman, M. L. The effects of anterior pituitary adrenocorticotropic hormone (ACTH) in myasthenia gravis with tumour of the thymus, J. Mt. Sinai Hosp., 15:73, 1948.

Soutter, L., Sommers, S., Relman, A. S., and Emerson, C. P. Problems in the surgical management of thymic tumors, Ann. Surg., 146: 424, 1957.

——— and Emerson, C. P. Elective thymectomy in the treatment of aregenerative anemia associated with monocytic leukemia, Am. J. Med., 28:609, 1960.

Viets, H. R. "Medical Progress: Myasthenia gravis," New England J. Med., 251:97, 1954.

——— Problems of myasthenia gravis, Am. J. Med., 19:697, 1955.

Walker, M. B. Treatment of myasthenia gravis with prostigmin, Lancet, 1:1200, 1934.

Weigert, C. Pathologisch Anatomischer Beitrag zur Erb-schen Krankheit (myasthenia gravis), Neurol. Centralb., 20:597, 1901.

Wilson, A., and Wilson, H., Jr. The thymus and myasthenia gravis, Am. J. Med., 19:697, 1955.

ESOPHAGUS

Carter, B. N., Stevenson, J., and Abbott, O. A. Transpleural esophagogastrostomy for carcinoma of the esophagus and for carcinoma of the cardiac portion of the stomach; report of two cases, Surgery, 8:587, 1940.

Dodge, O. G. The surgical pathology of gastro-oesophageal carcinoma, Brit. J. Surg., 49:121, 1961.

Eggers, C. Treatment of carcinoma of the esophagus, Surg., Gynec. & Obst., 63:54, 1936.

Faure, J. L. Cancer de la portion thoracique de l'oesophage. Extirpation du neoplasme par la voie mediastinale posterieure directe combinée à une incision cervicale, Rev. de chir., 27:401, 1903.

Meyer, W. Cancer of the esophagus from the standpoint of intrathoracic surgery; report of four resections, Surg., Gynec. & Obst., 15:639, 1912.

Ochsner, A., and DeBakey, M. Surgical aspect of carcinoma of the esophagus: Review of the literature and report of four cases, J. Thoracic Surg., 10:401, 1941.

Santy, P., Ballivert, M., and Berard, M. Thoracic esophagectomy for cancer; report of two successful cases, J. Thoracic Surg., 12:397, 1943.

Tuffier, M. Sur la résection de l'oesophage thoracique, Presse med., 11:364, 1903.

Turner, G. G. Excision of the thoracic oesophagus for carcinoma, with construction of the extrathoracic gullet, Lancet, 2:1315, 1933.

CONGENITAL ATRESIA OF THE ESOPHAGUS

Bigger, I. A. The treatment of congenital atresia of the esophagus with tracheo-esophageal fistula, Ann. Surg., 129:572–587, 1949.

Byron, F. X. Congenital atresia of the esophagus with hypoplasia or agenesis of the lower segment, Surgery, 24:841–845, 1948.

Dale, W. A., and Sherman, C. D., Jr. Late reconstruction of congenital esophageal atresia by intrathoracic colon transplantation, J. Thoracic Surg., 29:344, 1955.

Garlock, J. H. Re-establishment of esophagogastric continuity following resection of esophagus for carcinoma of middle third, Surg., Gynec. & Obst., 78:23–28, 1944.

Gross, R. E., and Scott, H. W., Jr. Correction of esophageal atresia and tracheo-esophageal fistula by closure of fistula and oblique anastomosis of esophageal segments, Surg., Gynec. & Obst., 82:518, 1946.

——— Surgery in Infancy and Childhood, London, Philadelphia, W. B. Saunders Co., 1953.

Gruenwald, P. Mechanism of abdominal development in the embryo, II. Embryonic development of malformations, Arch. Path., 44:398, 495, 1947.

Haight, C., and Townsley, H. A. Congenital atresia of esophagus with tracheo-esophageal fistula, Surg., Gynec. & Obst., 76:672–688, 1943.

——— Congenital atresia of esophagus with tracheo-esophageal fistula, Ann. Surg., 120: 623–655, 1944.

Congenital Atresia of the Esophagus (cont.)

——— Editorial, Surg., Gynec. & Obst., 84:504–506, 1947.

——— In discussion of paper by Lyon and Johnson, J. Thoracic Surg., 17:162–169, 1948.

——— Congenital tracheo-esophageal atresia, J. Thoracic Surg., 17:600, 1948.

——— Some observations of esophageal fistulas of congenital origin, J. Thoracic Surg., 34:141, 1957.

Humphreys, G. H., Hogg, B. M., and Ferrer, J. Congenital atresia of the esophagus, J. Thoracic Surg., 32:332, 1956.

Koop, C. E., Kiesewetter, W. B., and Johnson, J. Treatment of atresia of the esophagus by the transpleural approach, Surg., Gynec. & Obst., 98:687, 1954.

Ladd, W. E. Cited by Haight, Surg., Gynec. & Obst., 84:504–506, 1947.

——— and Swenson, O. Esophageal atresia and tracheo-esophageal fistula, Ann. Surg., 125:23, 1947.

Lanman, T. H. Congenital atresia of the esophagus; 32 cases, Arch. Surg., 41:1060–1083, 1940.

Leven, N. L. Congenital atresia of the esophagus with tracheo-esophageal fistula, J. Thoracic Surg., 10:648–657, 1941.

——— Varco, R. L., Lannin, B. G., and Tongen, L. A. The surgical management of congenital atresia of the esophagus and tracheo-esophageal fistula, Ann. Surg., 136:701, 1952.

Lewis, I. Surgical treatment of carcinoma of esophagus with special reference to new operation for growths of middle third, Brit. J. Surg., 34:18–31, 1946.

Longmire, W. P., Jr. Antethoracic jejunal transplantation for congenital esophageal atresia with hypoplasia of the lower esophageal segment, Surg., Gynec. & Obst., 93:310, 1951.

Lyon, C. E., and Johnson, S. G. Congenital esophageal atresia and tracheo-esophageal fistula, J. Thoracic Surg., 17:162–169, 1948.

Madden, J. L. Congenital atresia of the esophagus treated by a one-stage primary esophagogastrostomy employing a right transpleural approach, J. Thoracic Surg., 21:460, 1951.

Plass, E. D. Congenital atresia of the esophagus with tracheo-esophageal fistula, Johns Hopkins Hosp. Rep., 18:259, 1919.

Potts, W. J. Congenital atresia of the esophagus with tracheo-esophageal fistula, J. Thoracic Surg., 20:671, 1950.

——— Congenital atresia of the esophagus; antethoracic placement of stomach followed by intrathoracic transplantation, J. Thoracic Surg., 20:681, 1950.

Rienhoff, W. F., Jr. Antethoracic transplantation of the stomach in the treatment of congenital atresia of the thoracic esophagus, Bull. Johns Hopkins Hosp., 82:496, 1948.

Samson, P. C. Cited by Shaw, J. Thoracic Surg., 9:213–219, 1939.

Sandblom, P. Treatment of congenital atresia of the esophagus from a technical point of view, Acta chir. scandinav., 97:25, 1948.

Shaw, R. R. Surgical correction of congenital atresia of the esophagus with tracheo-esophageal fistula, J. Thoracic Surg., 9:213–219, 1939.

——— Paulson, D. L., and Siebel, E. K. Congenital atresia of the esophagus with tracheo-esophageal fistula, Ann. Surg., 142:204, 1955.

Singleton, A. O., and Knight, M. D. Congenital atresia of the esophagus with tracheo-esophageal fistula, Ann. Surg., 119:556–572, 1944.

Sweet, R. H. A new method of restoring continuity of the alimentary canal in cases of congenital atresia of the esophagus with tracheo-esophageal fistula not treated by immediate primary anastomosis, Ann. Surg., 127:757–768, 1948.

Swenson, O. End-to-end anastomosis of the esophagus for esophageal atresia, Surgery, 22:324–334, 1947.

Vogt, E. C. Congenital esophageal atresia, Am. J. Roentgenol., 22:463, 1929.

Wall, C. A., and Lucido, J. L. Congenital atresia of the esophagus with tracheo-esophageal fistula and duodenal atresia, Ann. Surg., 145:580, 1957.

Resection of Pharyngoesophageal Diverticulum

Adams, H. D. Diverticula of the thoracic esophagus, J. Thoracic Surg., 17:639–645, 1948.

Barrett, N. R. Diverticula of the thoracic esophagus, Lancet, 1:1009, 1933.

Bell, C. Surgical Observations, London, Longman, Rees, Orme, Brown & Green, 1816, pp. 64–70.

Bergmann, E. Ueber den Oesophagusdivertikel und seine Behandlung, Arch. klin. Chir., 43:1–30, 1892.

Bevan, A. D. Pulsion diverticulum of esophagus—cure by the Sippy-Bevan operation, Surg. Clin. Chicago, 1:449–457, 1917.

Crile, G. W., and Dinsmore, R. Diverticula of esophagus, S. Clin. North America, 4:863, 1924.

Crile, G., Jr., and Robnett, A. H. Treatment of pharyngoesophageal diverticulum by inversion of the sac, Cleveland Clin. Quart., 18:42, 1951.

Gants, R. T., and Cohen, A. A thyroidectomy type (transverse) incision for excision of pharyngoesophageal diverticula, Surg., Gynec. & Obst., 104:373, 1957.

Goldmann, E. E. Die zweizeitige Operation von Pulsiondivertikeln der Speiseroehre, Beitr. klin. Chir., 61:741–749, 1909.

Harrington, S. W. Pulsion diverticulum of the hypopharynx at pharyngoesophageal junction: surgical treatment in 140 cases, Surgery, 18:66, 1945.

Hill, W. Pharyngeal pouch treated by diverticulopexy, Proc. R. Soc. M. Lond. (Sect. Laryng.), 11:60, 1917–1918.

Kausel, H. W., and Lindskog, G. E. Epiphrenic diverticulum of the esophagus. A review of its surgical treatment and report of a case, Dis. of Chest, 21:334, 1952.

RESECTION OF PHARYNGOESOPHAGEAL DIVERTICULUM (cont.)

King, B. T. New concepts of the etiology and treatment of diverticula of the esophagus, Surg., Gynec. & Obst., 85:93, 1947.

Kocher, T. Das Oesophagus divertikel und dessen Behandlung, Cor.-Bl. f. schweiz. Aerzte, 22: 233–244, 1892.

Lahey, F. H. Technique of the two stage operation for pulsion oesophageal diverticulum, Surg., Gynec. & Obst., 43:359–365, 1926.

——— Esophageal diverticula, Arch. Surg., 41: 1118–1140, 1940.

——— Pharyngo-esophageal diverticulum; its management and complications, Ann. Surg., 124:617–636, 1946.

——— and Warren, K. W. Esophageal diverticula, Surg., Gynec. & Obst., 98:1–28, 1954.

Ludlow, A. Obstructed deglutition, from a preternatural dilatation of, and bag formed in, the pharynx, Med. Obs. Soc. Physicians, London, 3:85 101, 1762–1767.

McNealy, R. W., and McCallister, J. W. The surgical management of esophageal diverticula, S. Clin. North America, 31:71, 1951.

Negus, V. E. Pharyngeal diverticula. Observations on their evolution and treatment, Brit. J. Surg., 38:129–146, 1950.

Nicoladoni, K. Behandlung der Oesophagusdivertikel, Wien. med. Wschr., 27:606–607, 1877.

Niehans, cited by Zesas, G. Beitrag zur chirurgischen Behandlung des Speisenroehren-Divertikels, Deutsche Ztschr. f. Chir., 82:577, 1906.

Shallow, T. A., and Clerf, L. H. One stage pharyngeal diverticulectomy, Surg., Gynec. & Obst., 86:317, 1948.

Sweet, R. H. Pulsion diverticulum of the pharyngoesophageal junction: technic of the one-stage operation. A preliminary report, Ann. Surg., 125:41, 1947.

——— Thoracic Surgery, 2nd ed., Philadelphia, W. B. Saunders, 1954.

von Bergmann, E. Uber das Oesophagusdivertikel und seine Behandlung, Arch. f. klin. Chir., 43:1, 1892.

Warren, K. W. Am. J. Surg., 93:205–217, 1957.

Zenker, F. A., and Zeimssen, H. Krankheiten des Oesophagus, in Handbuch der speciellen Pathologie und Therapie, Leipzig, F. C. Vogel, Vol. 7 (supp.), pp. 50–87.

ESOPHAGOCARDIOMYOTOMY

Adams, C. W. M., Brain, R. H. F., Ellis, F. G., Kauntze, R., and Trounce, J. R. Achalasia of the cardia, Guy's Hospital Rep., 110:191, 1961.

Alvarez, W. C. A simple explanation for cardiospasm and Hirschsprung's disease, Gastroenterology, 13:442, 1949.

Barrett, N. R., and Franklin, R. H. Concerning the unfavourable late results of certain operations performed in treatment of cardiospasm, Brit. J. Surg., 37:194, 1949.

Browse, N. L., and Carter, S. J. The late results of Heller's operation in the treatment of achalasia, Brit. J. Surg., 49:59, 1961–62.

Effler, D. B., and Rogers, J. W. Megaesophagus, Arch. Surg., 71:551, 1955.

Frobese, A. S., Stein, G. N., and Hawthorne, H. R. Hiatal hernia as a complication of the Heller operation, Surgery, 49:599, 1961.

Gröndahl, N. B. Cardioplastik ved Cardiospasmus, Nord. med. Ark., 49:236, 1916.

Heller, E. Extramuköse Cardioplastik beim chronischen Cardiospasmus mit Dilatation des Oesophagus, Mitt. a. d. Grenzgeb. d. Med. u. Chir., 27:141–149, 1913.

Hertz, A. F. Case of achalasia of the cardia (socalled cardiospasm), Proc. Roy. Soc. Med., 8: 22, 1914–1915.

——— Achalasia of the cardia. Quart. J. Med. (Oxford), 8:300, 1915.

Heyrovsky, H. Casuistik und Therapie der idiopathischen Dilatation der Speiseröhre; Oesophagogastroanastomose, Arch. f. klin. Chir., 100: 703, 1913.

Laimer, E. Beitrag zur Anatomie des Oesophagus, Wien, Med. Jahrbucher, Jahrg., 333–338, 1883.

Lerche, W. The Esophagus and Pharynx in Action, Springfield, Charles C Thomas, 1950.

Maingot, R. Abdominal Operations, New York, Appleton-Century-Crofts, Inc., 1948, pp. 343–347.

——— Surgical treatment of cardiospasm, Postgrad. Med., 5:351, 1949.

Ochsner, A., and De Bakey, M. Surgical considerations of achalasia, Arch. Surg., 41:1146, 1940.

Olsen, A. M., Ellis, F. H., and Creamer, B. Cardiospasm (achalasia of the cardia), Am. J. Surg., 93:299, 1957.

Petrovsky, B. V. Cardiospasm and its surgical correction, Ann. Surg., 155:60, 1962.

Puppel, I. D. The role of esophageal motility in the surgical treatment of mega-esophagus, J. Thoracic Surg., 19:371, 1950.

Rake, G. W. On the pathology of achalasia of the cardia, Guy's Hosp. Rep., 77:141, 1927.

Sweet, R. H. A consideration of certain benign lesions of the esophagus, Surgery, 40:447, 1956.

Vinson, P. P. Diagnosis and treatment of cardiospasm, Postgrad. Med., 3:13–18, 1948.

von Mikulicz, J., Jr. Zur Pathologie und Therapie des Cardiospasms, Deutsche med. Wchnschr., 30:17, 1904.

Wangensteen, O. H. A physiologic operation for mega-esophagus (dystonia, cardiospasm, achalasia), Ann. Surg., 134:301, 1951.

——— Technique of achieving an adequate extramucosal myotomy in mega-esophagus (achalasia, cardiospasm, dystonia), Surg., Gynec. & Obst., 105:339, 1957.

Wendel, W. Zur Chirurgie des Oesophagus, Arch. f. klin. Chir., 93:311, 1910.

Wolf, S., and Almy, T. Experimental observations on cardiospasm in man, Gastroenterology, 13: 401, 1949.

Wooler, G. H. Cardiospasm, Thorax, 3:53, 1948.

Esophagectomy

Adams, H. A., Hare, H. F., Davis, W. T., Trump, J. C., and Granke, R. S. The treatment of carcinoma of the esophagus and cardia by resection and post-operative super voltage roentgen ray, Ann. Surg., 138:631, 1953.

Adams, W. E., and Phemister, D. B. Carcinoma of the lower thoracic esophagus: report of a successful resection and esophagogastrostomy, J. Thoracic Surg., 7:621, 1938.

Ariel, I. M. Left cervical, right thoracic approach for resecting carcinoma of the upper esophagus, J. Thoracic Surg., 32:103, 1956.

Berman, E. F. The experimental replacement of portions of the esophagus by a plastic tube, Ann. Surg., 135:337, 1952.

Brewer, L. A., III. One stage resection of carcinoma of the cervical esophagus with subpharyngeal esophagogastrostomy, Ann. Surg., 130:9, 1949.

Chauncey, L. R. Results of surgical treatment of carcinoma of the esophagus and gastric cardia. Follow up study, Arch. Surg., 68:872, 1954.

Conerly, D. B., Jr., Carlson, R. I., and Scott, H. W., Jr. The combined anterior surgical approach for carcinoma of the upper thoracic esophagus, Surg., Gynec. & Obst., 98:84, 1954.

Cooper, D. R., and Buxton, R. W. Gastrostomy: a statistical review of one hundred ninety-nine cases, Surgery, 23:821, 1948.

DeBakey, M. E., and Cooley, D. A. Palliative resection for carcinoma of the esophagus. Combined right thoracic, abdominal and cervical approach, Arch. Surg., 66:781, 1953.

Eggers, C. Treatment of carcinoma of the esophagus, Surg., Gynec., & Obst., 63:54, 1936.

Garlock, J. H. The surgical treatment of carcinoma of the thoracic esophagus: with a report of three successful cases, Surg., Gynec. & Obst., 66:534, 1938.

——— The surgical treatment of carcinoma of the esophagus, Surg., Gynec. & Obst., 70:556, 1940.

——— Re-establishment of esophagogastric continuity following resection of esophagus for carcinoma of middle third, Surg., Gynec. & Obst., 78:23, 1944.

——— Resection of thoracic esophagus for carcinoma located above arch of aorta: cervical esophagogastrostomy, Surgery, 24:1, 1948.

——— and Klein, S. H. The surgical treatment of carcinoma of the oesophagus and cardia, Ann. Surg., 139:19, 1954.

Harrison, A. W., and Pickett, W. H. One stage multiple approach operation for cancer of the upper and mid-thoracic esophagus, Surgery, 28: 771, 1950.

Hollingsworth, R. K. Further discussion of the right thoracic approach to esophageal lesions, J. Thoracic Surg., 24:201, 1952.

Humphreys, G. H., and Moore, R. L. Carcinoma involving the oesophagus, S. Clin. North America, 33:389, 1953.

Kent, E. M., and Harbison, S. P. The combined abdominal and right thoracic approach to lesions of the middle and upper third of the esophagus, J. Thoracic Surg., 19:559, 1950.

Kirklin, J. W., and Clagett, O. T. Some technical aspects of esophagogastrectomy for carcinoma of the lower part of the esophagus and cardiac end of the stomach, S. Clin. North America, 31: 959, 1951.

Krebs, C., Nielson, H., and Anderson, P. E. Rotation treatment of cancer of the esophagus, Acta radiol., 32:204, 1949.

Lawrence, G. H. Right thoracoabdominal approach to esophageal resection, Surg., Gynec. & Obst., 105:641, 1957.

Lewis, I. The surgical treatment of carcinoma of the esophagus, with special reference to growths of the middle third, Brit. J. Surg., 34:18, 1946.

MacManus, J. E. Combined left abdominal and right thoracic approach to resection of esophageal neoplasms, Surgery, 24:9, 1948.

Mustard, R. A., and Ibberson, O. Carcinoma of the esophagus, Ann. Surg., 144:927, 1956.

Nissen, R. Cervical esophagogastrostomy following resection of supra-aortic carcinoma of the esophagus, Ann. Surg., 130:21, 1949.

Ohsawa, T. The surgery of the esophagus, Arch. f. Jap. Chir., 10:605, 1933.

O'Shaughnessy, L., and Raven, R. W. Surgical exposure of the esophagus, Brit. J. Surg., 22:365, 1934.

Pomeranz, A. A., and Garlock, J. H. Primary melanocarcinoma of the esophagus, Ann. Surg., 142:296, 1955.

Ravitch, M. M., Bahnson, H. T., and Johns, T. N. P. Carcinoma of the oesophagus, J. Thoracic Surg., 24:256, 1952.

Robertson, R., and Sargeant, T. R. Reconstruction of oesophagus, J. Thoracic Surg., 20:689, 1950.

Scanlon, E. F., Morton, D. R., Walker, J. M., and Watson, W. L. The case against segmental resection for oesophageal carcinoma, Surg., Gynec. & Obst., 101:290, 1955.

Shedd, D. P., Crowley, L. G., and Lindskog, G. E. A ten year study of carcinoma of the esophagus, Surg., Gynec. & Obst., 101:55, 1955.

Strieder, J. W. Surgical management of carcinoma of the lower two-thirds of the esophagus and cardiac end of the stomach, J. Thoracic Surg., 17:143, 1948.

Sweet, R. H. Carcinoma of the superior mediastinal segment of the esophagus: a technique for resection with restoration of continuity of the alimentary canal, Surgery, 24:929, 1948.

——— The results of radical surgical extirpation in the treatment of carcinoma of the esophagus and cardia, Surg., Gynec. & Obst., 94:46, 1952.

Torek, F. The first successful case of resection of the thoracic portion of the esophagus for carcinoma, Surg., Gynec. & Obst., 16:614, 1913.

Turner, G. G. Carcinoma of the esophagus: the question of its treatment by surgery, Lancet, 230:67–72, 130–134, 1936.

Watson, W. L., and Pool, J. L. Cancer of the cervical esophagus, Surgery, 23:893, 1948.

——— Luomanen, R., and Goodner, J. T. Cancer of the upper thoracic esophagus, combined

Esophagectomy (cont.)

right thoracoabdominal approach, Surg., Gynec. & Obst., 98:45, 1955.

Wookey, H. Surgical treatment of carcinoma of pharynx and upper esophagus, Surg., Gynec. & Obst., 75:499, 1942.

——— The surgical treatment of carcinoma of the hypopharynx and the esophagus, Brit. J. Surg., 35:249, 1948.

Wylie, R. H., and Frazell, E. L. Cervical esophagogastric anastomosis following subtotal resection of the esophagus for carcinoma, Ann. Surg., 130:1, 1949.

Esophagocoloplasty

Björk, V. O., and Norberg, B. Absorption studies after the insertion of colon as a substitute for both the stomach and the esophagus, Ann. Surg., 152:1049, 1960.

Chrysospathis, P., Golematis B., and Campanis, N. One- or two-stage cervical esophagocolostomy or ileostomy for replacement of the esophagus, Surgery, 49:429, 1961.

Dale, W. A., and Sherman, C. D., Jr. Late reconstruction of congenital esophageal atresia by intrathoracic colon transplantation, J. Thoracic Surg., 29:344, 1955.

Goligher, J. D., and Robin, I. G. Use of left colon for reconstruction of pharynx and oesophagus after pharyngectomy, Brit. J. Surg., 42:1, 1954.

Gregorie, H. B., and Othersen, H. B., Jr. Total esophagectomy and esophagocoloplasty, Surg., Gynec. & Obst., 115:153, 1962.

Hacker, V. von. Ueber oesophagoplastik im allgemeinen und über den ersatz der speiserohre durch antethorakale haut-dickdarm-schlauchbildung im besonderen, Arch. f. klin. Chir., 105: 973, 1914.

Jianu, A. Gastrostomic und oesophagoplastik, Deutsche Ztschr. f. Chir., 118:383, 1912.

Kelling, G. Oesophagoplastik mit hilfe des querkolon, Zentralbl. f. Chir., 38:1209, 1911.

Kergin, F. G. Esophageal obstruction due to paraffinoma of mediastinum, Ann. Surg., 137:91, 1953.

Kummell, H., Jr. Ueber intrathorakale oesophagusplastik, Beitr. z. klin. Chir., 126:264, 1922.

Lafargue, P., Dufour, R., Cabanie, H., and Chavannaz, J. Iléo-colo-oesophagoplastie, Mém. Acad. chir., 77:420, 1951.

Lortat-Jacob, J. Oesophagoplastie isoperistaltique transthoraco-mediastinale avec le côlon transverse, Mém. Acad. chir., 77:586, 1951.

Le Roux, B. T. An analysis of 700 cases of carcinoma of the hypopharynx, oesophagus, and proximal stomach, Thorax, London, 16:226, 1961.

McBurney, R. P. Total esophagoplasty by utilizing the colon, Southern Med. J., 53:513, 1960.

Mahoney, E. B., and Sherman, C. D., Jr. Total esophagoplasty using intrathoracic right colon, Surgery, 35:937, 1954.

Maroney, J. Colonic replacement of the stomach, Lancet, 260:993, 1951.

Montenegro, E. B., and Cutait, D. E. Construction of a new esophagus by means of the transverse colon and its application for caustic atresia, carcinoma and varices of the esophagus, Surgery, 44:785, 1958.

Nardi, G. L., and Glotzer, D. J. Anastomotic ulcer of the colon following colonic replacement of the esophagus, Ann. Surg., 152:10, 1960.

Neville, W. E., and Clowes, G. H. A., Jr. Reconstruction of the esophagus with segments of the colon, J. Thoracic Surg., 35:2, 1958.

Orsoni, P., and Toupet, A. The use of the descending colon and left part of the transverse colon for préthoracic esophagoplasty, Presse méd., 58: 804, 1950.

Pories, W. J., Gerle, R. D., Sherman, C. D., and Hinshaw, J. R. The danger of esophageal replacement with antiperistaltic loops of small bowel, Ann. Surg., 156:68, 1962.

Rogers, F. A. A typical congenital atresia of the esophagus; Treatment of this anomaly by means of retrosternal colon transplant, Arch. Surg., 82:515, 1961.

Roux, C. L'oesophago-jejuno-gastrostomose nouvelle opération pour rétrécissement infranchissable de l'oesophage, Semaine méd., 27:37, 1907.

Rudler, J. C., and Monod-Broca, P. Un cas d'oesophagoplastie palliative retro-stenale avec l'iléocôlon droit, Mém. Acad. chir., 77:747, 1951.

Vulliet, H. De l'oesophagoplastik et des diverses modifications, Semaine méd., 31:529, 1911.

Watson, W. L., and Clifton, E. E. Total esophagoplasty using right colon, Cancer, 10:488, 1957.

Webb, B., and Woolsey, D. S. Lye burns of the esophagus, J.A.M.A., 141:384, 1949.

Wullstein, L. Ueber antethorakale oesophago-jejunostomie und operationem nach gleichen Prinzip, Deutsche med., Wchnschr., 30:734, 1904.

Esophageal Hiatus Hernia

Adler, R. H. Hiatal hernia and esophagitis, Surg., Gynec. & Obst., 116:1, 1963.

Allison, P. R. Reflux esophagitis, sliding hiatal hernia, and the anatomy of repair, Surg., Gynec. & Obst., 92:419, 1951.

——— Observations on conservative approach to nonmalignant lesions at the cardia, J. Thoracic Surg., 32:150, 1956.

Barrett, N. R. Benign structure in the lower esophagus, J. Thoracic & Cardiovasc. Surg., 43:703, 1962.

Bowden, L., and Miller, C. J. Massive hematemesis from hiatus hernia, Arch. Surg., 63:143, 1951.

Brick, I. B. Incidence of hiatus hernia and associated lesions diagnosed by roentgen rays, Arch. Surg., 58:419, 1949.

Carey, J. M., and Hollinshead, W. H. An ana-

ESOPHAGEAL HIATUS HERNIA (cont.)

tomic study of the esophageal hiatus, Surg., Gynec. & Obst., 100:196, 1955.

Dunhill, T. Diaphragmatic hernia, Brit. J. Surg., 22:475, 1935.

Effler, D. B., and Ballinger, C. S. Complications and surgical treatment of hiatus hernia and short esophagus, J. Thoracic Surg., 22:235, 1951.

——— and Groves, L. K. Short esophagus, Arch. Surg., 75:639, 1957.

Harrington, S. W. Diaphragmatic hernia in children, Ann. Surg., 115:705, 1942.

——— Surgical treatment of the more common types of diaphragmatic hernia; esophageal hiatus, traumatic, pleuroperitoneal hiatus, congenital absence and foramen of Morgagni. Report of 404 cases, Ann. Surg., 122:546, 1945.

——— Various types of diaphragmatic hernia treated surgically; report of 430 cases, Surg., Gynec. & Obst., 86:735, 1948.

——— Esophageal hiatal diaphragmatic hernia, Surg., Gynec. & Obst., 100:277, 1955.

Humphreys, G. H., II, Ferrer, J. M., Jr., and Wiedel, P. D. Esophageal hiatus hernia of the diaphragm. An analysis of surgical results, J. Thoracic Surg., 34:749, 1957.

Johnsrud, R. L. The repair of the phrenoesophageal ligament in surgical treatment of hiatal hernia, Surg., Gynec. & Obst., 103:708, 1956.

Kirklin, B. R. Roentgenologic diagnosis of diaphragmatic hernia, Postgrad. Med., 4:501, 1948.

Lam, C. R., and Kenny, L. G. The problem of the hiatus hernia of the diaphragm, J. Thoracic Surg., 27:1, 1954.

Lawlor, R. H., West, J. W., and Lawler, E. G. Treatment of diaphragmatic hernia in the newborn, Am. J. Dis. Child., 84:79, 1952.

Madden, J. L. Anatomic and technical considerations in the treatment of esophageal hiatal hernia, Surg., Gynec. & Obst., 102:187, 1956.

Merendino, K. A., Varco, R. L., and Wangensteen, O. H. Displacement of the esophagus into a new diaphragmatic orifice in the repair of paraesophageal and esophageal hiatus hernia, Ann. Surg., 129:185, 1949.

Miller, C. Carcinoma of thoracic esophagus and cardia: Review of 405 cases, Brit. J. Surg., 69: 507, 1962.

Morton, J. J. Herniation through the diaphragm, Surg., Gynec. & Obst., 68:257, 1939.

Neville, W. E., and Clowes, G. H. A., Jr. Surgical treatment of reflux esophagitis, Arch. Surg., 83: 534, 1961.

Olsen, A. M., and Harrington, S. W. Esophageal hiatal hernia of the short esophagus type: Etiologic and therapeutic considerations, J. Thoracic Surg., 17:189, 1948.

Plachta, A. Benign tumors of esophagus: Review of literature and report of 99 cases, Am. J. Gastroenterol, 38:639, 1962.

Pories, W. J., Gerle, R. D., Sherman, C. D., and Hinshaw, J. R. The danger of esophageal replacement with antiperistaltic loops of small bowel, Am. Surg., 1956:68, 1962.

Rives, J. D., and Baker, D. O. Anatomy of the attachments of the diaphragm. Their relation in the problems of the surgery of diaphragmatic hernia, Ann. Surg., 115:745, 1942.

Sweet, R. H. The repair of hiatus hernia of the diaphragm by the supradiaphragmatic approach. Technic and results, New England J. Med., 238:649, 1948.

——— Esophageal hiatus hernia of the diaphragm: The anatomical characteristics, technic of repair and results of treatment in 111 consecutive cases, Ann. Surg., 135:1, 1952.

——— Experience with 500 cases of hiatus hernia: a statistical survey, J. Thoracic & Cardiovas. Surg., 44:145, 1962.

Truesdale, P. E. Diaphragmatic hernia. Its varieties and surgical treatment of the hiatus type, Am. J. Surg., 32:204, 1936.

Wangensteen, O. H., and Leven, N. L. Gastric resection for esophagitis and stricture of acid-peptic origin, Surg., Gynec. & Obst., 88:560, 1949.

Young, D. Esophageal-hiatus hernia, Rev. Gastroenterol., 9:345, 1942.

EVENTRATION OF THE DIAPHRAGM

Arnheim, E. A. Congenital eventration of the diaphragm in infancy, Surgery, 35:809, 1954.

Beck, W. C. Etiologic significance of eventration of the diaphragm, Arch. Surg., 60:1154, 1950.

Butsch, W. L., and Leahy, L. J. A technique for the surgical treatment of congenital eventration of the diaphragm in infancy. Report of a case, J. Thoracic Surg., 20:968, 1950.

Chin, G. F. Surgery of eventration of the diaphragm, J. Thoracic Surg., 32:6, 1956.

Crastnopol, P. Surgical correction of eventration of diaphragm in patients with arthrogryposis, Arch. Surg., 70:114, 1955.

De Bord, R. A. Congenital eventration of diaphragm, J. Thoracic Surg., 31:731, 1956.

Laxdal, O. E. Congenital eventration of the diaphragm, New England J. Med., 250:401, 1954.

Neuman, H. W., Ellis, F. H., Jr., and Anderson, H. A. Eventration of the diaphragm, Proc. Staff Meet., Mayo Clin., 30:310, 1955.

Peck, G. A. Inversion of the stomach with eventration of the diaphragm, Am. J. Roentgenol., 67: 63, 1952.

Shellito, J. G., and Bartlett, W. C. Surgical correction of congenital eventration of the diaphragm, Am. Surgeon, 17:898, 1951.

RESECTION OF VAGUS NERVES

Beattie, A. D. Vagotomy and partial pylorectomy, Lancet, 1:525, 1950.

Coffey, R. J., and Lazaro, E. J. Vagotomy, hemi-

RESECTION OF VAGUS NERVES (cont.)

gastrectomy and gastroduodenostomy (Finney–Von Haberer) in the treatment of duodenal ulcer, Ann. Surg., 141:862, 1955.

Cooper, W. A. End results in the treatment of peptic ulcer by posterior gastroenterostomy, Surgery, 23:425, 1948.

Crile, G., Jr., Jones, T. E., and Davis, J. B. Surgical treatment of duodenal ulcer—comparison of results with and without vagotomy, Ann. Surg., 130:31, 1949.

Dragstedt, L. R., and Owens, F. M., Jr. Supra diaphragmatic section of the vagus nerves in the treatment of duodenal ulcer, Proc. Soc. Exper. Biol. & Med., 53:152, 1943.

——— Clarke, J. R., Harper, P. V., Jr., Woodward, E. R., and Tovee, E. B. Supra diaphragmatic section of the vagus nerves to the stomach in gastrojejunal ulcer, J. Thoracic Surg., 16:26, 1947.

——— Harper, P. V., Jr., Tovee, E. B., and Woodward, E. R. Section of the vagus nerves to the stomach in the treatment of peptic ulcer. Complications and end results after four years, Ann. Surg., 126:687, 1947.

——— Oberhelman, H. A., Jr., and Smith, C. A. Experimental hyperfunction of the gastric antrum with ulcer formation, Ann. Surg., 134: 332, 1951.

——— and Woodward, E. R. Appraisal of vagotomy for peptic ulcer after seven years, J.A.M.A., 145:11, 1951.

——— Oberhelman, H. A., Jr., and Woodward, E. R. Physiology of gastric secretion and its relation to the ulcer problem, J.A.M.A., 147:17, 1951.

——— Oberhelman, H. A., Jr., Evans, S. O., and Rigler, S. P. Antrum hyperfunction and gastric ulcer, Ann. Surg., 140:396, 1954.

——— Ragins, R., Dragstedt, L. R., II, and Evans, S. O., Jr. Stress and duodenal ulcer, Ann. Surg., 144:450, 1956.

Edkin, J. S. The chemical mechanism of gastric secretion, J. Physiol., 34:133, 1906.

——— and Tweedy, M. The natural channels of absorption evoking the chemical mechanism of gastric secretion, J. Physiol., 38:263, 1909.

Edwards, L. W., Herrington, J. L., Jr., Stephenson, S. E., Jr., Carlson, R. I., Phillips, R. J., Jr., Cote, W. R., Jr., and Scott, H. W., Jr. Duodenal ulcer: treatment by vagotomy and removal of gastric antrum, Ann. Surg., 145:738, 1957.

Farmer, D. A., Howe, C. W., Porell, W. S., and Smithwick, R. H. The effect of various surgical procedures upon the acidity of the gastric contents of ulcer patients, Ann. Surg., 134:319, 1951.

Grimson, K. S., Taylor, H. M., Trent, J. C., Wilson, D. A., and Hill, H. C. The effect of transthoracic vagotomy upon the functions of the stomach and upon the early clinical course of patients with peptic ulcer, South. M. J., 39:460, 1946.

——— Rowe, C. R., Jr., and Taylor, H. M. Results of vagotomy during seven years, Ann. Surg. 135:5, 1952.

Hartzell, J. B. The effect of section of the vagus nerves on gastric acidity, Am. J. Physiol., 91–92:161, 1929.

Hay, L. J., Varco, R. L., Code, C. F., and Wangensteen, O. H. The experimental production of gastric and duodenal ulcers in laboratory animals by the intramuscular injection of histamine in bees wax, Surg., Gynec. & Obst., 75: 170, 1942.

Hoerr, S. O., Brown, C. H., Ramsey, E. W., and Crile, G., Jr. Results of treatment of duodenal ulcer with vagus resection and gastroenterostomy, J.A.M.A., 149:16, 1952.

Hollander, F. The insulin test for the presence of intact nerve fibers after vagal operations for peptic ulcer, Gastroenterology, 7:607, 1946.

Klein, E. Left vagus section and partial gastrectomy for duodenal ulcer with hyperacidity, Ann. Surg., 90:65, 1929.

Latarjet, A. Note préliminaire sur l'innervation et l'énervation de l'estomac, Lyon méd., 130:166–167, 1921.

——— Résection des nerfs de l'estomac. Technique opératoire. Résultats Cliniques, Bull. Acad. de méd., Paris, 87:681, 1922.

MacKelvie, A. A. Vagal resection in treatment of duodenal ulcer, Brit. M. J., 1:321, 1957.

Mann, F. C., and Williamson, C. S. The experimental production of peptic ulcer, Ann. Surg., 77:409, 1923.

H. The technic and results of a dependent greater curvature gastroenterostomy, Ann. Surg., 134:844, 1951.

Moore, F. D., Chapman, W. P., Schulz, M. D., and Jones, C. M. Transdiaphragmatic resection of the vagus nerves for peptic ulcer, New England J. Med., 234:241, 1946.

——— Vagus resection for ulcer: an interim evaluation, I. Operative technique and hospital management, Arch. Surg., 55:164, 1947.

——— Vagus resection for ulcer: an interim evaluation, II. Clinical results, Ann. Surg., 126: 664, 1947.

Pavlov, I. P. The Work of the Digestive Glands, London, Charles Griffin and Co., Ltd., 1902.

Schiassi, B. The role of the pyloro-duodenal nerve supply in the surgery of duodenal ulcer, Ann. Surg., 81:939, 1925.

Walters, W., Neibling, H. A., Bradley, W. F., Small, J. T., and Wilson, J. W. A study of the results, both favorable and unfavorable, of section of the vagus nerves in the treatment of peptic ulcer, Ann. Surg., 126:679, 1947.

——— and Mobley, J. E. Five-to-ten-year follow up of 162 cases of duodenal ulcer treated by vagotomy with and without associated gastric operations, Ann. Surg., 145:753, 1957.

Wangensteen, O. H., Varco, R. L., Hay, L., Walpole, S., and Trach, B. Gastric acidity before and after operative procedures with special reference to role of pylorus and antrum; prelimi-

Resection of Vagus Nerves (cont.)

nary report of clinical and experimental study, Ann. Surg., 112:626, 1940.

Woodward, E. R., Bigelow, R. R. and Dragstedt, L. R. Effect of resection of antrum of stomach on gastric secretion in Pavlov pouch dogs, Am. J. Physiol., 162:99, 1954.

Patent Ductus Arteriosus

Blalock, A. Operative closure of the patent ductus arteriosus, Surg., Gynec. & Obst., 82:113, 1956.

Conklin, W. S., and Watkins, E., Jr. Use of the Potts-Smith-Gibson clamp for division of patent ductus arteriosus, J. Thoracic Surg., 19:361, 1950.

Donovan, M. S., Neuhauser, E. B. D., and Sosman, M. C. The roentgen signs of patent ductus arteriosus. A summary of 50 surgically verified cases, Am. J. Roentgenol., 50:293, 1943.

Eppinger, E. C., Burwell, C. S., and Gross, R. E. The effects of patent ductus arteriosus on the circulation, J. Clin. Investigation, 20:127, 1941.

Glenn, W. W. L., Bloomer, W. C., and Spear, H. C. Operative closure of the patent ductus arteriosus. A report of 110 operations without mortality, Ann. Surg., 143:471, 1956.

Graybiel, A., Strieder, J. W., and Boyer, N. H. An attempt to obliterate the patent ductus arteriosus in a patient with subacute bacterial endocarditis, Am. Heart J., 15:621, 1938.

Gross, R. E., and Hubbard, J. P. Surgical ligation of a patent ductus arteriosus; report of first successful case, J.A.M.A., 112:729 (Feb. 25), 1939.

——— Surgical management of patent ductus arteriosus, with summary of 4 surgically treated cases, Ann. Surg., 110:321, 1939.

——— Complete surgical division of the patent ductus arteriosus, Surg., Gynec. & Obst., 78:36, 1944.

——— Complete division for the patent ductus arteriosus, J. Thoracic Surg., 16:314, 1947.

——— and Longino, L. A. The patent ductus arteriosus. Observation from 412 surgically treated cases, Circulation, 3:125, 1951.

Jones, J. C. Complications of surgery of patent ductus arteriosus, J. Thoracic Surg., 16:305, 1947.

Kattus, A., Jr., and Muller, W. H. Patent ductus arteriosus with reversal of blood flow: report of a successful surgical closure and physiologic studies, Ann. Surg., 138:870, 1953.

Kennedy, J. A. A new concept of the cause of patency of the ductus arteriosus, Am. J. M. Sc., 204:570, 1952.

Keys, A., and Shapiro, M. J. Patency of the ductus arteriosus in adults, Am. Heart J., 25:158, 1943.

Krovetz, L. J., and Warden, H. E. Patent ductus arteriosus: An analysis of 515 surgically proved cases, Dis. Chest., 42:46, 1962.

Munro, J. C. Surgery of the vascular system. I. Ligation of the ductus arteriosus, Ann. Surg., 46:335, 1907.

Potts, W. J., Gibson, S., Smith, S., and Riker, W. L. Diagnosis and surgical treatment of patent ductus arteriosus, Arch. Surg., 58:612, 1949.

Scott, H. W., Jr. Closure of the patent ductus by suture-ligation technique, Surg., Gynec. & Obst., 90:91, 1950.

Shapiro, M. J., and Johnson, E. Results of surgery in patent ductus arteriosus, Am. Heart J., 33: 725, 1947.

Shumacker, H. B., Jr., and Luric, P. R. Patent ductus arteriosus with pulmonary venous drainage, Circulation 6:6, 1952.

Sirak, H. D., and Humphrey, G. H. The atypical ductus: physiological and technical considerations in its surgical therapy, Surgery, 41:112, 1957.

Touroff, A. S. W., and Vesell, H. Subacute *Streptococcus viridans* endarteritis complicating patent ductus arteriosus; recovery following surgical treatment, J.A.M.A., 115:1270, 1940.

Wangensteen, O. H., Varco, R. L., and Baronofsky, I. D. The technique of surgical division of patent ductus arteriosus, Surg., Gynec. & Obst., 88:62, 1949.

Tetralogy of Fallot

Abbott, M. E. Atlas of Congenital Cardiac Disease, New York, American Heart Association, 1936.

Blalock, A., and Taussig, H. B. The surgical treatment of malformations of the heart in which there is pulmonary stenosis or pulmonary atresia, J.A.M.A., 128:189 (May 19) 1945.

——— Surgical procedures employed and anatomical variations encountered in the treatment of congenital pulmonic stenosis, Surg., Gynec. & Obst., 87:385, 1948.

Brock, R. C. Direct cardiac surgery in the treatment of congenital pulmonary stenosis, Ann. Surg., 136:63, 1952.

Eisenmenger, V. Die Angeborenen Defecte der Kammer-Scheidewand des Herzens, Ztschr. f. klin. Med., 32 (Supplement) 1–28, 1897.

Fallot, A. Contribution a l'anatomic pathologique de la maladie bleue (cyanose cardiaque), Marseille méd., 25:77–93, 138–158, 207–223, 270–296, 341–354, 403–420, 1888.

Glenn, W. W. L., and Patino, J. F. Circulatory by-pass of right heart. 1. Preliminary observations on direct delivery of vena caval blood into pulmonary artery circulation: azygos vein-pulmonary artery shunt, Yale J. Biol. & Med., 27:147, 1954.

Humphreys, G. H., II. Diagnosis and treatment of congenital cyanotic heart disease, Bull. New York Acad. Med., 23:283, 1947.

Josephs, H. W. Mechanism of reduction of red cells and hemoglobin following operation for tetralogy of Fallot, Bull. Johns Hopkins Hosp., 86:1, 1950.

Keith, A. The Hunterian lectures on malformations of the heart, Lancet, 2:359, 1909.

Tetralogy of Fallot (cont.)

Paul, M. H., Miller, R. A., and Potts, W. J. Long term results of aortic-pulmonary anastomosis for tetralogy of Fallot, Circulation, 23:525, 1961.

Potts, W. J., Smith, S., and Gibson, S. Anastomosis of the aorta to a pulmonary artery, J.A.M.A., 132:627, 1946.

——— Aortic-pulmonary anastomosis for pulmonary stenosis, J. Thoracic Surg., 17:223, 1948.

——— Surgical treatment of congenital pulmonary stenosis, Ann. Surg., 130:342, 1949.

Redo, S. F. Shunting procedures for cyanotic congenital cardiac defects, Am. J. Surg., 107:469, 1964.

Sanger, P. W., Robicsek, F., Taylor, F. H., Ablaza, S. C., and Rees, T. T. Indications for surgical treatment in congenital heart disease, South. M. J., 54:1063, 1961.

Taussig, H. B. Diagnosis of tetralogy of Fallot and indications for operation, J. Thoracic Surg., 16:241, 1947.

——— Congenital malformations of the heart, New York, The Commonwealth Fund, 1947.

——— King, J. T., Bauersfeld, S. R., and Padbamat-Iyer, S. Results of operation for pulmonary stenosis and atresia (Report of 1000 cases), Tr. A. Am. Physicians, 64:67, 1951.

——— Crawford, H., Pelargonio, S., and Zachariondakis, S. Ten to thirteen year follow-up on patients after Blalock-Taussig operation, Circulation, 25:630, 1962.

Coarctation of the Aorta

Bahn, R. C., Edwards, J. E., and DuShane, J. Coarctation of the aorta as a cause of death in early infancy, Pediatrics, 8:192, 1951.

Bing, R. J., Handelsman, J. C., Campbell, J. A., Griswold, H. E., and Blalock, A. The surgical treatment and the physiopathology of coarctation of the aorta, Ann. Surg., 128:803, 1948.

Blalock, A., and Park, E. A. Surgical treatment of experimental coarctation of aorta, Ann. Surg., 119:445–456, 1944.

Bramwell, C., and Jones, A. M. Coarctation of the aorta: the collateral circulation, Brit. Heart J., 3:205, 1941.

Burford, T. H., and Carson, M. J. Visualization of the aorta and its branches by retroarterial diodrast injection, J. Pediat., 33:675, 1948.

Clagett, O. T. Coarctation of the aorta: surgical aspects, Proc. Staff Meet., Mayo Clin., 27:131–135, 1947.

Crafoord, C., and Nylin, G. Congenital coarctation of the aorta and its surgical treatment, J. Thoracic Surg., 14:437, 1945.

Friedman, M., Selzer, A., and Rosenblum, H. The renal blood flow in coarctation of the aorta, J. Clin. Investigation, 20:107, 1941.

Glenn, F., Keefer, E. B. C., Speer, D. S., and Dotter, C. T. Coarctation of the lower thoracic and abdominal aorta immediately proximal to celiac axis, Surg., Gynec. & Obst., 94:562, 1952.

Gross, R. E. Surgical correction for coarctation of the aorta, Surgery, 18:673, 1945.

——— and Hufnagel, C. A. Coarctation of the aorta. Experimental studies regarding its surgical correction, New England J. Med., 233: 287, 1945.

——— Coarctation of the aorta. Surgical treatment in one hundred cases, Circulation, 1:41, 1950.

——— Treatment of certain aortic coarctations by homologous grafts, a report of nineteen cases, Ann. Surg., 134:753, 1951.

Hamilton, W. F., and Abbot, M. E. Coarctation of the aorta of the adult type. II. A statistical study and historical retrospect of 200 recorded cases with autopsy of stenosis or obliteration of the descending arch in subjects above the age of two years, Am. Heart J., 3:574, 1928.

Holman, E. The obscure pathology of post-stenotic dilatation, J. Thoracic Surg., 28:109, 1954.

Johnson, J., Kirby, C. K., and Horn, R. C., Jr. The growth of preserved aorta homografts, Surgery, 31:141, 1952.

Kirklin, J. W., Burchell, H. B., Pugh, D. G., Burke, E. C., and Mills, S. D. Surgical treatment of coarctation of the aorta in a ten week old infant: report of a case, Circulation, 6:411, 1952.

Lewis, T. Material relating to coarctation of the aorta of the adult type, Heart, 16:205, 1933.

Railsbach, O. C., and Dock, W. Erosion of the ribs due to stenosis of the isthmus (coarctation) of the aorta, Radiology, 12:58, 1929.

Reifenstein, G. H., Levine, S. A., and Gross, R. E. Coarctation of the aorta, Am. Heart J., 33:146, 1947.

Scott, H. W., Jr., and Bahnson, H. T. Evidence for a renal factor in the hypertension of experimental coarctation of the aorta, Surgery, 30: 206, 1951.

Shumacker, H. B. Use of the subclavian artery in the surgical treatment of coarctation of the aorta, Surg., Gynec. & Obst., 93:491–495, 1951.

Pulmonary Valvotomy

Allanby, K. O., and Campbell, M. Congenital pulmonary stenosis with closed ventricular septum, Guy's Hosp. Rep., 98:18, 1949.

Blalock, A., and Kieffer, R. F., Jr. Valvulotomy for the relief of congenital valvular pulmonic stenosis with intact ventricular septum, Ann. Surg., 132:496, 1950.

Blount, S. G., Jr., McCord, M. C., Mueller, H., and Swan, H. Isolated valvular pulmonic stenosis. Clinical and physiologic response to open valvuloplasty, Circulation, 10:161, 1954.

Brock, R. C. Pulmonary valvulotomy for relief of congenital pulmonary stenosis, Brit. M. J., 1: 1121, 1948.

PULMONARY VALVOTOMY (cont.)

——— The surgery of pulmonary stenosis, Brit. M. J., 2:399, 1949.

——— Infundibular stenosis, Brit. Heart J., 12: 403, 1950.

——— Direct cardiac surgery in the treatment of congenital pulmonary stenosis, Ann. Surg., 136: 63, 1952.

Dow, J. W., Levine, H. D., Elkin, M., Haynes, F. W., Hellems, H. K., Whittenberger, J. W., Ferris, B. G., Goodale, W. T., Harvey, W. P., Eppinger, E. C., and Dexter, L. Studies of congenital heart disease IV. Uncomplicated pulmonary stenosis, Circulation, 2:481, 1950.

Engle, M. A., and Taussig, H. B. Valvular pulmonic stenosis with intact ventricular septum and patent foramen ovale, Circulation, 2:481, 1950.

Glover, R. P., Bailey, C. P., and O'Neil, T. J. E. Surgery of stenotic valvular disease of the heart, J.A.M.A., 144:1049, 1950.

——— O'Neil, T. J. E., Gontigo, H., McAuliffe, T. C., Wells, C. R. E. The surgery of infundibular pulmonic stenosis with intact ventricular septum (a type of "pure" pulmonic stenosis), J. Thoracic Surg., 28:481, 1954.

Greene, D. G., Baldwin, E. DeF., Baldwin, J., Himmelstein, A., Roh, C. E., and Cournand, A. Pure congenital pulmonary stenosis and idiopathic congenital dilatation of the pulmonary artery, Am. J. Med., 6:24, 1949.

Humphreys, G. H., II, Powers, S., Fitzpatrick, H., and Lanman, B. M. Pulmonary valvulotomy, results of operation in twenty-five cases, Surgery, 35:1, 1954.

Kirklin, J. W., Conolly, D. C., Ellis, F. H., Jr., Burchell, H. B., Edwards, J. E., and Wood, E. H. Problems in the diagnosis and surgical treatment of pulmonic stenosis with intact ventricular septum, Circulation, 8:849, 1953.

Lurie, P. R., and Shumacker, H. B. Hemodynamic effects of valvulotomy in pulmonic stenosis, Circulation, 8:345, 1953.

Muller, W. H., and Longmire, W. P., Jr. The surgical treatment of pure pulmonic stenosis, Surgery, 30:275, 1951.

Potts, W. J., Gibson, S., Riker, W. L., and Leininger, C. R. Congenital pulmonary stenosis with intact ventricular septum, J.A.M.A., 144:8, 1950.

——— and Riker, W. L. Surgical treatment of pulmonary stenosis with intact interventricular septum, Arch. Surg., 62:776, 1951.

Sellors, T. H. Surgery of pulmonic stenosis, Lancet, 1:988, 1948.

——— Surgery of congenital heart disease, Lancet, 2:71, 1948.

Swan, H., Cleveland, H. C., Mueller, H., and Blount, S. G., Jr. Pulmonic valvular stenosis, J. Thoracic Surg., 28:504, 1954.

——— Virtue, R. W., Blount, S. G., Jr., and Kircher, L. T., Jr. Hypothermia in surgery: analysis of 100 clinical cases, Ann. Surg., 142: 382, 1955.

MITRAL COMMISSUROTOMY

Allen, D. S., and Graham, E. A. Intracardiac surgery—new method: preliminary report, J.A.M.A., 79:1028, 1922.

——— Intracardiac surgery, Arch. Surg., 8:317, 1924.

Andrus, E. C., Blalock, A., and Melnor, W. R. Surgical treatment of mitral stenosis, Arch. Surg., 67:700, 1953.

Bailey, C. P., Glover, R. P., and O'Neill, T. J. E. The surgery of mitral stenosis, J. Thoracic Surg., 19:16, 1950.

——— Surgery of the Heart, Philadelphia, Lea & Febiger, 1955.

Baker, C., Brock, R. C., and Campbell, M. Valvulotomy for mitral stenosis, Brit. M. J., 1:1,283, 1950.

Beal, J. M., Longmire, W. P. Jr., and Leake, W. H. Resection of the auricular appendages, Ann. Surg., 132:517, 1950.

Bernheim, B. M. Experimental surgery of mitral valve, Bull. Johns Hopkins Hosp., 20:107, 1909.

Brock, R. C. The surgical and pathological anatomy of the mitral valve, Brit. Heart J., 14: 489, 1952.

Brunton, L. Preliminary note on possibility of treating mitral stenosis by surgical methods, Lancet, 1:352, 1902. See also editorial, Surgical operation for mitral stenosis, Lancet, 1:461, 1902.

Carrel, A., and Tuffier, T. Etude anatomopathologique et experimentale sur la chirurgie des orifices du coeur, Presse méd., 22:173, 1914.

Cooley, D. A., and De Bakey, M. E. The technique of mitral valvulotomy, Surgery, 32:923, 1952.

Cushing, H., and Branch, J. R. B. Experimental and clinical notes on chronic valvular disease in dog and possible relations to future surgery of cardiac valves, J. Med. Research, 12:471, 1907–1908.

Cutler, E. C., Levine, S. A., and Beck, C. S. Surgical treatment of mitral stenosis: experimental and clinical studies, Arch. Surg., 9:689, 1924.

——— and Beck, C. S. The present status of the surgical procedures in chronic valvular disease of the heart, Arch. Surg., 18:403, 1929.

Doyen, C. Chirurgie des malformations congenitales ou acquises du coeur, Presse méd., 21:860, 1913.

Gerbode, F., Holman, E., and Hultgren, H. Treatment of mitral stenosis by finger-fracture valvulotomy, Arch. Surg., 65:113, 1952.

Glover, R. P., Bailey, C. P., and O'Neill, T. J. E. The surgery of stenotic valvular disease of the heart, J.A.M.A., 144:1049, 1950.

Gorlin, R., Haynes, F. W., Goodale, W. R., Sawyer, C. G., Dow, J. W., and Dexter, L. Studies of the circulatory dynamics in mitral stenosis. Altered dynamics at best, Am. Heart J., 41:30, 1951.

Harken, D. E., Ellis, L. B., Ware, P. F., and Norman, L. R. The surgical treatment of mitral

Mitral Commissurotomy (cont.)

stenosis. I. Valvuloplasty, New England J. Med., 239:801, 1948.

——— Ellis, L. B., and Norman, L. R. The surgical treatment of mitral stenosis, J. Thoracic Surg., 19:1, 1950.

——— Dexter, L., Ellis, L. B., Farrand, R. E., and Dickson, J. F., III. The surgery of mitral stenosis. III. Finger-fracture valvuloplasty, Ann. Surg., 134:722, 1951.

Hurwitt, E. S., Bloomberg, A., Aaron, R., Jezer, A., and Young, D. An appraisal of the surgical treatment of mitral stenosis, Ann. Surg., 138: 219, 1953.

Janton, H. O., Glover, R. P., O'Neill, T. J. E., Gregory, J. E., and Froio, G. F. Results of surgical treatment for mitral stenosis. Analysis of one hundred consecutive cases, Circulation, 6: 321, 1952.

Keown, K. K., Grove, D. D., and Ruth, H. S. Anesthesia for commissurotomy for mitral stenosis, J.A.M.A., 146:446, 1951.

Longmire, W. P., Jr., Beal, J. M., and Leake, W. H. Resection of the auricular appendages, Dis. of Chest, 19:307, 1951.

Madden, J. L. Resection of the left auricular appendix, J.A.M.A., 140:769, 1949.

Morse, D. P., Hirose, T., and Bailey, C. P. Recurrent mitral stenosis: A study of sixty-six cases of recurrent mitral stenosis, their treatment and prophylaxis, Arch. Surg., 85:198, 1962.

Neptune, W. B., and Bailey, C. P. Mitral commissurotomy through the right thoracic approach, J. Thoracic Surg., 28:15, 1954.

Powers, J. H. Surgical treatment of mitral stenosis, Arch. Surg., 25:555, 1932.

Pribram, B. O. C. Die Operative Behandlung der Mitralstenose, Arch. f. klin. Chir., 142:458, 1926.

Samways, D. W. Cardiac peristalsis; its motions and effects, Lancet, 1:927, 1898.

Schepelmann, E. Herzklappen Chirurgie, Experimentelle Untersuchen, Deutsche Ztschr. f. Chir., 120:562, 1913.

Sellors, T. H. P. Finger-nail knife for commissurotomy in mitral stenosis, Lancet, 1:8, 448, 1951.

Smithy, H. G. An approach to the surgical treatment of chronic valvular disease of the Heart. XVI Annual Assembly of the Southeastern Surgical Congress, Hollywood, Florida, April 5–8, 1948.

——— Boone, J. A., and Stallworth, J. M. The surgical treatment of constrictive valvular disease of the heart, Surg., Gynec. & Obst., 90: 175, 1950.

Souttar, H. S. The surgical treatment of mitral stenosis, Brit. M. J., 2:603, 1925.

Sweet, R. H., and Bland, E. F. Surgical relief of congestion in the pulmonary circulation in cases of severe mitral stenosis, Ann. Surg., 130:384, 1949.

Cardiopericardiopexy

Beck, C. S., and Leighninger, D. S. Operation for coronary artery disease, Ann. Surg., 141:24, 1955.

——— and Leighninger, D. S. Coronary heart disease treated by operation, Arch. Surg., 85: 383, 1962.

——— and Leighninger, D. S. Anginal pain and fibrillating electricity-mobile components of coronary artery disease, J. Cardiovasc. Surg., 3: 337, 1962.

Bigelow, W. G., Basian, H., and Trusler, G. A. Internal mammary artery implantation for coronary heart disease: a clinical follow-up study one to eight years after operation, J. Thoracic & Cardiovasc. Surg., 45:67, 1963.

Block, W. J., Jr., Crumpacka, E. L., Dry, T. J., and Gage, R. P. Prognosis of angina pectoris, J.A.M.A., 150:259, 1952.

Effler, D. B., Groves, L. K., Sones, F. M., Jr., and Shirey, E. K. Increased myocardial perfusion by internal mammary artery implant: Vineberg's Operation, Ann. Surg., 158:526, 1963.

Gross, H., Bloomberg, A. E., Rosenblatt, M., Kantrowitz, A., Schein, C. J., and Ferreira, R. Failure of cardio-pericardiopexy to protect pigs against acute coronary occlusion, J. Thoracic Surg., 33:679, 1957.

Hahn, R. S., and Beck, C. S. Revascularization of the heart, Circulation, 6:801, 1952.

Master, A. M., Jaffe, H. C., and Dack, S. Treatment and immediate prognosis of coronary artery thrombosis: 267 attacks, Am. Heart J., 12:549, 1936.

Mautz, F., and Gregg, D. Dynamics of collateral circulation following chronic occlusion of coronary arteries, Proc. Soc. Exper. Biol. & Med., 36:797, 1937.

McAllister, F. F., Leighninger, D. S., and Beck, C. S. Revascularization of the heart by vein graft from aorta to coronary sinus, Ann. Surg., 133:153, 1951.

Thompson, S. A., and Raisbeck, M. J. Cardiopericardiopexy: The surgical treatment of coronary arterial disease by the establishment of adhesive pericarditis, Ann. Int. Med., 16:495, 1942.

——— and Raisbeck, M. J. The surgical rehabilitation of the coronary cripple, Ann. Int. Med., 31:1010, 1949.

——— and Plachta, A. Fourteen years' experience with cardiopexy in the treatment of coronary artery disease, J. Thoracic Surg., 27:64, 1954.

Sigler, L. H. Prognosis of angina pectoris and coronary occlusion: followup of 1,700 cases, J.A.M.A., 146:998, 1951.

Sones, F. M., Jr., and Shirey, E. K. Cine coronary arteriography, Mod. Concepts Cardiovasc. Dis., 31:725, 1962.

Stanton, E. J., Schildt, P., and Beck, C. S. The effect of abrasion of the surface of the heart upon intercoronary communications, Am. Heart J., 22:529, 1941.

Vineberg, A., Munro, D. D., Cohen, H., and Buller, W. Four years' clinical experience with

Cardiopericardiopexy (cont.)

internal mammary artery implantation in the treatment of human coronary artery insufficiency including additional experimental studies, J. Thoracic Surg., 29:1, 1955.

——— Coronary vascular anastomosis by internal mammary implantation, Canad. M. A. J., 78:871, 1958.

——— Experimental background of myocardial revascularization by internal mammary artery implantation and supplementary technics, with its clinical application in 125 patients: a review and critical appraisal, Ann. Surg., 159: 185, 1964.

Coronary Thromboendarterectomy

Absolon, K. B., Aust, J. B., Varco, R. L., and Lillehei, C. W. Surgical treatment of occlusive coronary artery disease by endarterectomy or anastomotic replacement, Surg., Gynec. & Obst., 103:180, 1956.

Beck, C. S. Personal communication.

Hallén, A., Björk, L., and Björk, V. O. Coronary thromboendarterectomy, J. Thoracic & Cardiovasc. Surg., 45:216, 1963.

Longmire, W. P. Personal communication.

May, A. M. Coronary endarterectomy. Curettement of coronary arteries in dogs, Am. J. Surg., 93:969, 1957.

Cardiac Resuscitation

Allen, C. R., Stuzman, J. W., and Meek, W. M. Production of ventricular tachycardia by adrenalin in cyclopropane anesthesia, Anesthesiology, 1:158, 1940.

Bailey, H. Cardiac massage for impending death under anesthesia, Brit. M. J., 2:84, 1941.

Barber, R. F., and Madden, J. L. Resuscitation of the heart, Am. J. Surg., 64:151, 1944.

——— and Madden, J. L. Historical aspects of cardiac resuscitation, Am. J. Surg., 70:135, 1945.

Beck, C. S., and Mautz, F. R. Control of heart beat by surgeon with special reference to ventricular fibrillation occurring during operation, Ann. Surg., 106:525–537, 1937.

——— Resuscitation for cardiac standstill and ventricular fibrillation occurring during operation, Am. J. Surg., 54:273–279, 1941.

Beecher, H. K. The Physiology of Anesthesia, Oxford Med. Publications, 1938.

Bohn, G. L. Artificial restoration of cardiac rhythm. Report of successful case, Brit. M. J., 2:725, 1939.

Burstein, C. L., Marangoni, B. A., De Graff, A. C., and Rovenstine, E. A. Laboratory studies on prophylaxis and treatment of ventricular fibrillation induced by epinephrine during cyclopropane anesthesia, Anesthesiology, 1:167–186, 1940.

Cole, S. L., and Corday, E. Four-minute limit for cardiac resuscitation, J.A.M.A., 161:1454–1458, 1956.

Condon, R. E. Pathophysiologic mechanisms in cardiac arrest, Surg. Gynec. & Obst., 114:8, 1962.

——— Acute circulatory arrest, Ann. Surg., 29:7, 1963.

Cook, L. Recovery after massage of the heart, Brit. M. J., 2:118, 1926.

Crafoord, C. Pulmonary ventilation and anesthesia in major chest surgery, J. Thoracic Surg., 9:237–253, 1940.

Crile, G., and Dolley, D. An experimental research into the resuscitation of dogs killed by anesthetics and asphyxia, J. Exper. Med., 8: 713, 1906.

D'Halluin. Resuscitation due coeur; la nie du coeur isale et le massage du coeur, These de Lille, No. 22, 1904.

——— Le massage du coeur, Presse Méd., 44: 345, 1904.

——— Contribution a l' étude du massage du coeur (suite): les tremulations fibrillaires, Paris et Lille, 1905.

Gildea E. F., and Cobb, S. The effects of anemia on the cerebral cortex of the cat, Arch. Neurol. & Psychiat., 23:877–903, 1930.

Glover, R. M. Recovery after massage of the heart, Brit. M. J., 2:342–343, 1926.

Green, T. A. Heart massage as a means of resuscitation in cases of apparent sudden death, Lancet, 2:1708, 1906.

Green, T. N. Cardiac arrest, Ann. Surg., 92:331–334, 1930.

Hinchey, P. R. Cardiac arrest—the most important disaster in the operating room, Arch. Surg., 74;365–380, 1957.

Hinton, J. W., Stephenson, H. E., Jr., and del Missier, P. A. Cardiac arrest: resumé of experimental and clinical data, J. Nat. M. A., 49:11–18, 1957.

Hookers, D. R. On the recovery of the heart in electric shock, Am. J. Physiol., 91:305–328, 1929.

——— Kouwenhoven, W. B., and Langworthy, O. R. The effect of alternating electrical currents on the heart, Am. J. Physiol., 103:444, 1933.

Hosler, R. M. Cardiac Arrest, Springfield, Ill., Charles C Thomas, 1954.

Hyman, A. S. Resuscitation of the stopped heart by intracardiac therapy; use of the artificial pacemaker, Arch. Int. Med., 50:283, 1932.

Igelsbrud, Quoted by Keen, Therap. Gaz., 28:217, 1904.

Johnson, J., and Kirby, C. K. Experimental study of cardiac massage, Surgery, 26:472–478, 1949.

——— and Kirby, C. K. Surgical treatment of ventricular fibrillation, Ann. Surg., 134:672–682, 1951.

——— and Kirby, C. K. Prevention and treatment of cardiac arrest, J.A.M.A., 154:291, 1954.

Kay, J. H., and Blalock, A. Use of calcium chlo-

CARDIAC RESUSCITATION (cont.)

ride in treatment of cardiac arrest in patients, Surg., Gynec. & Obst., 93:97–102, 1951.

Keen. A case of total laryngectomy (unsuccessful) and a case of abdominal hysterectomy (successful) in both of which massage of the heart for chloroform collapse was emphasized, with notes of 25 other cases of cardiac massage, Therap. Gaz., 28:217, 1904.

Kouwenhoven, W. B., Jude, J. R., and Knickerbocker, G. C. Closed-chest cardiac massage, J.A.M.A., 173:1064, 1960.

Lahey, F. H., and Ruzicka, E. R. Experience with cardiac arrest, Surg., Gynec. & Obst., 90:108–118, 1950.

Lee, W. E., Downs, T. McK. Resuscitation by direct massage of the heart in cardiac arrest, Ann. Surg., 80:555, 1924.

Martin, J. T., and Tarrow, A. B. Review of cardiac resuscitation, Anesth. & Analg., 35:147–164, 1956.

Mautz, F. R. Reduction of cardiac irritability by the epicardial and systemic administration of drugs as a protection in cardiac surgery, J. Thoracic Surg., 5:612–628, 1936.

McQueen, E. M. Recovery of heart beat after massage for an hour and a quarter, Med. J. Australia, 2:341, 1938.

Nicholson, J. C. Cardiac massage, Brit. M. J., 1:385–386, 1942.

Nickel, S. N., and Gale, H. H. Altered prognosis with cardiac massage; cardiac resuscitation in acute myocardial infarction—Report of two successfully treated cases, J.A.M.A., 170:23, 1959.

Prevost, J. L., and Batelli, F. Sur quelques effects des discharges electriques sur le coeur des maniferes, Compt. rend. Acad. d. sc., 129:1267, 1899.

Primrose, W. B. Cardiac resuscitation by heart massage, Brit. M. J., 2:540, 1935.

Rivkin, L. M., Roe, B. B., and Gardner, R. E. Closed chest cardiac resuscitation, Am. J. Surg., 104:283, 1962.

Robinson, E. C., and Bredeck, J. L. Ventricular fibrillation in man with cardiac recovery, Arch. Int. Med., 20:725–738, 1917.

Schull, L. C. A review of the cases of cardiac arrest at Vanderbilt Hospital and Thayer Veterans Hospital, South. M. J. 52:143, 1959.

Seidman, J., Parsonnet, V., Evers, W., Applebaum, I., and Kern, M. L. Cardiac arrest occurring outside the operating room, J.A.M.A., 170:1053, 1959.

Simpson, R., Abrams, B., and Gordon, A. S. Cardiac monitor for detection and differentiation of cardiac standstill, ventricular fibrillation, or peripheral vascular collapse during surgery, Surg., Gynec. & Obst., 104:110–113, 1957.

Starling, E. A., and Lane, W. A. Minutes of meeting of society of anesthetists, Lancet, 2:1397, 1902.

Stephenson, H. E., Reid, L. C., and Hinton, J. W. Some common denominators in 1200 cases of cardiac arrest, Ann. Surg., 137:731–744, 1953.

——— Reid, L. C., and Hinton, J. W. Pitfalls, precautions and complications in cardiac resuscitation; study of 1200 cases, Arch. Surg., 69: 37–53, 1954.

——— Cardiac Arrest and Resuscitation, St. Louis, C. V. Mosby, 1958, p. 32.

Stewart, G. H., Guthrie, C. C., Burns, R. L. and Pike, F. A. Studies in resuscitation, J. Exper. Med., 8:289, 1906.

Tuffier, T. La chirurgie du coeur, Cinquieme Congress de la Societe Internationale de Chirurgie, Paris, pp. 66–75, July 19–23, 1920.

Weale, F. E., and Rothwell-Jackson, R. L. Efficiency of cardiac massage, Lancet, 1:990, 1962.

Weinberger, L. W., Gibbon, M. H., and Gibbon, J. H., Jr. Temporary arrest of the circulation to the central nervous system. I. Physiologic effects, Arch. Neurol. & Psychiat., 43:615, 1940.

West, J. P. Cardiac arrest during anesthesia and surgery. Analysis of 30 cases, Ann. Surg., 140: 623–629, 1954.

White, C. S. The role of heart massage in surgery, Surg., Gynec. & Obst., 9:388, 1909.

Wiggers, C. J. Cardiac massage followed by countershock from fibrillation due to coronary occlusion, Am. J. Physiol., 116:161, 1936.

Wrede, L. Ueber direkte Herzmassage, Arch. f. klin. Chir., 100:833, 1913.

PERICARDIECTOMY

Andrews, G. W. S., Pickering, G. W., and Sellors, T. H. The aetiology of constrictive pericarditis with special reference to tuberculous pericarditis, together with a note on polyserositis, Quart. J. Med., 17:291, 1948.

Bigelow, W. G., Dolan, F. G., Wilson, D. R., and Gunton, R. W. Subtotal pericardiectomy for constrictive pericarditis, Surgery, 41:102, 1951.

Bishop, C. A., and Lipin, R. J. A technique of pericardiectomy, J. Thoracic Surg., 31:686, 1956.

Blakemore, W. S., Zinsser, H. F., Kirby, C. K., Whitaker, W. B., and Johnson, J. Pericardiectomy for relapsing pericarditis and chronic constrictive pericarditis, J. Thor. & Cardiovasc. Surg., 39:26, 1960.

Blalock, A., and Burwell, C. S. Chronic pericardial disease: report of 28 cases of constrictive pericarditis, Surg., Gynec. & Obst., 73:433, 1941.

——— and Ravitch, M. M. Consideration on nonoperative treatment of cardiac tamponade resulting from wounds of the heart, Surgery, 14: 157, 1943.

Churchill, E. D. Decortication of the heart (Delorme) for adhesive pericarditis, Arch. Surg., 19:1457, 1929.

——— Pericardial resection in chronic constrictive pericarditis, Ann. Surg., 104:516, 1936.

Cooper, F. W., Stead, E. A., and Warren, J. V. Beneficial effect of intravenous infusions in acute pericardial tamponade, Ann. Surg., 120: 822, 1944.

PERICARDIECTOMY (cont.)

Dalton, J. C., Pearson, F. R., Jr., and White, P. D. Constrictive pericarditis review and long term follow-up of 78 cases, Ann. Int. Med., 45:445, 1956.

Delorme, E. Sur un traitement chirurgical: De la symphyse cardopericardique, Gaz. des hop., 71: 1150, 1898.

Deterling, R. A., Jr., and Humphreys, G. H., II. Factors in the etiology of constrictive pericarditis, Circulation, 12:30, 1955.

de Vernejoul, R., Buisson, P., Courbier, R., and Tricot, R. Les pericardites contrictives post-traumatiques, Presse. med., 65:241, 1957.

Ehrenhaft, J. L., and Taber, R. E. Homopericardium and constrictive pericarditis, J. Thoracic Surg., 24:355, 1952.

Elkin, D. C. Suturing wounds of the heart, Ann. Surg., 95:573, 1932.

——— and Campbell, R. E. Cardiac tamponade, treatment by aspiration, Ann. Surg., 133:623, 1951.

Farringer, J. L., Jr., and Carr, D. Cardiac tamponade, Ann. Surg., 141:437, 1955.

Glenn, F., and Diethelm, A. G. Surgical treatment of constrictive pericarditis, Ann. Surg., 155:883, 1962.

Griswold, R. A., and Drye, J. C. Cardiac wounds, Ann. Surg., 139:783, 1954.

Heuer, G. J., and Stewart, H. J. The surgical treatment of chronic constrictive pericarditis, Surg. Clin. North America, 477, 1946.

Holman, E. The recognition and correction of constrictive pericarditis, J. Thoracic Surg., 18: 643, 1949.

——— Surgical treatment of tuberculous pericarditis, Arch. Surg., 61:266, 1950.

——— and Willett, F. The surgical correction of constrictive pericarditis, Surg., Gynec. & Obst., 89:129, 1949.

——— and Willett, F. Results of radical pericardiectomy for constrictive pericarditis, J.A.M.A., 157:789, 1955.

Isaacs, J. P. Sixty penetrating wounds of the heart: clinical and experimental observations, Surgery, 45:606, 1959.

Johnson, J., and Kirby, C. K. A new incision for pericardiectomy, Ann. Surg., 133:540, 1951.

Maynard, A. De L., Cordice, N. W. V., and Naclerio, E. A. Penetrating wounds of the heart: A report of 81 cases, Surg., Gynec. & Obst., 94:605, 1952.

Ravitch, M. M., and Blalock, A. Aspiration of blood from pericardium in treatment of acute cardiac tamponade after injury: further experience with report of cases, Ann. Surg., 58:463, 1949.

Rehn, L. Zur experimentellen Pathologic des Herzbeutels, Arch. f. klin. Chir., 102:1, 1913.

——— Die Chirurgie des Herzene und des Herzbeutels, Berl. klin. Wchschr., 50:241, 1913.

——— Uber perikardiale Verwachsungen, Med. Klin., 16:999, 1920.

Schmieden, V., and Westermann, H. H. The operative management of fibrous constricting pericarditis, Surgery, 2:350, 1937.

Sellors, T. H. Constricitve pericarditis, Brit. J. Surg., 33:215, 1945.

Uglov, F. G. Diagnosis and surgical treatment of constrictive pericarditis, Surgery, 47:247, 1960.

Volhard, F., and Schmieden, V. Uber Erkennung und Behandlung der Umklammerung des Herzens durch schwillige Parikarditis, Klin. Wchnschr., 2:5, 1925.

White, P. D., Alexander, F., Churchill, E. D., and Sweet, R. H. Chronic constrictive pericarditis over the left heart chambers and its surgical relief, Am. J. M. Sc., 216:378, 1948.

AORTIC EMBOLECTOMY

Blum, L. Consideration of technique of aortic embolectomy, Arch. Surg., 70:52, 1955.

Brock, R. Late arterial embolectomy, J. Cardiovasc. Surg., 3:39, 1962.

Burgess, C. M., and Hartwell, A. S. Removal of saddle embolus of aorta, J.A.M.A., 141:387, 1949.

Cranley, J. J., Krause, R. J., Strasser, E. S., Hafner, G. D., and Fogarty, T. J. Peripheral arterial embolism: Changing concepts, Surgery, 55:57, 1964.

Dale, W. A., and Mahoney, E. B. Aortic "saddle" embolism, Arch. Surg., 76:930, 1958.

Danzis, M. Arterial embolectomy, Ann. Surg., 98: 249 (Aug.); 422 (Sept.) 1933.

Griffiths, D. L. Arterial embolism: study of eight cases, Lancet, 2:1339, 1938.

Hesse, E. Ueber die Embolie und Thrombose der Aorta abdominalis und ihre operative Behandlung, Arch. f. klin. Chir., 115:812, 1921.

Holden, W. D. Arteriosclerosis obliterans of the abdominal aorta, Arch. Surg., 53:456, 1946.

Keeley, J. L. Saddle embolus of the aorta: report of successful embolectomy, Ann. Surg., 128: 257, 1948.

Key, E. Ueber Embolectomie als Behandlungs Methode bei embolischen Zirculations-storungen der Extremitaten, Acta. chir. Scandinav., 54: 339, 1921–1922.

——— Embolectomy in the treatment of circulatory disturbances in the extremities, Surg., Gynec. & Obst., 36:309, 1923.

Linton, R. R. Arterial embolism: simplified technique for removal of saddle embolus at bifurcation of aorta with report of successful case, Surg., Gynec. & Obst., 80:509, 1945.

Lord, J. W., and Burke, G. Comprehensive surgical management of aortic saddle emboli, Surgery, 33:294, 1953.

Lund, C. C. Treatment of embolism of greater arteries, Ann. Surg., 106:880, 1937.

Madden, J. L. Resection of the left auricular appendix. A prophylaxis for recurrent arterial emboli, J.A.M.A., 140:769, 1949.

——— Technique for aortic embolectomy, Surg., Gynec. & Obst., 93:167, 1951.

McClure, R. D., and Harkins, H. N. Recent ad-

AORTIC EMBOLECTOMY (cont.)

vances in the treatment of peripheral arterial embolism, Surgery, 14:747, 1943.

McGarity, W. C., and Robertson, R. L. Arterial embolism with notes on operative and anticoagulant therapy, Surg., Gynec. & Obst., 96: 522, 1953.

McKechnie, R. E., and Allen, E. V. Sudden occlusion of the arteries of the extremities. A study of 100 cases of embolism and thrombosis, Surg., Gynec. & Obst., 63:231, 1936.

Murray, G. Aortic embolectomy, Surg., Gynec. & Obst., 77:157, 1943.

Nystrom, G. Embolism of arteries, in Lectures on Embolism and Other Surgical Subjects, Baltimore, Williams & Wilkins Co., 1936.

Ravdin, I. S., and Wood, F. C. The successful removal of a saddle embolus of the aorta, eleven days after acute coronary occlusion, Ann. Surg., 114:834, 1941.

Reich, N. E. Occlusion of the abdominal aorta: a study of sixteen cases of saddle embolus and thrombosis, Ann. Int. Med., 19:36, 1943.

Reynolds, J. T., and Jirka, F. J. Embolic occlusion of major arteries, Surgery, 16:485, 1944.

Shaw, R. S. A method for the removal of the adherent distal thrombus, Surg., Gynec. & Obst., 110:225, 1960.

Taylor, F. W. Saddle embolus of the aorta, Arch. Surg., 62:38, 1951.

Thiessen, N. W., and Marxen, N. L. Successful direct aortic embolectomy, Am. J. Surg., 84: 358, 1952.

Warren, R., and Linton, R. The treatment of arterial embolism, New England J. Med., 238: 421, 1948.

Weismann, R. E., and Ellsworth, W. J., Jr. Saddle emboli requiring multiple embolectomies. Report of two successful cases, Ann. Surg., 147:75, 1958.

Wilson, H. Aortic embolectomy: successful removal of saddle embolus by transabdominal route, J.A.M.A., 141:389, 1949.

ANEURYSM OF THE THORACIC AORTA

Adams, H. D., and van Geertruyden, H. H. Neurologic complications of aortic surgery, Ann. Surg., 144:574, 1956.

Bahnson, H. T. Definitive treatment of saccular aneurysms of the aorta with excision of the sac and aortic suture, Surg., Gynec. & Obst., 96:383, 1953.

——— Surgical treatment of thoracic aneurysms, International Symposium on Cardiovascular Surgery, Philadelphia, W. B. Saunders Co., 1955, pp. 434–447.

Brock, R. C., and Graham, A. J. P. Resection of combined aneurysm and coarctation of the aorta with insertion of a homograft, Guy's Hosp. Rep., 101:207, 1952.

Clatworthy, H. W., Jr., and Varco, R. L. A small bore polythene shunt to prevent mechanical shock after prolonged cross-clamping of the thoracic aorta, Proc. Soc. Exper. Biol. & Med., 74:434, 1950.

Cooley, D. A., and De Bakey, M. E. Surgical considerations of excisional therapy for aortic aneurysms, Surgery, 34:1005, 1953.

——— and De Bakey, M. E. Resection of the thoracic aorta with replacement by homograft for aneurysms and constrictive lesions, J. Thoracic Surg., 29:66, 1955.

——— Mahaffey, D. E., and De Bakey, M. E. Total excision of the aortic arch for aneurysm, Surg., Gynec. & Obst., 101:667, 1955.

——— De Bakey, M. E., and Morris, G. C., Jr. Controlled extracorporeal circulation in surgical treatment of aortic aneurysms, Ann. Surg., 146:473, 1957.

De Bakey, M. E., Creech, O., Jr., and Morris, G. C., Jr. Aneurysm of thoracoabdominal aorta involving the celiac, superior mesenteric, and renal arteries. Report of four cases treated by resection and homograft replacement, Ann. Surg., 144:549, 1956.

——— Crawford, E. S., Cooley, D. A., and Morris, G. C. Successful resection of fusiform aneurysm of aortic arch with replacement by homograft, Surg., Gynec. & Obst., 105:657, 1957.

——— Cooley, D. A., Crawford, E. S., and Morris, G. C., Jr. Aneurysms of the thoracic aorta; analysis of 179 patients treated by resection, J. Thoracic Surg., 36:393, 1958.

——— Henly, W. S., Cooley, D. A., Crawford, E. S., and Morris, G. C., Jr. Surgical treatment of dissecting aneurysms of the aorta; analysis of 72 cases, Circulation, 24:290, 1961.

Ellis, F. H., Jr., Kirklin, J. W., and Bruwer, A. J. Surgical experiences in the treatment of aneurysms of the thoracic aorta, Surg., Gynec. & Obst., 106:179, 1958.

Gerbode, F., Braimbridge, M., Osborn, J. J., Hood, M., and French, S. Traumatic thoracic aneurysms: Treatment by resection and grafting with the use of an extracorporeal by-pass, Surgery, 42:975, 1957.

Glendy, R. E., Castleman, B., and White, P. D. Dissecting aneurysm of aorta; Clinical and anatomical analysis of nineteen cases (thirteen acute) with notes on differential diagnosis, Am. Heart J., 13:129, 1937.

Gore, I., and Siewart, V. J. Dissecting aneurysm of the aorta; pathologic aspects; an analysis of 85 fatal cases, Arch. Path., 53:121, 1952.

Gross, R. E. Coarctation of the aorta, Circulation, 7:757, 1953.

Groves, L. K. Experience with thirteen cases of resection of aneurysms of the descending thoracic aorta, Cleveland Clin. Quart., 28:176, 1961.

Hufnagel, C. A., and Conrad, P. W. Dissecting aneurysms of the ascending aorta: Direct approach to repair, Surgery, 51:84, 1962.

Hume, D. M., and Porter, R. R. Acute dissecting aortic aneurysms, Surgery, 53:322, 1963.

Lam, C. R., and Aram, H. H. Resection of descending thoracic aorta for aneurysm: report of

ANEURYSM OF THE THORACIC AORTA (cont.)

use of homograft in case and an experimental study, Ann. Surg., 134:743, 1951.

Schafer, P. W., and Hardin, C. A. The use of temporary polythene shunts to permit occlusion, resection and frozen homologous graft replacement of vital vessel segments, Surgery, 31:186, 1952.

Stranahan, A., Alley, R. D., Sewell, W. H., and Kausel, H. W. Aortic arch resection and grafting for aneurysm employing an external shunt, J. Thoracic Surg., 29:54, 1955.

Swan, H., Maaske, C., Johnson, M., and Grover, R. Arterial homografts: II. Resection of thoracic aortic aneurysm using a stored human arterial transplant, Arch. Surg., 61:732, 1950.

Warren, W. D., Beckwith, J., and Muller, W. H., Jr. Problems in the surgical management of acute dissecting aneurysm of the aorta, Ann. Surg., 144:530, 1956.

ANEURYSM OF THE ABDOMINAL AORTA

Bahnson, H. T. Considerations in the excision of aortic aneurysms, Ann. Surg., 138:377, 1953.

Barry, K. G., Cohen, A., and LeBlanc, P. Mannitolization. I. The prevention and therapy of oliguria associated with cross-clamping of the abdominal aorta, Surgery, 50:335, 1961.

Beall, A. C., Jr., Holman, M. R., Morris, G. C., Jr., and DeBakey, M. E. Mannitol-induced osmotic diuresis during vascular surgery: renal hemodynamic effects, Arch. Surg., 86:34, 1963.

——— Cooley, D. A., Morris, G. C., Jr., and De Bakey, M. E. Perforation of arteriosclerotic aneurysms into inferior vena cava, Arch. Surg., 86:809, 1963.

Blakemore, A. H. The surgical aspects of aneurysm of the aorta, Ann. Surg., 126:841, 1947.

Brock, R. C. Discussion of reconstructive arterial surgery, Proc. Royal Soc. Med., 46:115, 1953.

Cooley, D. A., and De Bakey, M. E. Ruptured aneurysms of abdominal aorta, excision and homograft replacement, Postgrad. Med., 16: 334, 1954.

De Bakey, M. E., and Cooley, D. A. Surgical treatment of aneurysm of abdominal aorta by resection and restoration of continuity with homograft, Surg., Gynec. & Obst., 97:257, 1953.

——— Cooley, D. A., and Creech, O., Jr. Surgical considerations of acquired diseases of the aorta, Ann. Surg., 139:763, 1954, and 140:290, 1954.

Deterling, R. A., and Bhonslay, S. B. An evaluation of synthetic materials and fabrics suitable for blood vessel replacement, Surgery, 38:71, 1955.

Dubost, C., Allary, M., and Oeconomos, N. Resection of an aneurysm of the abdominal aorta: re-establishment of the continuity by a preserved human arterial graft, with result after five months, Arch. Surg., 64:405, 1952.

Edwards, W. S., and Tapp, J. S. Chemically treated nylon tubes as arterial grafts, Surgery, 38:61, 1955.

Estes, J. E., Jr. Abdominal aortic aneurysm: a study of one hundred and two cases, Circulation, 2:258, 1950.

Hesse, F. G., and Kletschka, H. D. Rupture of abdominal aortic aneurysm: control of hemorrhage by intraluminal balloon tamponade, Ann. Surg., 155:320, 1962.

Hufnagel, C. A. The use of rigid and flexible plastic prostheses for arterial replacement, Surgery, 37:165, 1955.

Humphries, A. W., Young, J. R., de Wolfe, V. G., and Le Fevre, F. A. Complications of abdominal aortic surgery. I. Aortoenteric Fistula, Arch. Surg., 86:43, 1963.

Javid, H., Dye, W. S., Grove, W. J., and Julian, O. C. Resection of ruptured aneurysms of the abdominal aorta, Ann. Surg., 142:613, 1955.

Julian, O. C., Grove, W. J., Dye, W. S., Olwin, J. H., and Sadove, M. S. Direct surgery of arteriosclerosis. Resection of abdominal aorta with homologous aortic graft replacement, Ann. Surg., 138:387, 1953.

Kirklin, J. W., Waugh, J. M., Grindlay, J. H., Openshaw, C. R., and Allen, E. V. Surgical treatment of arteriosclerotic aneurysms of the abdominal aorta, Arch. Surg., 67:632, 1953.

Leriche, R., and Morel, A. The syndrome of thrombotic obliteration of the aortic bifurcation, Ann. Surg., 127:193, 1948.

Merendino, K. A. Ruptured abdominal aneurysm —transthoracic control, Surg., Gynec. & Obst., 103:639, 1956.

Morton, J. J., and Scott, W. J. M. Ligation of the abdominal aorta for aneurysm, Ann. Surg., 119: 457, 1944.

Oudot, J. Deux cas de greffe de la bifurcation aortique pour syndrome de Leriche par thrombose arterique, Mem. Acad. de chir., 77:642, 1951.

——— and Beaconsfield, P. Thrombosis of the aortic bifurcation treated by resection and homograft replacement: report of 5 cases, Arch. Surg., 66:80, 1953.

Perdue, G. D., and Lowry, K. Arterial insufficiency to colon following resection of abdominal aortic aneurysms, Surg., Gynec. & Obst., 115: 39, 1962.

Sautot, J., Jr. The resection of the aortic bifurcation in one stage for thrombosis, Lyon chir., 46:206, 1951.

Savage, C. R. Trans-thoracic aortic control in the management of acute rupture of an abdominal aortic aneurysm, Brit. J. Surg., 47:257, 1959.

Schafer, P. W., and Hardin, C. A. The use of temporary polythene shunts to permit occlusion, resection and frozen homologous graft replacement of vital vessel segments, Surgery, 31:186, 1952.

Schatz, I. J., Fairbairn, J. F., II, and Juergens, J. L. Abdominal Aortic Aneurysms: Reappraisal, Circulation, 26:200, 1962.

Shumacker, H. B., Jr., Harris, E. J., and Siderys, H. Pliable plastic tubes as aortic substitutes, Surgery, 37:80, 1955.

ANEURYSM OF THE ABDOMINAL AORTA (cont.)

Stallworth, J. M., Price, R. G., Jr., Hughes, J. C., III, and Parker, E. F. Surgical treatment of ruptured abdominal aortic aneurysms, Ann. Surg., 155:711, 1962.

Stump, M. M., Jordan, G. L., Jr., DeBakey, M. E., and Halpert, B. The endothelial lining of homografts and dacron prostheses of the canine aorta, Am. J. Path., 40:487, 1962.

Szilagyi, D. E., Smith, R. F., Macksood, A. J., and Eyler, W. R. Abdominal aortography: its value and its hazards, Arch. Surg., 85:25, 1962.

Voorhees, A. B., Jaretzki, A., III, and Blakemore, A. H. The use of tubes constructed from Vinyon "N" cloth in bridging arterial defects, Ann. Surg., 135:332, 1952.

Wesolowski, S. A., Fries, C. C., Karlson, K. E., DeBakey, M. E., and Sawyer, P. N. Porosity: Primary determinant of ultimate fate of synthetic vascular grafts, Surgery, 50:91, 1961.

Wylie, E. J., and McGuinness, J. F. The recognition and treatment of arteriosclerotic stenosis of major arteries, Surg., Gynec. & Obst., 97: 425, 1953.

Young, J. R., Britton, R. C., DeWolfe, V. G., and Humphries, A. W. Intestinal ischemic necrosis following abdominal aortic surgery, Surg., Gynec. & Obst., 115:615, 1962.

——— Humphries, A. W., de Wolfe, V. G., and LeFevre, F. A. Complications of abdominal aortic surgery. II. Intestinal ischemia, Arch., Surg., 86:51, 1963.

ANEURYSM OF THE POPLITEAL ARTERY

Austin, D. J., and Thompson, J. E. Excision and arterial grafting in surgical management of popliteal aneurysms, South. M. J., 51:43, 1958.

Blakemore, A. H. Restorative endoaneurysmorrhaphy by vein graft inlay, Ann. Surg., 126:841, 1947.

Crawford, E. S., Creech, O., Jr., Cooley, D. A., and DeBakey, M. E. Treatment of arteriosclerotic occlusive disease of the lower extremities by excision and graft replacement or by-pass, Surgery, 38:981, 1955.

——— DeBakey, M. E., and Cooley, D. A. Surgical considerations of peripheral arterial aneurysms, Arch. Surg., 78:226, 1959.

Eastcott, H. H. G. Arterial grafting for the ischemic lower limb, Ann. Roy. Coll. Surgeons, England, 13:177, 1953.

Gerbode, F., Holman, E., Dickenson, E. H., and Spencer, F. C. Anteriovenous fistulas and arterial aneurysms, Surgery, 32:259, 1952.

Gifford, R. W., Jr., Hines, E. A., Jr., and Janes, J. M. An analysis and follow-up study of 100 popliteal aneurysms, Surgery, 32:284, 1953.

——— Tarkin, T. W., and Janes, J. M. Atherosclerotic popliteal aneurysm in a man 35 years old, Circulation, 9:363, 1954.

Hufnagel, C. A. The use of rigid and flexible plastic prostheses for arterial replacement, Surgery, 37:165, 1955.

Hunter, J. A., Julian, O. C., Hushang, J., and Dye, S. Arteriosclerotic aneurysms of the popliteal artery, J. Cardiovasc. Surg., 2:404, 1961.

Janes, J. M., and Ivens, J. C. A method of dealing with arteriosclerotic popliteal aneurysms, Surgery, 29:398, 1951.

Johnson, J., Kirby, C. K., Griefenstein, F. E., and Castillo, A. The experimental and clinical use of vein grafts to replace defects of large arteries, Surgery, 26:945, 1949.

Julian, O. C., Dye, W. S., Olwin, J. H., and Jordan, P. H. Direct surgery of arteriosclerosis, Ann. Surg., 136:459, 1952.

——— Dye, W. S., Javid, H., and Grove, W. J. The use of vessel grafts in the treatment of popliteal aneurysms, Surgery, 38:970, 1955.

Linton, R. R. The arteriosclerotic aneurysm: a report of 14 patients treated by preliminary lumbar sympathetic ganglionectomy and aneurysmectomy, Surgery, 26:41, 1949.

——— Some practical considerations in the surgery of blood vessel grafts, Surgery, 38:817, 1955.

Matas, R. Endoaneurysmorrhaphy, Surg., Gynec., & Obst., 30:456, 1920.

McAllister, F. F. Experiences with replacement of segments of diseased femoral and popliteal arteries, Surgery, 38:964, 1955.

Pringle, J. H. Two cases of vein grafting for the maintenance of direct arterial circulation, Lancet, 1:1795, 1913.

Rob, C. G., and Eastcott, H. H. G. Arterial grafting, Brit. Surg. Progress, Supplement to Brit. Surg. Practice, London, Butterworth & Co., Ltd., 1953, p. 1.

Sauvage, L. R., and Weslowski, S. A. The healing and fate of arterial grafts, Surgery, 38: 1090, 1955.

Silverman, J. J., and Hurwitt, E. S. Subcutaneous rupture of a popliteal aneurysm with a diagnostic roentgen sign, Arch. Int. Med., 100:34, 1957.

Watts, S. H. The suture of blood vessels, implantation and transplantation of vessels and organs. An historical and experimental study, Bull. Johns Hopkins Hosp., 18:153, 1907.

ANEURYSM OF COMMON CAROTID ARTERY

Albright, H. L., and VanHale, L. A. Traumatic aneurysms: Study of 43 cases in overseas general hospital, Surgery, 20:452, 1946.

Beall, A. C., Jr., Crawford, E. S., Cooley, D. A., and DeBakey, M. E. Extracranial aneurysms of carotid artery: report of seven cases, Postgrad. Med., 32:93, 1962.

Brackett, C. E. The complications of carotid artery ligation in the neck, J. Neurosurg., 10:91, 1953.

Conley, J. J., and Pack, G. T. Surgical procedure for lessening hazard of carotid bulb excision, Surgery, 31:845, 1952.

Dorrance, G. M. Ligation of the great vessels of the neck, Ann. Surg., 99:721, 1934.

Elkin, D. C., and Campbell, J. L. Aneurysm: A

Aneurysm of Common Carotid Artery (cont.)

review of sixty-two cases, Am. J. Surg., 24:611, 1934.

Ellis, F. H., Jr., and Whisnant, J. P. Occlusions and aneurysms of the cervical carotid arteries, Surg., Gynec. & Obst., 43:1145, 1963.

Inui, F. K., Shannon, J., and Howard, J. M. Arterial injuries in the Korean conflict. Experiences with 111 consecutive injuries, Surgery, 37:850, 1955.

Kirby, C. K., Johnson, J., and Donald, J. G. Aneurysm of the common carotid artery, Ann. Surg., 130:913, 1949.

Mahorner, H., and Spencer, R. Shunt grafts, Ann. Surg., 139:439, 1954.

Matas, R. Discussion on vascular surgery with special reference to surgery of the carotid tracts, Am. J. Surg., 24:692, 1934.

——— Classified summary of 620 operations on the blood vessels for all causes, Tr. Am. S. A., 58:335, 1940.

Pilcher, C., and Thuss, C. Cerebral blood flow. Cerebral effects of occlusion of the common or internal carotid arteries, Arch. Surg., 29:1024, 1934.

Rogers, L. Ligature of arteries, with particular reference to carotid occlusion and circle of Willis, Brit. J. Surg., 35:43, 1947.

Shea, P. C., Glass, L. F., Reid, W. A., and Harland, A. Anastomosis of common and internal carotid arteries following excision of mycotic aneurysm, Surgery, 37:829, 1955.

Spencer, F. C. Aneurysm of the common carotid artery treated by excision and primary anastomosis, Ann. Surg., 145:254, 1957.

Sweet, W. H., and Bennett, H. S. Changes in internal carotid pressure during carotid and jugular occlusion and their clinical significance, J. Neurosurg., 5:178, 1948.

Whalley, N. Traumatic aneurysm of the common carotid artery associated with massive infarction of the brain, Brit. J. Surg., 33:400, 1946.

Williams, M. H. Accidental incision of aneurysm of the left common carotid artery. Treatment by thoracocervical excision with recovery, Ann. Surg., 135:267, 1952.

Reconstructive Arterial Surgery

Bazy, L. A propos du procès-verbel sur l'endarteriectomie désobliterante, Mém. Acad. de chir., 74:109, 1948.

——— Huguier, J., Reboul, H., and Laubry, R. Technique des "endartériectomies" pour artérites oblitérantes chroniques des membres inférieurs, des iliaques et de l'aorte abdominale inférieure, J. de chir., 65:196, 1949.

Cannon, J. A., and Barker, W. F. Successful management of obstructive femoral arteriosclerosis by endarterectomy, Surgery, 38:48, 1955.

Carrel, A. The surgery of blood vessels, Bull. Johns Hopkins Hosp., 18:18, 1907.

Cockett, F. B., and Maurece, B. A. Evolution of direct surgery for claudication and ischemia of legs, Brit. M. J., 1:353, 1963.

Connolly, J. E., Harris, E. J., and Mills, W., Jr. Autogenous in situ saphenous vein for by-pass of femoral-popliteal obliterative disease, Surgery, 55:144, 1964.

Cranley, J. J. Clinical grading of the severity of obliterative arterial disease of the lower extremities, Surgery, 38:928, 1955.

Crawford, E. S., Creech, O., Cooley, D. A., and DeBakey, M. E. Treatment of arteriosclerotic occlusive disease of the lower extremities by excision and graft replacement or by-pass, Surgery, 38:981, 1955.

——— and DeBakey, M. E. The by-pass operation in the treatment of arteriosclerotic occlusive disease of the lower extremities, Surg., Gynec. & Obst., 101:529, 1955.

——— DeBakey, M. E., Morris, G. C., and Garrett, E. Evaluation of late failures after reconstructive operations for occlusive lesions of the aorta and iliac, femoral and popliteal arteries, Surgery, 47:79, 1960.

Dale, W. A., DeWeese, J. A., and Scott, W. J. M. Autogenous venous shunt grafts. Rationale and report of 31 for atherosclerosis, Surgery, 46: 145, 1959.

Darling R. C., and Limton, R. R. Aortoiliofemoral endarterectomy for atherosclerotic occlusive disease, Surgery, 55:184, 1964.

Dos Santos, J. C. Sur la désobstruction des thromboses artérielles anciennes, Mém. Acad. de chir., 73:409, 1947.

Eastcott, H. H. G. Arterial grafting for the ischemic lower limb, Ann. Roy. Coll. Surgery, England, 13:177, 1953.

Edwards, E. A., and LeMay, M. Occlusion patterns and collaterals in arteriosclerosis of the lower aorta and iliac arteries, Surgery, 38:950, 1955.

——— Late occlusion of femoral and popliteal fabric arterial grafts, Surg., Gynec. & Obst., 110:714, 1960.

Fontaine, R., Buck, P., Riveaux, R., Kim, M., and Hubinot, J. Treatment of arterial occlusion, comparative value of thrombectomy, thromboendarterectomy, arteriovenous shunt, and vascular grafts: fresh venous autografts, Lyon chir., 46:73, 1951.

Hafner, C. D., Fogarty, T. J., and Cranley, J. J. Nonsuture anastomosis of small arteries using a tissue adhesive, Surg., Gynec. & Obst., 116: 417, 1963.

Harrison, J. H., and Davalos, P. A. Influence of porosity on synthetic grafts, Arch. Surg., 82:8, 1961.

Hershey, F. B., and Spencer, A. D. Autogenous vein grafts for repair of arterial injuries, Arch. Surg., 86:836, 1963.

Holden, W. D. Reconstruction of the femoral artery for arteriosclerotic thrombosis, Surgery, 27:417, 1950.

Hoye, S. J., and Warren, R. Follow-up studies of iliofemoral arterial reconstruction in arterioscle-

RECONSTRUCTIVE ARTERIAL SURGERY (cont.)

rosis obliterans, New England J. Med., 254: 102, 1956.

Inui, F., Shannon, J., and Howard, J. Arterial injuries in the Korean conflict, Surgery, 37:850, 1955.

Julian, O. C., Dye, W. S., Olwin, J. H., and Jordan, P. H. Direct surgery of arteriosclerosis, Ann. Surg., 136:459, 1952.

——— and Dye, W. S. Treatment of peripheral vascular disease: modern concepts, S. Clin. North America, 32:263, 1952.

Kunlin, J., Bitory-Boely, C., Valne, and Beaudry. Le traitement de l'ischemic arteritique par la greffe veineuse longue, Rév. de chir., Paris, 89: 206, 1951

Lemaire, A., Reboul, H., and Loeper, J. Endarteriectomie désobliterantes de l'aorte, Bull. Soc. méd. hosp., 65:656, 1949.

Leriche, R. Quatorze essais de thrombectomie arteriel suivant la methode de Jean Cid dos Santos, Thrombo-endarteriectomie desobstruante, Mém. Acad. de chir., 74:100, 1948.

Lewis, F. J. Cardiovascular surgery, Surg., Gynec. & Obst., 116:131, 1963.

Linton, R. R. Some practical considerations in the surgery of blood vessel grafts, Surgery, 38:817, 1955.

McAllister, F. F. Experiences with replacement of segments of diseased femoral and popliteal arteries, Surgery, 38:964, 1955.

Mustard, W. T., and Bull, C. A reliable method for relief of traumatic vascular spasm, Ann. Surg., 155:339, 1962.

Phillips, C. E., Jr., DeWeese, J. A., and Carpet, F. C. Comparison of peripheral arterial grafts, Arch. Surg., 82:38, 1961.

Shaw, R. E., and Wheelock, F. Blood vessel grafts in the treatment of chronic occlusive disease in the femoral artery, Surgery, 37:94, 1955.

——— Reconstructive vascular surgery, New England J. Med., 266:339, 1962.

Shucksmith, H. S., and Addison, N. V. Late results of arterial reconstructive surgery, Brit. M. J., 2:1144, 1962.

Spencer, F. C., and Grewe, R. J. The management of arterial injuries in battle casualties, Ann. Surg., 141:304, 1955.

Szilagyi, D. E., Smith, R. F., and Esfahani, A. Arterioplasty for severe ischemia of the lower limbs: indications and results, Surgery, 49:242, 1961.

——— Whitcomb, J. G., and Smith, R. F. Anteromedial approach to the popliteal artery for femoropopliteal arterial grafting, Arch. Surg., 78:647, 1959.

Vogelfanger, I. J., Beattie, W. G., Brown, F. M., Devitt, J. E., Scobie, T. K., and Scobie, D. H. The problem of small vessel anastomosis, Surgery, 52:354, 1962.

Warren, R. Evaluation of thromboendarterectomy for arteriosclerosis obliterans of the femoral artery, Surg., Gynec. & Obst., 104:571, 1957.

Wylie, E. J. Thromboendarterectomy for arteriosclerotic thrombosis of major arteries, Surgery, 32:275, 1952.

——— and McGuinness, J. F. The recognition and treatment of arteriosclerotic stenosis of major arteries, Surg., Gynec. & Obst., 97:425, 1953.

CAROTID THROMBOENDARTERECTOMY AND CAROTID ARTERIAL BYPASS GRAFT

Adams, J. E., Smith, M. C., and Wylie, E. J. Cerebral blood flow and hemodynamics in extracranial vascular disease: effect of endarterectomy, Surgery, 53:449, 1963.

Arnulf, G. Pathologie et chirurgie des carotides, Paris, Masson, 1957, p. 540.

Bahnson, H. T., Spencer, F. C., and Quattelbaum, J. K. Surgical treatment of occlusive disease of the carotid artery, Ann. Surg., 149:711, 1959.

Broadbent, W. H. Absence of pulsation in both radial arteries, vessels being full of blood, Tr. Clin. Soc., London, 8:165, 1875.

Bull, J. W. D., Marshall, J., and Show, D. A. Cerebral angiography in the diagnosis of acute stroke, Lancet, 1:562, 1960.

Chiari, H. Ueber das Verhaltan des Teilungswinkels der Carotis Cummunis bei der Endarteritis Chronica deformans, Verhandl. deutsch. path. Gesellsch., 9:326, 1905.

Crawford, E. S., DeBakey, M. E., Fields, W. S., Cooley, D. A., and Morris, G. C., Jr. Surgical treatment of atherosclerotic occlusive lesions in patients with cerebral arterial insufficiency, Circulation, 20:168, 1949.

Davis, J. R., Grove, W. J., and Julian, O. C. Thrombotic occlusion of the branches of the aortic arch, Martorell's Syndrome: report of a case treated surgically, Ann. Surg., 144:124, 1956.

DeBakey, M. E., Crawford, E. S., Cooley, D. A., and Morris, G. C. Surgical considerations on occlusive diseases of innominate, carotid, subclavin, and vertebral arteries, Ann. Surg., 149: 690, 1959.

——— Crawford, E. S., Morris, G. C., and Cooley, D. A. Surgical considerations of occlusive disease of the innominate, carotid, subclavian and vertebral arteries, Ann. Surg., 154: 698, 1961.

Eastcott, H. H. G., Pickering, G. W. P., and Rob, C. G. Reconstruction of internal carotid artery, Lancet, 2:944, 1954.

Freeman, T. R., and Lippitt, W. H. Carotid artery syndrome, Ann. Surg., 150:1041, 1959.

Fróvig, A. G. Bilateral obliteration of the common carotid artery, thromboangiitis obliterans?, ACTA Psychiatrica et Neurologica, Suppl. 39, p. 1, 1946.

Girard, P. F., Aimard, G., and Bourrat, C. A clinical and anatomical study of thromboses of the internal carotid, J. Cardiovasc. Surg., 2:269, 1961.

Hunt, J. R. The role of the carotid arteries in the

CAROTID THROMBOENDARTERECTOMY AND CAROTID ARTERIAL BYPASS GRAFT (cont.)

causation of vascular lesions of the brain, with remarks on certain special features of the symptomatology, Am. J. M. Sc., 147:704, 1914.

Hurwitt, E. S., Carton, C. A., Fell, S. C., Kessler, L. A., Seidenberg, B., and Shapiro, J. H. Critical evaluation and surgical correction of obstructions in the branches of the aortic arch, Ann. Surg., 152:472, 1960.

Kinney, J. R. Pulseless disease, Am. J. Med., 22: 231, 1957.

Lewis, T., and Stokes, J. A curious syndrome with pulse of neck and arm lost, Brit. Heart J., 4:57, 1942.

Lyons, C., and Galbraith, G. Surgical treatment of atherosclerotic occlusion of the internal carotid artery, Ann. Surg., 146:487, 1957.

Martorell, F., and Fabré, J. El sindrome de obliteración de los troncos supraaórticos, Medicina Clinica, 2:26, 1944.

——— El sindrome de obliteración de los troncos supraaórticos, Angiologia, 11:301, 1959.

——— The syndrome of occlusion of the supraaortic trunks, J. Cardiovasc. Surg., 2:291, 1961.

Moniz, E., Lima, A., and de Lacerda, R. Hemiplegies par thrombose de la carotide interne, Presse Med., 45:977, 1937.

——— Thrombosis y otras obstrucciones de las carótidas, manuales de Medicina Práctica, Salvat Editores, Barcelona, 1941.

Paillas, J., Christophe, L., Bonnal, J., and Thiry, S. Les thromboses de la carotide interne et de ses branches, Rapport présenté à la reunion annuelle de la Société de Neurochirurgie de la langue française, Masson, E., 108, 1955.

Penzolot, F. Über thrombose der carotis, Deutsches Arch. klin. Med., 28:60, 1881.

Powers, S. R., Jr., Drislane, T. M., and Iandoli, E. W. The surgical treatment of vertebral artery insufficiency. Successes and failures, Arch. Surg., 86:60, 1963.

Rob, C. G. The surgical treatment of stenosis and thrombosis of the extracranial portions of the carotid arteries, J. Cardiovasc. Surg., 2:336, 1961.

——— and Wheeler, E. B. Thrombosis of the internal carotid artery treated by arterial surgery, Brit. Med. J., 2:264, 1957.

Ross, R. S., and McKusick, V. A. Aortic arch syndrome, Arch. Int. Med., 92:701, 1953.

Savory, W. S. Case of a young woman in whom the main arteries of both upper extremities and of the left side of the neck were throughout completely obliterated, Med. Chir. Trans., 39: 205, 1856.

Skipper, E., and Flint, F. J. Symmetrical arterial occlusion of upper extremities, head, and neck: a rare syndrome, Brit. Med. J., 2:9, 1952.

Strully, K. J., Hurwitt, E. S., and Blankenberg, H. W. Thrombo-endarterectomy; for thrombosis of the internal carotid artery in the neck, J. Neurosurg., 10:474, 1953.

Takayasu, M. A case of strange anastomosis of the central vessel of the retinae, J. Jap. Ophthal. Soc., 12:554, 1908.

Thompson, J. E., and Austin, D. J. Surgical treatment of arteriosclerotic occlusions of the carotid artery in the neck, Surgery, 51:74, 1962.

Warren, R., and Friedman, L. J. Pulseless disease and carotid-artery thrombosis, Surgical Considerations, New England J. Med., 257:685, 1957.

Wertheimer, P., and Sisteron, A. A radiological study of obstruction of the extracranial carotid arteries, J. Cardiovasc. Surg., 2:284, 1961.

CAROTID GLOMECTOMY

Nakayama, K. Surgical removal of carotid body for bronchial asthma, Dis. Chest., 40:595, 1961.

——— The surgical significance of the carotid body in relation to bronchial asthma, J. Inter. Coll. Surg., 39:374, 1963.

Overholt, R. H. Glomectomy for asthma, Dis. Chest., 40:605, 1961.

——— Resection of carotid body (cervical glomectomy) for asthma, J.A.M.A., 180:809, 1962.

——— Glomectomy for asthma, New York State Med., 63:3372, 1963.

Plangger, V. E., and Ritz, W. The extirpation of the glomus caroticum as a surgical therapy of bronchial asthma, Wien. med. Wchnschr., 111: 182, 1961.

RENAL HYPERTENSION

Anson, B. J., Richardson, G. A., and Minear, W. L. Variations in the number and arrangement of the renal vessels; a study of blood supply of four hundred kidneys, J. Urol., 36:211, 1936.

DeBakey, M. E., Morris, G. C., Jr., Morgen, R. O., Crawford, E. S., and Cooley, D. A. Lesions of the renal artery. Surgical technic and results, Am. J. Surg., 107:84, 1964.

DeCamp, P. T., and Birchell, R. Recognition and treatment of renal arterial stenosis associated with hypertension, Surgery, 43:134, 1958.

Dustan, H. P., Page, I. H., and Poutasse, E. F. Renal hypertension, New England J. Med., 261: 647, 1959.

——— and Page, I. H. Renal hypertensive suspect: clinical characteristics, Am. J. Surg., 107: 35, 1964.

Goldblatt, H., Lynch, G., Hanzel, R. F., and Summerville, W. W. Studies on experimental hypertension: production of persistent elevation of systolic blood pressure by means of renal ischemia, J. Exper. Med., 59:374, 1934.

——— Experimental observations on surgical treatment of hypertension, Surgery, 4:483, 1938.

——— Experimental hypertension induced by renal ischemia; Harvey Lectures, Bull. N. Y. Acad., 14:523, 1938.

——— Studies on experimental hypertension pro-

Renal Hypertension (cont.)

duction of malignant phase of hypertension, J. Exper. Med., 67:809, 1938.

——— The renal origin of hypertension, Physiol. Rev., 27:120, 1947.

——— Hypertension of renal origin. Historical and experimental background, Am. J. Surg., 107:21, 1964.

Howard, J. E., Berthrong, M., Gould, D. M., and Yendt, E. R. Hypertension resulting from unilateral renal vascular disease and its relief by nephrectomy, Bull. Johns Hopkins Hosp., 94: 51, 1954.

——— and Connor, T. B. Use of differential renal function studies in the diagnosis of renovascular hypertension, Amer. J. Surg., 107:58, 1964.

Hurwitt, E. S., Seidenberg, B., Haimovici, H., and Abelson, D. S. Splenorenal arterial anastomoses, Circulation, 14:532, 1956.

Lauler, D. P., and Harrison, J. H. Ureteral catheterization measurements in renal hypertension, Am. J. Surg., 107:67, 1964.

Luke, J. C., and Levitan, B. A. Revascularization of the kidney in hypertension due to renal artery stenosis, Arch. Surg., 79:269, 1959.

——— The useful splenic artery, Surg., Gynec. & Obst., 110:633, 1960.

Margolin, E. G., Merrill, J. P., and Harrison, J. H. Diagnosis of hypertension due to occlusion of renal artery, New England J. Med., 256: 581, 1957.

Morris, G. C., DeBakey, M. E., Cooley, D. A., and Crawford, E. S. Surgical treatment of renal hypertension, Ann. Surg., 151:854, 1960.

——— Surgical treatment of renovascular hypertension, A.M.A. Arch. Surg., 82:723, 1961.

——— Experience with 200 renal artery reconstructive procedures for hypertension or renal failure, Circulation, 27:346, 1963.

Pick, J. W., and Anson, B. J. Renal vascular pedicle: anatomical study of 430 body halves, J. Urol., 44:411, 1940.

Poutasse, E. F., Humphries, A. W., McCormack, L. J., and Corcoran, A. C. Bilateral stenosis of renal arteries and hypertension treated by arterial homografts, J.A.M.A., 161:419, 1956.

——— Surgical treatment of renal hypertension: results in patients with occlusive lesions of renal arteries, J. Urol., 82:403, 1959.

——— Surgical treatment of renal hypertension, Am. J. Surg., 107:97, 1964.

Rob, C. Place of direct surgery in treatment of obliterative arterial disease, Brit. M. J., 2:1027, 1956.

Robertson, C. W. Retrograde aortography in the study of renal lesions, Am. J. Surg., 107:78, 1964.

Spencer, F. C., Stamey, T. A., Bahnson, H. T., and Cohen, A. Diagnosis and treatment of hypertension due to occlusive disease of the renal artery, Ann. Surg., 154:674, 1961.

Stewart, B. H., DeWeese, M. S., Conway, J., and Correa, R. J., Jr. Renal hypertension: An appraisal of diagnostic studies and of direct operative treatment, Arch. Surg., 85:617, 1962.

Thompson, J. E., Austin, D. J., and Wheeler, C. G. Renal artery reconstruction for hypertension, Surgery, 55:42, 1964.

Wylie, E. J., Perloff, D., and Wellington, J. S. Fibromuscular hyperplasis of renal arteries, Ann. Surg., 156:592, 1962.

Ligation of the Superficial Femoral Vein

Anlyan, W. G., Delaughter, G. D., Jr., Fabrikant, J. I., Sullenberger, J. W., and Weaver, W. T. Management of acute venous thromboembolism, J.A.M.A., 168:725, 1958.

Barker, W. F. The management of venous thrombosis and pulmonary embolism, Surgery, 45: 198, 1959.

Butcher, H. R. Anticoagulant drug therapy for thrombophlebitis in the lower extremities: Valuation. Arch. Surg., 80:864, 1960.

Dale, W. A., and Scott, H. W. Grafts of the venous system, Surgery, 53:52, 1963.

De Weese, J. A., and Niguidula, F. The replacement of short segments of veins with functional autogenous venous grafts, Surg., Gynec. & Obst., 110:303, 1960.

Edwards, W. S. Observations on the Pathogenesis and Management of massive venous occlusion, Surgery, 43:153, 1958.

Fontaine, R. Venous thrombosis and its sequelae, Surgery, 41:6, 1957.

Fuller, C. H., Robertson, C. W., and Smithwick, R. H. Management of thromboembolic disease, New England J. Med., 263:983, 1960.

Griffith, G. C., Zinn, W. J., Engelberg, H., Dooley, J. V., and Anderson, R. Heparin versus heparin-bishydroxycoumarin anticoagulant therapy, J.A.M.A., 174:1151, 1960.

Haller, J. A., Jr., and Abrams, B. L. Use of thrombectomy in the treatment of acute iliofemoral venous thrombosis in forty-five patients, Ann. Surg., 158:561, 1963.

John, H. T., and Shepherd, R. C., and Warren, R. Replacement of venous defects, Brit. J. Surg., 48:677, 1961.

Laufman, H. Superiority of heparin over prothrombin depressants in the treatment of thrombophlebitis and its sequelae, S. Clin. North America, 44:195, 1964.

Mahorner, H., Castleberry, J. W., and Coleman, W. A. Attempts to restore function in major veins which are the site of massive thrombosis, Ann. Surg., 146:510, 1957.

——— Treatment of venous thrombosis and its sequelae, Arch. Surg., 85:355, 1962.

Palma, E., and Esperon, R. Vein transplants and grafts in the surgical treatment of the postphlebitic Syndrome, J. Cardiovasc. Surg., 1:94, 1960.

Schauble, J. F., Anlyan, W. G., and Postlethwait, R. W. A study of grafts in the venous system, Arch. Surg., 78:288, 1959.

Ligation of the Inferior Vena Cava

Allen, A. W., Linton, R. R., and Donaldson, G. A. Thrombosis and embolism, Ann. Surg., 118: 728, 1943.

——— Interruption of the deep veins of the lower extremities in the prevention and treatment of thrombosis and embolism, Surg., Gynec. & Obst., 84:519–527, 1947.

——— Management of thromboembolic disease in surgical patients, Surg., Gynec. & Obst., 96: 107, 1953.

Anlyan, W. G., Campbell, F. H., Shingleton, W. W., and Gardner, C. E., Jr. Pulmonary embolism following venous ligation, Arch. Surg., 64:200, 1952.

Bowers, R. F., and Leb, S. M. Late results of inferior vena cava ligation, Surgery, 37:622, 1955.

Boyd, J. F., and Smith, G. Gangrene due to acute massive venous occlusion of a limb, Brit. J. Surg., 44:179, 1956.

Clain, A., and Nussbaum, L. L. Puerperal gangrene, Lancet, 2:290, 1950.

Clifton, E. E., and Neel, J. C. Ligation of the vena cava in extending thrombophlebitis, Arch. Surg., 59:1122, 1949.

Connerley, M. C., and Heintzelman, J. H. C. Treatment and prophylaxis of pulmonary embolism by vein interruption, New England J. Med., 240:830, 1949.

Crutcher, R. R., and Daniel, R. A. Pulmonary embolism—a correlation of clinical and autopsy studies, Surgery, 23:47, 1948.

Dale, W. A. Ligation of the inferior vena cava for thromboembolism, Surgery, 43:24, 1958.

Davies, O. G., and Grimes, O. F. Pseudo-embolic phlebitis (phlegmasia cerulea dolens): a report of two cases, Am. J. Surg., 86:480, 1953.

De Bakey, M. E., and Ochsner, A. Gangrene associated with thrombophlebitis, phlegmasia cerulea dolens, Surgery, 26:16, 1949.

——— A critical evaluation of the problem of thromboembolism, Internat. Abst. Surg., 98:1, 1954.

De Takats, G. Anticoagulant treatment in surgery, J.A.M.A., 142:527, 1950.

Duff, I. F., Linman, J. W., and Birch, R. The administration of heparin, Surg., Gynec. & Obst., 93:343, 1951.

Edwards, W. S. Observations on the pathogenesis and management of massive venous occlusion, Surgery, 43:153, 1958.

Ellis, S. T., and Windham, S. W. Acute massive venous occlusion in the lower extremity, Ann. Surg., 135:262, 1952.

Fogarty, T. J., Cranley, J. J., Krause, R. J., Strasser, E. S., and Hafner, C. D. Surgical management of phlegmasia cerulea dolens, Arch. Surg., 86:256, 1963.

Gage, M. Thromboembolic phenomenon—local process with regional spread and systemic complications, Ann. Surg., 137:577, 1953.

Gibbs, N. M. Venous thrombosis of the lower limbs with particular reference to bed-rest, Brit. J. Surg., 45:15, 1957.

Grant, R. R., and Deddish, M. R. Phlegmasia cerulea dolens and gangrene, New York State J. Med., 52:584–585, 1952.

Grégoire, R. La phlébite bleue (phlegmatia caerulea dolens), Presse méd., 46:1313–1315, 1938.

Haimovici, H., and Suffness, G. Gangrene of the extremities of venous origin: report of a case, Am. J. M. Sc., 215:278–281, 1948.

——— Gangrene of the extremities of venous origin: review of the literature with case reports, Circulation, 1:225–240, 1950.

Halligan, E. J., Costello, J. L., and Lewis, T. F. Acute massive venous occlusion of the lower extremity, Ann. Surg., 137:543–547, 1953.

Hampton, A. O., and Castleman, B. Correlation of chest teleroentgenograms with autopsy findings, Am. J. Radiol., 43:305, 1940.

Homans, J. Thrombosis of the deep veins of the lower leg causing pulmonary embolism, New England J. Med., 211:993, 1934.

——— Venous thrombosis, Surgery, 26:8, 1949.

Kirtley, J. A., Jr., Riddell, D. H., and Hamilton, E. C. Indications and late results of ligation of inferior vena cava, Ann. Surg., 141:653, 1955.

Madden, J. L. Ligation of the inferior vena cava, Ann. Surg., 140:200, 1954.

——— Venous thrombosis and thromboembolism, Am. J. Surg., 87:909, (June) 1954.

Mahorner, H. A new method of management of thrombosis of deep veins of the extremities: thrombectomy, restoration of the lumen and heparinization, Am. Surgeon, 20:487, 1954.

Manheimer, L. H., and Levin, L. M. Phlegmasia cerulea dolens. Report of two cases and discussion of pathogenesis, Angiology, 5:472, 1954.

McLachlin, J., and Paterson, J. C. Some basic observations on venous thrombosis and pulmonary embolism, Surg., Gynec. & Obst., 93:1, 1951.

——— Richards, T., and Paterson, J. C. Evaluation of clinical signs in diagnosis of venous thrombosis, Arch. Surg., 85:738, 1962.

Miles, R. M. Phlegmasia cerulea dolens. Successful treatment by vena cava ligation, Surgery, 30:718, 1951.

Moore, R. F., and Scott, G. B. D. Gangrene of venous origin, Brit. J. Surg., 43:591, 1956.

Moses, W. R. Ligation of the inferior vena cava or iliac veins: a report of thirty-six operations, New England J. Med., 235:1, 1946.

Murray, G. Anticoagulants in venous thrombosis and the prevention of pulmonary embolism, Surg., Gynec. & Obst., 84:665, 1947.

Northway, R. O., and Buxton, R. W. Caval ligation in phlebothrombosis, Surgery, 18:85, 1945.

Núñez Núñez, A., Milanés, B., De La Vega, L. M., Vázquez, G., and Iñigo, J. R. Acute massive venous occlusion of the lower extremities. Report of two cases, Angiology, 3:386–391, 1952.

Oaks, W., and Hawthorne, H. Pseudo-embolic phlebitis with ligation of the inferior vena cava. A case report, Ann. Surg., 127:1247, 1948.

LIGATION OF THE INFERIOR VENA CAVA (cont.)

Ochsner, A., and De Bakey, M. E. Thrombophlebitis and phlebothrombosis, South. Surgeon, 8:269–290, 1939.

——— and De Bakey, M. E. Thrombophlebitis: the role of vasospasm in the production of clinical manifestations, J.A.M.A., 114:117, Jan. 13, 1940.

——— and De Bakey, M. E. Therapeutic considerations of thrombophlebitis and phlebothrombosis, New England J. Med., 225:207–227, 1941.

Osius, E. A. Acute massive venous occlusion, Arch. Surg., 65:19–30, 1952.

Owens, F. M., Jr. Vena cava ligation in thromboembolic disease, Arch. Surg., 65:600, 1952.

Payne, J. T. Indications for ligation of the inferior vena cava in venous thrombosis, Arch. Surg., 67:902, 1953.

Perlow, S. Phlegmasia cerulea dolens—massive venous thrombosis associated with shock, J.A.M.A., 144:1257, 1950.

Proceedings of First International Congress on Thrombosis and Embolism, Basel, 1954, Basel, Schwabe, 1955.

Rasmussen, J. A., Potter, S. E., and Best, R. R. The management of acute massive venous occlusion, Surgery, 40:387, 1956.

Ravdin, I. S., and Kirby, C. K. Experiences with ligation and heparin in thromboembolic disease, Surgery, 29:334, 1951.

Ray, C. T., and Burch, G. Vascular responses in man to ligation of the inferior vena cava, Arch. Int. Med., 80:587, 1947.

Robinson, J. R., and Moyer, C. A. Comparison of late sequelae of common and superficial femoral vein ligation, Surgery, 35:690, 1954.

Shea, P. C., Jr., and Robertson, R. L. Late sequelae of inferior vena cava ligation, Surg., Gynec. & Obst., 93:153, 1951.

Spencer, F. C., Quattlebaum, J. K., Quattlebaum, J. K., Jr., Sharp, E. H., and Jude, J. R. Plication of inferior vena cava for pulmonary embolism: report of 20 cases, Ann. Surg., 155: 827, 1962.

Thebaut, B. R., and Ward, C. S. Ligation of the inferior vena cava in thromboembolism; report of 36 cases, Surg., Gynec. & Obst., 84:385, 1947.

Thompson, N. Surgical treatment of chronic lymphodema of the lower limb; with preliminary report of new operation, Brit. M. J., 2:1566, 1962.

Tilley, J. H. Gangrene of the extremities in peripheral thrombophlebitis, Am. J. Obst. & Gynec., 36:157, 1938.

Trémolières, F., and Véran, P. Syndrome d'oblitération artérielle du membre inferieur droit apparu au cours d'une phlébite superficielle et profonde avec embolies pulmonaires. Effec thérapeutique de l'acetylcholine, Bull. méd., Paris, 43:1101–1105, 1929.

Veal, J. R., Hussey, H. H., and Barnes, E. Ligation of the inferior vena cava in thrombosis of the deep veins of the lower extremities, Surg., Gynec. & Obst., 84:605, 1947.

——— Dugan, T. J., Jamison, W. C., and Bauersfeld, R. S. Acute massive venous occlusion of the lower extremities, Surgery, 29:355, 1951.

Veith, F. J., Marshall, D. C., and Crane, C. A Technique for ligation of the inferior vena cava, Surg., Gynec. & Obst., 119:109–112, 1964.

Young, R. L., and Derbyshire, R. C. Ligation of the inferior vena cava during pregnancy, Ann. Surg., 131:252, 1950.

Zollinger, R., and Teachnor, W. A. Late results of inferior vena caval ligations, Arch. Surg., 65:31, 1952.

CIRCUMFERENTIAL VEIN LIGATION

Andersen, N. N., and McDonald, K. E. Results of surgical therapy of sever stasis ulceration of the legs, Ann. Surg., 157:281, 1963.

Bauer, G. The patho-physiology and treatment of the lower leg stasis syndrome, Angiology, 1:1, 1950.

Madden, J. L., and Kim, M. Circumferential venous ligation in the treatment of the postphlebitic ulcer, Surgery, 53:90, 1963.

PORTAL HYPERTENSION, PORTACAVAL AND SPLENORENAL SHUNTS

Arcari, F. A., and Lynn, H. B. Bleeding esophageal varices in children, Surg., Gynec. & Obst., 112:101, 1961.

Baronofsky, I. D. Portal hypertension with special reference to the acid-peptic factor in the causation of hemorrhage and extensive gastric resection in its treatment, Surgery, 25:135, 1949.

Berman, J. K., and Hull, J. E. Hepatic, splenic and left gastric arterial ligations in advanced portal cirrhosis, Arch. Surg., 65:37, 1952.

Blakemore, A. H., and Lord, J. W., Jr. The technic of using vitallium tubes in establishing portacaval shunts for portal hypertension, Ann. Surg., 122:476, 1945.

——— Indications for portacaval anastomosis—analysis of cases, Surg., Gynec. & Obst., 84:645, 1947.

——— Portacaval shunting for portal hypertension, Surg., Gynec. & Obst., 94:443, 1952.

Blalock, A. The use of shunt or by-pass operations in the treatment of certain circulatory disorders including portal hypertension and pulmonic stenosis, Ann. Surg., 125:129, 1947.

Boerema, I. Chirurgische Hulp By Bloedingen uit Varices van de Oesophagus By Lever-Cirrhose on By Het Syndrom van Banti, Arch. chir., neerl., 1:4174, 1949.

Britton, R. C., Brown, C. H., and Shirey, E. K. Intrahepatic veno-occlusive disease in cirrhosis with chronic ascites: diagnosis by hepatic phlebography and results of surgical treatment, Ann. Surg., 158:370, 1963.

Chalmers, T. C., Zamcheck, N., Curtins, G. W., and White, F. W. Fatal gastrointestinal hemorrhage: clinicopathologic correlations in 101 pa-

Portal Hypertension, Portacaval and Splenorenal Shunts (cont.)

tients, Am. J. Clin. Path., 22:634, 1952.

Child, C. G., III. The Hepatic Circulation and Portal Hypertension, Philadelphia, W. B. Saunders Co., 1954.

——— Eck's fistula, Surg., Gynec. & Obst., 96:375, 1953.

——— Portal circulation, New England J. Med., 252:837, 1955.

Cooley, D. A. Side-to-side splenorenal anastomosis with splenic preservation for portal hypertension, Surg., Gynec. & Obst., 116:626, 1963.

Crile, G., Jr. Transesophageal ligation of bleeding esophageal varices, Arch. Surg., 61:654, 1950.

——— Treatment of esophageal varices by transesophageal obliteration, Surg., Gynec. & Obst., 96:537, 1953.

Crosby, R. C., and Cooney, E. A. Surgical treatment of ascites, New England J. Med., 235: 581, 1946.

DeMartel, M. F. Report of an Eck fistula in a woman, Rev. de chir., Paris, 42:1181, 1910.

Dock, W. The role of increased hepatic arterial flow in the portal hypertension of cirrhosis, Tr. A. Am. Physicians, 77:302, 1942.

Douglas, B. E., and Snell, A. M. Portal cirrhosis: an analysis of 444 cases with notes on the modern methods of treatment, Gastroenterology, 15:407, 1950.

Dumont, A. E., and Mulholland, J. H. Alterations in thoracic duct lymph flow in hepatic cirrhosis: significance in portal hypertension, Ann. Surg., 156:668, 1962.

Eck, N. V. K. voprosu o perevyaskie vorotnois veni. Predvaritelnoye soobshtshjenye (Ligature of the portal vein), Voen. med. J., St. Petersburg, 130(2):1–2, 1877.

Ekman, C. A. Portal hypertension, Acta. Chir. Scan., supp. 222, 1957.

Ferguson, D. J. Hemodynamics in surgery for portal hypertension, Ann. Surg., 158:383, 1963.

Fine, J., Seligman, A. M., and Frank, H. A. On specific role of liver in hemorrhagic shock: report of progress to date, Ann. Surg., 126:1002, 1947.

Hallenbeck, G. A., Comess, M. S., Wollaeger, E. E., and Gage, R. P. Bleeding varices due to cirrhosis: survival after (1) non-surgical treatment, (2) splenectomy with or without omentopexy, and (3) portacaval and splenorenal shunts, Arch. Surg., 78:774, 1959.

——— Wollaeger, E. E., Adson, M. A., and Gage, R. P. Results after porta-systemic shunts in 120 patients with cirrhosis of the liver, Surg., Gynec. & Obst., 116:435, 1963.

Hamilton, J. E. The management of bleeding esophageal varices associated with cirrhosis of the liver, Ann. Surg., 141:637, 1955.

Herrick, F. C. An experimental study into the cause of the increased portal pressure in portal cirrhosis, J. Exper. Med., 9:93, 1907.

Imanaga, H., Yamamoto, S., and Kuroyanagi, Y. Surgical treatment of portal hypertension according to the state of intrahepatic circulation, Ann. Surg., 155:42, 1962.

Johns, T. N. P. A comparison of suture with nonsuture methods for the anastomosis of veins, Surg., Gynec. & Obst., 84:939, 1947.

Kelty, R. H., Baggenstoss, A. H., and Butt, H. R. The relation of the regenerated hepatic nodule to the vascular bed in cirrhosis, Proc. Staff Meet., Mayo Clin., 25:17, 1950.

Krook, H. Circulatory studies in liver cirrhosis, Acta. Med. Scan., supp. 318, 1956.

Large, A., Johnston, C. G., and Preshaw, D. E. The portacaval venous shunt, Ann. Surg., 135: 22, 1952.

Lempke, R. E., Kaiser, G. C., King, R. D., and King, H. Autogenous ascitic infusion in the management of cirrhotic surgical patient, J.A.M.A., 183:347, 1963.

Linton, R. R., Jones, C. M., and Volwiler, W. Portal hypertension: treatment by splenectomy and splenorenal anastomoses with preservation of kidney, S. Clin. North America, 27:1162, 1947.

——— Hardy, I. B., Jr., and Wade, V. Portacaval shunts in the treatment of portal hypertension, Surg., Gynec. & Obst., 87:129, 1948.

——— The selection of patients for portacaval shunts, Ann. Surg., 134:433, 1951.

——— and Warren, R. The emergency treatment of massive bleeding from esophageal varices by transesophageal suture of these vessels at the time of acute hemorrhage, Surgery, 33:243, 1954.

——— Ellis, D. S., and Geary, J. E. Critical comparative analysis of early and late results of splenorenal and direct portacaval shunts performed in 169 patients with portal cirrhosis, Ann. Surg., 154:446, 1961

Longmire, W. P., Jr., Mulder, D. G., Mahoney, P. S., and Mellinkoff, S. W. Side-to-side portacaval anastomosis for portal hypertension, Ann. Surg., 147:881, 1958.

Madden, J. L. Ligation of the hepatic and splenic arteries in the treatment of cirrhosis of the liver, Surg., Gynec. & Obst., 96:594, 1953.

——— Loré, J. M., Gerold, F. P., and Ravid, J. M. The pathogenesis of ascites and a consideration of its treatment, Surg., Gynec. & Obst., 99:385, 1954.

——— End-to-side portacaval shunt, Arch. Surg., 74:978, 1957.

——— The pathogenesis of ascites and its surgical treatment, J. Louisiana M. Soc., 115:157, 1963.

Mahoney, E. B., and Hogg, L., Jr., Congenital stricture of the portal vein, Arch. Surg., 61: 713, 1950.

Markowitz, J., Rappaport, A. M., and Scott, A. C. Prevention of liver necrosis following ligation of hepatic artery, Proc. Soc. Exper. Biol. & Med., 20:305, 1949.

McDermott, W. V., Jr., Adams, R. D., and Riddell, A. G. Ammonia metabolism in man, Ann. Surg., 140:539, 1954.

——— The double portacaval shunt in the treat-

Portal Hypertension, Portacaval and Splenorenal Shunts (cont.)

ment of cirrhotic ascites, Surg., Gynec. & Obst., 110:457, 1960.

McIndoe, A. H. Vascular lesions of portal cirrhosis, Arch. Path., 5:23, 1928.

Mikkelsen, W. P., Turrill, F. L., and Pattison, A. C. Portacaval shunt in cirrhosis of the liver: Clinical and hemodynamic aspects, Am. J. Surg., 104:204, 1962.

Murray, J. F., and Mulder, D. G. The effects of retrograde portal venous flow following side-to-side portacaval anastomosis: a comparison with end-to-side shunts, J. Clin. Invest., 40: 1413, 1961.

Nachlas, M. M., O'Neil, J. E., and Campbell, A. J. A. The life history of patients with cirrhosis of the liver and bleeding esophageal varices, Ann. Surg., 141:10, 1955.

Orloff, M. J. A comparative study of emergency transesophageal ligation and non-surgical treatment of bleeding esophageal varices in unselected patients with cirrhosis, Surgery, 52: 103, 1962.

Patek, A. J., Jr., Post, J., Ratnoff, O. D., Mankin, H. D., and Hillman, R. W. Dietary treatment of cirrhosis of the liver. Results in one hundred and twenty-four patients observed during a ten-year period, J.A.M.A., 138:543, 1948.

Patton, T. B., and Johnston, C. G. A method of control of bleeding from esophagal varices, Arch. Surg., 59:502, 1949.

Phemister, D. B., and Humphries, E. M. Gastro-esophageal resection and total gastrectomy in treatment of bleeding varicose veins in Banti's Syndrome, Ann. Surg., 126:397, 1947.

Phillips, E. G., Schwartz, R., Gabuzda, G. J., and Davidson, C. S. Syndrome of impending hepatic coma in patients with cirrhosis of liver given certain nitrogenous substances, New England J. Med., 274:239, 1952.

Ratnoff, O. D., and Patek, A. J., Jr. The natural history of Laennec's cirrhosis of the liver. An analysis of 386 cases, Medicine, 21:207, 1942.

Reinhoff, W. F. Ligation of the hepatic and splenic arteries in the treatment of portal hypertension with a report of six cases, Bull. Johns Hopkins Hosp., 88:368, 1951.

——— and Woods, A. C., Jr. Ligation of the hepatic and splenic arteries in the treatment of cirrhosis with ascites, J.A.M.A., 152:687, 1953.

Reynolds, T. B., Mikkelsen, W. P., Redecker, A. G., and Yamahiro, H. S. The effects of a side-to-side portacaval shunt on hepatic hemodynamics in cirrhosis, J. Clin. Invest., 41:1242, 1962.

Riddell, A. C., Kopple, P. N., and McDermott, W. V., Jr. Etiology of "meat intoxication" in Eck fistula. Dog. Surgery, 36:675, 1954.

——— and Jones, W. K. Studies in portal hypertension, Brit. M. J., 1:928, 1961.

Ripstein, C. B. Experiences with portacaval anastomosis in the treatment of portal hypertension, Surgery, 34:571, 1953.

Rosenstein, P. Über die Behandlung der Leber Cirrhose durch Aulegung einer Eck'schen Fistul, Arch. klin. Chir., 98:1082, 1912.

Rousselot, L. M. The role of congestion (portal hypertension) in so-called Banti's Syndrome, J.A.M.A., 107:178, 1937.

——— Congestive splenomegaly (Banti's Syndrome), the medical-surgical splenopathies, Bull. New York Acad. Med., 2nd Series, 15: 188, 1939.

——— The late phase of congestive splenomegaly (Banti's Syndrome) with hematemesis but without cirrhosis of the liver, Surgery, 8:34, 1940.

Rowntree, L., Zimmerman, E. F., Todd, M. H., and Ajac, J. Intraesophageal venous tamponage, J.A.M.A., 135:630, 1947.

Sengstaken, R. W., and Blakemore, A. H. Balloon tamponage for the control of hemorrhage from esophageal varices, Ann. Surg., 131:781, 1950.

Smith, R. M., and Farber, S. Splenomegaly in children with early hematemesis, J. Pediat., 7:585, 1935.

Som, M. L., and Garlock, J. H. New approach to the treatment of esophageal varices, J.A.M.A., 135:628, 1947.

Turunen, M., Pasila, M., and Sulamaa, M. (Helsinki). Supradiaphragmatic transposition of the spleen for portal hypertension: a clinical study, Ann. Surg., 157:127, 1963.

Vidal, M. E. Discussion of deMartel's case, Rev. de Chir., Paris., 42:1181, 1910.

Voorhees, A. B., and Blakemore, A. H. Clinical experience with the superior mesenteric vein-inferior vena caval shunt in the treatment of portal hypertension, Surgery, 51:35, 1962.

Walshe, J. M. Effect of glutamic acid on coma of hepatic failure, Lancet, 1:1075, 1953.

Warren, W. D., Restrepo, J. E., Respess, J. C., and Muller, W. H. The importance of hemodynamic studies in management of portal hypertension, Ann. Surg., 158:387, 1963.

Welch, C. S. Portal hypertension, New England J. Med., 243:598, 1950.

——— Ligation of esophageal varices by the transabdominal route, New England J. Med., 255:677, 1956.

——— Kiley, J. E., Reeve, T. S., Goodrich, E. O., and Welch, H. F. Treatment of bleeding from portal hypertension in patients with cirrhosis of liver, New England J. Med., 254:493, 1956.

——— Welch, H. F., and Carter, J. H. The treatment of ascites by side-to-side portacaval shunt, Ann. Surg., 150:428, 1959.

Whipple, A. O. The problem of portal hypertension in relation to the hepato-splenopathies, Ann. Surg., 122:449, 1945.

Transaxillary, Transpleural Sympathetic Ganglionectomy

Adson, A. W., and Brown, G. E. The treatment of Raynaud's disease by resection of the upper thoracic and lumbar sympathetic ganglia and trunks, Surg., Gynec. & Obst., 48:577, 1929.

Transaxillary, Transpleural Sympathetic Ganglionectomy (cont.)

Atkins, H. J. B. Peraxillary approach to the stellate and upper thoracic sympathetic ganglia, Lancet, 2:1152, 1949.

——— Sympathectomy by the axillary approach, Lancet, 1:538, 1954.

Barcroft, H., and Hamilton, G. T. C. Results of sympathectomy of the upper limb, with special reference to Raynaud's disease, Lancet, 1:441, 1948.

Barnes, R. The role of sympathectomy in the treatment of causalgia, J. Bone & Joint Surg., 35–B:172, 1953.

Crandell, W. B., and Bosien, W. R. Transaxillary approach for upper thoracic sympathetic ganglionectomy, Ann. Surg., 142:28, 1955.

Fulton, J. F. Physiology of the Nervous System. New York, Oxford, 1938.

Goetz, R. H., and Marr, J. A. S. The importance of the second thoracic ganglion for the sympathetic supply of the upper extremities with a description of two new approaches for its removal, Clin. Proc., Cape Town, 3:102, 1944.

——— Collective Review: the surgical physiology of the sympathetic nervous system with special reference to cardiovascular disorders, Surg., Gynec. & Obst., Int. Abst. Surg., 87: 417, 1948.

——— Diagnosis and treatment of vascular disease, Brit. J. Surg., 37:146, 1949.

Guttman, L. The distribution of disturbances of sweat secretion after extirpation of certain sympathetic cervical ganglia in man, J. Anat., 74: 537, 1940.

Hoffman, H. H. An analysis of the sympathetic trunk and rami in the cervical and upper thoracic region in man, Ann. Surg., 145:94, 1957.

Kuntz, A. Distribution of the sympathetic rami to the brachial plexus, Arch. Surg., 15:871, 1927.

——— Alexander, W. F., and Furculo, C. L. Complete sympathetic denervation of the upper extremity, Ann. Surg., 107:25, 1938.

——— and Dillon, J. B. Preganglionic components of the first thoracic nerve; their role in the sympathetic innervation of the upper extremity, Arch. Surg., 44:772, 1942.

Livingston, W. K. Pain Mechanisms: A Physiologic Interpretation of Causalgia and its Related States. New York, Macmillan, 1943.

Mayfield, F. H., and Devine, J. W. Causalgia, Surg., Gynec. & Obst., 80:631, 1945.

Palumbo, L. T. New surgical approach for upper thoracic sympathectomy, A.M.A. Arch. Surg., 76:807, 1958.

——— Anterior transthoracic approach for upper thoracic sympathectomy, A.M.A. Arch. Surg., 72:659, 1956.

——— A new concept of the sympathetic pathways to the eye. A new technique to avoid a Horner's Syndrome, Surgery, 42:740, 1957.

Peddie, G. H., and Longmore, D. B. The treatment of hyperhidrosis by upper dorsal sympathectomy through an axillary approach, Am. Surg., 24:959, 1958.

Ray, B. S. Sympathectomy of the upper extremity, J. Neurosurg., 10:624, 1953.

Sheehan, D. On the innervation of the blood vessels of the upper extremity: Some anatomical considerations, Brit. J. Surg., 20:412, 1933.

Shumacker, H. B., and Abramson, D. I. Posttraumatic vasomotor disorders: with particular reference to late manifestations and treatment, Surg., Gynec. & Obst., 88:417, 1949.

Simmons, H. T., and Sheehan, D. The causes of relapse following sympathectomy of the arm, Brit. J. Surg., 27:234, 1939.

Smithwick, R. H. Modified dorsal sympathectomy for vascular spasm (Raynaud's disease) of the upper extremity, preliminary report, Ann. Surg., 104:339, 1936.

——— The problem of producing complete and lasting sympathetic denervation of the upper extremity by preganglionic section, Ann. Surg., 112:1085, 1940.

Telford, E. D. The technique of sympathectomy, Brit. J. Surg., 23:448, 1935.

White, J. C., Smithwick, R. H., and Simeone, F. The Autonomic Nervous System: Anatomy, Physiology and Surgical Application, 3rd ed. New York, Macmillan, 1952, p. 569.

Lumbar Sympathetic Ganglionectomy

Atlas, L. N. Lumbar sympathectomy in the treatment of selected cases of peripheral arteriosclerotic disease, Am. Heart J., 22:75, 1941.

——— The growth of collateral arterial circulation in the sympathectomized arteriosclerotic leg—an oscillometric study, Surgery, 33:268, 1953.

Beaconfield, P. Effect of exercise on muscle blood flow in normal and sympathectomized limbs: B. Collateral circulation before and after sympathectomy, Ann. Surg., 140:786, 1954.

Bergan, J. J., and Trippel, O. H. Arteriograms in ischemic limbs worsened after lumbar sympathectomy, Arch. Surg., 85:643, 1962.

Berry, R. E. L., Flotte, C. T., and Coller, F. A. A critical evaluation of lumbar sympathectomy for peripheral arteriosclerotic vascular disease, Surgery, 37:115, 1955.

Blain, A. III, Zadeh, A. T., Teves, M. L., and Bing, R. J. Lumbar sympathectomy for arteriosclerosis obliterans, Surgery, 53:164, 1963.

De Bakey, M. E., Creech, O., and Woodhall, J. P. Evaluation of sympathectomy in arteriosclerotic peripheral vascular disease, J.A.M.A., 144: 1227, 1950.

De Takats, G., Fowler, E. F., Jordan, P., and Risley, T. C. Sympathectomy in the treatment of peripheral vascular sclerosis, J.A.M.A., 131: 495, 1946.

LUMBAR SYMPATHETIC GANGLIONECTOMY (cont.)

Edwards, E. A., and Crane, C. Lumbar sympathectomy for arteriosclerosis of the lower extremities, New England J. Med., 244:199, 1951.

Flothow, P. E. Anterior extraperitoneal approach to lumbar sympathetic nerves, Am. J. Surg., 29:23, 1935.

Freeman, N. E., Leeds, F. H., and Gardner, R. E. Sympathectomy for obliterative arterial disease; Indications and contraindications, Ann. Surg., 126:873, 1947.

Grimson, K. S., D'Angelo, G. J., Zavaleta, A. A., and Hustead, A. P. Lower thoracic and lumbar sympathectomy for arteriosclerotic obliterative disease of the lower aorta or the iliac arteries, Surgery, 37:146, 1955.

Julian, O. C., and Shabart, E. J. Lumbar sympathectomy in peripheral vascular disease, Arch. Surg., 61:804, 1950.

Lilly, G. D., Smith, D. W., Biggane, C. F., Jr., and Jana, J. T., Jr. An evaluation of "high" lumbar sympathectomy in arteriosclerotic circulatory insufficiency of the lower extremities, Surgery, 35:1, 1954.

Lindstrom, B. L. The effect of high lumbar sympathectomy in patients with organic arterial disease of the lower limb, previously treated with low lumbar sympathectomy, Act. chir. Scandinav., 103:370, 1952.

Luke, J. C. Value of lumbar sympathectomy in intermittent claudication, Surgery, 41:165, 1957.

Mackenzie, D. D., and Lowenthal, J. Lumbar sympathectomy and claudification distance, Surg., Gynec. & Obst., 115:303, 1962.

Madden, J. L. Technic for lumbar sympathetic ganglionectomy, Am. J. Surg., 83:695, 1952.

Nelson, A. R., and Trimble, I. R. A critique on the therapeutic value of lumbar sympathectomy, Surgery, 39:797, 1956.

Palumbo, L. T., and Lulu, D. J. Lumbar sympathectomy in peripheral vascular diseases, Arch. Surg., 86:512, 1963.

Pearl, F. L. Muscle-splitting extraperitoneal lumbar ganglionectomy, Surg., Gynec. & Obst., 65: 107, 1937.

——— and Michels, L. M. Lumbar sympathectomy for advanced occlusive peripheral arteriosclerosis, J. Internat. Coll. Surgeons, 18:422, 1952.

Pratt, G. H. Surgical sympathectomy for obliterative vascular disease, N. Y. State J. Med., 54: 3357, 1954.

Royle, N. D. The treatment of spastic paralysis by sympathetic ramisection. Experimental basis and clinical results, Surg., Gynec. & Obst., 39: 701, 1924.

Simmons, H. T., and Sheehan, D. An inquiry into "relapse" following sympathectomy, Lancet, 2: 788, 1937.

Smith, R. G., Gullickson, M., and Campbell, D. A. Some limitations of lumbar sympathectomy in arteriosclerosis obliterans, Arch. Surg., 64:103, 1952.

Smithwick, R. H. The rationale and technique of sympathectomy for the relief of vascular spasm of the extremities, New England J. Med., 222: 699, 1940.

——— Lumbar sympathectomy in the treatment of obliterative vascular disease of the lower extremities, Surgery, 42:415–430; 567–578, 1957.

Telford, E. D., and Simmons, H. T. Sympathectomy in peripheral arteriosclerosis, Brit. M. J., 1:386, 1946.

Tracy, G. D., and Cockett, F. B. Pain in lower limb after sympathectomy, Lancet, 1:12, 1957.

Yeager, G. H., and Cowley, R. A. Anatomical observation on the lumbar sympathetics with evaluation of sympathectomies in organic peripheral vascular disease, Ann. Surg., 127:953, 1948.

MODIFIED KONDOLÉON OPERATION

Aird, I. Treatment of chronic oedema of the leg, Proc. Roy. Soc. Med., 43:1052, 1950.

Allen, E. V. Lymphedema of the extremities. Classification, etiology and differential diagnosis. A study of three hundred cases, Arch. Int. Med., 54:606–624, 1934.

Auchincloss, H. A new operation for elephantiasis, Puerto Rico J. Pub. Health & Trop. Med., 6: 149–150, 1930.

Boyd, A. M. Treatment of chronic oedema of the leg, Proc. Roy. Soc. Med., 43:1045, 1950.

Carnochan, J. M. Elephantiasis arabum of the right inferior extremity, successfully treated by ligature of the femoral artery. Part First, New York J. Med., 9:162–169, 1852.

Drinker, C. K., Field, M. E., and Homans, J. The experimental production of edema and elephantiasis as a result of lymphatic obstruction, Am. J. Physiol., 108:509–520, 1934.

——— Field, M. E., Ward, H. K., and Lyons, C. Increased susceptibility of local infection following blockage of lymph drainage, Am. J. Physiol., 112:74–81, 1935.

——— The Relation of Lymph Circulation to Streptococcic Infection. Medical Papers Dedicated to Henry Asbury Christian, Baltimore, Waverly Press, Inc., 1936, pp. 705–710.

Ghormley, R. K., and Overton, L. M. The surgical treatment of severe forms of lymphedema (elephantiasis) of the extremities: a study of end results, Surg., Gynec. & Obst., 61:83–89, 1935.

Gibson, T., and Tough, J. S. Surgical correction of chronic lymphedema of legs, Brit. J. Plastic Surg., 7:159, 1954.

Gillies, H., and Fraser, F. R. Treatment of lymphoedema by plastic operation. (A preliminary report), Brit. M. J., 1:96–98, 1935.

——— The lymphatic wick, Proc. Roy. Soc. Med., 43:1054, 1950.

Modified Kondoléon Operation (cont.)

Halsted, W. S. The swelling of the arm after operations for cancer of the breast. Elephantiasis chirurgica—its cause and prevention, Bull. Johns Hopkins Hosp., 32:309–313, 1921.

Handley, W. S. Lymphangioplasty: a new method for the relief of the brawny arm of breast-cancer and for similar conditions of lymphatic oedema, Lancet, 1:783–785, 1908.

Homans, J., Drinker, C. K., and Field, M. E. Elephantiasis and the clinical implications of its experimental reproduction in animals, Ann. Surg., 100:812–832, 1934.

——— The treatment of elephantiasis of the legs. A preliminary report, New England J. Med., 215:1099–1104, 1936.

Keysser. Zur operativen Behandlung der Elephantiasis, Deutsche Ztschr. f. Chir., 203:356–375, 1927.

Kinmonth, J. B., and Taylor, G. W. The lymphatic circulation in lymphedema, Ann. Surg., 139: 129, 1954.

Kondoléon, E. Die operative Behandlung der Elephantiastischen Oedeme, Zentralbl. f. Chir., 39: 1022, 1912.

——— Die chirurgische Behandlung der elefantiastischen Oedeme durch eine neue methode der Lymphableitung, München. med. Wchnsch., 59:2726, 1912.

Macey, H. B. A new surgical procedure for lymphedema of the extremities: report of a case, Proc. Staff Meet., Mayo Clin., 15:49–52, 1940.

——— A surgical procedure for lymphedema of extremities—follow-up report, J. Bone & Joint Surg., 30A:339, 1948.

Matas, R. The surgical treatment of elephantiasis and elephantoid states dependent upon chronic obstruction of the lymphatic and venous channels, Am. J. Trop. Dis. & Prev. Med., 1:60–85, 1913.

McIndoe, A. H. Treatment of chronic oedema of the leg, Proc. Roy. Soc. Med., 43:1043, 1950.

Poth, E. J., Barnes, S. R., and Ross, G. T. A new operative treatment for elephantiasis, Surg., Gynec. & Obst., 84:642, 1947.

Pratt, G. H., and Wright, I. S. Surgical treatment of chronic lymphoedema (elephantiasis), Surg., Gynec. & Obst., 72:244, 1941.

Reichert, F. L. Circulator disturbances of the extremities. With special reference to thromboangiitis obliterans and elephantoid conditions, California & West. Med., 31:233–237, 1929.

Sistrunk, W. E. Elephantiasis treated by Kondoléon operation, Surg., Gynec. & Obst., 26: 388–393, 1918.

——— Results obtained in elephantiasis, Ann. Surg., 85:185, 1927.

Unna, P. G. The Histopathology of the Disease of the Skin, Edinburgh, William F. Clay, 1896, pp. 492, 493.

Watson, J. Chronic lymphoedema of the extremities and its management, Brit. J. Surg., 41:31, 1953.

Repair of Traumatic Laceration of the Inferior Vena Cava

Fitzsimons, L. E., and Garvey, F. K. Inferior vena caval injury: case report, J. Urol., 83:285, 1959.

Fraser, R. W. Laceration of inferior vena cava requiring ligation; report of case, Bull. U.S. Army Med. Dept., 5:357, 1946.

Hartzell, J. B. Suture of stab wound of inferior vena cava, Ann. Surg. 111:659, 1940.

Kidd, H. A. Suture of laceration of inferior vena cava due to bomb splinter, Brit. J. Surg., 32:508, 1945.

Ochsner, J. L., Crawford, E.S., and De Bakey, M. E. Injuries of the vena cava caused by external trauma, Surgery, 49:397, 1961.

Rack, F. J. Laceration of the inferior vena cava with delayed hemorrhage and primary suture, Am. J. Surg., 80:807, 1950.

Starzl, T. E., Broadway, R. K., Dever, R. C., and Reams, G. B. The management of penetrating wounds of the inferior vena cava, Am. Surg., 23:455, 1957.

——— Kaupp, H. A., Jr., Beheler, E. M., and Freeark, R. J. Penetrating injuries of the inferior vena cava, Surg. Clin. North America, 43:387, 1963.

Taylor, D. C. Two cases of penetrating wounds of the abdomen involving the inferior vena cava, Lancet, 2:60, 1916.

Excision of Cylindroma of the Trachea

Adkins, P. C., and Icawa, E. Resection of tracheal cylindroma using cardiopulmonary bypass, Arch. Surg., 88:405, 1964.

Clagett, O. T., Grindlay, J. H., and Moersch, H. J. Resection of the trachea: an experimental study and a report of a case, Arch. Surg., 57: 253, 1948.

——— Grindlay, J. H., and Moersch, H. J. Intrathoracic tracheal tumors: development of surgical technics for their removal, Ann. Surg., 136: 520, 1952.

Culp, O. S. Primary carcinoma of trachea, J. Thoracic Surg., 7:471, 1938.

D'Aunoy, R., and Zoeller, A. Primary tumors of the trachea: report of a case and review of the literature, Arch. Path., 11:589, 1931.

Ellman, P., and Whittaker, H. Primary carcinoma of the trachea, Thorax, 2:153, 1947.

Ferguson, D. J., Wild, J. J., and Wangensteen, O. H. Experimental resection of trachea, Surgery, 28:597, 1950.

Goodner, J. T., Berg, J. W., and Watson, W. L. The nonbenign nature of bronchial carcinoids and cylindromas, Cancer, 14:539, 1961.

Kergin, F. G. Carcinoma of the trachea, J. Thoracic Surg., 23:164, 1952.

Payne, W. S., Ellis, H. F., Woolner, L. B., and Moersch, H. J. The surgical treatment of cylindroma, J. Thoracic Surg., 38:709, 1959.

Tauxe, W. N., McDonald, J. R., and Devine, K. D. A century of cylindromas, Arch. Otolaryngol., 75:364, 1962.

Weiss, L., and Ingram, M. Adenomatous bronchial tumors, Cancer, 14:161, 1961.

INDEX

Achalasia of the esophagus, 100-108
Allison technic for repair of esophageal hiatus hernia, 170, 171
Aneurysm of
  abdominal aorta, excision of and graft replacement, 276-289
    clinical case history, 288
    discussion of, 282, 284
  common carotid artery, excision of and insertion of autogenous vein graft, 298-303
    author's comment, 302
    discussion of, 302
  popliteal artery, excision of and graft replacement, 290-295
    choice of graft, 296, 297
    discussion of, 294, 296, 297
  thoracic aorta, excision of and graft replacement, 264-275
    discussion of, 274
    with partial cardiopulmonary bypass, 274, 275
    with shunt bypass graft, 270, 271
Angle of His, 102, 174
Aorta
  abdominal, aneurysm of, 276-289
  thoracic
    aneurysm of, 264-275
    coarctation of, 212-223
Aortic embolectomy, 258-263
  author's comment, 258
  autochthonous thrombi, 258
  discussion of, 260
Aortorenal bypass graft, 342-345
Autochthonous thrombi, 258

Band of Low, 162
Blalock operation for tetralogy of Fallot, 204, 208-211
Brock, Sir Russell C.
  method for thoracotomy, 12, 13
  operation for pulmonary valve stenosis, 224-229

Cardiac arrest, 24, 25, 246, 247
Cardiac massage, 24, 25, 246, 247
Cardiac resuscitation, 246, 247
Cardiopericardiopexy, 238-241
  discussion of, 238, 240
Carotid arterial bypass graft (dacron), 312-317
  choice of materials for bypass, 316
  clinical case history, 312
  discussion of, 314, 316
Carotid glomectomy, 318-321
  discussion of, 320
  incision preferred, 320
Carotid thromboendarterectomy, 304-311
  choice of anesthesia in, 304, 306
  choice of incision, 310
  discussion of, 306, 308, 310
Cervical esophageal diverticulum, 94
Circumferential venous ligation for postphlebitic ulcer, 362, 363
Clagett operation for coarctation of aorta, 220, 221
Coarctation of aorta, 212-223
  alternate methods for resection and anastomosis, 218, 219, 220, 221
    graft replacement, 218, 219
    technic of Clagett, 220, 221
    technic of Dubost, 222, 223
    technic of Gross and Hufnagel, 218, 219
  discussion of, 212, 214, 216, 218, 220, 222
Congenital atresia of esophagus, 88-93
  with hypoplasia of lower esophageal segment, 92, 93
    discussion of, 92
    treatment by primary right transpleural esophagogastrostomy, 92, 93
  with tracheoesophageal fistula, 88-89
    choice of operation, 90
    discussion of, 90, 91
    Haight "telescoping" technic of end-to-end anastomosis, 88, 89
Constrictive pericarditis, 248-257
  causes of, 248, 252
  treatment of, 248-257
Coronary thromboendarterectomy, 242, 243
  clinical case history, 242, 244
  discussion of, 244, 245
Crisis
  cholinergic, 82, 84
  myasthenic, 82, 84
Cylindroma of trachea, excision of, 32-35
  clinical case history, 32
  discussion of, 32, 34

Diaphragm
  esophageal hiatus hernia of, 162-181
  eventration of, 182-187
Diverticula
  esophageal, 94
    cervical, 94
    epiphrenic, 94
  pharyngoesophageal, 94
  pulsion, 94
  traction, 94
Dubost's operation for coarctation of aorta, 212, 213
Ductus arteriosus, patent, 196-201. *See also* Patent ductus arteriosus.
Duval-Barasty, longitudinal sternal splitting incision, 80, 81, 230, 231, 248, 249

Eck fistula, 388
Embolectomy, 258-263
Epiphrenic diverticula, 94
Esophageal diverticula, 94
  cervical, 94
  epiphrenic, 94
Esophageal hiatus hernia, 162-181
  anatomic aspects, 162, 163
  angle of His, 174
  author's comments, 172, 174, 176
  band of Low, 162
  discussion of, 162, 164, 166, 168, 170, 172, 180, 181
  transabdominal approach for repair of, 178, 179
  transthoracic approach for repair of, 162-176
    Allison technic utilizing phrenoesophageal ligament, 170, 171
    Johnsrud technic, 172
    modified Allison technic, 172, 173
    Sweet's method, 170, 171
Esophagectomy
  and colon transplant (esophagocoloplasty), 138-161
    substernal transplant, 156-157
    transabdominal, transpleural (right), transcervical (right) approach, 138-155
      discussion of, 140, 142, 144, 156
      left colon, 158-161
      right colon, 138-157
  combined right cervical, right thoracic, and left abdominal approach with cervical esophagogastrostomy, 118-133
    discussion of, 126, 128
  left transpleural, transdiaphragmatic approach, 110-117
    discussion of, 114, 116
    with infraaortic esophagogastrostomy, 116, 117
    with supraaortic esophagogastrostomy, 114-117
  right transpleural approach with intrapleural esophagogastrostomy, 134-137
Esophagocardiomyotomy (Heller), 100-108
  transabdominal approach, 100-102
    discussion of, 100, 102
  transthoracic approach, 104-108
    discussion of, 104, 106, 108
Esophagocoloplasty, 138-161
Esophagogastrostomy
  cervical, 118, 119, 132, 133, 156, 157
  infraaortic, 116, 117
  supraaortic, 114-117
Esophagus
  atresia of, 88
  congenital atresia of, 88-93
  diverticula of, 94
  resection of, 110-161
Eventration of the diaphragm, 182-187
  clinical case history, 186
Excision of
  aneurysm
    abdominal aorta, 276-289
    common carotid artery, 298-303
    popliteal artery, 290-295
    thoracic aorta, 264-275
Excision of (cont.)
  cylindroma of trachea, 32-35
  pharyngoesophageal diverticulum, 94-98

Fallot's tetralogy, 202-2211. *See also* Tetralogy of Fallot.
Femoral thromboendarterectomy, 330-333
  discussion of, 332
  in Hunter's canal, 332, 333
  extension into popliteal artery, 334, 335

Gastrojejunostomy, antecolic with resection of the vagus nerves, 188-195

Haight "telescoping" technic of end-to-end anastomosis in treatment of congenital atresia of esophagus, 88, 89
Halsted mattress sutures, 148, 149
Heller operation (esophagocardiomyotomy), 100-103
Hernia, esophageal hiatus, 162-181
His, angle of, 102, 174
Hunter's canal, 332, 333

Incisions
  combined thoracoabdominal, right, 16-23
  thoracic
    anterior, 2-5
    Duval-Barasty (sternal splitting), 80, 81, 230, 231, 248, 249
    posterior (prone), 6-9
    posterolateral, 10-15
      Brock method, 12
    sternal splitting (Duval-Barasty), 80, 81, 230, 231, 248, 249
    transaxillary, 390-397
    transsternal cross-bow, 229, 230, 231
Inferior vena cava, 352-361
  ligation of, 352-359
    discussion of, 354, 358
    ligation in continuity, 354-357
    ligation in continuity and transection, 358, 359
    incision preferred, 358
  repair of traumatic laceration of, 360, 361
    clinical case history, 360

Johnsrud technic for repair of esophageal hiatus hernia, 172

Kocher maneuver, 378, 379
Kondoléon operation, modified, 406-417
  author's comment
  classification of lymphedema, 410, 412
  discussion of, 408
  historical aspects, 408, 410, 412, 414

Laceration (traumatic) of inferior vena cava, 360, 361
Lee mesenteric coapting suture, 144, 145

Lembert sutures, 140, 141
Lembert-Cushing sutures, 152, 153
Ligation of
  inferior vena cava, 352-359
  patent ductus arteriosus, 196-201
  superficial femoral vein, 348-351
Lobectomy, pulmonary
  combined right middle and lower lobes, 42-49
    discussion of, 44, 46, 48
  left lower lobe, 66-71
    discussion of, 66, 68, 70
  left upper lobe, 58-65
    clinical case history, 58
    discussion of, 58, 60, 62, 64
  right upper lobe, 36-41
    discussion of, 36, 38, 40
Lymphedema, 406-417

Marion (Pierre) shunt operation for portal hypertension, 374
Mitral commissurotomy, 232-235
  discussion of, 236, 237
Mitral stenosis, 232-235
Mestinon (pyridostigmine bromide), 80, 84, 86
Mytelase (ambenonium chloride), 80

Patent ductus arteriosus, 196-201
  choice of incision, 196
  discussion of, 196, 198, 200, 201
  methods of treatment, 196, 198, 199, 201
    ligation in continuity, 196, 198, 199, 201
    transection and suture ligation, 198, 199
  recurrent laryngeal nerve as anatomic landmark for, 196
Pericardiectomy, 248-257
  choice of incision, 252
  clinical case history, 248
  control of cardiac arrhythmia during, 254, 256
  discussion of, 250, 252, 254, 256
  results of, 256
Peripheral arterial continuity, restoration of, 322-327
  clinical case history, 326
  discussion of, 326
  resection and graft (vein) replacement, 322-325
    choice of material for graft, 326
  shunt bypass, 326, 327
    choice of material for bypass, 326
  varied types of blood vessel anastomoses, 324, 325
Pharyngoesophageal diverticulum, 94
  age incidence, 94
  choice of incision, 96
  classification, 94
  discussion of, 96, 98
  introduction, 94
  resection of, one stage, 94-98
  sex ratio, 94
Phrenoesophageal ligament, 166-168, 170-174
Pneumomectomy, total
  left, 72-79
    discussion of, 74, 76, 78
  right, 50-55
    discussion of, 50, 52, 54, 56, 57

Popliteal artery
  aneurysm of, excision and graft replacement, 290-295
  thromboendarterectomy of, 334, 335
Popliteal vessels, surgical exposure of
  in popliteal space, 334, 335
  in upper third of leg, 328, 329
Portacaval shunts, for portal hypertension, 376-389
  end-to-side, 376-381
    choice of incision, 376, 377, 385
    discussion of, 376, 378, 380, 383, 384, 385
    general considerations in, 376
    three parts (steps) of operation, 378, 380, 383
  side-to-side, 386-389
    direct, 386-389
    discussion of, 388
    Eck fistula, 388
    incision preferred, 388
    indirect, through interposed autogenous vein (H) graft, 388, 389
Portal hypertension, operations for
  Marion shunt operation, 374
  portacaval shunt
    end-to-side anastomosis
    side-to-side anastomosis
      direct, 386-389
      indirect, through interposed autogenous vein (H) graft, 388, 389
  splenectomy and end-to-side splenorenal shunt, 364-371
Posterior (prone) thoracic incision, 6-9
Posterolateral thoracic incision, 10-15
Postphlebitic ulcer, circumferential venous ligation for, 362, 363
  discussion of, 362
Potts' operation for tetralogy of Fallot, 204-207, 210, 211
Prostigmine (neostigmine bromide), 80, 84, 86
Pulmonary valvotomy, 224-231
  closed or indirect method (Brock), 224-229
  discussion of, 224, 226
  open or direct method (Swan), 230-231
    choice of incisions, 230, 231
      Duval-Barasty longitudinal, sternal splitting, 230, 231
      transsternal cross-bow, 224, 230, 231
Pyloroplasty, 190

Renal hypertension
  operations for, 336-347
    aortorenal bypass graft, 342-345
      discussion of, 344
    discussion of, 340, 344, 346
    incision preferred, 346
    segmental resection of renal artery and primary anastomosis, 346, 347
      discussion of, 346
    splenorenal arterial anastomosis, 346, 347
      discussion of, 346
    thromboendarterectomy, renal artery, 336-341
      clinical case history, 336
      discussion, 340

Renal thromboendarterectomy, 336-341
  clinical case history, 336
  discussion, 340
Resuscitation of the heart, 24, 25, 246, 247

Scalenotomy, 24-27
  discussion of, 24, 26
Sliding hernia, 162-181
Splenectomy and end-to-side splenorenal shunt, 364-371
  choice of incision, 364, 365, 368, 374, 375
  discussion of, 368, 370, 372, 373, 374, 375
  indications for the operation, 374
  the three steps of the operation, 368, 370, 372, 373
Splenorenal shunt, end-to-side, for portal hypertension, 364-371
Superficial femoral vein, ligation of, 348-351
  choice of anesthesia,
  discussion of, 350
Surgical exposure of popliteal vêssels and posterior tibial nerve in upper third of leg, 328, 329
  author's comment, 328
Sutures
  Halsted mattress, 148, 149
  Lee mesenteric coapting, 144, 145
  Lembert, 140, 141
  Lembert-Cushing, 152, 153
Sweet's method for repair of esophageal hiatus hernia, 170, 171
Sympathectomy, 390-405. *See also* Sympathetic ganglionectomy
  lumbar, 398-405
  thoracic, 390-397
Sympathetic ganglionectomy
  lumbar, 398-405
    discussion of, 398, 400, 402
    left, 398-403
    right, 404, 405
  thoracic, 390-397
    transaxillary, transpleural approach, 390-397
      discussion of, 394
      Horner's syndrome in,
      left, 396, 397
      right, 390-395

Tensilon (edrophonium chloride), 82, 84
  test, 82
Tetralogy of Fallot, 202-211
  author's comment, 208
  Blalock operation for, 204, 208, 209, 210, 211
  discussion of, 208, 210
  Potts operation for, 204, 205, 206, 207, 210, 211
Thoracic incisions
  anterior, 2-5
    discussion of, 6
  Duval-Barasty (sternal splitting), 80, 81, 230, 231, 248, 249
  posterior (prone), 6-9
    discussion of, 8
  posterolateral, 10-15
    Brock method, 12
    discussion of, 6, 8
  sternal splitting (Duval-Barasty), 80, 81, 230, 231, 248, 249
  transaxillary, 390-397
  transsternal cross-bow, 224, 230, 231
Thoracoabdominal, right, 16-23
  author's comment, 16
  discussion of, 8
Thromboendarterectomy
  carotid artery, 304-311
  coronary artery, 242, 243
  femoral artery, 330-333
  popliteal artery, 334, 335
  renal artery, 336-341
Thrombi, autochthonous, 258
Thymectomy, 80-87
  clinical case history, 80
  cholinergic crisis, 82, 84
    differentiation from myasthenic crisis, 82
    treatment of, 82, 84
  discussion of, 82, 84, 86
  mestinon (pyridostigmine bromide), 80, 84, 86
  myasthenic crisis, 82, 84
    differentiation from cholinergic crisis, 82
    treatment of, 82, 84
  mytelase (ambenonium chloride), 80
  postoperative management, 84, 86
  prostigmine (neostigmine bromide), 80, 84, 86
  tensilon (edrophonium chloride), 82, 84
    test, 82
  tracheostomy in, 80, 82, 86
Tracheostomy, 28-31
  discussion of, 28
Transsternal cross-bow incision, 224, 230, 231

Vagus nerves, resection of, 188-195
  discussion of, 188, 190, 192, 194
  transperitoneal (infradiaphragmatic) approach and antecolic gastrojejunostomy, 188-195
  transthoracic approach, 418-421
Vena cava, inferior, 352-361
  laceration of, 360, 361
  ligation of, 354-357
  transection of, 358